Trauma Management

This book is dedicated to **Alfredo Gomez Peraza,**
a wise man,

and to the memory of **Joseph Mathias Naughton,**
a friend

Contents

Contributing Authors

Raymond H. Alexander, M.D.
Professor and Associate Chairman, Department of Surgery, University of Florida College of Medicine, Gainesville; Chairman of Surgery, University Hospital of Jacksonville, Jacksonville

Jeffrey S. Augenstein, M.D., Ph.D., F.A.C.S.
Associate Professor of Surgery and Anesthesiology and Director, Medical Computer Systems Laboratory, University of Miami School of Medicine, Miami

Christopher C. Baker, M.D.
Associate Professor of Surgery, Yale University School of Medicine; Director of Trauma Center, Department of Surgery, Yale-New Haven Hospital, New Haven

Deborah Blacker, M.D.
Clinical Fellow in Psychiatry, Harvard Medical School; Chief Resident, Acute Psychiatry Service, Massachusetts General Hospital, Boston

Hooshang Bolooki, M.D.
Professor of Surgery, University of Miami School of Medicine; Attending Surgeon and Director, Adult Cardiac Surgery and Cardiac Transplant, Department of Surgery, University of Miami–Jackson Memorial Hospital, Miami

William L. Buntain, M.D., F.A.C.S.
Professor of Surgery, University of Tennessee College of Medicine; Director, Division of Pediatric Surgery, University of Tennessee Medical Center, Knoxville

Patricia M. Byers, M.D.
Clinical Assistant Professor of Surgery and Medicine, University of Miami School of Medicine; Section Chief, Nutritional Support Service, Department of Surgery, University of Miami Hospital and Clinics–Jackson Memorial Hospital, Miami

Alexander S. Cass, M.B., B.S., F.R.C.S.
Associate Professor of Urologic Surgery, University of Minnesota Medical School; Chief, Division of Urology, Hennepin County Medical Center, Minneapolis

Howard R. Champion, F.R.C.S. (Edin.), F.A.C.S.
Clinical Associate Professor of Surgery and Chief, Division of Trauma Surgery, Uniformed Services University of Health Sciences, Bethesda; Senior Attending Surgeon; Chief, Trauma Service; and Director, Surgical Critical Care Services, Washington Hospital Center, Washington, D.C.

Joseph M. Civetta, M.D.
Professor and Chief, Division of Surgical Intensive Care, Department of Surgery, University of Miami School of Medicine, Miami

Linda C. Degutis, M.S.N.
Lecturer and Trauma Coordinator, Yale University School of Medicine, New Haven

Frank J. Eismont, M.D.
Professor of Orthopaedics, University of Miami School of Medicine; Co-Director, Acute Spinal Cord Injury Unit, Department of Orthopaedics, Jackson Memorial Hospital, Miami

John A. Elefteriades, M.D.
Assistant Professor of Surgery, Yale University School of Medicine; Attending Surgeon, Department of Cardiothoracic Surgery, Yale-New Haven Hospital, New Haven

Timothy C. Fabian, M.D.
Associate Professor of Surgery, University of Tennessee College of Medicine, Memphis; Medical Director of Trauma, Regional Medical Center at Memphis, Memphis

Evan R. Geller, M.D.
Assistant Professor of Surgery, State University of New York at Stony Brook; Assistant Chief, Division of Trauma, The University Hospital at Stony Brook, Stony Brook

Gerardo A. Gomez, M.D.
Associate Professor of Clinical Surgery, University of Miami School of Medicine; Attending Surgeon, Assistant Chief of Trauma Services, and Section Chief of Surgical Emergency Room, Jackson Memorial Hospital; Medical Director, Metro-Dade Fire Rescue, Miami

Barth A. Green, M.D.
Professor, Neurological Surgery, University of Miami School of Medicine; Attending Neurosurgeon, Jackson Memorial Hospital, Miami

Frederick L. Grover, M.D.
Professor, Division of Cardiothoracic Surgery, The University of Texas Health Science Center at San Antonio; Chief, Cardiothoracic Surgery Section, Audie L. Murphy Memorial Veterans Hospital, San Antonio

Jeffrey S. Hammond, M.D.
Assistant Professor of Surgery, University of Miami School of Medicine; Co-Director, Burn Center, University of Miami–Jackson Memorial Hospital, Miami

Scott H. Kitchel, M.D.
Spine Consultant, Orthopedic and Fracture Clinic, Eugene; Staff Orthopedic Surgeon, Sacred Heart General Hospital, Eugene

Stuart N. Kline, D.D.S.
Professor of Oral Surgery, University of Miami School of Medicine; Chief, Division of Oral and Maxillofacial Surgery, Jackson Memorial Hospital, Miami

David J. Kreis, Jr., M.D., F.A.C.S.
Associate Professor of Clinical Surgery, State University of New York at Stony Brook; Chief, Division of Trauma and Director, Program in Emergency Medicine, The University Hospital at Stony Brook, Stony Brook

Larry C. Martin, M.D.
Instructor in Clinical Surgery, University of Miami School of Medicine; Attending Surgeon, Jackson Memorial Hospital, Miami

James Maurer, M.D.
Trauma/Critical Care Fellow, State University of New York at Stony Brook; The University Hospital at Stony Brook, Stony Brook

J. Wayne Meredith, M.D.
Assistant Professor of Surgery, Bowman Gray School of Medicine of Wake Forest University; Attending Surgeon and Director of Trauma, Department of Surgery, North Carolina Baptist Hospitals, Winston-Salem

Martin L. Milgrom, M.D., Ph.D.
Assistant Professor of Surgery, University of Miami School of Medicine; Attending Surgeon, Transplant Services, Jackson Memorial Hospital, Miami

O. LaWayne Miller, M.D.
Clinical Assistant Professor of Surgery, Texas Tech University Health Sciences Center School of Medicine, Amarillo

Peter Mucha, Jr., M.D., F.A.C.S.
Associate Professor of Surgery, Mayo Medical School; Consultant, Department of Surgery, Mayo Clinic, Rochester, Minnesota

Loren D. Nelson, M.D., F.A.C.S.
Associate Professor of Surgery and Anesthesiology, Vanderbilt University School of Medicine; Director, Surgical Intensive Care Unit, Vanderbilt University Medical Center, Nashville

Scott H. Norwood, M.D., F.A.C.S.
Assistant Professor of Surgery, University of Illinois College of Medicine at Urbana-Champaign; Director, Critical Care and Trauma Services, Carle Foundation Hospital, Urbana

Thomas A. Noto, M.D.
Professor of Pathology, University of Miami School of Medicine; Director, Transfusion Service, University of Miami–Jackson Memorial Hospital, Miami

C. Richard Patterson, M.D.
Assistant Professor of Surgery, University of Tennessee College of Medicine, Memphis; Chief of Surgical Services, Regional Medical Center at Memphis, Memphis

David B. Pilcher, M.D.
Professor of Surgery, University of Vermont College of Medicine; Attending Surgeon and Director of Trauma Service, Medical Center Hospital of Vermont, Burlington

Christina Rehm, M.D.
Trauma Fellow, Department of Surgery, Emory University School of Medicine, Atlanta

Michael J. Savini, Jr., M.D.
Trauma Fellow, Department of Surgery, Division of Trauma Services, University of Miami–Jackson Memorial Hospital, Miami

Roger Sherman, M.D.
Professor of Surgery, Emory University School of Medicine; Chief of Surgery and Chief of Trauma Service, Grady Memorial Hospital, Atlanta

Joseph J. Tepas, III, M.D.
Associate Professor of Pediatric Surgery, University of Florida College of Medicine, Gainesville; Director, Pediatric Trauma Services and Co-Chairman, Department of Surgery, University Hospital of Jacksonville, Jacksonville

George E. Tesar, M.D.
Instructor in Psychiatry, Harvard Medical School; Director, Acute Psychiatry Service, Massachusetts General Hospital, Boston

Donald D. Trunkey, M.D.
Chairman and Professor of Surgery, Oregon Health Sciences University School of Medicine, Portland

Philip A. Villanueva, M.D.
Assistant Professor of Surgery (Neurosurgery), University of Miami School of Medicine; Attending Surgeon, Jackson Memorial Hospital, Miami

Alexander J. Walt, M.B., Ch.B., M.S. (Minn.), F.R.C.S.(E), F.R.C.S.(C), F.A.C.S.
Chairman, Department of Surgery, Wayne State University School of Medicine; Chief of Surgery, Harper-Grace Hospitals, Detroit

C. Gillon Ward, M.D.
Associate Professor of Surgery, University of Miami School of Medicine; Director of Burn Center, University of Miami–Jackson Memorial Hospital, Miami

George M. Watkins, M.D., F.A.C.S.
Clinical Professor of Surgery, Hahnemann University School of Medicine, Philadelphia; Director, Department of Surgery, Easton Hospital, Easton

A. Enrique Whittwell, M.D.
Trauma Fellow, Department of Surgery Division of Trauma Service, University of Miami School of Medicine–Jackson Memorial Hospital, Miami

Gregory A. Zych, D.O.
Associate Professor of Orthopaedics, University of Miami School of Medicine; Attending Surgeon and Chief, Orthopaedic Trauma, Jackson Memorial Hospital, Miami

Foreword

And Cain talked with Abel, his brother; and it came to pass, when they were in the field, that Cain rose up against his brother and slew him.

Genesis 4:8 (4004 B.C.)

So began trauma in recorded human history. Death most likely resulted from blunt trauma produced by a farm implement, as Cain was "a tiller of the ground." The late Edward D. Churchill, a former professor of mine, said that surgery began with trauma and congenital anomalies and therein shall it end. I think it more likely that surgery will end with trauma alone, since mankind will continue to find ways to injure itself, whereas congenital anomalies will be prevented by genetic engineering or increasingly treated or repaired in utero.

This book, co-edited by Drs. Kreis and Gomez, is a compendium of what is known and what can be done but goes beyond mere technical recitations to the epidemiology of injury and the systems and organization of care. Specialists have been brought together to share their particular expertise and to indicate the relationship to trauma of fields such as psychiatry, transplantation, blood banking, geriatrics, and pediatrics. It is truly a comprehensive bible for those who work in the vineyard of trauma. I am particularly pleased to participate in a book co-edited by my former student and resident at Yale, Dr. David Kreis. His interest, expertise, and research in and his dedication to trauma care have been an immense contribution.

I would like now to write a few words of encouragement about the prevention of injury. Recently Foege, from the Carter Center of Emory University, wrote: "And now in an impressive display of overriding the scientific evidence, Congress has voted to kill more of its constituents by allowing the states to reconsider the 55-mph speed limit. The March of Folly continues." The weak controls on handguns and inability of Congress to buck the lobbying efforts of the gun people lead to the deaths of many, including law enforcement officers.

Drunken drivers are another problem that society has not faced squarely. Colquitt et al. recently found that one-third of automobile accidents were associated with intoxication. Few of these patients were referred either to alcoholism-rehabilitation programs or to the courts for prosecution. They, and I, urge that physicians become active in implementing these programs in the best interest of their patients.

Industrial accidents, dangerous environments, MTVs (multiple terrain vehicles), the repeal of helmet laws, the lack of a coherent trauma care system, and many other problems all cry out for active involvement of those who best know the price of these injuries to individuals and society. Premature death and premature disability from gunshot wounds are as final and as expensive as from arteriosclerosis.

You are learning to be, or are already, experts in the care of injury. What are you doing to put yourself out of business? Isn't that, after all, the purpose of surgery? James Baldwin said that not everything that is faced can be changed but that nothing can be changed until it is faced.

And the Lord asked Cain, "Where is Abel, thy brother?" And Cain replied, "I know not. Am I my brother's keeper?"

Arthur E. Baue, M.D.

Preface

Trauma continues to be the leading cause of death in the first four decades of life and accounts for 150,000 deaths each year in the United States. This is a staggering number, for it is three times the total number of American combat-related deaths in the entire Vietnam War. Approximately 30 percent of these deaths are caused by motor vehicle accidents and 22 percent by the violence of gunshot wounds. The total economic consequence of trauma to the American society is $100 billion annually.

These poignant facts demonstrate clearly that trauma in America remains a major uncorrected public health problem. In general, the solution for decreasing the mortality from injury lies in three major areas: prevention, treatment, and education. Prevention and public education concerning simple and inexpensive maneuvers such as wearing a seat belt, using a child restraint, and abstaining from driving while under the influence of psychotropic drugs or alcohol would decrease the incidence of these fatal injuries. Treatment of severely injured patients requires a systems approach. Data to support this approach has come in part from numerous preventable trauma deaths studies. In general, the most common causes of preventable deaths are a delay to definitive surgery or the lack of performance of indicated surgery.

Trauma Management was conceived in order to provide a comprehensive yet practical guide to a systems approach to trauma care. The text is written primarily for practicing surgeons, emergency medicine physicians, and critical care physicians. Resident physicians, nurses, and other health care professionals concerned with the injured patient should find the organized approach to trauma care presented in the text helpful in their clinical practice.

The editors wish to thank the contributing authors for their thoughtfulness in providing the reader a useful discussion of the important principles of trauma management. We would also like to thank Susan Pioli and Katherine Arnoldi of Little, Brown and Company for their most professional assistance and encouragement throughout the development and production of this book. Jane Brown and Sadie Hernandez of Miami, Florida and Patricia Cellini and Carol Povolny of Stony Brook, New York have provided outstanding staff support for which the editors are most grateful.

D.J.K.
G.A.G.

Trauma Management

Notice

The indications and dosages of all drugs in this book have been recommended in the medical literature and conform to the practices of the general medical community. The medications described do not necessarily have specific approval by the Food and Drug Administration for use in the diseases and dosages for which they are recommended. The package insert for each drug should be consulted for use and dosage as approved by the FDA. Because standards for usage change, it is advisable to keep abreast of revised recommendations, particularly those concerning new drugs.

1

Trauma: A Major Public Health Problem

J. Wayne Meredith
Donald D. Trunkey

Trauma is accidental or intentional injury. It is caused by the transfer of energy (usually mechanical but sometimes thermal or chemical) to a victim. Trauma represents a major public health problem. Injuries are the leading cause of death during half of the human life span. About 8 million Americans alive today can be expected to die from trauma. One death in every twelve in the United States results from injuries. Injuries are the fourth leading cause of death, claiming more than 160,000 lives each year [1]. For every 100,000 Americans, 40 can be expected to die in motor vehicle accidents annually, and 9.5 can be expected to die from homicide. Worldwide, the accident death rate ranges from 17.8 per 100,000 population to 69.1 per 100,000 population (Table 1-1).

Tragically, trauma concentrates its devastation upon the young and accounts for the loss of more working years of life than all other causes. Annually, there are more than 4 million potential years of life lost prematurely because of injuries, compared to less than 2 million each for cancer and heart disease. Epidemiologists estimate that more than 1 percent of persons aged 10 to 34 alive in 1985 will die of injury by the year 2000 [2]. A white boy aged 15 years in 1985 has a 1 in 110 estimated risk of dying of a motor vehicle–related injury by the time he is 30 years old. A black man aged 20 years has a 1 in 50 estimated risk of dying by homicide by the time he is 35 years old. Overall, in 1985 for children aged 5 to 9 years, the estimated risk of dying of injury by the year 2000 is 2.6 times the risk of dying from all other causes combined [2].

The actual cost of accidents to society is staggering. The National Safety Council [3] estimated the total cost of accidents in 1984 to have been $96.9 billion annually or $265,000,000 daily. This cost includes wage

Table 1-1. Motor Vehicle Deaths by Nation

Nation	Year	Deaths	Rate	Nation	Year	Deaths	Rate
Syrian Arab Rep.	1981	155	1.7	Cuba	1977	1,484	14.7
Egypt	1978	854	2.1	Hungary	1982	1,636	15.3
Peru	1978	889	5.0	East Germany	1976	2,746	16.4
Paraguay	1982	207	5.6	Canada	1982	4,073	16.5
Nicaragua	1978	168	7.0	El Salvador	1981	851	17.0
Uruguay	1978	207	7.2	Ireland	1980	567	17.2
Israel	1983	436	8.2	Spain	1979	6,562	17.7
Dominican Rep.	1982	541	8.3	Italy	1978	10,354	18.3
Hong Kong	1982	471	9.0	West Germany	1983	11,209	18.3
Sweden	1982	801	9.6	Switzerland	1983	1,180	18.4
Chile	1982	1,167	10.2	Panama	1980	351	19.1
Norway	1983	428	10.3	Greece	1982	1,925	19.7
England, Wales	1982	5,241	10.6	UNITED STATES	1982	45,779	19.8
Japan	1983	12,708	10.6	Costa Rica	1979	434	20.0
Czechoslovakia	1982	1,668	10.9	France	1981	11,033	20.4
Bulgaria	1983	989	11.0	Ecuador	1978	1,817	21.8
Finland	1982	557	11.4	New Zealand	1982	709	21.8
Singapore	1981	281	11.5	Australia	1981	3,287	22.0
Netherlands	1983	1,689	11.7	N. Ireland	1978	345	22.4
Puerto Rico	1982	487	12.3	Belgium	1976	2,463	25.1
Scotland	1983	639	12.4	Austria	1983	1,954	25.7
Denmark	1982	633	13.0	Portugal	1981	3,340	33.2
Thailand	1982	6,355	13.5	Kuwait	1982	535	34.2
Argentina	1978	3,853	14.6	Venezuela	1978	4,822	36.7

Rate is deaths per 100,000 population.
Source: *Accident Facts 1985*. Chicago: National Safety Council, 1985.

loss, medical expense, insurance administration cost, and property damage from moving motor vehicle accidents but does not include the cost of public agencies such as fire and police departments, courts, indirect losses to employers due to off-the-job accidents or the value of cargo lost in commercial vehicles, and damages awarded in excess of direct losses (Table 1-2).

EPIDEMIOLOGY

Trauma can be categorized according to the mechanism of injury or as intentional or unintentional. The term *accidental* has fallen out of favor because it implies that nothing can be done to prevent it. Unintentional trauma occurs from a wide variety of mechanisms. The most important are auto accidents, falls, and burns. Drowning, frostbite, electrocution,

Table 1-2. Certain Costs[a] of Accidents by Class, 1984 ($ Billions)

Cost	Total[b]	Motor Vehicle	Work	Home	Public Non–motor Vehicle
Total	$96.9	$47.6	$33.0	$10.8	$7.2
Wage loss	28.8	15.2	6.8	4.0	4.1
Medical expense	13.8	4.7	4.3	3.2	2.0
Insurance administration	13.4	8.9	4.3	0.1	0.1
Fire loss	6.7	c	2.2	3.5	1.0
Motor vehicle property damage	18.8	18.8	c	c	c
Indirect work loss	15.4	c	15.4	c	c

[a]Cost estimates are not comparable with those of previous years. As additional or more precise data become available, they are used from that year forward, but previously estimated figures are not revised. Wage loss estimating procedures were revised for the 1985 edition.
[b]Duplications between work and motor vehicle and home and motor vehicle are eliminated in the totals.
[c]Not included.
Source: National Safety Council estimates.

poisoning, railroad and aviation injuries, machinery injuries, and others also occur. Of unintentional injuries, automotive accidents account for the most deaths. In 1984, 46,200 victims died from motor vehicle accidents. Motor vehicle accidents accounted for 1.7 million injuries that resulted in either temporary or permanent disability. These accidents cost $47.6 billion [3]. Most at risk for motor vehicle accidents are white males aged 13 to 35 years. Death rates from motor vehicle crashes vary tremendously by race and per capita income. Native Americans have the highest death rates from all types of motor vehicle crashes combined, being 51 per 100,000, compared to 24 per 100,000 for whites. Death rates from motor vehicle accidents are higher in low-income neighborhoods. The death rate in counties where the annual per capita income is less than $3000 is more than double the rate in counties where the average income is $6000 or more. This may be due to variations in the occupant death rate, which is almost three times as high in low-income areas. Motor vehicle death rates are more than twice as high among residents in rural areas as in cities of a million or more [1].

Falls are the second most common cause of unintentional injury and death and account for nearly 12,000 deaths per year in the United States. Death rates are equally distributed between males and females [3]. Almost 30 percent of all deaths from falls occur among people aged 85 or older, although this age group makes up only 1 percent of the population. More than half of all fatal falls involve people 75 or older [1]. In the majority of cases where the place of injury is specified, the injury occurs at home. About 1800 fatal falls are known to occur each year in residential institutions such as nursing homes [1]. Children are also at high risk of fall injury, but their death rate is low.

Fires and burns account for 5200 deaths per year, with about a 3:2 male-to-female ratio [3]. Death rates are highest among children and the elderly, in part because of the difficulty in escaping burning buildings. In addition, these groups have a higher risk of dying from a given severity of burn. Death rates are more than twice as high in areas of low per capita income. There is a pronounced geographic pattern in house fire deaths, with high death rates in the East, especially the Southeast, which may be attributable to kerosene heaters and other space-heating equipment, which are more common in these regions [1].

In 1984, there were 1.9 million disabling injuries incurred at work and 11,500 deaths. These account for $33 million direct cost to the nation [3]. Of some 1500 machinery-related deaths annually, more than half involve farm equipment (55 percent). Cranes, forklifts, and lifting machinery account for 16 percent. The highest death rates from nonfarm machinery occur at ages 20 to 24, whereas farm machinery deaths are lowest at this age group and highest at ages 65 to 74 [1].

Intentional injuries generally include deaths by homicides and suicides. Homicides account for 22,000 deaths per year, while suicides account for 28,000 deaths per year [2]. Many suicides are not traumatic but are rather overdoses and poisoning, making these data difficult to interpret when considering only injuries as cause of death. For the ages 15 to 34, only unintentional injuries surpass homicide as a cause of death. Among blacks aged 20 to 34, homicide is the leading cause of death. Firearms are used in two-thirds of homicides, and cuttings and stabbings account for another 22 percent. The majority of homicides take place in the home and involve friends or family members of the victim. Homicide rates are highest for 25- to 29-year-old men. Assaults by strangers are most important among teenagers and the elderly but never account for more than about one-fourth of all homicides. Hospital data indicate that many more people are assaulted with sharp instruments than with firearms, yet the ratio of deaths to injuries is roughly five times as great for shootings. The homicide rate is four times as great for shootings. The homicide rate is four times as high among people in cities of a million or more as among people who do not live in large cities. Half of all homicides occur on Friday, Saturday, and Sunday, with the largest number, 20 percent, occurring on Saturday. Alcohol has been shown to be involved in a large proportion of killings [1].

THE SOLUTION

It can be concluded from the data cited that trauma represents the number one health and social problem in the country today. This fact is overlooked or underestimated by many, if not most, citizens. The problem will not solve itself; as a society we need to address the issue of trauma. The solution revolves around four important areas: prevention, patient care, education, and research.

Prevention

There are three general strategies available for the prevention of injuries. The first is to persuade persons at risk of injury to alter their behavior for increased self-protection, the second is to require individual behavior change by law or administrative rule, and the third is to provide automatic protection by product or environmental design [1]. Each of these approaches is helpful and should be applied to the problem.

Injury prevention by persuasion and education requires voluntary behavior change and has had disappointingly poor results. The most injury-prone populations are the very groups least likely to respond to such programs. However, it is likely that such programs can heighten public awareness of safety issues and thereby generate support for more efficacious legislation and better funding of research.

The second approach, laws and regulations mandating behavior change, has been shown to be more effective than voluntary approaches. For example, only about 50 percent of motorcyclists will voluntarily wear helmets, but helmet laws result in nearly 100-percent use [1].

The third and most successful approach to injury prevention is the alteration of our environment so that potential victims are automatically protected. Successful examples include improved automobile design, automatic water sprinkler systems in buildings, and fire-retardant clothing.

Many motor vehicle accident deaths could be prevented. We need legislation to get the drunk off the highway, uniform seat belt requirements that are well enforced, uniform helmet legislation for motorcycles, and mandatory restraints for children in automobiles. The United States has the highest civilian death rate from handguns in the world. This is unacceptable. There are 120 million guns in the possession of American civilians. Handgun control is a controversial issue that must be addressed. At the least, strict registration for the purchase of ammunition should be advocated. Regulations regarding stairway installation, lighting, and handrails as well as bed rails and bed height in nursing homes would prevent many falls and deaths. The technology and resources for these and many other preventive measures are available but are underutilized because of lack of public awareness and support.

Patient Care

Data from several parts of the country show that death from trauma has a trimodal distribution when the death rate is plotted as a function of time after injury [4]. The first peak is characterized as immediate deaths, which occur within minutes of injury and are related to laceration of the brain, brain stem, spinal cord, heart, or major blood vessel. Only a fraction of the patients in this group can be saved even under the most favorable medical conditions, although a few can and have been saved by early and rapid transport to appropriate trauma care facilities. The second peak, characterized as early deaths, represents people who die within the first few hours after an injury. These deaths are usually caused by major internal hemorrhages of the head or thoracic or abdominal organs or by multiple lesser injuries resulting in severe blood loss. Almost all injuries of this type are considered treatable by currently available medical procedures. The interval between injury and definitive treatment, however is critical to the probability of recovery. The third peak, characterized as late deaths, represents people who die days or weeks after an injury. Eighty percent of these deaths are caused by infection or multiple organ systems failure.

Many of these deaths can be prevented by timely and appropriate surgical care. Kreis and associates [5] found in Dade County, Florida that 21 percent of deaths from non–central nervous system trauma were preventable. Sixty percent of these were due to a delay in getting to surgery or failure to perform surgery. Lowe and coworkers [6], in Portland, Oregon, found 34 of 135 trauma deaths to be potentially preventable. The average response time of surgeons was 1.26 hours to get to the hospital after being called to the case. Cales [7], in Orange County, California, found the preventable death rate fell from 34 percent prior to institution of a trauma system to 4 percent when patients were treated in a designated trauma facility. Clearly, part of the solution to the trauma problem is the development of an effective regional trauma system. For a trauma system to be most effective, it requires excellence in four phases of patient care: (1) availability of the trauma system to the patient, (2) prehospital patient management, (3) hospital patient management, and (4) rehabilitation.

The first of these phases, access to care, requires general public awareness of methods for entry into the trauma system, including standardized emergency telephone numbers and recognized designated trauma care centers. Access to care also requires modern communications technology. Some countries have unique problems in this regard. For example, in Queensland, Australia, there are huge land masses that are sparsely populated. This requires the use of special radio transmitters in vehicles that start transmitting a signal upon impact. This allows prompt recognition of an accident and also can lead rescuers to the area.

The second phase, prehospital care, is extremely variable. Some countries have very sophisticated rescue ambulances, including fixed-wing aircraft and helicopters. Other countries have highly advanced paramedics or physicians who travel to the scene of an accident, institute resuscitation, and rapidly transport the patient to the nearest trauma center. The West German system is an excellent one, with trauma centers located at various intervals up and down the autobahn. It is estimated that no patient in Germany is more than 30 minutes from a designated trauma center [8]. Unfortunately, in many countries and in many parts of this country, the patient is merely transported to the nearest hospital, and no consideration is given as to whether the personnel or equipment is available at this hospital for the proper management of the patient. The available resources may vary from region to region, but in most circumstances the first responder should be an emergency medical technician (EMT) with at least basic life support training and an appropriately equipped ambulance. The EMT should be in direct communication with and under direct supervision of medical control whenever possible. Ideally, previously established categorizations will have identified those institutions with facilities and personnel best able to manage patients with specific injuries. Predefined triage criteria regarding the patient's physiologic status (trauma score) and mechanism of injury should be utilized to direct the patient to an appropriate institution for management. The seriously injured patient should be taken directly to the center most appropriately equipped and staffed to handle this specific patient's needs, bypassing those facilities not committed to the immediate management of the trauma patient.

The in-hospital management of the trauma patient is an exhaustive topic, which will be covered in the remaining chapters. Suffice it to say that the management of serious trauma should be in those institutions that have demonstrated the commitment not only in the surgical disciplines, but also involving the entire medical staff as well as hospital administration and board of trustees.

The final phase of patient care is rehabilitation. The goal of trauma care is the return of a functional patient to a useful position in society, and proper rehabilitation is important to this goal. In 1984, 330,000 patients suffered permanent disabilities as a consequence of injuries [3]. It is estimated that one in ten of these patients uses a rehabilitation facility. There are only 15 spinal cord injury rehabilitation centers in the United States, and less than 10 percent of the 7500 persons with new spinal cord injuries every year have access to one of these centers [1]. Proper rehabilitation facilities are also needed for patients with amputations, severe musculoskeletal injuries, permanent disability and deformity, peripheral nerve injuries, and burns, including a number of psychosocial issues.

Education

Trauma is so ubiquitous in our society that most physicians will be called on to care for a trauma victim sometime during their career. Everyone graduating from medical school should have at least a basic exposure to trauma management. A recent study conducted by one of the authors sent a survey to deans of medical schools inquiring about trauma education. This survey revealed that, in many institutions, medical students received little or no formal instruction in trauma during the preclinical years. Special courses in advanced trauma life support were required in very few of the medical schools that responded. Just as all physicians should have a basic understanding of trauma, surgeons should have in-depth training in trauma management. Trauma is a surgical disease with impact on society equal to other major diseases of our time. Nonetheless, a recent survey [4] addressed to surgery program directors revealed that, in most institutions, trauma represents a small part of the surgical resident's total operative experience. A recent review of applications to the American Board of Surgery revealed that 47 percent of applications handled fewer than 20 trauma cases in their training [4]. Proper management of the trauma patient requires education also of the various support personnel involved in the trauma patient's management. These include paramedics, communications officers, intensive care unit nurses, operating room nurses, and emergency room nurses. These individuals and groups of individuals play a key role in the successful salvage of trauma victims and require a thorough understanding of the principles of management of shock and injuries as well as the prevention and management of sepsis.

Education in trauma should extend beyond

health professionals. It is important to have outreach programs to the lay community in terms of trauma prevention. An excellent example of this is the group called Mothers Against Drunk Driving (MADD). This group represents a grass roots attempt to reduce the carnage caused by drunk drivers. It is somewhat embarrassing that this had to begin at a lay level and not as a result of medical initiatives. In addition to education regarding the impact and prevention of trauma, the public at large needs education in terms of access to the trauma system.

Research

Trauma-related research is critical in the further understanding of many areas of trauma management. Presently, only 43 of the 350 surgical programs in the country today have ongoing trauma-related research, most of which is funded from professional fee income [9]. Less than 3 percent of surgical faculty members in the United States are involved in basic trauma-related research. Less than 1 percent of all surgical residents in the United States participate in trauma-related research. In fiscal year 1984, the number of trauma and burn centers in program projects numbered 10, for a total encumbered budget of $4.161 million. Presently, there is insufficient information concerning the epidemiology of trauma. Most of the available information is based on trauma death data, and there is little information based on incidence of accidents or on disability for nondeath trauma incidents. Further information must be gathered regarding the costs of trauma management and improving our cost-effectiveness as well as our resources for providing health services for society. Clearly, the most cost-efficient method of managing the trauma problem is better trauma prevention, and further research in this area is badly needed. Sepsis is an important cause of death in those patients who survive beyond 48 hours. Much more information is needed regarding the incidence and etiology of sepsis, its prevention, and the management of multiple organ failure that ensues. Head injuries account for a significant portion of prehospital and early hospital trauma deaths. The exact mechanisms of and potential preventive measures of cerebral edema are presently poorly understood. Our present preventive and therapeutic maneuvers are somewhat rudimentary. A simple and effective method of preventing or treating cerebral edema would save many lives. Spinal cord injuries account for thousands of serious disabilities annually. Further research needs to be done in the biomechanics of rehabilitating these patients, including the new research on nerve regeneration as well as computerized models for helping these patients become more ambulatory, functional, and self-sufficient. Several authors, including the National Research Council's document "Trauma: The Neglected Disease of Modern Society," as well as presidential addresses to the American Trauma Society by Dr. Adams Cowley and to the American Association of Surgery of Trauma by Dr. George Sheldon [9], have recommended the formation of a trauma institute that would be part of the National Institutes of Health. This could serve as a focal point for the administration and direction of trauma research throughout the country. Presently, the allocation of research dollars is unproportionately small compared to the an-

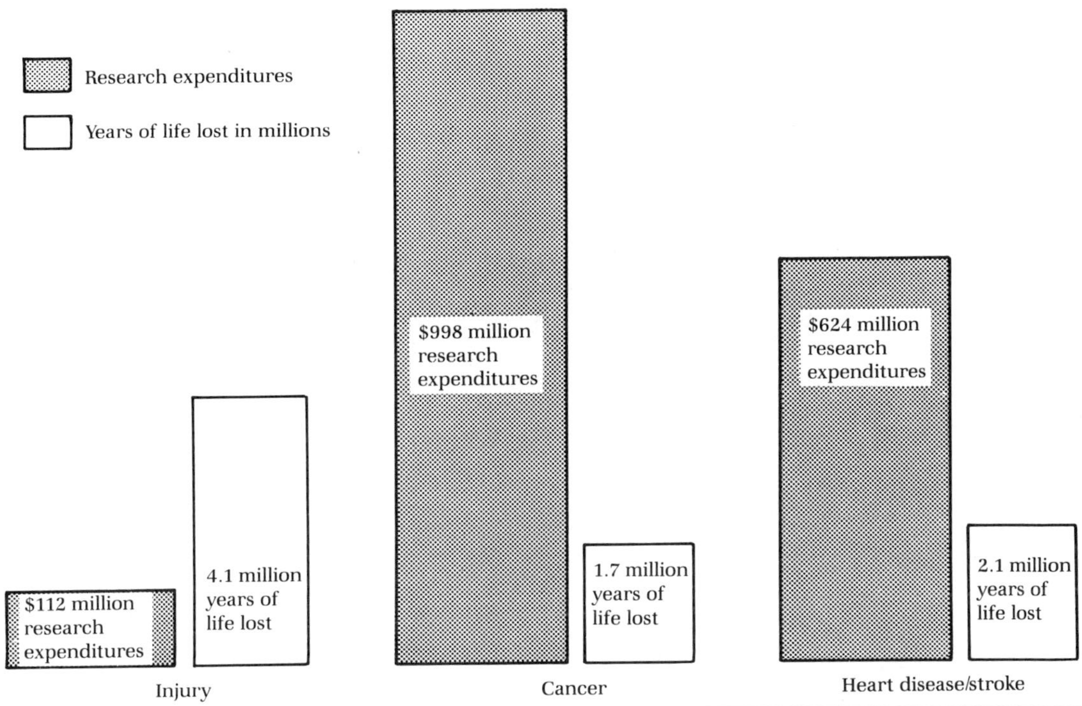

Fig. 1-1. Relationship of research dollars allocated and potential years of life lost annually for three diseases. (Modified from *Injury in America: A Continuing Public Health Problem.* Washington, D.C.: National Academy Press, 1985.)

nual loss of pre-retirement years of life (Fig. 1-1). Without this research and progress in our further understanding of trauma, the injured patient will continue to be a drain on our society and a tragic loss of human productivity.

REFERENCES

1. Balzer, S. P., O'Neil, B., and Karpf, R. S. *The Injury Fact Book.* Lexington, Mass.: D. C. Heath, 1984.
2. Budnick, L. D. The probability of dying of injuries by the year 2000. *J.A.M.A.* 254:3350.
3. *Accident Facts 1985.* Chicago: National Safety Council, 1985.
4. Trunkey, D. D. Presidential address: On the nature of things that go bang in the night. *Surgery* 92:123, 1982.
5. Kreis, D. J., Jr., et al. Preventable trauma deaths: Dade County, Florida. *J. Trauma* 26:649, 1986.
6. Lowe, D. K. Patterns of death, complication, and error in the management of motor vehicle accident victims: Implications for regional system of trauma care. *J. Trauma* 23:503, 1983.
7. Cales, R. H. Trauma mortality in Orange County: The effect of implementation of a regional trauma system. *Ann. Emerg. Med.* 13:15, 1984.
8. Trunkey, D. D. Trauma. *Sci. Am.* 249:28, 1983.
9. Sheldon, G. F. Presidential address: Medical education and the trauma surgeon—The role of the A.A.S.T. *J. Trauma* 25:727, 1985.

2

Organization of Trauma Care

Howard R. Champion

THE PROBLEM

Approximately 160,000 people a year die from injury [1]. Of these, some 50,000 deaths are related to automobile accidents, and approximately 30,000 are due to ballistic weapons, predominantly handguns [1]. Injury is the leading cause of years of lost life in the United States, surpassing cancer and cardiovascular disease combined. In terms of economic impact, trauma is second only to cancer. In 1966, the National Academy of Sciences characterized trauma as "the neglected disease of modern society" [2]. In 1985, in a monograph entitled *Injury in America,* the National Academy of Sciences identified continuing major deficiencies and apathy approaching negligence in our approach to the disease [3]. Many deficiencies remain in the acute care system.

During the past 10 years, some 50 studies on preventable deaths identified that, on average, 19.3 percent of injury-related deaths in the hospital are preventable. Thus, approximately 20,000 deaths a year from injury can be prevented. The usual cause of preventable death is related to timeliness of surgical intervention or lack of surgery when surgery is needed. There is little doubt that an appropriately configured and focused acute health care system can substantially reduce the mortality of major injury, as well as the morbidity and societal costs, which in 1985 exceeded $107 billion [1]. In configuring the acute health care system for injury, it is essential to recognize the fundamental factors that influence the logistics of the provision of care to trauma victims.

1. *The time-critical nature of the disease.* Approximately 50 percent of those who die from injury do so before reaching the hospital. Of those who reach the hospital alive, 60 percent of deaths from hemorrhage occur

within the first 4 hours; 40 percent of deaths from central nervous system–related injuries also occur within the first 4 hours. Thus, if a measurable reduction in trauma mortality is to be achieved, it is important to provide the necessary intervention as close to the time of injury and as promptly as possible.

2. *The time of day at which mobilization of health care resources is required.* Trauma tends to be a nocturnal disease, with peak occurrences at night and on weekends. Normally, during these times, hospitals are "geared down"; consequently, many of the elements of the health care system that function smoothly and promptly during the workweek are not necessarily available to provide interventions for life-threatening injuries.

3. *The relatively small fraction of patients with severe injuries.* There are approximately 3.7 million hospital discharges each year for injury [1]. Forty to fifty percent of the 80 million emergency department visits would also fall under this rubric but are minor in nature. Thus, the number of individuals with severe or life-threatening injuries is relatively small. Where such population-based statistics are available, it would appear that the number of patients with an injury severity score [4] of 15 or more requiring trauma center care each year is in the region of 550 patients per million per year [5]. Only about 350 patients per million per year require intensive care for trauma [6]. Approximately 60 percent of patients treated in trauma centers in the United States have injury severity scores of 10 or less [7]. Thus, by any computation, there are no more than 200,000 cases of severe or multiple injuries in the United States each year, which is just over 5 percent of those patients who require hospitalization for injury.

4. *Triage.* Identifying those who are at risk of early death from injury can be very difficult. Many methods currently in use have not been subjected to scientific scrutiny.

5. *Lack of insurance.* A large proportion (over 30 percent) of urban trauma patients are not covered by any health insurance scheme. Thus, hospitals treating these patients often bear the significant financial burden for their care.

Only by recognizing and responding to these factors that influence the configuration and operation of the trauma system can appropriate adjustments be made to an emergency medical health care system for those patients suffering from severe injury.

THE REGIONAL TRAUMA SYSTEM

The problem of providing timely, prompt delivery of care to patients at risk of dying from injury has led to the development of regional systems for trauma care. The concept behind these systems is that a restrictive and focused health care system is needed for patients at risk of dying from injury. Effective prehospital care is ensured by appropriate protocols and triage guidelines. Prompt access to the trauma center is provided by communications and transport systems. The hub of a regional trauma system is the trauma center, a hospital with specialized capabilities available 24 hours a day to provide the highest level of care possible to victims of serious injury. The whole system is rounded off by the presence

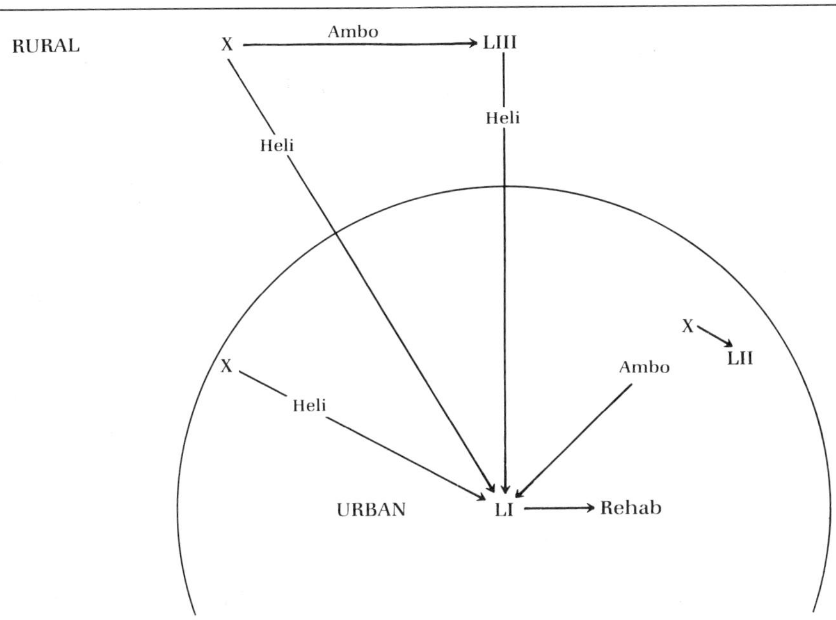

Fig. 2-1. Configuration of a regional trauma system. Modes of transport utilized by an EMS system to triage critically injured patients to level I trauma centers depend on the region (urban vs. rural) and distance to the center. X = site of accident; Heli = helicopter transport; Ambo = ambulance transport; LI = ACS level I center; LII = ACS level II center; LIII = ACS level III center (community hospital); Rehab = rehabilitation hospital/services.

of rehabilitation pre- and posthospital discharge that helps the trauma victim attain maximal functioning capabilities and aids in reintegration into normal living routines (Fig. 2-1).

Each component of a regional trauma system will be discussed briefly, followed by a discussion of the internal organization of the trauma center. The basic organizational structure reflects an urban/suburban population mix. Appropriate qualifiers should be considered for addressing rural trauma.

Prehospital Care System

Prehospital trauma care is an integral component of an emergency medical services (EMS) system that provides a specific focus on identifying, treating, and transporting victims of major injury.

Many EMS systems throughout the country were developed without a specific focus on the urgent needs of the victims of major injury. Many prehospital treatments are implemented by protocol, resulting in their automatic application to injury victims, without evaluation of potential benefits on a case-by-case basis. Often, application of a specific intervention results in unnecessary delay in transport of the victim to a hospital environment. Basic prehospital treatment modalities routinely applied to the trauma victim that merit brief mention are listed below.

Airway Management
Adequate airway management is the single most important therapy needed by a victim of severe injuries. Establishing and maintaining an adequate airway require maneuvers to clear the airway and ensure adequate ventilation and oxygenation by using simple techniques such as oral airway, bag-mask techniques, or for the unconscious victim or patient in shock, endotracheal intubation.

Intravenous Lines
There is currently considerable debate about the efficacy of intravenous lines (IVs) for the urban trauma victim because of the length of time often required to establish an IV [8]. Repeated unsuccessful attempts to establish an IV often result in delayed transport to a hospital where multiple IVs could be quickly established and more sophisticated therapies could be promptly initiated. There is great concern that these delays are detrimental to the patient's condition.

IVs are certainly warranted where long transport times will occur because of the geographic distance between the accident site and the hospital or where the patient is entrapped, extrication is required, and a delay in initiating transport will result. However, growing concern with apparently unwarranted transport delays has resulted in physician-initiated modifications to prehospital protocols. Consequently, in many urban environments now, it is not permissible to delay transport of a severely injured trauma victim to a trauma center for the sole purpose of inserting an IV.

MAST
While Military Anti-Shock Trousers (MAST) probably are beneficial because of their tamponade effect for venous intra-abdominal pelvic bleeding, their application to prehospital trauma care has yet to be fully researched, and limits for their use have yet to be defined.

Neck and Spinal Immobilization and Fracture Immobilization
Minimizing further damage from unstable spinal or other fractures is vital in prehospital care. Thus, it is essential that steps be taken to minimize the amount of continued motion that can occur in the neck, spine, and fracture sites during extrication and transport that might otherwise be deleterious to the patient. Despite the need to take time to immobilize potential fractures, there is a general consensus that excessive prehospital treatment is of little value, especially if it will result in delayed hospital access.

Triage
Prehospital identification of those at risk of dying from their injuries has received inadequate attention. Yet, such identification is critical because it determines the pace and level of care that a trauma victim will receive. The American College of Surgeons has promulgated a set of guidelines that may aid in the early identification of patients at risk of dying from injury (Fig. 2-2). The intent of these

guidelines is to cull the 5 percent of those with severe, life-threatening injuries from the total population of injured victims. It is not possible to cast a net around this 5 percent without capturing other patients for whom transport to trauma centers was not warranted. Nonetheless, such overtriage is necessary. To ensure that severely injured patients are not misssed, it is quite acceptable to include 10 percent of injured patients (an actual overtriage rate of 100 percent) in an attempt to minimize the number of patients dying from injury without access to the regional trauma system.

Prehospital Transport

Recognition of the pathophysiology of injury and the dynamic and deteriorating nature of the sequelae of energy transfer to the human body dictate that the primary purpose of the prehospital care system be to expedite the identification and definitive hospital care of patients at risk of dying. In this context, the primary contribution of the prehospital care system is rapid transport to the source of definitive care. Advanced life support maneuvers that can be provided without delaying access to definitive care are really temporizing measures that buy time until definitive care can be instituted.

The choice of transport system is between an ambulance and a helicopter and depends on both the time-distance to the appropriate trauma center and the level of care that needs to be rendered en route. The spectrum of care available on both ambulances and helicopters varies widely. For example, on ambulances, care can range from basic life support (BLS) through advanced life support (ALS). In helicopters, the care may range from first responder level on some multipurpose police force helicopter systems to the availability of a critical care nurse or emergency physician with advanced trauma life support (ATLS) training in some hospital-based helicopter systems.

Helicopters

There is little doubt that the helicopter is an instrument that can reduce the mortality, morbidity, and cost of trauma. Cost-effective application, however, can only be ensured through careful integration of the helicopter into regional EMS trauma systems, deployment based solely on medical reasons, and ongoing and thorough monitoring. Recommendations for equipment standards already exist [9]. Program standards for urban air ambulance operations should work to increase efficiency of the service, ensure that patients are transported to the most appropriate facility, and thus maximize use of health care dollars. The following standards are proposed.

Standard 1. Urban air ambulances should complement (not compete with) existing regional EMS systems. In most cities where air ambulance services are operational, there are existing EMS systems. Most EMS systems began with a basic life support program; each echelon of more sophisticated care and technology (e.g., advanced life support, telemetry) was built on that foundation. Duplicating and competing EMS systems in a region produce conflicts, confusion, and increased costs. Territorial and turf disputes deter from maximal patient care potential. Whether it is a private ambulance service, a military air ambulance,

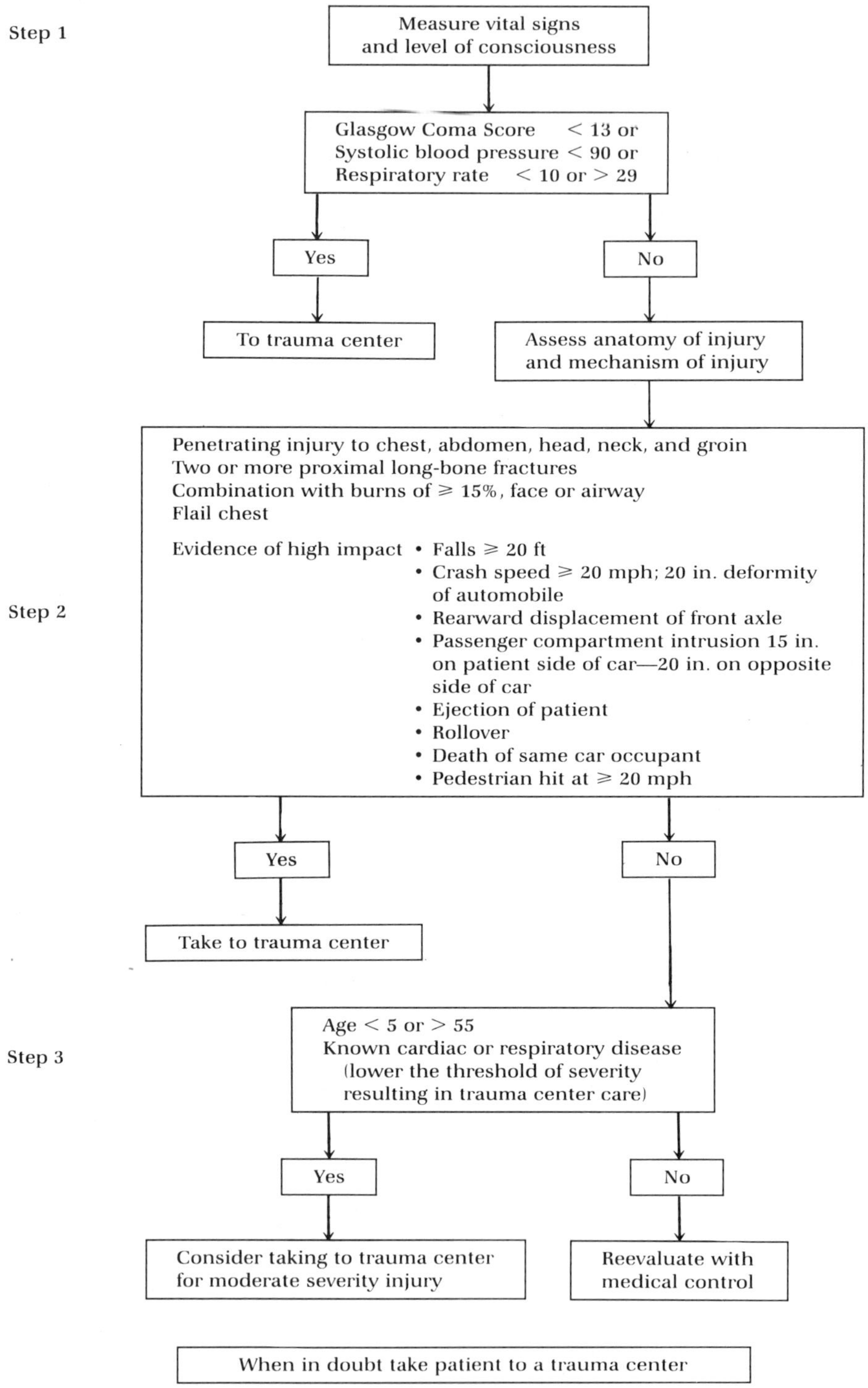
Step 1
Measure vital signs and level of consciousness
Glasgow Coma Score < 13 or
Systolic blood pressure < 90 or
Respiratory rate < 10 or > 29
Yes
No
To trauma center
Assess anatomy of injury and mechanism of injury
Step 2
Penetrating injury to chest, abdomen, head, neck, and groin
Two or more proximal long-bone fractures
Combination with burns of ⩾ 15%, face or airway
Flail chest
Evidence of high impact
• Falls ⩾ 20 ft
• Crash speed ⩾ 20 mph; 20 in. deformity of automobile
• Rearward displacement of front axle
• Passenger compartment intrusion 15 in. on patient side of car—20 in. on opposite side of car
• Ejection of patient
• Rollover
• Death of same car occupant
• Pedestrian hit at ⩾ 20 mph
Yes
No
Take to trauma center
Step 3
Age < 5 or > 55
Known cardiac or respiratory disease (lower the threshold of severity resulting in trauma center care)
Yes
No
Consider taking to trauma center for moderate severity injury
Reevaluate with medical control
When in doubt take patient to a trauma center

or a private hospital-based air ambulance service, activities of dispatch, protocol, audit, and utilization should be subject to regional EMS policies.

Standard 2. Urban air ambulances should be designated for medical purposes only. Multipurpose vehicles (e.g., used for police, rescue, EMS, weather observation, traffic control), either air or ground, cannot provide the optimal resources and personnel needed to complete each of the differing targeted tasks. Demographic data review can provide information as to the optimal number and distribution of medical care vehicles (air and/or ground) and personnel.

Standard 3. Urban air ambulance personnel should have advanced life support capability and responsibility for training, dispatch, and review under the direction of a designated medical director. Freestanding noncoordinated air ambulance services are expensive and have no documented health care advantages in the medical literature. The greatest documented advantage of the air ambulance is its ability to transport personnel with increased medical capability, skill, and judgment to the accident site or transferring hospital. Thus, air ambulance services should provide, as a minimum, advanced life support capability, especially endotracheal intubation [9].

Standard 4. Periodic quality assurance audits should be performed by an advisory panel to assure that this more costly system is being used for documentable medical reasons and is having a positive effect on the patient and the health care system.

Fig. 2-2. American College of Surgeons guidelines for triage of trauma victims.

Aeromedical transport has recently experienced phenomenal growth. In 1982, there were only 55 hospital-based helicopter programs; by March 1986, 117 programs were operating 136 helicopters [10]. With the proliferation of helicopter programs, however, has come a significant rise in the number of helicopter accidents. Presently, hospital-based helicopter programs are experiencing an accident rate three times greater and a fatal accident rate five times greater than that of all general aviation turbine helicopters [10]. Although the cause of these accidents has often been attributed to "pilot error," such characterization often masks the underlying cause. Flying in adverse conditions, inadequate consideration of flight safety prior to lift-off, lack of current pilot instrument rating, and pilot fatigue have been cited as the actual causes of fatal accidents. It is clear that the issue of helicopter safety must be addressed for aeromedical transport programs to continue. Further, those establishing new programs must include flight safety as a program component of the transport service.

In addition, several items should be considered by the regional EMS medical director when an air ambulance service is proposed.

1. Will the proposed air ambulance service serve only one hospital, or is it a regional/resource service?
2. What are the specific medical/surgical criteria for determining when an air ambu-

lance (versus ground ambulance) should be used?

3. What are the realistic time-distance relationships for that region that would justify use of the air ambulance?
4. How many helicopters (and/or competing helicopter services) should be allowed to operate in a geographic catchment area? Each helicopter can effectively transport 600 to 800 patients a year before availability becomes a problem.

These proposed standards for urban air ambulance operations should increase the efficiency of the service, provide coordination with existing ground ambulance services, and ensure that patients with emergency conditions are transported to the most appropriate facility, thus making better use of limited health care dollars.

Ambulances

Although there is a proliferation of helicopter systems, in part prompted by the need to expedite care to the trauma victim, the vast majority of those who suffer major injury are transported from the scene of the accident by ground transport. This remains the transport mode of choice in the urban environment where transport times to a level I or level II trauma center should not exceed 15 minutes and where total prehospital time should not exceed 30 minutes, unless entrapment or unusual impediments to egress exist.

Choice of Transport

The choice of transport mode should be made on the basis of the most expeditious method of getting the patient with multiple injuries to definitive care. This choice should be made by the highest available medical authority, preferably incorporating input of the specially trained physician prehospital director.

URBAN TRAUMA SYSTEMS

Urban systems in the northeastern United States have very little call for helicopters to expedite care for trauma victims. Most of these trauma systems have wide access to tertiary care teaching hospitals meeting level I or level II American College of Surgeons trauma center standards. In such cities, helicopters should be reserved for (1) expediting care where egress or access to the site is impeded by traffic or other problems, (2) bringing physicians or critical care nurses to the scene where victims are entrapped or where delayed transport from the scene will likely occur, and (3) distributing multiple casualties with severe injuries throughout a number of trauma centers. In other cities where the surface area is large and the concentration of hospitals is generally in one area, helicopters may be necessary to expedite care to distant parts of the city. Houston, with a surface area of over 160 square miles, is a good example of an urban environment where helicopters have proved to be useful.

Just as one should not delay transport to bring an advanced life support ambulance to the scene when a basic life support vehicle is available, one should not delay transport to bring a helicopter to the scene of an accident when an ambulance is available and can be en route to the hospital.

SUBURBAN TRAUMA SYSTEMS

With a greater distance between appropriate facilities in suburban areas, helicopters are of some value in expediting care. Their selection, however, should be under medical control with one guideline being that total prehospital time should be shortened as a result of the use of a helicopter.

RURAL ENVIRONMENT

In the rural environment, it is likely that too much time will elapse before the helicopter can arrive at the scene of the injury. It is in the patient's interest that this time be spent en route to a hospital that will expedite both immediate care and if necessary transfer to a definitive care facility.

Medical Control

The quality of the prehospital triage, treatment, and transport systems is largely based on the ability of those systems to be responsive to state-of-the-art medical direction. Further, medical control can aid in the correct identification of individuals who need trauma center care, as well as in the correct use of helicopters to expedite their transport. A standard of excellence is emerging in systems where individuals trained in effective and expeditious prehospital care have the responsibility of directing and monitoring the trauma system of care. Unfortunately, these systems are rare. In a study prepared in the Metropolitan Washington, D.C. area, it was found that medical control and public guidelines were able to reduce the mistriages by about 50 percent.

It is still possible to find prehospital systems without medical surveillance or control spending significant amounts of time placing IVs and doing cardiopulmonary resuscitation on patients who have cardiac arrest following injury rather than focusing on expediting patient transport to the hospital. It is unfortunate that patients can deteriorate to an irreversible point in the prehospital care system when appropriate medical control and surveillance are not instituted. All prehospital care systems need a knowledgeable person to provide surveillance of trauma care and ensure that only necessary and potentially beneficial maneuvers are rendered without sacrificing expedited transport.

Hospitals

Of the 6640 hospitals in the United States, between 100 and 150 legitimately functioned as trauma centers in 1986. These trauma centers cover approximately 25 percent of the population. There is little disagreement now that death and disability from injury can be substantially reduced if patients receive timely care in hospitals that have demonstrated a special commitment to 24-hour availability of trauma care. The American College of Surgeons has promulgated guidelines that characterize this commitment and classify trauma centers as level I, level II, or level III [11].

Generally, level I trauma centers provide a community with 24-hour, immediately available care by in-hospital surgeons and other on-call physicians. These hospitals have a significant research and teaching commitment to the community and provide leadership in regional trauma system development. Level II trauma centers may be academic centers or community, suburban hospitals with a special commitment to trauma care by immediately available on-call attending physicians. Level II centers provide 24-hour available care by in-hospital and on-call physicians.

Level III hospitals provide prompt assessment, resuscitation, and stabilization followed by surgical treatment or interhospital transfer. There is little use for level III trauma centers in the urban environment, but they do provide a valuable function in the more sparsely populated rural or outer suburban communities where it may be in the patient's interest to be evaluated in-hospital prior to transfer to definitive care.

Verification and Designation

In addition to defining the criteria by which hospitals can measure their commitment to trauma care, the American College of Surgeons also provides a mechanism for trauma center designation to occur, which is multidisciplinary team evaluation of a hospital against the trauma center criteria. This verification process is vastly different from designation of trauma centers on the basis of local politics, which unfortunately has occurred in several jurisdictions in the United States. In these jurisdictions, efforts to ensure high-quality trauma care are sacrificed to the political or jurisdictional considerations of the reviewing agency. There is a sharp contrast between a facility that meets the rigorous trauma center criteria of the American College of Surgeons and one that meets less exacting state-devised standards.

Given that both the methods and the mechanism exist for fair and impartial trauma center assessment and designation, health planners should focus their efforts on appropriate configuration of regional trauma systems. Specifically, the following factors should be taken into account:

1. Geographic characteristics and distance between hospitals.
2. Transport resource capabilities, including helicopter and fixed wing available for distances in excess of 50 km and 150 km, respectively.
3. Distribution of level I, level II, and level III hospitals in the community.
4. Population density.
5. Willingness of hospitals to function as trauma centers.
6. Medical politics, where competing tertiary care institutions believe they must provide a trauma service.
7. Training and research.
8. Patient volume: There is no doubt that certain benefits accrue from concentrating personnel and equipment resources in a limited number of institutions. If patient volume at these institutions subsequently increases, the in-hospital system of trauma care improves, and the ability develops to provide concentrated training and much-needed research. This is possible in certain areas where medical politics among multiple institutions are not too disabling. Unfortunately, this is not so in most urban areas because of the increasing competition to receive the accolade of "trauma center" for the purpose of attracting patients. There is little doubt that high-technology, multidisciplinary care is on a volume curve and that institutions require a minimum exposure to sustain proficiency [12]. For

trauma, a minimum exposure per trauma center is 600 severely injured patients a year, thus allowing the number of trauma patients treated by a given surgeon covering the service to exceed a minimum of 50 per year. In many parts of the country, this may not be possible as a result of population density. However, whenever the population exists, this standard should be aspired to.

Patient Volume

Projecting the likely volume of trauma patients for a given population is an important factor in determining the distribution of trauma centers. In Maryland, it was computed that the number of patients hospitalized with an injury severity score of greater than 15 was approximately 550 patients per million per year. Of those, only 350 patients per million per year require care in an intensive care unit. There are others whose morbidity can be limited by treatment or assessment in trauma centers. The total number who should be triaged to trauma center care is probably in the region of 1000 patients per million per year. Nationwide, the number of patients who require trauma center care is estimated to be 240,000 per year; of these, approximately 80,000 (30 percent) will die in-hospital.

In-Hospital Organization of Acute Care

Level I Trauma Center

By definition, a level I trauma center is a tertiary care community trauma resource with a research and teaching commitment. The minimum level of the available expertise must be an attending emergency physician and a senior resident in surgery. The in-hospital response should be organized as a team response system that is activated for all patients who meet entry triage guidelines at the emergency room door. The triage guidelines used at the Washington Hospital Center for the past 10 years are shown in Table 2-1; the configuration of the trauma team is shown in Table 2-2. Many teaching institutions now believe that care to the trauma victim is substantially improved by the presence of attending surgeons who have completed their boards in surgery and who may or may not have specialized for 1 year in trauma care. A number of leading trauma centers in the United States have at least 24-hour attending availability.

The level I trauma center is also able to mobilize additional resources when necessary to receive additional patients and can offer the immediate availability of 24-hour operating capabilities and extensive blood banking resources. Since the level I trauma center has a teaching commitment, it should receive at least 1000 patients a year to maintain state-of-the-art techniques to satisfy the teaching commitment to residents in training and to conduct clinical research.

The level I trauma center has the responsibility of establishing quality assurance programs for the regional trauma program. It must therefore provide the political interface with the jurisdictional government to ensure a continuing political commitment to the regional trauma system, as well as to implement regional quality assurance guidelines and provide professional and public education of the system.

Table 2-1. Interhospital Triage Criteria

The following list identifies patients at a particularly high risk of dying from multiple and severe injuries. Ideally, such patients should be treated in a high-level trauma center where continued exposure to such problems by multidisciplinary team systems may afford a patient an optimum outcome. Such patients should be considered for transfer to high-level centers wherever possible.

- Central nervous system
  - Head injury
    - Penetrating injury
    - Depressed skull fracture
    - Open injury
    - CSF leak
    - Severe coma (GCS <10)
    - Deterioration in GCS of 2 or more
    - Lateralizing signs
  - Spinal cord injury
- Chest
  - Wide superior mediastinum
  - Major chest wall injury
  - Cardiac injury
  - Patients who may require protracted ventilation
- Pelvis
  - Pelvic ring disruption with shock, more than 5 units transfusion, evidence of continued hemorrhage, and compound (open) pelvic injury or pelvic visceral injury
- Multiple system injury
  - Severe face injury with head injury
  - Chest injury with head injury
  - Abdominal or pelvic injury with head injury
  - Burns with head injury
- Secondary deterioration (late sequelae)
  - Patient requiring mechanical ventilation
    - Sepsis
    - Single or multiple organ system failure (deterioration in CNS, cardiac, pulmonary, hepatic, renal, or coagulation systems)
    - Osteomyelitis

Table 2-2. Configuration of a Trauma Team

- Trauma attending
- Trauma fellow
- Team leader—Resident-4
- Resident-2
- Resident-1
- Trauma nurse
- Responder nurse, critical care
- Respiratory therapist
- Anesthesiologist
- Cardiovascular technician
- Blood bank technician
- X-ray technician

Level II Trauma Center

The rationale behind the level II trauma center is that it should be able to deliver the same care as a level I center, but without the teaching, research, and community leadership commitments and obligations of level I centers. Consequently, level II trauma centers are those teaching hospitals that have chosen not to develop all of the resources required for level I trauma care but that, nonetheless, have certain obligations to the community for providing trauma care. Alternatively, they may be community hospitals that have a limited teaching commitment and man the trauma service with on-call surgeons. Such institutions, again, should focus their ability to provide acute care on the basis of a team response. The coordinator of the team in these instances is often the emergency department physician, who should be, at a minimum, ATLS-certified and in-hospital 24 hours a day. Other surgeons should be immediately available on-call and certainly no more than 20 minutes away. Often, it is demanded that these individuals be in-house or at least en route to the hospital when the patient's condition is called in from the prehospital system.

The chief of the trauma service at a level II center is usually a part-time appointment. Such an individual, however, must also have a role in establishing and sustaining prehospital protocols of trauma care. Ideally, there should be some relationship between this individual and an academic trauma center for exposure to state-of-the-art techniques, technology, and continuing education opportunities.

Unfortunately, the criteria used to designate level II trauma centers widely vary throughout the country. Furthermore, it must be realized that a busy surgeon's commitment to the nocturnal demands of trauma care often begins to give way as his or her private practice becomes more successfully established. Unless the surgeon has the ability to divest him- or herself of other responsibilities, the system often fails when patient needs are most critical or when multiple patients need treatment. The level II trauma center can and often does provide the level of commitment that can substantially reduce the unnecessary deaths, and provided it is linked into a quality of care assessment system, the level II trauma center will be the future linchpin in the effort to provide widespread availability of trauma center care in the United States.

Level III Trauma Center

While there is little rationale for level III trauma centers in urban communities, level III centers may expedite advanced life support and prompt triage of patients in certain suburban areas of the United States. The most important role of these institutions, however, is to provide trauma care in the rural environments. As such, the emergency physician and attending surgeon should at least be ATLS-certified and be able to provide initial resuscitation and evaluation of patients with traumatic injuries. These individuals not only provide initial care but, more importantly, identify patients whose injuries are either beyond the capabilities of the level III center or whose morbidity could be reduced by transport to a level I or level II institution. In such instances, the level III trauma center can provide resuscitation while plans are finalized to transport the patient in as stable a mode as possible. There is still residual concern among many level I trauma centers that initial transport of patients to level III institutions results in unnecessary delay. These concerns have grown out of instances where the level III hospital has focused greater attention on processing numerous x-rays instead of on prompt resuscitation and transfer. It is extremely distressing for a level I trauma center to receive a hypovolemic patient, accompanied by numerous x-rays of limbs, the taking of which clearly was not warranted as a matter of priority. Often, in these cases, the half hour gained in expediting care, at the expense of x-rays, would be more beneficial for the patient.

Factors Important in Sequencing and Continuum of Care of the Major Trauma Victim

Emergency Entrance

Immediately upon arrival, triage of the patient must occur. Patients with potentially life-threatening injuries should be identified and channeled into a special system of hospital care. In many institutions, there is a discrete separation of patients with major injuries and mobilization of a specific team response that provide additional resources to the emergency environment. This has the effect of providing significant resources to those severely injured as soon as possible while not detracting from the care that is required by other patients in the emergency department. The team response system was developed by Dr. William Gissane in 1932 at Birmingham Accident Hospital and has been successfully adopted in many leading trauma centers.

Quality assessment of the initial care received by patients in this environment is essential. All deaths should be routinely scrutinized, as should all patients whose initial evaluation takes in excess of 2 hours (including x-ray).

X-ray

Unnecessary x-rays and delay in x-ray have been cited as frequent problems of trauma care. It is often more practical to keep the patient in the controlled environment of the emergency department or resuscitation area and take portable x-rays as part of identifying the treatment priorities, rather than to take the patient to the x-ray department, where control may be forfeited. Often, however, the need for a computed tomographic (CT) scan or angiography mandates that the patient be taken to the radiology department. In these cases, it is essential that a coordinated system be developed whereby ventilator and pharmacologic support be continued, if necessary. It is this multidisciplinary high-technology support throughout the continuum of care that is likely to result in lives saved. X-rays should be read by appropriate senior individuals. It is important that CT scan interpretation not be left to junior residents in radiology but rather be completed by senior personnel.

Operating Room

Immediate operating room capability should be available 24 hours a day in level I and level II trauma centers. When the operating room is occupied, other teams should be brought into the hospital so that expedited management of a second patient can occur. Nearly 20 percent of multiple trauma victims, whether they have blunt or penetrating wounds, require multiple surgical teams [13]. Anesthesia time can be shortened with multiple operating teams; the exposure of patients to massive transfusion and hypothermia is likely to be reduced.

Intensive Care

The trauma surgeon should acquire and maintain state-of-the-art knowledge of intensive care management. In all levels of trauma centers, 24-hour in-hospital physician coverage for trauma patients in the intensive care unit is mandatory. Here again, a coordinated multidisciplinary team approach is important in patient care; systematic multiple use of consultants is much less satisfactory.

Surgical Ward

The trauma service of a level I trauma center should have a discrete postoperative non–intensive care unit ward, where patients are managed by the trauma teams. These units require a higher nurse-patient ratio than that required in normal general surgical wards. In the intensive care unit, the nurse-patient ratio is often 1:1 or 1:2. It is advisable that the postoperative ward have a general availability of nurses in a ratio of about 1:4 to 1:6. Detection and management of cardiopulmonary deterioration, early signs of sepsis, and orthopedic or neurologic sequelae of injury all require increased nursing care.

Rehabilitation

Sadly, the integration of current state-of-the-art rehabilitative capabilities into the acute care of the trauma victim is often lacking. The techniques and technology in this discipline have rapidly advanced over the past 10 years. As a result, early integration of rehabilitation medicine into the management of patients with multisystem injuries, particularly neurologic, soft tissue, or orthopedic injuries, can substantially reduce residual disability, maximize patient capabilities, and shorten the time that it takes the patient to return to maximum postinjury capability.

The MedSTAR Trauma Service at the Washington Hospital Center is fortunate to have a tertiary care rehabilitation facility on the same campus. This enables rehabilitative care to be integrated directly into the acute phases of management. Rehabilitation department personnel perform trauma rounds on a weekly basis with the trauma service and are involved in the intensive care and step-down unit phases of patient care.

Currently, much rehabilitative care of the comatose patient is directed toward undoing the sequelae and complications that have ensued during the acute care phase. Only by actively integrating the rehabilitative medicine technologies and techniques into acute care on a systematic basis can these sequelae and their associated costs be minimized.

Referral Centers

Spinal Cord

The National Spinal Cord Injury Association has established criteria for spinal cord injury centers. Unfortunately, many of these are not associated with trauma centers; consequently, it is possible for patients with multisystem diffuse blunt injury to be triaged to such centers without prior adequate multisystem evaluation. Wherever possible, the regional trauma system should designate the leading level I trauma center or another level I or level II trauma center with a special commitment to spinal cord injury to be the referral point for all patients with spinal cord injury. There is no doubt that these patients can benefit from specifically focused multidisciplinary care, involving neurosurgery, orthopedics, rehabilitation medicine, and general trauma surgery. The objective of this focused care is to ensure that the patient has a multisystem evaluation and appropriate hospital intensive care management with early fixation of the spinal column, so that rehabilitation can be instituted as promptly as possible. Ideally, such patients should be in a rehabilitation mode within 3 weeks of injury. Total rehabilitation time in state-of-the-art centers is about 60 days for paraplegics and about 90 days for quadriplegics, at which point these individuals should be able to make progress toward reintegration into society.

Pediatric Trauma

There is some debate as to the need for pediatric trauma centers. Suffice it to say that where the community resources exist, it may be of benefit to triage all pediatric trauma patients to a facility with those commitments. Although trauma is the leading cause of death in children, the frequency and incidence are not great enough for more than a handful of pediatric surgeons to become facile with the management of injury as a discipline. Pediatric trauma centers probably require a population base in excess of 2 to 3 million. Where such a referral base does not exist, it is preferable to treat the patient at an adult trauma center, where they are afforded the skills of an experienced trauma surgeon, and then provide additional pediatric intensive care backup and psychosocial rehabilitative resources.

Organ Replantation

The trauma system must have the ability to replant digits and distal upper limbs. This requires a two-team multidisciplinary approach and availability of specific personnel, resources, and organization.

Transplantation

A regional trauma system should act as an adjunct to a regional transplantation system. Individuals with irreversible brain damage are the most likely source of organs for donation. There is an increasing need to recognize and respond to the increasing demands of the transplantation services and provide kidneys, hearts, livers, and so on.

Economics

There are significant threats to the economic viability of regional trauma systems. These result from several forces. Many urban trauma centers are located in downtown areas, with the result that many patients with penetrating injuries requiring significant medical resources are indigent. Consequently, many urban trauma centers often provide a high proportion of uncompensated care. In addition, such institutions often act as a referral point for private hospitals that choose not to treat patients whose care cannot be reimbursed. Thus, the urban trauma center often assumes an unfair load of indigent care, some of which commands significant resource utilization. About 50 percent of such care is currently uncompensated, amounting to a $1 billion national problem.

Further, the prospective payment system, based on diagnosis-related groups (DRGs), cannot equitably compensate hospitals for their costs in caring for trauma patients. DRGs have several structural weaknesses, the most significant of which are as follows: (1) the DRG system does not account for severity mix within a DRG grouping; (2) the DRG for traumatic injury poorly describes multiple injuries and does not account for the additive effect of multiple injuries on treatment required; and (3) with injuries that result in severe coma, there is no mechanism for ensuring reimbursement of care for long hospitalization.

Although DRG-based reimbursement was initiated for Medicare patients, many states are moving to implement prospective reimbursement for Medicaid patients based on the DRG system. Further, many private insurance companies are evaluating the efficacy of such reimbursement. There is no doubt that should the DRG system for trauma be adopted by all insurance companies, it would have significant negative impact on the ability of an institution to provide state-of-the-art care.

REFERENCES

1. *Accident Facts 1986.* Chicago, National Safety Council, 1986 Chicago:
2. National Academy of Sciences/National Research Council. *Accidental Death and Disability: The Neglected Disease of Modern Society.* Washington, D.C.: National Academy Press, 1966.
3. National Academy of Sciences/National Research Council. *Injury in America: A Continuing Health Problem.* Washington, D.C.: National Academy Press, 1985.
4. Baker, S. P., O'Neill, B., Haddon, W., and Long, W. B. The injury severity score: A method for describing patients with multiple injuries and evaluating emergency care. *J. Trauma* 14:187, 1974.
5. San Diego Hospital Association. *Annual Report of the San Diego Trauma System.* San Diego: Department of Health Services, 1987.
6. American College of Surgeons Committee on Trauma. Field categorization of trauma patients. *Am. Coll. Surg. Bull.* 71(10): 17–21, 1986.
7. Champion, H. R., Copes, W. S., et al. *The Major Trauma Outcome Study.* Submitted for publication.
8. Champion, H. R., and Lewis, F. Report on the Conference on Injury Severity Scoring and Triage. U.S. Army Medical Research and Development Command, Contract No. DAMD17-83-G-9529, Washington, D.C., 1983.
9. Commission on Emergency Medical Services. *Air Ambulance Guidelines.* Washington, D.C.: U.S. Department of Transportation, February 1981.
10. Collett, H. M. Risk management and the aeromedical helicopter. *Emerg. Care Q.* 2(3):31, 1986.
11. Committee on Trauma of the American College of Surgeons. Hospital and pre-hospital resources for optimal care of the injured patient. *Am. Coll. Surg. Bull.* 71(10):4 1986.
12. Luft, H. S., Bunker, J. P., and Enthoven, A. C. Should operations be regionalized? The empirical relation between surgical volume and mortality. *N. Engl. J. Med.* 301:1364, 1979.
13. Champion, H. R., and Rupp M. *Use of Surgical Resources in the Treatment of Major Trauma.* Submitted for publication.

3

Trauma and Shock

David J. Kreis, Jr.

Shock is a common clinical problem. This is particularly true today as emergency medical services have been modernized in many communities throughout the United States over the past 20 years. With appropriate prehospital care, many severely injured patients are successfully being transported alive to hospitals for definitive care. It is important for all physicians involved with treating the injured patient to understand the different causes of shock following injury so that a rational and effective therapeutic plan can be instituted.

The first use of the term *shock* is credited to James Lotta in 1795 [1]. Throughout the nineteenth century, shock was thought to result from a primary dysfunction of the central nervous system. This interpretation was popularized by both Goltz and Crile. Henderson in 1908 introduced the acapnia theory of shock, namely that shock was caused by the hypocarbia that results from the hyperventilation seen commonly in shock. Cannon and Bayliss in 1919 thought that shock was a direct result of a circulating depressant factor.

Alfred Blalock was the first to classify shock based on modern physiologic principles [2,3]. He outlined four major causes of shock as follows: (1) hematogenic shock, due to decreased blood volume; (2) cardiogenic shock, due to pump failure; (3) vasogenic shock, due to vasodilatation secondary to humoral agents; and (4) neurogenic shock, due to vasodilatation secondary to altered vascular tone. This original classification system will be updated in the subsequent section.

Regardless of the etiology of shock, shock may best be defined as a clinical syndrome that results from circulatory insufficiency and inadequate tissue perfusion. It is this deficit in sufficient tissue perfusion and not hypotension per se that best characterizes the essential concept of shock.

This chapter will describe the major causes of shock that can occur in the injured patient.

ETIOLOGY

Blalock's classification of shock can be updated. It is known that vasogenic and neurogenic shock are due primarily to alterations in total peripheral vascular resistance. Neurogenic shock can thus be considered a subset of vasogenic shock. There exist, therefore, three main causes of shock: hematogenic, cardiogenic, and vasogenic (Table 3-1). These three major etiologies of shock correspond to the three major components of the circulatory system. The circulation should be regarded as a closed-loop system comprising the blood volume, the heart, and the blood vessels. A defect in the normal functioning of any or all of these vital components may cause shock. In the trauma patient, it is not uncommon for more than one cause of shock to be present simultaneously. For example, a patient in shock following a motor vehicle accident may have both bleeding (hematogenic shock) and a tension pneumothorax (cardiogenic shock). It is paramount for the physician to identify the life-threatening conditions causing shock during the initial evaluation of the patient.

Table 3-1. Causes of Shock

Blalock	Update
Hematogenic Decrease in blood volume	Hematogenic
Cardiogenic Pump failure	Cardiogenic
Vasogenic Vasodilatation due to humoral agents	Vasogenic Altered peripheral vascular resistance
Neurogenic Vasodilatation due to altered vascular tone	Neurogenic Septic Anaphylactic

In common practice, physicians recognize five clinical forms of shock. These clinical forms occur mainly because of one of the above three causes of shock. These clinical forms are hemorrhagic or hypovolemic shock (hematogenic shock), cardiogenic shock, neurogenic shock (vasogenic shock), septic shock (vasogenic shock), and anaphylactic shock (vasogenic shock). As outlined in this classification scheme, neurogenic shock, septic shock, and anaphylactic shock are all subsets of vasogenic shock because the primary defect in each of these clinical conditions involves changes in total peripheral vascular resistance regardless of whether these changes are due to blood-borne factors or alterations in nervous system control over vascular tone.

It is practical to characterize early and late causes of shock in the trauma patient. Early causes, occurring soon after injury, usually involve either hemorrhagic shock, cardiogenic shock, or neurogenic shock. A late cause of shock, usually occurring days after injury, is septic shock. Sepsis is the most common late cause of death following injury. Anaphylactic shock is rare in the trauma patient unless the patient has an unpredictable anaphylactic reaction to an administered medication.

It is clear that, during the initial resuscitation of the critically injured patient, it is vital to rule out whether any or all of the early causes of shock are present. Is the patient bleeding? Is there a pneumothorax or cardiac tamponade? Is a spinal cord injury present? These are some of the crucial questions that need to be answered promptly.

DIAGNOSIS

Shock after injury is usually easily recognized. The classic clinical findings include hypotension, a weak and rapid pulse, shallow and rapid respirations, altered mental status, skin pallor and coldness, decreased urine output, and acidemia. There are deviations from this usual picture in the occasional patient.

In the adult, hypotension is usually defined as a systolic blood pressure of less than 90 mm Hg. In a previously hypertensive patient, a decrease in systolic blood pressure of 50 mm Hg would also signify hypotension. This is particularly true in the geriatric population. Alterations in mental status are common and are due to abnormalities in cerebral perfusion or hypoxemia. These changes may be manifest as anxiety, confusion, combativeness, stupor, or coma. The effects of intoxication with alcohol or psychotropic drugs may also be contributory.

The heart rate in shock is variable, although the majority of patients have tachycardia. This is a compensatory response to improve cardiac output. An occasional patient in shock may have bradycardia. This may be seen if the patient has sustained a myocardial contusion or a myocardial infarction. Most patients will be hyperventilating, which is the normal response to sympathoadrenal stimulation and anxiety.

A detailed discussion of the various causes of shock in the trauma patient will follow. It is important, however, to outline how one should be able to differentiate the major cause of shock that occurs soon after injury. If the patient is in shock and has tachycardia and flat neck veins, then the most likely cause is bleeding (hemorrhagic shock). If the patient has tachycardia and distended neck veins, then the most likely cause is tension pneumothorax or pericardial tamponade (cardiogenic shock). If the patient has a normal pulse rate, flat neck veins, and paralysis, then the most likely cause is a spinal cord injury (neurogenic shock). These clinical judgments should be made rapidly during the initial assessment of all trauma patients in shock. In general, these diagnostic maxims hold true unless there are other concurrent causes for shock.

HEMORRHAGIC SHOCK

Hemorrhagic shock is a common cause of shock after injury and is due to an acute decrease in blood volume. The bleeding may be obvious, as in a gunshot wound of the femoral artery, or cryptic, such as in a retroperitoneal hematoma. The normal adult blood volume is 4.0 to 4.5 liters (67 ml/kg) in the female and 5.0 to 5.5 liters (75 ml/kg) in the male.

There are four classes of hemorrhage following injury [4]. Class I represents an acute blood loss of up to 15 percent (750 ml) of the blood volume. These patients have a normal physical examination. Class II hemorrhage is caused by an acute loss of 15 to 30 percent (750–1500 ml) of the blood volume. These patients have a normal blood pressure; however,

Table 3-2. Classes of Hemorrhage

Class	Blood loss	Physical examination	Therapy
I	15% (750 ml)	Normal	Crystalloid
II	15–30% (750–1500 ml)	Normal BP Tachycardia + Refill test Anxious	Crystalloid
III	30–40% (1500–2000 ml)	Hypotension Tachycardia + Refill test Confused/combative	Crystalloid and blood
IV	40% (2000 ml)	Hypotension Tachycardia + Refill test Comatose	Crystalloid and blood

they are tachycardic, have a positive capillary refill test, and are anxious. The capillary refill test involves pressing on the nail beds and noting the time it takes for subungual reperfusion. This normally occurs in less than 2 seconds. A prolonged refill test signifies circulatory insufficiency. Class III hemorrhage involves an acute decrease of 30 to 40 percent (1500–2000 ml) of the blood volume. These patients are in obvious shock. They are hypotensive and tachycardic, have a positive capillary refill test, and are confused or combative. Class IV hemorrhage is caused by an acute loss of greater than 40 percent (2000 ml) of the blood volume. These patients are in profound shock. They are hypotensive and tachycardic, have a positive capillary refill test, and are stuporous or comatose (Table 3-2).

This classification system of hemorrhage provides a rapid clinical way to assess how much blood the patient may have lost at the time of initial evaluation. It serves as a guideline as to whether blood should be administered early in the resuscitation effort. Class I and II hemorrhages can usually be treated with crystalloid infusions. Class III and IV hemorrhages invariably also require blood transfusions and usually surgery to obtain hemostasis.

Pathophysiology

Cardiac output (CO) equals the product of heart rate (HR) times stroke volume (SV):

$$CO = HR \times SV$$

The normal cardiac output for the adult is 5.6L/min or 3.0 ± 0.5L/min/m^2 (cardiac index). Stroke volume is the volume of blood ejected by the heart per cardiac contraction. The normal stroke volume for the adult is about 70 ml or 40 ± 7 ml/m (stroke index). The regulation of cardiac output is mainly achieved through regulation of stroke volume. Stroke volume is controlled by the cardiac preload (amount of stretch put on the cardiac muscle before contraction), cardiac afterload (the resistance to forward blood flow caused by aortic pressure and vascular resistance), and the contractile state of the myocardium.

The factors that can affect the cardiac preload include blood volume, body position, intrathoracic pressure, intrapericardial pressure, venous tone, pumping action of skeletal muscle, and atrial contraction. An acute decrease in blood volume will directly decrease the cardiac preload and subsequently will effect a decrease in stroke volume and cardiac output. Since blood pressure equals the product of cardiac output times the total peripheral vascular resistance, the acute decrease in cardiac output caused by a class III or IV hemorrhage will result in hypotension.

The above changes can be viewed schematically. The relationship between cardiac preload and strength of cardiac contraction is known as the Frank-Starling relationship. This relationship can be expressed as a ventricular function curve relating preload to cardiac performance (Fig. 3-1). The preload of the right ventricle is estimated clinically by measuring the central venous pressure (CVP). The preload of the left ventricle is estimated by measuring the mean pulmonary artery occlusion pressure (PAOP). In general, as preload increases, so does cardiac performance. This

Fig. 3-1. The ventricular function curve is a graphic way of portraying cardiac performance as a function of preload. Factors affecting preload: blood volume, body position, intrathoracic pressure, intrapericardial pressure, venous tone, atrial contraction, and pumping action of skeletal muscle. (From D. J. Kreis, Jr., Shock [Part I]: Pathophysiology. *Curr. Rev. Respir. Ther.* 6:60, 1983.)

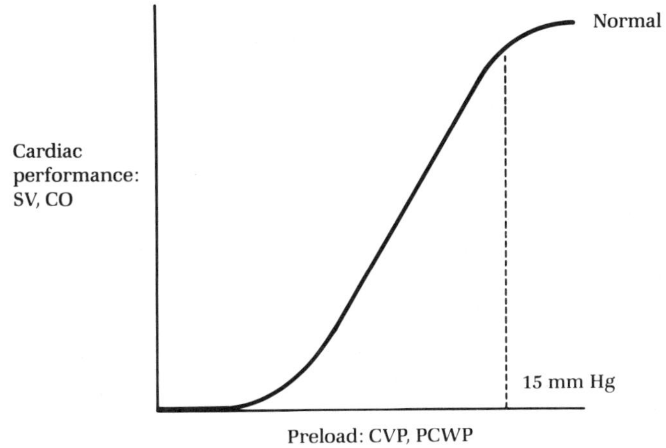

linear relationship reaches a plateau starting at a PAOP of 10 to 12 mm Hg.

The ventricular function curve is a graphic way to portray the effect of preload on cardiac performance. The reverse relationship, called the systemic function curve, exists as well [5,6]. It portrays venous return function and the effect of cardiac performance on preload (Fig. 3-2). In general, as cardiac output increases, cardiac preload decreases. Using a simple analogy, a pump that increases its pumping will lower the level of its reservoir priming the pump and vice versa. The main factors that influence the position of the systemic function curve are the blood volume and the vascular resistance.

The axes of the systemic function curve may be arbitrarily reversed (Fig. 3-3) so that both function curves can be plotted on the same graph (Fig. 3-4). A decrease in blood volume causes the systemic function curve (venous return curve) to shift downward and to the left (from equilibrium point *A* to new point *B*) (Fig. 3-5). There is an acute decrease in cardiac output and blood pressure. How does the body adjust to this loss of blood volume?

There are three major homeostatic mechanisms following hemorrhage: hemodynamic adjustments, hormonal adjustments, and volume adjustments. The hemodynamic adjustments involve activation of the sympathoadrenal axis so that total peripheral vascular resistance, cardiac contractility, and heart rate are increased. Water and salt are conserved by the actions of antidiuretic hormone and aldosterone. Interstitial fluid moves rapidly into the intravascular space. This process

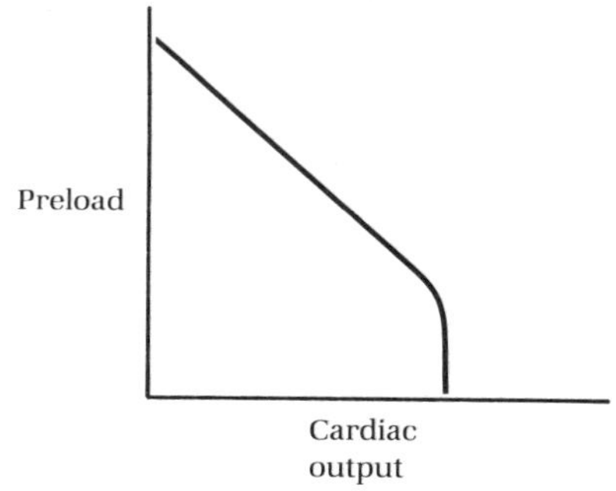

Fig. 3-2. The systemic function curve is a graphic way to portray venous return. It relates the functional dependence of preload on cardiac output. (From D. J. Kreis, Jr., Shock [Part I]: Pathophysiology. *Curr. Rev. Respir. Ther.* 6:61, 1983.)

of plasma refill may approach 1 liter in the first hour following severe hemorrhage and accounts for the low hematocrits that may be obtained soon after injury. The function of these compensatory mechanisms in concert is to increase the effective blood volume, increase cardiac output, and increase blood pressure.

These homeostatic improvements in blood volume will shift the systemic function curve toward normal. In a similar manner, the homeostatic changes in contractility and heart rate will improve the position of the ventricular function curve. The resulting new equilibrium point, *C*, is an improved hemodynamic position compared with point *B* (Fig. 3-5). If the acute blood loss is severe, then these normal compensatory mechanisms may fail unless the appropriate therapy is begun promptly.

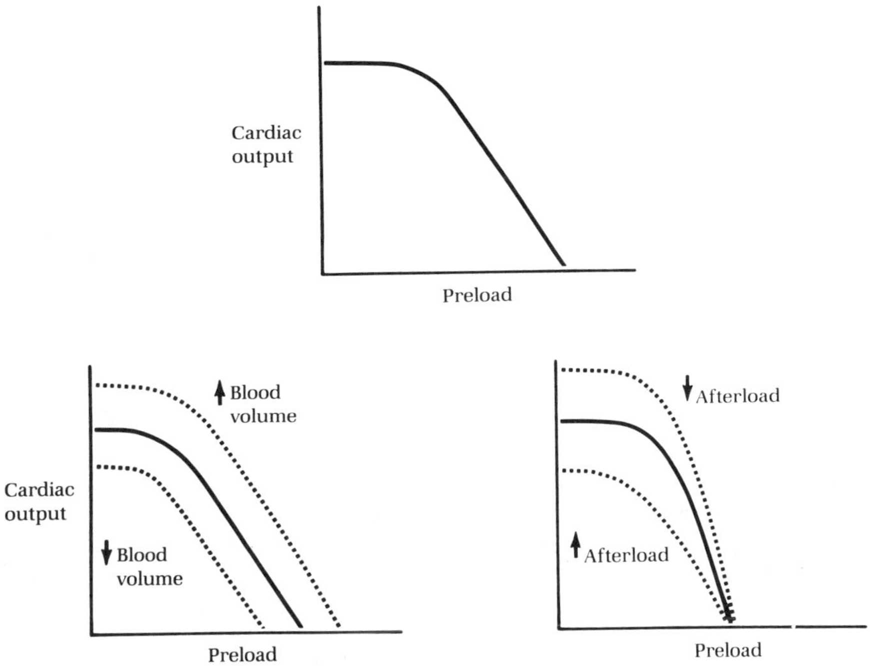

Fig. 3-3. The axes of the systemic function curve may be reversed so that they are similar to the ventricular function curve. The blood volume and vascular resistance are the main factors that influence the position of the systemic function curve. (From D. J. Kreis, Jr., Shock [Part I]: Pathophysiology. *Curr. Rev. Respir. Ther.* 6:62, 1983.)

Treatment

As in all resuscitation efforts certain priorities must be followed in the treatment of hemorrhagic shock. These priorities are known as the ABCs of resuscitation: airway, breathing, and circulation (Table 3-3).

The oropharynx should be cleared of all debris, blood, or vomitus. If the patient is in respiratory distress, then an airway must be secured immediately. This is usually accomplished by performing an endotracheal intubation while an assistant holds the head and cervical spine in-line. The patient is placed on 100% oxygen and is hand-ventilated using an Ambu bag. If the patient has sustained massive maxillofacial injury, intubation may be impossible, and a cricothyroidotomy should be performed. This can usually be accomplished in less than 1 minute. A formal tracheostomy should not be done emergently, since even in experienced hands, it may take well over 5 minutes to effect.

Once the airway and breathing are estab-

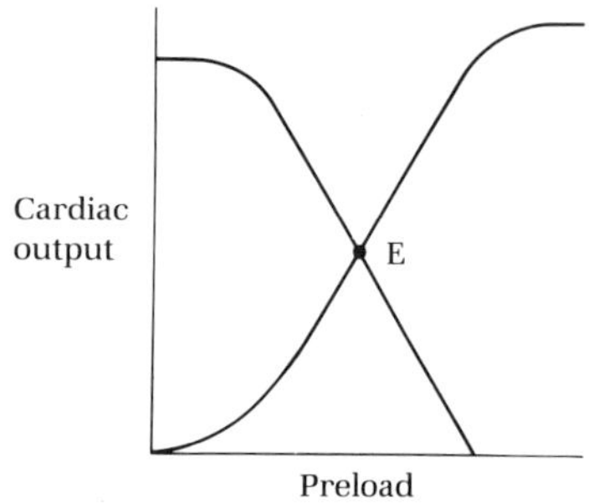

Fig. 3-4. The ventricular and systemic function curves can be integrated on the same graph. The point of intersection (*E*) represents the equilibrium point in overall cardiovascular function at any given time. Homeostatic mechanisms tend to maintain a steady state about this point. (From D. J. Kreis, Jr., Shock [Part 1]: Pathophysiology. *Curr. Rev. Respir. Ther.* 6:61, 1983.)

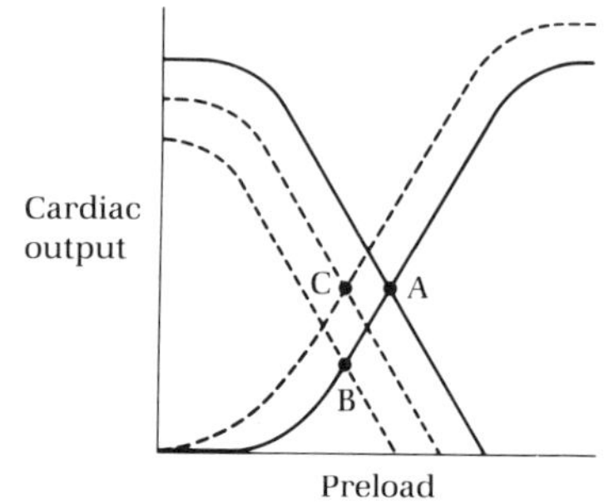

Fig. 3-5. In hemorrhagic shock, there is an acute decrease in blood volume. The systemic function curve shifts downward and to the left (point *A* to point *B*). Homeostatic mechanisms shift the systemic function curve upward and to the right and the ventricular function curve upward and to the left. The new compensated equilibrium point (*C*) represents an improved hemodynamic state over point *B*. (From G. R. Kelman, *Applied Cardiovascular Physiology.* Woburn, Mass.: Butterworth, 1979. P. 125.)

lished, the next priority is to control all external bleeding points. This is best accomplished using direct digital pressure. Often this task is being done by another assistant simultaneously as the airway is being secured. Blind clamping must be avoided. If there is massive bleeding following major amputation at the forearm or leg level, then it is reasonable to apply a tourniquet to stop the bleeding prior to operative exploration. The Military Anti-Shock Trouser (MAST) suit is not adequate in stopping major hemorrhage from an open leg wound. Patients may bleed several units of blood between the skin and the leg portion of the MAST suit. In this situation, direct digital pressure over the bleeding leg wound is the best therapy.

Once all external major bleeding points are controlled, the next priority is directed further at the circulation. Two large-bore (14- or 16-gauge in adults) intravenous catheters should be placed in the upper extremities. A central venous line is unnecessary in the acute resuscitation unless peripheral access is impossible or a CVP measurement is required to prove coexistent cardiac tamponade. More fluid may be administered in less time through peripheral catheters than through central catheters of similar size. Occasionally a saphenous venous cutdown will be required if the above access is impossible. Blood samples should be collected through the initial intravenous cannula at the time of insertion. Of all the samples collected, the most important is the blood for type and cross matching. This must be properly la-

Table 3-3. ABCs of Resuscitation

Airway
1. Remove all debris, blood, or vomitus from oropharynx
2. Secure airway: endotracheal intubation
3. Cricothyroidotomy if required
Breathing
1. 100% oxygen
2. Ambu bag manual ventilation
Circulation
1. Digital pressure on all external bleeding sites
2. Insert two large-gauge IVs
3. Volume load with Ringer's lactate:
2 L in 10 min (adult)
20 ml/kg in 10 min (child)
4. Blood transfusions
5. Consider MAST suit
6. Surgical intervention
7. Inotropic/vasopressor agents if required

beled and preferably hand-delivered to the blood bank by runner. The patient in severe hemorrhagic shock after trauma should be typed and cross matched for 6 units of blood.

In the adult in hemorrhagic shock, 2 liters of Ringer's lactate should be administered in the initial 10 to 15 minutes of the resuscitation. The dosage in children is 20 ml/kg, and this may be repeated once prior to commencing transfusion therapy. Therapy with Ringer's lactate has three functions: it replaces both intravascular and interstitial volume losses, it allows time for proper cross matching of type-specific blood, and it serves as an indicator of continuing hemorrhage. For example, if the blood pressure and pulse improve toward normal following the above fluid challenges, then it is probable that the bleeding has abated. On the other hand, if after the above fluid therapy the patient remains in shock, then ongoing hemorrhage is most likely, transfusion therapy should be started, and the need for operative intervention should be determined.

Ringer's lactate offers several advantages over normal saline in the resuscitation of the trauma patient in hemorrhagic shock: (1) the electrolyte composition of Ringer's lactate more closely approximates that of plasma, (2) the pH of Ringer's lactate is 6.5, whereas that of normal saline is 5.0, and (3) Ringer's lactate offers some buffering power, since 50 percent of the 28 mEq/L of lactate is metabolically available for conversion to bicarbonate by the liver. The argument that Ringer's lactate therapy may augment the lactic acidemia of shock is unfounded, as shown in clinical studies during the Vietnam War [7]. By improving circulatory volume, cardiac output, and tissue perfusion, Ringer's lactate actually corrects the acidemia of shock. It should be emphasized too that transfusion requirements are less when crystalloid solutions are part of volume therapy.

In class III or IV hemorrhage, transfusion therapy is required. It is unusual to have to resort to administering universal donor blood. Most blood banks should be able to supply type-specific blood within approximately 10 minutes. Fresh whole blood (< 24 hours old) is ideal but rarely available. In general, component therapy is the usual transfusion method. Packed red blood cells should be administered, with the estimated blood loss in mind. The hematocrit should be maintained at approximately 30. Raising the hematocrit above this level has little effect on the oxygen-carrying capacity of blood. Furthermore, the rheologic properties of blood are actually optimized at this level due to decreases in blood viscosity. During massive transfusion (> 10 units), dilution of clotting factors and platelets may cause a coagulopathy. This potential scenario makes the surgeon's job all the more difficult. It is important to consider fresh frozen plasma and platelet transfusions as part of the usual therapy of the massively bleeding trauma patient.

All trauma patients in hemorrhagic shock should be resuscitated with Ringer's lactate, blood products, and any indicated surgery. There is little if any role for the use of colloid solutions in the treatment of hemorrhagic shock. Colloid therapy is expensive and offers no proven advantage over the other treatments. There are five types of colloid solutions available for clinical use: fresh frozen plasma, albumin, plasma protein fraction (PPF) (Plasmanate, Plasmatein), dextran, and hetastarch.

Fresh frozen plasma carries a hepatitis risk and should be reserved to treat dilutional coagulopathy conditions following massive transfusion. Albumin is available either as a 5% or 25% solution in saline. The 5% solution is equivalent to its volume of plasma, whereas the 25% solution is equivalent to five times its volume of plasma. PPF is also available as a 5% solution. Dextran is a glucose polymer that is available as either dextran 40 (increases plasma volume by twice the volume given) or dextran 70 (increases plasma volume only slightly). Dextran should not be used in hemorrhagic shock since it interferes with blood cross matching, can cause an increased bleeding tendency with prolonged use by decreasing platelet adhesiveness, carries a risk of anaphylaxis, and can damage renal tubular cells in large doses.

Trendelenburg's position is sometimes used in the initial resuscitation of the patient in hemorrhagic shock. This should be avoided, since this positioning may increase carotid sinus flow and pressure and cause an undesired peripheral vasodilatation [8]. Although elevation of the patient's legs may cause a small autotransfusion of blood, this is a dangerous maneuver as well in the trauma patient in shock since there may be present an associated spine, pelvic, or lower extremity fracture.

The MAST suit has been used in the initial treatment of the civilian trauma patient in shock since 1973 [9]. It is routine for paramedic personnel to apply this garment at the scene of an injury if the patient is in shock. The MAST suit works mainly by increasing total peripheral vascular resistance (and thus blood pressure) rather than by increasing venous return as originally thought [10,11]. Although prospective randomized data concerning its proven usefulness are sparse, it is commonly used as an adjunct in shock following trauma [12]. It should be emphasized, however, that if inflation of the MAST suit is required to attain an adequate blood pressure, then it should, in general, remain inflated while the initial hospital resuscitation and diagnostic workup is undertaken and the patient is transported to the operating room.

Other measures that are routine procedure in the resuscitation of the trauma patient in shock include insertion of a Foley catheter (unless blood is noted at the urethral meatus or the prostate is floating on rectal examination), insertion of a nasogastric tube (unless there is a basilar skull fracture), splinting all fractures, obtaining a chest x-ray and other indicated radiographs, obtaining an electrocardiogram (ECG), arterial blood gas analysis, urine analysis, tetanus booster (if indicated), and antibiotics (if indicated).

In summary, the treatment of hemorrhagic shock after injury includes (1) securing the airway and breathing, (2) controlling all external bleeding sites with direct pressure, (3) volume therapy with Ringer's lactate and blood, and (4) the prompt determination of whether emergent surgery is needed.

CARDIOGENIC SHOCK

Cardiogenic shock results from the heart failing to pump blood effectively. The heart fails to produce an adequate cardiac output. There are two main causes of cardiogenic shock: primary (intrinsic) causes and secondary (extrinsic) causes (Table 3-4).

Primary causes of cardiogenic shock in the trauma patient include cardiac contusion, myocardial infarction, coronary air embolization, and cardiac arrhythmias. Secondary causes of cardiogenic shock in the trauma patient result from a mechanical obstruction to blood flow. This is sometimes called obstructive shock and may be caused by tension pneumothorax or pericardial tamponade.

Table 3-4. Causes of Cardiogenic Shock in Trauma

Primary
Cardiac contusion
Myocardial infarction
Coronary air embolization
Cardiac arrhythmias
Secondary
Tension pneumothorax
Pericardial tamponade

Pathophysiology

Cardiogenic shock is caused by a markedly decreased cardiac output. Since cardiac output is the product of heart rate times stroke volume, cardiogenic shock may result from abnormalities in either or both of these variables.

In cardiac contusion and myocardial infarction, there occurs actual structural damage to the myocardium. If this damage is severe, the heart will not function normally as a pump, and myocardial contractility will decrease. It has been estimated [13,14] that when cardiogenic shock complicates myocardial infarction, at least 40 percent of the myocardium has been infarcted. The cardiac effects of coronary air embolization are much like myocardial infarction in that there is an acute obstruction of normal coronary artery blood flow. Malignant arrhythmias may also occur either from hypoxemia or as effects of the other primary causes of cardiogenic shock.

Tension pneumothorax and pericardial tamponade both cause a decrease in the cardiac preload by greatly increasing intrathoracic and intrapericardial pressures, respectively. These pressure changes in effect prevent adequate venous return to the heart. Since preload is one of the major determinants of stroke volume, the stroke volume acutely decreases, as do the cardiac output and blood pressure subsequently.

Cardiac Contusion

Cardiac contusion is usually caused by a steering wheel or steering column impact on the anterior chest over the sternum. These patients usually do not present in shock. The key to the diagnosis is to maintain a high index of suspicion, especially when informed by the paramedics that the steering wheel was bent or when there is an obvious precordial contusion or abrasion on physical assessment. More common than extensive cardiac necrosis in this entity is the ever present danger of developing a fatal cardiac arrhythmia, such as ventricular tachycardia or fibrillation. These arrhythmias may develop without premonitory signs. Sternal tenderness is present in all patients; however, actual sternal fracture may be lacking.

All patients with suspected cardiac contusion should be monitored in either an intensive care unit or a telemetry unit, depending on the presence of associated injuries. Serial ECGs should be obtained as well as serial measurements of serum creatine kinase isoenzymes (CK-MB). Cardiac ultrasonography may be helpful in identifying associated wall motion abnormalities or pericardial effusions. The key to success is expectant observation in an appropriate environment [15].

Myocardial Infarction

Myocardial infarction can occur secondary to prolonged hypoxemia or other causes of shock in the trauma patient. It is not uncommon for severe hemorrhagic shock to be complicated by myocardial infarction, particularly in the older age group. Likewise, it is possible that the patient suffered the myocardial infarction prior to the injury. Most awake patients with myocardial infarction complain of substernal chest pain. This pain may radiate to the neck, arm, jaw, back, or epigastrium.

The ECG is nondiagnostic in 20 percent of cases. It is important to monitor the patient in the intensive care unit. Serial ECGs and CK-MB studies usually provide a definitive diagnosis. Oxygen therapy and prophylactic antiarrhythmic therapy with lidocaine are routine.

Patients in cardiogenic shock due to a myocardial infarction all have cardiac indices less than $2.2 L/min/m^2$ by definition [16]. Some patients may be hypovolemic. This is especially true if the infarction complicated a massive hemorrhage. These patients would therefore benefit from volume therapy because of the positive effects of improving preload on improving stroke volume. On the other hand, some patients may be hypervolemic and actually manifest signs of pulmonary congestion, namely dyspnea and rales. These patients have an elevated PAOP of greater than 18 mm Hg and usually require diuretic therapy, inotropic agents, and vasodilating agents both to decrease pulmonary congestion and to improve tissue perfusion.

Coronary Air Embolization

Coronary air embolization is a rare condition that may cause cardiogenic shock in the trauma patient. A lacerated lung from a fractured rib may cause air to escape into the pulmonary venous circulation. This air can then travel both to the coronary arteries and to the cerebral arteries. The result is the combined picture of sudden cardiogenic shock and seizures. Definitive therapy involves exploratory thoracotomy and occlusion of the hilum of the affected lung to prevent further air embolism.

Cardiac Arrhythmias

Cardiac arrhythmias causing shock in the trauma patient are usually a result of hypoxemia or myocardial contusion or infarction. About 90 percent of patients with myocardial infarction develop a disturbance in cardiac rhythm. Furthermore, over 90 percent of patients who die within 1 hour of infarction have ventricular fibrillation. For these reasons, oxygen therapy and appropriate antiarrhythmic agents should be instituted early.

Tension Pneumothorax

Tension pneumothorax is one of the most common causes of shock in the trauma patient. The pathophysiology involves a laceration of the visceral pleura such that, with each breath, air escapes and is trapped within the pleural space. As the intrapleural pressure increases, the great veins of the chest become compressed. This subsequently blocks venous return. Cardiac preload decreases, as do stroke volume, cardiac output, and blood pressure.

These patients present with hypotension, tachycardia, and diminished breath sounds on the affected side. There may be palpable subcutaneous emphysema, a shift of the trachea to the opposite side, and distended neck veins. A tension pneumothorax may cause death if not treated promptly. A temporary measure is to insert an 18- or 16-gauge cannula in the second intercostal space at the midclavicular line. This will in effect remove the tension component of the pneumothorax. The definitive treatment is tube thoracostomy. Pneumothorax following trauma usually has an associated hemothorax component. For this reason, it is customary when inserting a chest tube for tension pneumothorax to use a 36 or 40 Fr tube in the adult. It is inserted at the fifth or sixth intercostal space at the midaxillary line and directed posterior toward the chest apex.

Tension pneumothorax is a clinical diagnosis. Therapy must be immediate and should not depend on x-ray confirmation. Indeed, the chest x-ray in this situation should be obtained after the tube is inserted, to verify tube position and to rule out other possible thoracic abnormalities.

Pericardial Tamponade

Pericardial tamponade is usually due to penetrating cardiac injuries. As bleeding occurs into the pericardial space, the intrapericardial pressure increases. This increase in pressure effectively prevents venous return and adequate cardiac preload. The result is a decrease in stroke volume, cardiac output, and blood pressure.

Patients in pericardial tamponade are hypotensive and tachycardic and have muffled heart sounds and distended neck veins. Measuring a CVP value in this setting is helpful and usually registers greater than 25 to 30 cm H_2O. Since one of the major defects in this condition is inadequate cardiac preload, volume loading is an essential first step in the resuscitation of these patients. Pericardiocentesis may be lifesaving with the removal of as little as 50 ml of blood. Since tamponade is due to cardiac trauma, definitive therapy involves exploring the heart either through median sternotomy or thoracotomy.

Treatment

The ABCs of resuscitation should be applied to any critically injured patient regardless of the specific etiologies of shock. Airway and breathing are the first priorities. If the patient is noted to have a tension pneumothorax on initial survey, this must be treated immediately by either needle or chest tube decompression. In general, the therapy of cardiogenic shock following trauma involves preventing ventricular arrhythmias or treating existing arrhythmias, establishing normovolemia, and improving cardiac performance. Invasive procedures, such as tube thoracostomy, pericardiocentesis, or thoracotomy, may be required as part of the resuscitation depending on the etiology of cardiogenic shock.

If cardiogenic shock following injury fails to respond to adequate volume therapy and any indicated procedure as above, then therapy should be directed at improving the contractility of the heart and vascular tone (Table 3-5).

Dopamine is the initial sympathomimetic amine used to treat shock that is refractory to volume. Low doses improve renal and mesenteric blood flow, moderate doses improve cardiac contractility, and high doses cause generalized vasoconstriction. The initial infusion rate should be low, since the desired physiologic effect can be titrated. Dobutamine acts mainly on the beta-adrenergic receptors to improve cardiac contractility and is an excellent alternative in this setting. Side effects are rare. Epinephrine is a mixed alpha- and beta-adrenergic agonist. Its main use is in patients needing inotropic support who are refractory to dopamine or dobutamine. Amrinone is a newer class of inotropic agent that is a phosphodiesterase inhibitor. Its hemodynamic effects are similar to dobutamine; however, it is unclear what role it will play in the resuscitation of cardiogenic shock in trauma. Isoproterenol should be avoided, since it is very arrhythmogenic and decreases blood flow to ischemic areas of myocardium. Norepinephrine has its major effect on the alpha receptor and causes generalized vasoconstriction. Its use may accelerate tissue ischemia. Phenylephrine is a pure alpha agent used to increase peripheral vascular resistance.

If shock remains refractory to inotropic support, the vascular resistance is elevated, and the patient is adequately volume loaded, then the use of an agent that decreases total

Table 3-5. Commonly Used Inotropic and Vasoactive Drugs

Drug	Dosage (IV)
Dopamine	Low: 0.5–2.0 μg/kg/min Moderate: 2–10 μg/kg/min Large: 10–20 μg/kg/min High: 20–50 μg/kg/min
Dobutamine	2–10 μg/kg/min
Amrinone	5–10 μg/kg/min
Epinephrine	1–15 μg/min
Isoproterenol	1–20 μg/min
Nitroglycerin	10–400 μg/min
Nitroprusside	0.5–10.0 μg/kg/min
Norepinephrine	1–4 μg/min
Phenylephrine	0.5–5.0 μg/kg/min

peripheral vascular resistance is indicated. Sodium nitroprusside is commonly used for this purpose. It is both a vasodilator and venodilator. Afterload and preload are decreased. Intravenous nitroglycerin can also be used for this purpose and acts mainly as a venodilator.

It should be mentioned that severe shock is accompanied by acidemia. Acidemia may by itself decrease the heart's responsiveness to inotropic agents. For this reason, it is prudent to administer 1 to 2 ampuls (50–100 mEq) of sodium bicarbonate during the resuscitation of the patient in severe shock. Subsequent bicarbonate therapy can be based on arterial blood gas analysis.

NEUROGENIC SHOCK

Spinal cord trauma may cause neurogenic shock. A patient who presents with paraplegia or quadriplegia following trauma must be suspected of having a spinal cord injury. Shock developing in this setting may be due to the neurologic injury; however, it is of primary importance to rule out coexisting hemorrhagic or cardiogenic etiologies. Patients with isolated neurogenic shock present with altered spinal cord function, hypotension, a normal or slowed pulse, and warm, dry skin. Sometimes the skin actually appears flushed.

Pathophysiology

When the spinal cord is severed, all motor, sensory, and reflex function below the level of injury is abolished. There occurs paralysis of muscle function, anesthesia of skin, and loss of spinal reflexes. Bladder and rectal function are lost. In addition, there is abolition of all sympathetic vasomotor control below the level of injury. This results in vasodilatation of the arteriolar resistance vessels and venodilatation of venous capacitance vessels. Total peripheral vascular resistance decreases, as do cardiac preload and subsequently cardiac output. Since blood pressure is directly related to the product of cardiac output and vascular resistance, the patient becomes hypotensive and presents in neurogenic shock.

Treatment

The therapy of neurogenic shock complicating spinal cord injury involves volume loading with Ringer's lactate and the judicious use of vasopressor agents. Ringer's lactate can be administered using boluses of 250 ml. A CVP or Swan-Ganz catheter may assist as a useful guide for volume therapy in this situation. Phenylephrine is the alpha-adrenergic agent of choice and causes a marked increase in peripheral vascular resistance. It does so by a direct effect on the alpha receptor as well as by causing a release of endogenous norepinephrine. Reflex bradycardia may occur; however, this can be blocked by atropine. The infusion rate may be titrated to the hemodynamic response.

SEPTIC SHOCK

Septic shock is usually a late cause of shock in trauma [17]. It usually results from intra-abdominal abscess, peritonitis, or pneumonia; however, iatrogenic infections, such as catheter-related sepsis, may also be the cause. The mortality of septic shock is approximately 50 percent. The bacterial family Enterobacteriaceae cause most cases of septic shock in the trauma patient. Included in this family is *Escherichia coli, Klebsiella, Enterobacter, Serratia,* and *Proteus* species. *Pseudomonas aeruginosa* and *Bacteroides* species are also common gram-negative causes. Gram-positive organisms, especially *Staphylococcus aureus,* as well as *Candida* species can cause septic shock as well.

Most patients with septic shock present with fever, chills, and hypotension. Hypothermia may be noted in the geriatric patient. Two of the earliest manifestations of sepsis are hyperventilation and alterations in mental status such as confusion or obtundation. Skin lesions may occur. The lesions of ecthyma gangrenosum may occur in *Pseudomonas* and *Aeromonas* sepsis. These lesions consist of a necrotic center surrounded by erythema and are located usually in the axilla and anogenital areas. Other findings may include the adult respiratory distress syndrome, renal insufficiency, hepatic dysfunction, and coagulation abnormalities, including thrombocytopenia and disseminated intravascular coagulation syndrome.

Pathophysiology

There are two main clinical syndromes of septic shock. In warm septic shock (early sepsis), the patient has warm, dry, pink skin, normal mental status, and adequate urine output despite hypotension. Hemodynamically, this state is characterized by a normal or elevated cardiac output and a lowered total peripheral vascular resistance. In cold septic shock (late sepsis), the patient has cold, moist skin, altered mental status, decreased urine production, and hypotension. Hemodynamically, this state is characterized by a decreased cardiac output and a markedly increased vascular resistance. In general, septic shock should be viewed as a spectrum between the warm and cold types. Some patients may present initially with warm sepsis and then deteriorate into a cold septic state. Other patients may present initially with cold sepsis, which represents profound circulatory failure due to infection.

Although studied extensively [17–20], the details of warm and cold septic shock are but partially understood. In gram-negative septic shock, the hemodynamic abnormalities are probably due to the effects of endotoxin. The cell wall of the gram-negative bacterium is composed of a lipopolysaccharide. The polysaccharide moiety of the outer membrane is responsible for type O somatic antigenicity. The lipid A moiety is responsible for the endotoxic effects of the bacterium and is released during lysis of the cell wall. Endotoxin is known to activate the complement system, the coagulation cascade, the plasmin-fibrinogen system, and the kinin system among others. This effects many of the changes seen in gram-negative sepsis (Table 3-6).

Treatment

The therapy of septic shock involves supporting the respiratory and cardiovascular systems and treating the infection. Most patients in septic shock are hypovolemic, and therefore, volume therapy is important. These patients must be monitored and treated in an intensive care unit. Ventricular filling pressures should be optimized using a pulmonary artery catheter.

The source of the infection must be ascer-

Table 3-6. Effects of Endotoxin

Complement system	
	Inflammatory response: tissue damage
	Mast cell: histamine, hypotension
Coagulation system	
	Coagulopathy
	Thrombocytopenia
	Disseminated intravascular coagulation
Fibrinolytic system	
	Fibrinolysis
	Fibrin split products
	Coagulopathy
Kinin system	
	Bradykinin, hypotension

tained. Surgery may be required. Antibiotics play an important but adjunct role in this setting. If the specific causative organism is unknown, then it is important to start antibiotics that are effective against both gram-positive and gram-negative organisms. A reasonable combination includes a penicillinase-resistant penicillin (oxacillin) and an aminoglycoside (gentamicin or tobramycin). If an anaerobic infection is suspected, then either clindamycin or metronidazole should be added. It remains to be seen what the exact role of the newer numerous third-generation cephalosporins and beta-lactam antibiotics will be in the initial treatment of sepsis in the trauma patient. The role of corticosteroid therapy remains controversial [21].

REFERENCES

1. Kreis, D. J., and Baue, A. E. *Clinical Management of Shock.* Baltimore: University Park Press, 1984.
2. Shires, G. T., Carrico, C. J., and Canizaro, P. C. *Shock.* Philadelphia: Saunders, 1973.
3. Shires, G. T., and Shires, G. T., III. Classification and Clinical Signs. In G. T. Shires (ed.), *Shock and Related Disorders.* New York: Churchill Livingstone, 1984. Pp. 3–11.
4. *Advanced Trauma Life Support Manual.* Chicago: American College of Surgeons, 1984. Pp. 179–191.
5. Guyton, A. C., and Young, D. B. (eds.). *Cardiovascular Physiology.* Baltimore: University Park Press, 1979.
6. Holcroft, J. W. Impairment of venous return in hemorrhagic shock. *Surg. Clin. North Am.* 62:17, 1982.
7. Carey, L. C., Lowery, E. D., and Cloutier, C. T. Hemorrhagic shock. *Curr. Probl. Surg.,* January 1971, Pp. 3–48.
8. Baue, A. E. Recent developments in the study and treatment of shock. *Surg. Gynecol. Obstet.* 127:849, 1968.
9. Kaplan, B. C., Civetta, J. M., Nagel, E. L., et al. The Military Anti-Shock Trouser in civilian pre-hospital emergency care. *J. Trauma* 13:843, 1973.
10. Gaffney, F. A., Thal, E. R., Taylor, W. F., et al. Hemodynamic effects of the medical anti-shock trousers (MAST garment). *J. Trauma* 21:931, 1981.
11. Hoffman, J. R. External counterpressure and the MAST suit: Current and future roles. *Ann. Emerg. Med.* 9:419, 1980.
12. Pepe, P. E., Bass, R. R., and Mattox, K. L. Clinical trials of the pneumatic antishock garment in the urban prehospital setting. *Ann. Emerg. Med.* 15:1407, 1986.
13. Opie, L. H. Myocardial infarct size: Part I. Basic considerations. *Am. Heart J.* 100:355, 1980.
14. Alonso, D. R., Scheidt, S., Post, M., et al. Pathophysiology of cardiogenic shock: Quantification of myocardial neurosis, clinical, pathologic and electrocardiographic correlations. *Circulation* 48:588, 1973.
15. Tenzer, M. L. The spectrum of myocardial contusion: A review. *J. Trauma* 25:620, 1985.
16. Forrester, J. S., Diamond, G., Chatterjee, K., et al. Medical therapy of acute myocardial infarction by application of hemodynamic subsets. *N. Engl. J. Med.* 295:1356, 1976.
17. Carmona, R., Catalano, R., and Trunkey, D. D.

Septic shock. In G. T. Shires (ed.), *Shock and Related Problems.* New York: Churchill Livingstone, 1984. Pp. 156–177.
18. Lefer, A. M. Leukotrienes as mediators of ischemia and shock. *Biochem. Pharmacol.* 35:123, 1986.
19. Lefer, A. M. Eicosanoids as mediators of ischemia and shock. *Fed. Proc.* 44:275, 1985.
20. Filkins, J. P. Monokines and the metabolic pathophysiology of septic shock. *Fed. Proc.* 44:300, 1985.
21. Sprung, C. L., Caralis, P. V., Marcial, E. H., et al. The effects of high-dose corticosteroids in patients with septic shock: A prospective, controlled study. *N. Engl. J. Med.* 311:1137, 1143, 1984.

4

The Workup of the Trauma Patient

Gerardo A. Gomez
Michael J. Savini, Jr.

The American College of Surgeons Committee on Trauma has recommended an organized approach to the initial assessment of trauma patients. During the primary survey, a quick assessment is made of the ABCs—airway maintenance with cervical spine control, breathing, circulation with hemorrhage control, and the D and Es—disability (neurologic status), and complete exposure. In the resuscitation phase, shock management is initiated, patient oxygenation and hemorrhage control are reevaluated, and life-threatening conditions are monitored. The secondary survey, a more detailed head-to-toe evaluation, utilizes physical examination and special procedures to plan the formal workup of the trauma patient. Finally, in the definitive care phase, disposition is made as to whether the patient needs immediate therapeutic intervention, admission to the intensive care unit, or transfer to a trauma center [1].

The workup of a trauma patient is directed toward the identification of injuries using accurate diagnostic modalities so appropriate therapy can be implemented. A good history and an orderly physical examination are the basic elements in the diagnosis of injuries, hence an important part of the workup. They also provide information to support the need for a particular diagnostic test.

CENTRAL NERVOUS SYSTEM

During the secondary survey, the head is inspected and palpated for contusions, external evidence of skull fractures, and active hemorrhage. Periorbital ecchymosis (racoon eyes) and ecchymosis over the mastoid process (Battle's sign) are suggestive of basilar skull fractures. The Glasgow Coma Scale (Table 4-1) continues to be an accurate tool not only to assess the level of consciousness but also when obtained serially to indicate improve-

Table 4-1. Glasgow Coma Scale

Factor	Response	Score
Eye opening response	Spontaneous	4
	To voice	3
	To pain	2
	None	1
Best verbal response	Oriented	5
	Confused	4
	Inappropriate	3
	Incomprehensible sounds	2
	None	1
Best motor response	Obeys commands	6
	Localizes pain	5
	Withdraws (pain)	4
	Flexion (pain)	3
	Extension (pain)	2
	None	1
	Total	3–15

ment or deterioration of central nervous system (CNS) function [2,3].

The eyes are inspected to evaluate the size of the pupils and reactivity to light. The cervical, thoracic, and lumbar spine need to be palpated and inspected for tenderness, ecchymosis, and deformities. Reflexes should be checked as well as motor and sensory response. The absence of sphincter tone may be the initial finding suggestive of spinal cord injury.

The cross-table lateral cervical spine x-ray showing all seven vertebrae continues to be an excellent diagnostic tool for cervical spine injuries. Multiple-trauma patients should have their cervical spine immobilized until injuries have been ruled out by radiologic examination.

Computed tomography (CT), initially introduced in the early 1970s [4], has become not a luxury but a necessity in the workup of the head trauma patient. While in the past diagnostic burr holes were performed in a semiblind setting, presently the new generation of CT scanner will accurately produce both anatomic location and extent of head injuries to guide neurosurgeons in their management [5].

In stable trauma patients who require surgical intervention for non-CNS injuries but who may have head injuries, CT scan should be performed before surgery when possible, since if head injuries amenable to surgical therapy are identified, their management can be accomplished simultaneously with other surgical procedures.

The use of skull x-ray series has become a lower priority in patients with head trauma. Indications for skull x-ray in trauma patients are basically similar to those for CT scan, and information provided by the latter overwhelm the former. The finding of a linear skull fracture or basilar skull fracture alone may not change the management. Skull x-ray may be helpful for quick determination of the path of a gunshot wound or the location of foreign bodies (e.g., bullet, knife) [6].

NECK TRAUMA

Penetrating Neck Trauma

Since the management and workup of penetrating neck trauma may be different according to the anatomic location of the injury, it is important to discuss the anatomic zones of the neck. We use the classifications of zones proposed by Roon [7] and supported by Thal [8] defining zone I below the cricoid cartilage,

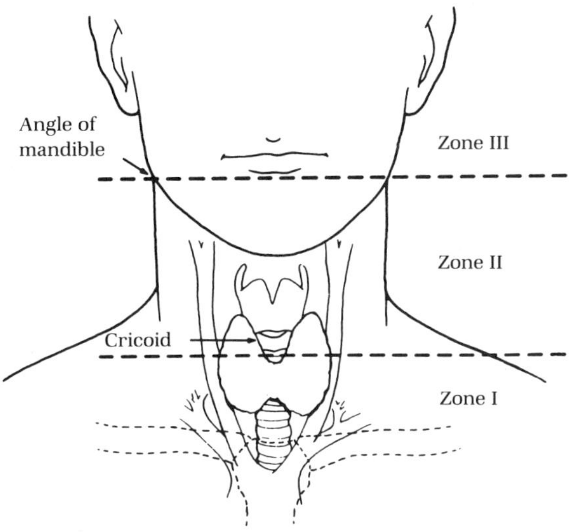

Fig. 4-1. Anatomic zones of the neck. (From E. R. Thal [8] by permission of Appleton & Lange.)

zone II between the angle of the mandible and the cricoid cartilage, and zone III above the angle of the mandible (Fig. 4-1).

Most authors would agree that injuries to zones I and III should be worked up before surgical intervention, particularly with the use of arteriography. In these two zones, arteriography not only detects the injuries but also allows the trauma surgeon to plan the operative approach, particularly in regard to proximal and distal control of vascular structures. Arteriography in some instances can also be used as a therapeutic modality in very selective cases by the use of embolization as suggested by Sclafani [9].

For zone I injuries, a Gastrografin swallow combined with panendoscopy (esophagoscopy and bronchoscopy) is recommended to rule out esophageal and/or tracheobronchial tree injuries if proximity to these structures is suspected.

Controversy still exists in the management of zone II injuries in stable patients. In 1956, Fogelman [10] recommended mandatory neck exploration if the platysma muscle was violated. This approach, supported by others [11,12], was questioned based on a high negative exploration rate, and a selective approach was proposed [13,14], suggesting arteriography, panendoscopy, and Gastrografin swallow. Patients with positive studies would undergo surgery, and those with negative workup would be observed. More recent reports [15,16] go back to recommend mandatory exploration for all zone II injuries where the platysma is violated, based not only on the accuracy and safety of the procedure but also on the claim that the cost of mandatory exploration is similar to or less than using the selective approach.

In conclusion, it seems that both approaches are comparable in accuracy, safety, and cost. The rationale in using mandatory exploration or the selective approach in stable patients with zone II penetrating injuries will depend in part on both the availability of diagnostic tests and the expertise of the people performing them.

Blunt Neck Trauma

Before any workup is begun, adequate airway control and proper ventilation as well as stabilization of the cervical spine should have first priority in blunt neck injuries.

The history of the mechanism of injury is useful in establishing a thought process to direct the workup in patients with blunt neck trauma. A motor vehicle accident can result in hyperextension of the neck, exposing the trachea and larynx, smashing the neck on the steering wheel or instrument panel during deceleration [17], and crushing the thyroid and cricoid cartilages against the cervical vertebra [18]. Other examples of blunt cervical trauma include strangulation, hanging, and garrote injuries. The clothesline injury [19] can cause direct impact on the neck by a stretched, horizontal cable, causing damage to the pharynx, larynx, trachea, esophagus, and/or cervical spine. This type of injury can occur during a multitude of activities, including waterskiing, trail bike riding, sledding, and snowmobiling. Also, direct blows to the neck in other sports can cause significant injuries.

Physical examination may reveal deformity of the neck with loss of cartilaginous landmarks, subcutaneous emphysema, supraclavicular retraction, cervical hematoma, blood present in the pharynx, diminished or absent pulses, and motor and/or sensory deficits. If the patient is conscious, pain may be present on palpation. Other signs and symptoms suggestive of laryngotracheal or esophageal injuries include dyspnea, dysphagia, hoarseness, hemoptysis, hematemesis, and stridor.

Establishment of an airway if necessary is the first priority in the management of blunt cervical trauma. If laryngotracheal injury is suspected, tracheostomy and not intubation is the procedure of choice [20,21], although orotracheal intubation may be carefully undertaken under direct visualization [22,23]. Cricothyroidotomy should be avoided if laryngeal trauma is present, as this may contribute to or worsen the injury [24].

The cervical spine must be immobilized until all seven cervical vertebrae have been visualized on a lateral cervical spine x-ray. A soft-tissue lateral view of the neck is also helpful in demonstrating subcutaneous emphysema, retropharyngeal air, or loss of continuity of prevertebral fascia [25].

A chest roentgenographic study is obtained to evaluate the mediastinum for air. Also, this study is helpful to evaluate tracheal tube placement if necessary.

Indirect laryngoscopy was the mainstay of preoperative examination to evaluate the larynx and trachea, and laryngograms and laryngeal tomography were employed as adjuvant diagnostic aids [26,27]. Presently, direct laryngoscopy and flexible fiberoptic nasopharyngeal endoscopy are considered useful [24].

Esophagoscopy should be part of the regimen in the assessment and workup of blunt cervical trauma, as blunt injuries to the cervical esophagus have been reported and if missed cause significant morbidity and mortality. An esophogram with Gastrografin should be the first contrast study performed, and if not conclusive, then a thin barium study can be obtained [28].

Computed tomography can be used to evaluate nondisplaced and displaced fractures of the cartilaginous structures of the larynx [29,30], the cervical spine [31], soft tissues of the neck [32], and hematomas. Dynamic scanning with contrast can demonstrate major vascular structures of the neck, but fine details are not appreciable.

Vascular injuries caused by blunt trauma secondary to fractures, dislocations, contusions, and traction are uncommon but if suspected must be evaluated by angiography. The carotid or vertebral artery can be injured directly by compression or indirectly by stretching, causing an intimal tear with resultant thromboembolism. The vessels must be studied by four-vessel angiography and an arch aortogram demonstrating the origin of the arteries [33].

Duplex scanning of the major vessels of the neck is on the horizon, but its place in the evaluation of the trauma patient has not yet been defined.

CHEST TRAUMA

Penetrating Chest Trauma

Penetrating trauma to the chest necessitates rapid assessment and management of respiratory compromise and circulatory collapse. Rapid decompression of hemothorax, pneumothorax, or tension pneumothorax and aggressive resuscitation with crystalloid solutions and blood are cornerstones in the initial management [34]. Needle thoracostomy and pericardiocentesis are temporizing but lifesaving measures that may be rapidly carried out while awaiting definitive surgical management, that is, chest tube thoracostomy and thoracotomy.

The type of weapon and the pathway of the weapon and/or missile, accompanied by a thorough knowledge of anatomy in general, will suggest the possible injuries present, directing the initial management and workup of the patient [35].

Conventional chest roentgenogram should be the initial diagnostic tool, but stabilization and management of the patient must never be delayed to confirm a suspected injury radiographically. This is particularly important in patients with suspected cardiac tamponade, tension pneumothorax, or massive hemothorax who are unstable or in respiratory distress.

Clinical evidence of cardiac tamponade includes hypotension, tachycardia, elevated central venous pressure, and pulsus paradoxus. Beck's triad—distant heart sounds, distended neck veins, and arterial hypotension—may not be evident since it occurs in only two-thirds of these patients [36,37]. Pericardiocentesis in patients with penetrating chest trauma may be diagnostsic as well as therapeutic. A long needle placed into the pericardial sac by the subxiphoid approach may yield nonclotting blood (diagnostic) followed by hemodynamic improvement (therapeutic). Aspiration of as little as 10 ml of blood can relieve tamponade and may be repeated as necessary as a temporizing measure prior to definitive operative treatment [38–40]. It must be noted that failure to obtain blood on aspiration does not rule out the possibility of tamponade [41–43]. False-positive and false-negative results may occur, and clotted blood is commonly found when performing emergency pericardiocentesis [37]. There is a school of thought that believes there is no place for pericardiocentesis as a diagnostic or a therapeutic procedure [44].

Needle thoracostomy that demonstrates the characteristic "whoosh" of air on insertion followed by clinical improvement definitively diagnoses the presence of a tension pneumothorax [45]. An anteroposterior chest roentgenogram obtained after initial stabilization will provide a significant amount of information such as subcutaneous emphysema, pneumothorax, hemothorax, widened or displaced mediastinum, pneumomediastinum, pulmonary contusion, enlarged cardiac silhouette, rib fractures, sternal fractures, and the position of chest tubes and central lines. In gunshot wound patients, a metallic marker should be taped to the entrance and exit wounds to give an idea of the path of the bullet.

Management of transmediastinal gunshot wounds in stable patients is unique among penetrating chest trauma. The selective approach to transmediastinal gunshot wounds consists of emergency angiographic examination of the aortic arch, descending aorta, and the great vessels of the arch and water-soluble contrast esophagography accompanied by esophagoscopy and bronchoscopy in the operating room [46]. Subxiphoid pericardial window is also a very useful diagnostic tool in the workup of these patients [46].

Pericardial windows provide a safe but very rapid means of diagnosing cardiac injuries in patients with equivocal signs of cardiac injuries. In a study of 104 patients (51 stab wounds, 45 gunshot wounds, and 8 blunt injuries), 7 patients had a positive window but no clinical signs of tamponade [47].

Blunt Chest Trauma

A comprehensive history to ascertain the magnitude of kinetic energy imparted to the victim by deceleration should be obtained. This should include mechanism of injury, speed of the vehicle, use of seat belt restraints, location of the victim, the height from which the patient fell, and so on. Deceleration force is responsible for pulmonary contusion and aortic or tracheobronchial disruption. Fixed intrathoracic structures decelerate faster than nonfixed structures, resulting in laceration. A contrecoup mechanism may also be responsible for pulmonary contusion as well as direct trauma [35,48,49]. In addition to deceleration, shearing forces with oblique stress applied to the chest in a motor vehicle accident can produce aortic rupture [50]. Compression directly on the rib cage may cause rib fractures resulting in hemothorax, lung lacerations, and tension pneumothorax. Compression directly by the thoracic cage onto the mediastinal structures trapping the esophagus, tracheobronchial tree, or heart can result in contusion or rupture. Compression of the abdominal cavity can cause diaphragmatic rupture.

An anteroposterior chest roentgenogram, as in penetrating injuries, should be the initial test, but again it should not delay the treatment of any life-threatening conditions. The film may detect the presence of rib fractures, sternal fractures, subcutaneous emphysema, pneumothorax, hemothorax, widened or displaced mediastinum, pneumomediastinum, tracheal deviation, abnormal displacement of a nasogastric tube, or intrathoracic abdominal contents. Most chest roentgenograms are taken in the supine position, but if the patient can be placed in the upright position, the diagnostic accuracy for hemothorax, pneumothorax, and evaluation of mediastinal width is increased. Aortic knob blurring is a sensitive indicator of ruptured aorta [51]. Cervical emphysema can occur with esophageal and tracheobronchial rupture even if pneumomediastinum is not evident [28]. Pulmonary contusion is evident 2 to 24 hours postinjury and varies from small patchy infiltrates to total lobe opacification [52]. Rib fractures that are located posteriorly are more evident than those located anteriorly and laterally. Sternal fractures are not that obvious on anteroposterior supine films and require lateral chest films and sometimes sternal tomograms for diagnosis [49]. Lateral films may show a retrosternal soft tissue density representing a fracture hematoma in sternal fractures [53]. Fractures of the first rib, especially if the posterior portion of the rib is displaced downward and the anterior portion is forced upward, should be an indication for aortogram [54].

Arterial blood gas determinations are not initially indicative of the magnitude of lung contusion. As the injury progresses, hypoxia becomes evident, particularly in those injuries causing significant decrease in pulmonary volume or abnormal mechanical function.

Electrocardiography may aid in identifying myocardial contusion, by detecting arrhythmias, conduction defects, ST-segment and T-wave changes, and a pathologically long Q–T interval [55]. Seat-shoulder restraints may produce an increase in the incidence of myocardial contusion [56].

Aortography should be considered if there is clinical evidence for potential rupture of the thoracic aorta or if chest x-ray criteria are encountered. The clinical evidence includes history of high-speed deceleration accident, ejection from the vehicle, upper limb hypertension, pulse pressure differential between right and left arms, precordial or paravertebral systolic murmur, sternal fracture by palpation, cardiac contusion, or unexplained hypotension. The chest x-ray criteria for aortogram include widened mediastinum, left hemothorax, apical pleural cap, depression of left main stem bronchus, deviation of nasogastric tube to the right, loss of normal aortic knob, fractures of first or second ribs, and obliteration of paravertebral pleural reflection [57]. The mortality of aortic disruption is directly related to the amount of time elapsed between injury and surgical repair. Most patients with aortic disruption (80–90 percent) die before reaching the hospital. Of those admitted alive, 30 percent die within 6 hours and 50 percent within 24 hours without surgical intervention [58–60].

Even though CT scan of the chest is being used in patients with suspected ruptured thoracic aorta, angiography continues to be the ideal diagnostic modality in these patients.

Pericardiocentesis is considered as a diagnostic and/or temporizing maneuver in a patient demonstrating venous hypertension accompanied by arterial hypotension. If necessary, this procedure may be repeated [35].

Needle thoracostomy with a large-bore intravenous catheter placed through the second intercostal space at the midclavicular line should be performed immediately whenever the diagnosis of tension pneumothorax is considered [1]. After this lifesaving temporizing maneuver, the formal insertion of a chest tube should be carried out.

Emergency department thoracotomy is rarely indicated for blunt trauma. The chest tube is monitored, and if massive air leak persists or massive hemorrhage or inability to reexpand the lung is demonstrated, urgent thoracotomy in the operating room setting may be indicated.

Computed tomography can accurately define defects in the diaphragm and identify which organ(s) are present within the thoracic cavity [57].

ABDOMINAL TRAUMA

The workup of a patient who has sustained abdominal trauma should be intended not only to diagnose intra-abdominal injuries, but most of all to determine whether emergency surgical intervention is indicated. The workup of these patients is different depending on the mechanism of injury.

Blunt Abdominal Trauma

The most common causes of blunt abdominal trauma include motor vehicle accidents in more than 50 percent of the cases, assaults in 13 to 22 percent, and falls in 8 to 22 percent [61,62]. The diagnostic accuracy of intra-abdominal injuries requiring surgical intervention on the basis of clinical evaluation alone has been reported to range from 42 to 84 percent [63–66].

Blunt abdominal trauma patients with obvious peritoneal signs during the initial assessment are the exception, and missed intra-abdominal injuries are not an infrequent cause of preventable trauma death [67–69].

Diagnostic peritoneal lavage (DPL), introduced by Root and associates [70], and CT scan of the abdomen, supported by Federle and coworkers [71], are the two most commonly used diagnostic modalities in patients with blunt abdominal trauma.

Diagnostic peritoneal lavage has an overall accuracy rate of 97.8 percent with a complication rate of 1.9 percent [62]. Data from a literature review (Table 4-2) including 5715 patients in whom the "standard criteria" (Table 4-3) for positive and negative DPL was used showed an accuracy rate of 97.5 percent in 1744 patients with positive DPL and 98 percent in 3971 patients with negative DPL [62,64,72–77].

In regard to the standard criteria for positive DPL, we use an elevated amylase level selectively as an indication for emergency laparotomy. High levels of amylase in the lavage fluid are usually due to enteric perforation. Surgery is clearly indicated in these cases. However, if the elevated lavage amylase level may be due to traumatic pancreatitis then exploratory laparotomy may not be required unless a major ductal injury is present. Presently, stable patients with either serum amylase or DPL amylase elevations undergo CT scan of the abdomen. Patients with a normal pancreas by CT are observed. Patients with either an abnormal pancreas or a nondiagnostic study undergo an endoscopic retrograde pancreatogram. If major ductal injury is documented, emergency laparotomy is performed. If the ductal system is intact, then a period of observation is indicated.

Overall DPL is a safe, inexpensive, easy to perform, and accurate adjunctive diagnostic tool in the workup of a patient with blunt abdominal trauma. Limitations of DPL include the fact that DPL does not detect injuries to retroperitoneal organs and diaphragmatic injuries may be missed. Supporters of CT scanning feel that DPL is an invasive method with potential serious complications including perforation of hollow viscus and major vessels in the abdomen. There are no absolute contraindications to DPL; however, in pa-

Table 4-2. Literature review on the use of diagnostic peritoneal lavage in patients with blunt abdominal trauma based on standard criteria (series of 100 patients)

Authors	Year	Number	True ⊕	False ⊕	Accuracy ⊕	True ⊖	False ⊖	Accuracy ⊖	Overall ⊖	Complication Rate (%)
Perry and Strate [72]	1972	401	116	3	98	280	2	99	99	0.5
Thal and Shires [73]	1973	287	84	10	89	184	9	95	93	4.5
Engrav et al. [64]	1975	1465	505	6	99	935	19	98	98	1.0
Ahmad and Polk [74]	1976	252	104	6	95	136	6	96	95	0.8
Drew and Perry [75]	1977	230	72	1	99	156	1	99	99	0.8
Fischer et al. [76]	1978	2586	755	6	99	1793	32	98	98	1.7
Gruenberg et al. [77]	1982	356	37	10	79	303	6	98	96	4.1
Gomez et al. [62]	1987	138	28	1	97	108	1	99	99	0.0
Totals		5715	1701	43	97.5	3895	76	98	97.8	1.9

Table 4-3. Criteria for positive peritoneal lavage in blunt abdominal trauma

Free aspiration of blood (5 ml or greater)
Red blood cell count of 100,000/mm^3 or greater
White blood cell count of 500/mm^3 or greater
Presence of bile, bacteria, or food particles
Lavage fluid exits through Foley catheter or chest tube

tients with previous abdominal surgery, pelvic fractures, pregnancy, or in children the open technique is recommended.

Even though in our institution we have been using DPL as the initial diagnostic tool of choice, as our experiences have progressed we have started to use the CT scan more often in selected patients. The first requirement in using CT scanning is the patient must be hemodynamically stable. In hypotensive patients, particularly victims of multiple trauma or with pelvic fractures, even if they respond to fluid resuscitation, an intra-abdominal source of hemorrhage should be ruled out immediately. The most appropriate test in this setting is DPL.

In terms of workup, patients with blunt abdominal trauma are divided into three categories (Fig. 4-2):

1. Patients with obvious evidence of acute abdomen on physical examination or pneumoperitoneum on plain x-ray—need no further workup, and emergency exploratory laparotomy is indicated.
2. Patients with a negative abdominal physical examination who have altered pain response due to alcohol intoxication, drugs, head trauma, or spinal cord injury; have hypotension of unclear origin; and require surgical intervention under general anesthesia for other injuries—need either DPL or CT scan of the abdomen to rule out intra-abdominal injuries before undergoing surgery.
3. Patients who have sustained blunt abdominal trauma, who are awake and alert without convincing signs of an acute abdomen, but whose abdominal examination is not completely negative—need DPL or CT scan of the abdomen.

All patients with negative DPL should be admitted for a minimum of 24 hours' observation, whereas those with positive lavage should undergo exploratory laparotomy.

Patients with blunt abdominal trauma should have routine chest and pelvic x-rays. The chest x-ray may be helpful in detecting a diaphragmatic rupture by showing elevation of a hemidiaphragm or by showing the nasogastric tube going upward into the left chest. The pelvic x-ray will detect pelvic fractures, sometimes even in asymptomatic victims. Also, in our institution, the pelvic x-ray will direct the technique to be used in performing DPL. If no pelvic fractures are present, the percutaneous technique is utilized; in patients with pelvic fractures, a supraumbilical open technique is used.

In patients with hematuria, even though controversial, we still recommend intravenous pyelogram (IVP) except when CT scan of the abdomen is indicated to rule out intra-abdominal injuries, since the CT scan provides similar or better information than the

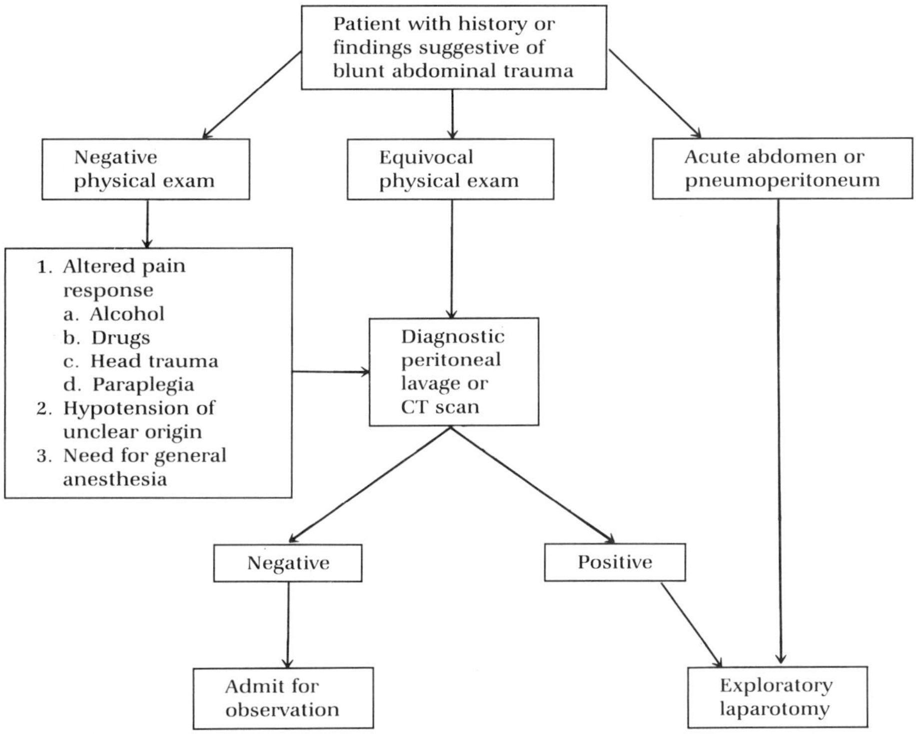

Fig. 4-2. Approach to the patient with blunt abdominal trauma.

IVP. When urethral or bladder disruption is suspected, a cystourethrogram is indicated. We insist that a minimum of 400 ml of contrast material be injected to obtain maximum distention of the bladder.

Penetrating Abdominal Trauma

To direct the workup in patients with penetrating abdominal trauma, it is important to define anatomic landmarks: (1) anterior abdomen—fourth intercostal space superiorly, anterior axillary line laterally, and symphysis pubis and inguinal ligaments inferiorly; (2) flanks—sixth intercostal space superiorly, anterior axillary line anteriorly, posterior axillary line posteriorly, and iliac crest inferiorly; and (3) back—both posterior axillary lines laterally, tip of scapulas superiorly, and iliac crest inferiorly (Figs. 4-3 and 4-4).

In patients with penetrating abdominal trauma, the initial workup is intended to determine whether an emergency exploratory laparotomy is indicated. Patients presenting with hypotensive, shock, evisceration, upper or lower gastrointestinal hemorrhage, pneumoperitoneum or obvious peritonitis on physical examination should be considered for immediate laparotomy.

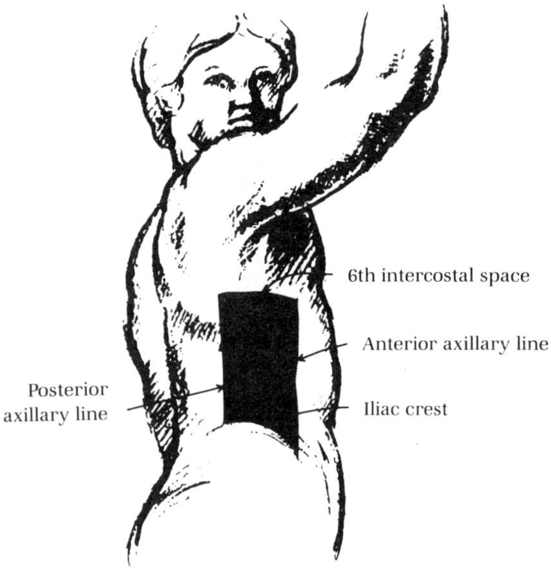

Fig. 4-3. Anatomic landmarks of the flank. (From *J. Trauma,* September 1979.)

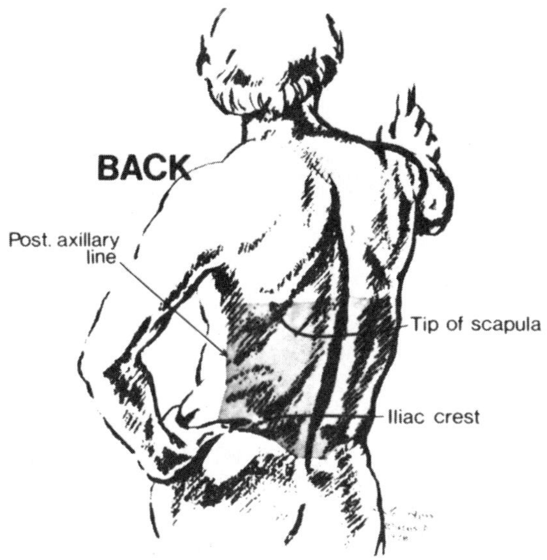

Fig. 4-4. Anatomic landmarks of the back. (From *J. Trauma,* September 1979.)

Victims of gunshot wounds, regardless of location—anterior abdomen, flank, or back—should be considered for immediate laparotomy if the bullet or missile has penetrated the peritoneal cavity. In patients with only one wound (entrance), penetration of the peritoneal cavity can be estimated by plain anteroposterior and lateral x-ray of the abdomen. Stable patients with gunshot wounds to the lower chest in whom it is unclear whether or not the missile has penetrated the peritoneal cavity may be worked up by either CT scan or the abdomen, DPL [78], or close observation. For gunshot wounds to the back and flank where there is a question of peritoneal penetration, CT scan of the abdomen is the diagnostic modality of choice [79], although admission with close observation has also been advocated [80].

Stab wounds to the anterior abdomen in stable patients should be explored under local anesthesia. If the anterior fascia is intact, the patient may be discharged if no other indications for admission are present. If the fascia is violated or the depth of the wound is unclear, DPL is indicated. If the stab wound is located in the lower chest (from the fourth intercostal space to the costal margin), local wound exploration is not recommended and DPL is performed (Fig. 4-5).

Stab wounds to the flank and back are worked up best by CT scanning of the abdomen with triple contrast [79]. Criteria for positive diagnostic peritoneal lavage in penetrat-

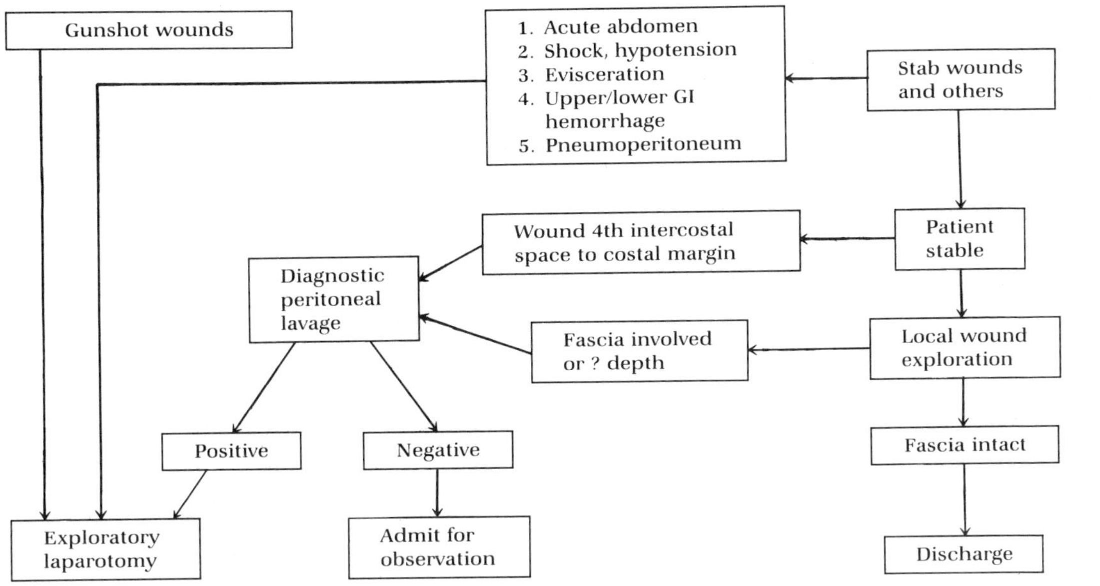

Fig. 4-5. Approach to the patient with penetrating abdominal trauma.

ing trauma have been less consistent than those for blunt abdominal trauma, particularly in regard to the red blood cell count, ranging from 1000 [81] to 100,000 [6,82]. At our institution, we have been using a red blood cell count of 20,000 as a positive lavage criterion and have maintained an accuracy rate of 96 to 98 percent.

In patients with either gunshot wounds or stab wounds in proximity to the kidney or ureter, we recommend the use of a preoperative one-shot IVP. The IVP will determine the presence of both kidneys, will give information about renal function, and may detect leakage of contrast if genitourinary injury is present.

EXTREMITY TRAUMA

Blunt and penetrating trauma of the extremities require an accurate and timely assessment. The injured extremity must be evaluated structurally, angiodynamically, and neurologically.

A careful history to identify the mechanism of injury and the surrounding events is of paramount importance. The amount of force involved, the type of weapon employed, the amount of blood present at the scene, and the nature of the bleeding, as well as the maneuvers necessary to control the injury, all interact in the planning of the diagnostic workup.

The physical examination of the traumatized extremity on inspection reveals ecchymosis, angulation and/or deformity, lack of movement, loss of continuity of the skin, and nature of the wound. A fairly accurate assessment of vascular injury in an extremity can be made by inspection of the wound, examination of the peripheral pulses, and a careful neurologic examination [83].

Most vascular injuries secondary to penetrating wounds are easily diagnosed by characterizing the bleeding, evaluating the hematoma dimensions, and determining pulse changes, neurologic deficits, and the presence or absence of hypotension [84]. A bruit or thrill may be present if an arteriovenous fistula or pseudoaneurysm is present [85,86]. It must be kept in mind that the absence of these findings does not rule out vascular injury.

The classic signs of ischemia of an extremity are the "five *P*s": pain, paresthesia, paralysis, pallor, pulselessness. Prolongation of the capillary refill times in fingers and toes greater than 3 seconds indicates some degree of ischemia [86]. The earliest signs of ischemia in the lower extremity usually appear in the distribution of the peroneal nerve, which is limited to the dorsum of the base of the first and second toes [87]. The deterioration of motor function is a very late sign of ischemia.

The most reliable sign of blunt or penetrating arterial trauma is absent or diminished pulses [88,89]. A transient (waxing and waning) unilateral pulse loss is as significant as a persistent loss [90]. Normal pulses may be evident distal to an arterial injury in approximately 25 percent of patients [91,92].

An expanding hematoma may originate from a lacerated artery or from transection of a major vein [93]. The pulsatile nature of the hematoma will differentiate the etiology as arterial or venous.

Radiologic evaluation of the extremities to include the pelvis and chest is helpful in evaluating trauma to extremities. The presence of fractures, dislocations, bullets/projectiles, or fragments indicating a bullet path is very useful in planning a diagnostic workup and management.

Vascular injury is the most serious problem in both blunt and penetrating trauma of the extremity. Blunt injury causing dislocation of the knee posteriorly can result in thrombosis of the popliteal artery [94]. The thrombosis is the result of arterial occlusion caused by a tear in the artery itself or only the intima.

Arteriography is indicated selectively in trauma of the extremity [95] and should not delay definitive surgical management of an obvious injury [96]. If the diagnosis of vascular trauma is in doubt and the patient is hemodynamically stable, an arteriogram is indicated [84]. In patients with injuries in proximity to a major vascular structure, especially those caused by high-velocity projectiles, but with no clinical signs of vascular injury, the use of arteriography is recommended by many authors [97–101]. The routine use of arteriography in the evaluation of patients without clinical findings of vascular trauma has resulted in a high percentage of negative arteriograms [98,101–103]. For this reason, a controversy has developed, and some investigators [104,105] have demonstrated no major arterial injuries in clinically asymptomatic patients, with the only indication for arteriography being proximity to a major vascular structure. In one study, 72 patients with penetrating trauma were subjected to arteriography for proximity injury only. Gunshot wounds accounted for 91.7 percent of patients, and a normal arteriogram was found in 76.4 percent of patients. The remaining 23.6

percent had arteriographic abnormalities that did not warrant surgical correction [104]. Overall, arteriography has a sensitivity of 97 percent, a specificity of 90 percent, and an accuracy of 92 percent [101].

Digital subtraction angiography is less invasive than conventional contrast angiograms [106]. The accuracy of intravenous digital subtraction angiography was studied in 270 patients with extremity trauma (90 percent penetrating). Twenty-one abnormal vessels were identified, and one false-negative and two false-positive results were encountered. No further angiographic evaluation was required in 94 percent of patients studied by intravenous digital subtraction angiography [107].

Intra-arterial digital subtraction angiography and conventional contrast angiography were compared prospectively in 50 patients with extremity trauma. Both procedures demonstrated a sensitivity of 100 percent, and specificity was 94 percent for intra-arterial digital subtraction angiography and 97 percent for conventional contrast angiography. Intra-arterial digital subtraction angiography was better for demonstration of extravasation, and conventional contrast angiography was better in demonstrating pathology involving intimal dissection [108].

Any decrease in the ankle brachial index is indicative of arterial injury until proved otherwise [95]. Ankle systolic blood pressure should be greater than or equal to brachial systolic blood pressure. Ankle brachial index less than 0.5 indicates significant decrease in blood flow [109].

Contrast venograms can aid in the diagnosis of venous injuries and demonstrate venous anatomy and pathology [110].

REFERENCES

1. Committee on Trauma. *Advanced Trauma Life Support Instructor's Manual.* Chicago: American College of Surgeons, 1984.
2. Jennett, B., and Bond, M. Assessment of outcome after severe brain damage: A practical scale. *Lancet* 1:480, 1975.
3. Jennett, B., and Teasdale, G. Aspects of coma after severe head injury. *Lancet* 878, 1977.
4. Sclafani, S. J. A. Advances in Trauma Radiology. In K. I. Maull, H. C. Cleveland, G. O. Strauch, and C. C. Wolferth (eds.), *Advances in Trauma,* Vol. 1 Chicago: Year Book, 1986.
5. Saul, T. G. Beyond Central Nervous System Monitoring. In K. I. Maull, H. C. Cleveland, G. O. Strauch, and C. C. Wolferth, (eds.), *Advances in Trauma,* Vol. II. Chicago: Year Book, 1987.
6. Moore, E. E. Resuscitation and Evaluation of the Injured patient. In G. D. Zuidema, R. B. Rutherford, and W. F. Ballinger (eds.), *The Management of Trauma.* Philadelphia: Saunders, 1985.
7. Roon, A. J., and Christensen, N. Evaluation and treatment of penetrating cervical injuries. *J. Trauma* 19:391, 1979.
8. Thal, E. R. Injury to the Neck. In K. L. Mattox, E. E. Moore, and D. V. Feliciano (eds.), *Trauma.* Norwalk, Conn.: Appleton & Lange, 1988.
9. Sclafani, S. J. A., Panetta, T., Goldstein, A. S., et al. The management of arterial injuries caused by penetration of zone III of the neck. *J. Trauma* 25:871, 1985.
10. Fogelman, M. J., and Stewart, R. D. Penetrating wounds of the neck. *Ann. Surg.* 91:581, 1956.
11. Markey, J. C., Hines, J. L., and Nance, F. C. Penetrating neck wounds: A review of 218 cases. *Am. Surg.* 41:71, 1975.
12. Saletta, J. D., Lowe, R. J., Lim, L. T., et al. Penetrating trauma of the neck. *J. Trauma* 16:579, 1976.
13. Broniatowski, M., and Tucker, H. M. Penetrating injuries of the neck: Emergency evaluation and management. *Postgrad. Med.* 80:155, 1986.
14. Cohen, E. S., Breaux, C. W., Johnson, P. N., and Leitner, C. A. Penetrating neck injuries: Experience with selective exploration. *South. Med. J.* 80:26, 1987.
15. Meyer, J. P., Barrett, J. A., Schuler, J. J., and Flanigan, P. Mandatory vs. selective exploration for

penetrating neck trauma. *Arch. Surg.* 122:592, 1987.
16. Noyes, L. D., McSwain, N. E., and Markowitz, I. P. Panendoscopy with arteriography vs. mandatory exploration of penetrating wounds of the neck. *Ann. Surg.* 204:21, 1986.
17. Butler, R. M., Moser, F. H. The padded dash syndrome: Blunt trauma of the larynx and trachea. *Laryngoscope* 78:1172, 1968.
18. Ballenger, J. J. (ed.). Trauma of the Larynx. In *Diseases of the Nose, Throat and Ear* (12th ed.). Philadelphia: Lea & Febiger, 1977. Pp. 371–388.
19. Nahum, A. M. Immediate care of acute blunt laryngeal trauma. *J. Trauma* 9:112, 1969.
20. Fitz-Hugh, G. S., and Powell, J. B. Management of laryngotracheal injuries. *Va. Med.* 97:490, 1970.
21. Schaefer, S. D. Primary management of laryngeal trauma. *Ann. Otol. Rhinol. Laryngol.* 91:399, 1982.
22. Sheely, C. H., Mattox, K. L., and Beall, A. C. Management of acute cervical tracheal trauma. *Am. J. Surg.* 128:805, 1974.
23. Yarrington, C. T. Trauma involving the air and food passages. *Otolaryngol. Clin. North Am.* 12:321, 1979.
24. Gussack, G. S., Jurkovich, G. J., and Luterman, A. Laryngotracheal trauma: A protocol approach to a rare injury. *Laryngoscope* 96:660, 1986.
25. Fischer, R. P. Cervical radiographic evaluation of alert patients following blunt trauma. *Ann. Emerg. Med.* 13:904, 1984.
26. Harris, H. H., and Tobin, H. A. Acute injuries of the larynx and trachea in 49 patients. *Laryngoscope* 80:1376, 1970.
27. Olson, N. R., and Miles, W. K. Treatment of acute blunt laryngeal injuries. *Ann. Otol. Rhinol. Laryngol.* 80:704, 1971.
28. Glatterer, M. S., Toon, R. S., Ellestad, C., et al. Management of blunt and penetrating external esophageal trauma. *J. Trauma* 25:784, 1985.
29. Maceri, D. R., Mancuso, A. A., and Canalis, R. F. Value of computed axial tomography in severe laryngeal injury. *Arch. Otolaryngol.* 108:449, 1982.
30. Stanley, R. B. Value of computed tomography of the injured larynx. *Radiology* 133:139, 1979.
31. Brown, B. M., Brant-Zawadzki, M., and Cann, C. E. Dynamic CT scanning of spinal column trauma. *A.J.R.* 139:1177, 1982.
32. Gentry, L. R., Manor, W. F., Turski, P. A., and Strother, C. M. High resolution CT analysis of facial struts in trauma: 2. Osseous and soft-tissue complications. *A.J.R.* 140:533, 1983.
33. Dragon, R. Blunt injuries to the carotid and vertebral arteries. *Am. J. Surg.* 141:497, 1981.
34. Karrel, R., Shaffer, M. A., and Franaszek, J. B. Emergency diagnosis, resuscitation and treatment of acute penetrating trauma. *Ann. Emerg. Med.* 11:504, 1982.
35. Jurkovich, G. J., and Moore, E. E. Thoracic trauma. *Trauma Q.* 1:37, 1984.
36. Demetriades, D. Cardiac penetrating injuries: Personal experience of 45 cases. *Br. J. Surg.* 71:95, 1984.
37. Evans, J., Gray, L. A. Rayner, A., and Fulton, R. L. Principles for the management of penetrating cardiac wounds. *Ann. Surg.* 189:777, 1979.
38. Kaye, W. Invasive Therapeutic Techniques. In K. M. McIntyre and A. J. Lewis (eds.), *Advanced Cardiac Life Support.* Dallas: American Heart Association, 1981.
39. Sherman, M. M., Saini, V. K., Yarnoz, M. D., et al. Management of penetrating heart wounds. *Am. J. Surg.* 135:553, 1978.
40. Siemans, R., Polk, H. C., Gray, L. A., et al. Indications for thoracotomy following penetrating thoracic trauma. *J. Trauma* 17:493, 1977.
41. Kaushik, V. S., Mandal, A. K., Awariefe, O. E., et al. Early thoracotomy for stab wounds of the heart. *J. Cardiovasc. Surg.*, 20:423, 1979.
42. Oprah, S. S., and Mandal, A. K. Penetrating stab wounds of the chest: Experience with 200 consecutive cases. *J. Trauma* 16:868, 1976.
43. Sugg, W. S., Rea, W. J., Ecker, R. R., et al. Penetrating wounds of the heart: An analysis of 459 cases. *J. Thoroc. Cardiovasc. Surg.* 56:531, 1968.
44. Demetriades, D. Cardiac wounds: Experience with 70 patients. *Ann. Surg.* 203:315, 1986.
45. Glinz, W. Chest trauma: Diagnosis and management. Berlin: Springer-Verlag, 1984.
46. Richardson, J. D., Flint, L. M., Snow, N. J., et al. Management of transmediastinal gunshot wounds. *Surgery* 90:671, 1981.
47. Miller, F. B., Sheldon, S. J., Shumate, C. R., et al. Diagnostic pericardial window: A safe alterna-

tive to exploratory thoracotomy for suspected heart injury. *Arch. Surg.* 122:605, 1987.
48. Dieter, R. A., Hamouda, F., Asselmeier, G. H., et al. Traumatic disruption of the thoracic aorta: A community hospital experience. *Milit. Med.* 148:502, 1983.
49. Glintz, W. Priorities in diagnosis and treatment of blunt chest injuries. *Injury* 17:318, 1986.
50. Newman, R. J., and Rastogi, S. Rupture of the thoracic aorta and its relationship to road traffic accident characteristics. *Injury* 15:296, 1984.
51. Shaikh, K. A., Schwab, C. W., and Camishon, R. C. Aortic rupture in blunt trauma. *Am. Surg.* 52:47, 1986.
52. Levine, S. D., and Hopkins, R. L. Blunt chest trauma in children. *La. State Med. Soc. J.* 137:54, 1985.
53. Blank, N. Non-penetrating thoracic trauma: Emphasis on plain film findings. *Postgrad. Radiol.* 4:5, 1984.
54. Phillips, E. H., Rogers, W. F., and Gaspar, M. R. First rib fracture: Incidence of vascular injury and indications for angiography. *Surgery* 89:42, 1981.
55. Kettunen, P. Cardiac damage after blunt chest trauma diagnosed using CK-MB enzyme and electrocardiogram. *Int. J. Cardiol.* 6:355, 1984.
56. Muwanga, C. L., Cole, R. P., Sloan, J. P., et al. Cardiac contusion in patients wearing seat belts. *Injury* 17:37, 1986.
57. Mulder, D. S., Shennib, B. H., and Angood, P. Thoracic Injuries. In K. I. Maull, H. C. Cleveland, G. O. Strauch, and C. C. Wolferth (eds.), *Advances in Trauma,* Vol. 1. Chicago: Year Book, 1986.
58. Beel, T., and Harwood, A. L. Traumatic rupture of the thoracic aorta. *Ann. Emerg. Med.* 9:483, 1980.
59. Schmidt, C. A., and Jacobson, J. G. Thoracic aortic injury: A ten year experience. *Arch. Surg.* 119:1244, 1984.
60. Stiles, Q. R., Cohlmia, G. S., Smith, J. H., et al. Management of injuries of the thoracic and abdominal aorta. *Am. J. Surg.* 150:132, 1985.
61. Goldstein, A. S., Sclafani, S. J. A., Kupperstein, N. H., et al. The diagnostic superiority of computerized tomography. *J. Trauma* 25:938, 1985.
62. Gomez, G. A., Alvarez, R., Plasencia, G., et al. Diagnostic peritoneal lavage in the management of blunt abdominal trauma: A reassessment. *J. Trauma* 27:1, 1987.
63. Danto, L. A. Paracentesis and Diagnostic Peritoneal Lavage. In F. W. Blaisdell and D. D. Trunkey (eds.), *Trauma Management.* Vol. 1. Abdominal Trauma. New York: Thieme-Stratton, 1982.
64. Engrav, L. H., Benjamin, C. I., Strate, R. G., et al. Diagnostic peritoneal lavage in blunt abdominal trauma. *J. Trauma* 15:854, 1975.
65. Olsen, W. R., Redman, H. C., and Hildreth, D. H. Abdominal paracentesis and peritoneal lavage in blunt abdominal trauma. *J. Trauma* 11:824, 1971.
66. Perry, J. F., DeMeules, J. E., and Root, H. D. Diagnostic peritoneal lavage in blunt abdominal trauma. *Surg. Gynecol. Obstet.* 131:742, 1970.
67. Foley, R. W., Harris, L. S., and Pilcher, D. B. Abdominal injuries in automobile accidents: Review of care of fatally injured patients. *J. Trauma* 17:611, 1977.
68. Kreis, D. J., Plasencia, G., Augenstein, D., et al. Preventable trauma deaths: Dade County, Florida. *J. Trauma* 26:649, 1986.
69. Neuman, T. S., Bockman, M. A., Moody, P., et al. An autopsy study of traumatic deaths: San Diego, 1979. *Am. J. Surg.* 144:722, 1982.
70. Root, H. D., Hauser, C. W., McKinley, C. R., et al. Diagnostic peritoneal lavage. *Surgery* 57:633, 1965.
71. Federle, M. P., Crass, R. A., Jeffrey, R. B., and Trunkey, D. D. Computed tomography in blunt abdominal trauma. *Arch. Surg.* 117:645, 1982.
72. Perry, J. F., and Strate, R. G. Diagnostic peritoneal lavage in blunt abdominal trauma: Indication and results. *Surgery* 71:898, 1972.
73. Thal, E. R., and Shires, G. T. Peritoneal lavage in blunt abdominal trauma. *Am. J. Surg.* 125:64, 1973.
74. Ahmad, W., and Polk, H. C. Blunt abdominal trauma: A prospective study with selective peritoneal lavage. *Arch. Surg.* 111:489, 1976.
75. Drew, R., and Perry, J. F. The expediency of peritoneal lavage in blunt trauma in children. *Surg. Gynecol. Obstet.* 145:885, 1977.
76. Fischer, R. P., Beverlin, B. C., Engrav, L. H., et al. Diagnostic peritoneal lavage: Fourteen years and 2,586 patients later. *Am. J. Surg.* 136:701, 1978.

77. Gruenberg, J. C., Brown, R. S., Tallbert, J. G., et al. The diagnostic usefulness of peritoneal lavage in penetrating trauma: A prospective evaluation and comparison with blunt trauma. *Am. Surg.* 48:402, 1982.
78. Merlotti, G. J., Dillon, B. C., Lange, D. A., et al. Peritoneal lavage in penetrating thoracoabdominal trauma. *J. Trauma* 28:17, 1988.
79. Hauser, C. J., Huprich, J. E., Bosco, P., et al. Triple-contrast computed tomography in the evaluation of penetrating posterior abdominal injuries. *Arch. Surg.* 122:1112, 1987.
80. Demetriades, D., Rabinowitz, B., Sofianos, C., et al. The management of penetrating injuries of the back: A prospective study of 230 patients. *Ann. Surg.* 207:72, 1988.
81. Oreskovich, M. R., and Carrico, C. J. Stab wounds of the anterior abdomen: Analysis of a management plan using local wound exploration and quantitative peritoneal lavage. Ann. Surg. 198:411, 1983.
82. Thal, E. R. Evaluation of peritoneal lavage and local exploration in lower chest and abdominal stab wounds. *J. Trauma* 17:642, 1977.
83. Saide, R. Jacobsen, D. C., Bloch, J. H., et al. Management of peripheral vascular trauma. *Am. Surg.* 47:729, 1981.
84. Sitzmann, J. V., and Ernst, C. B. Management of arm arterial injuries. *Surgery* 96:895, 1984.
85. Graham, J. M. Subclavian, Axillary, and Brachial Artery Injuries. In E. E. Moore, B. Eiseman, and C. W. VanWay (eds.), *Critical Decisions in Trauma.* St. Louis: Mosby, 1984.
86. Meyer, J. P., Davenport, K., and Flanigan, D. P. Penetrating extremity trauma. *Trauma Q.* 1:67, 1985.
87. Rutherford, R. B. Trauma to the Peripheral Vascular System. In G. R. Schwartz, P. Safer, J. H. Stone, et al. (eds.), *Principles and Practices of Emergency Medicine.* Philadelphia: Saunders, 1978.
88. Sirnek, K. R., Gaskill, H. V., Oittman, W. L., et al. Exclusion angiography for patients with possible vascular injury of the extremities: A better use of trauma center resources. *Surgery* 94:598, 1983.
89. Smith, P. L., Lim, W. N., Ferris, E. J., et al. Emergency arteriography in extremity trauma: Assessment of indications. *Am. J. Roentgenol.* 137:803, 1981.
90. Perry, M. O. *The Management of Acute Vascular Injuries.* Baltimore: William & Wilkins, 1981.
91. Orcutt, M. B., Levine, B. A., Gaskill, H. V., et al. Civilian vascular trauma of the upper extremity. *J. Trauma* 26:63, 1986.
92. Pasch, A. R., Bishara, R. A., Lim, L. T., et al. Optimal limb salvage in penetrating civilian vascular trauma. *J. Vasc. Surg.* 3:189, 1986.
93. Bole, P. V., Purdy, R. T., Munda, R. T., et al. Civilian arterial injuries. *Ann. Surg.* 183:12, 1976.
94. Welling, R. E., Kakkaseril, J., and Craney, J. J. Complete dislocations of the knee with popliteal vascular injury. *J. Trauma* 21:450, 1981.
95. Soderstrom, C. A., and Wasserman, D. H. Vascular injuries. *Emerg. Clin. North Am.* 2:853, 1984.
96. Turcotte, J. K., Towne, J. B., and Bernhard, V. M. Is angiography necessary in the management of vascular trauma of the extremities. *Surgery* 84:557, 1978.
97. McCready, R. A., Procter, C. D., and Hyde, G. L. Subclavian-axillary vascular trauma. *J. Vasc. Surg.* 3:24, 1986.
98. Menzoian, J. O., Doyle, J. E., Logerfo, F. W., et al. Evaluation and management of vascular injuries of the extremities. *Arch. Surg.* 118:93, 1983.
99. O'Gorman, R. B., Feliciano, D. V., Bitondo, C. G., et al. Emergency center arteriography in the evaluation of suspected peripheral vascular injuries. *Arch. Surg.* 119:568, 1984.
100. Rich, N. M., Hobson, R. W., and Collins, G. J. Elective vascular reconstruction after trauma. *Am. J. Surg.* 130:712, 1975.
101. Snyder, W. H., Thal, E. R., Bridges, R. A., et al. The validity of normal arteriography in penetrating trauma. *Arch. Surg.* 113:424, 1978.
102. McCormick, T. M., and Burch, B. H. Routine angiographic evaluation of neck and extremity injuries. *J. Trauma* 19:384, 1979.
103. McDonald, E. J., Goodman, P. C., and Winestock, D. P. The clinical indications for arteriography in trauma to the extremity. *Radiology* 116:45, 1975.
104. Gomez, G. A., Kreis, D. J., Ratner, L., et al. Suspected vascular trauma of the extremities: The role of angiography in proximity injuries. *J. Trauma* 26:1005, 1986.
105. McCorkell, S. J., Harley, J. D., Morishima, M. S., et al. Indications for angiography in extremity trauma. *Am. J. Roentgenol.* 145:1245, 1985.

106. Ricketts, J. M., and Seutter, W. M. Digital subtraction angiography: Principles and potential applications in emergency medicine. *Ann. Emerg. Med.* 14:41, 1985.
107. Gavant, M. L., Gold, R. E., Fabian, T. C., et al. Vascular trauma to the extremities and lower neck: Initial assessment with intravenous digital subtraction angiography. *Radiology* 158:755, 1986.
108. Sibbitt, R. R., Palmaz, J. C., Garcia, F., et al. Trauma of the extremities: Prospective comparison of digital and conventional angiography. *Radiology* 160:179, 1986.
109. Greer, G. W. Popliteal artery injuries: A review. *Milit. Med.* 148:351, 1983.
110. Gerlock, A. J., Thal, E. R., and Snyder, W. H. Venography in penetrating injuries of the extremities. *Am. J. Roentgenol.* 126:1023, 1976.

5

Treatment of the Trauma Patient: Overview

Raymond H. Alexander

As the role of the trauma physician becomes established in our profession and trauma becomes almost a subspecialty of surgery, orthopedics, or emergency medicine, one could easily conclude that the treatment of trauma focuses surgical and medical skills to a small, concentrated area. This concept could be nothing further from the truth. The trauma physician, instead of narrowing his scope, has actually expanded it, gaining expertise in surgery, orthopedics, neurosurgery, prehospital care, endoscopy, and emergency department care. In that sense, the trauma physician is almost a return to the "renaissance physician." The trauma surgeon, particularly, has an expanded role in the trauma center. This fact will be emphasized throughout the chapter. To describe the scope of the trauma physician's responsibilities, I shall divide the chapter into several sections. The first of these will be the role of the trauma physician in *prehospital care.* The importance of the prehospital course, as to the eventual outcome of the patient and how this care greatly influences how viable a patient the surgeon inherits, will be emphasized. The next section will consider aspects of *aeromedical transport,* particularly rotorcraft transport. As these capabilities expand throughout the nation, particularly in the hospital-based services, physicians are becoming more and more involved with prehospital care as administered by helicopter transport teams. Treatment in the *emergency department* and the surgeon's role as the leader of the trauma team will next be considered. The importance of a protocol approach to emergency department care will be emphasized, as will the speed of the resuscitation. Considerations of "ER bypass," resulting in the patient being taken directly to the operating room, will also be mentioned. *Operative care,* operative priorities, and operating room techniques will next be considered. The role of the surgeon in the *intensive care unit* and his treatment of the trauma patient in this area will be discussed next. Finally, *public education, physician outreach programs,* and *trauma prevention* will be presented as one of the important characteristics of the trauma surgeon and one of his most important responsibilities.

PREHOSPITAL CARE

Beginning in the early 1970s, ambulance companies across the country were replaced by prehospital specialists who fall into two broad categories. The most basic level of prehospital life support team is the emergency medical technician (EMT). EMTs receive approximately 40 hours of training, as described in the Department of Transportation (DOT) curriculum, that results in skills in basic first aid, cardiopulmonary resuscitation, immobilization, and extrication [1]. Some states allow the use of Military Anti-Shock Trousers (MAST) and some type of respiratory support, such as the esophageal airway. Other states, such as Florida, are allowing EMTs to monitor, but not start, intravenous (IV) fluids. Recently, there has been a move to allow EMTs to defibrillate patients.

A more advanced level of life support is given by paramedics. These individuals are trained in the use of advanced cardiac resuscitation techniques such as drug administration, establishing IV routes, and administering IV fluids. More importantly, they are trained to give advanced respiratory support through endotracheal intubation. Paramedics have the basic EMT skills, which include extrication, immobilization, and splinting. As the first life support units were initially instituted for the care of cardiac patients, many of the traditions have been carried over to other forms of care. One of the strong traditions, which is associated with advanced cardiac life support, is "on-scene stabilization." In such a scenario, paramedics arrive at the scene, start IV routes, administer drugs, and defibrillate. Only after a rhythm has been achieved and the patient has been stabilized is transport carried out. An important exception to this is, if no response to resuscitation is evident, the paramedics may transport, supporting with cardiopulmonary resuscitation. Currently, controversy rages within the prehospital community, and it centers on whether or not such on-scene stabilization is appropriate for the trauma victim. Many surgeons feel that a "swoop and scoop" or "scoop and run" serves the patient better in the field. They argue that derangements experienced by the trauma patient, mainly those of hemorrhage, cannot be adequately addressed in a field situation. These two divergent philosophies basically establish the need for surgical input into the prehospital system with reference to the trauma patient. As one might guess, studies vary on which approach produces the greater survivability and the least morbidity. Before reaching a consistent philosophy on such matters, it is incumbent on one to review some of the studies concerning prehospital trauma care. Gervin and Fischer [2] retrospectively studied the response of EMTs versus paramedics, with reference to the mortality of penetrating heart wounds. These investigators found patients who were managed by scoop and run, spending an average of 9 minutes on the scene, had an 83-percent survival. The group of patients treated by on-scene stabilization spent an average of 20 minutes on the scene. There were no survivors in this group. The authors concluded that on-scene stabilization resulted in an unacceptable mortality in patients with potential cardiac wounds. Aprahamian and colleagues [3] studied 112 patients with intra-abdominal vascular trauma. No difference in mortality could be found between on-scene stabilization and scoop and run in those patients with initial blood pressures greater than 60 mm Hg recorded in the emergency department. On the other hand, patients with blood pressures less than 60 mm Hg benefitted from the administration of advanced life support (ALS) techniques. The ALS group had a 50-percent mortality, whereas the scoop and run patients experienced an 86-percent mortality. Jacobs and coworkers [4] studied two groups of patients within the Boston emergency medical services (EMS) system. Those who were delivered by EMTs and received no ALS were compared to those patients delivered by an ALS team. The two groups were matched according to their severity scores as described by Champion and associates [5] (Table 5-1). It was found that, in the midtrauma score ranges, that is, from approximately 6 to 12, patients generally did better with ALS than with basic life support (BLS) only. Individuals with very high and very low scores experienced little benefit from ALS. Patients transported by BLS personnel experienced little change in their trauma score at the scene as compared to that computed in the emergency department. Patients transported by ALS teams had a significant increase in trauma score in the midtrauma score ranges, indicating a decrease in expected mortality.

Pons and coworkers [6] have prospectively studied critical penetrating wounds of the thorax and abdomen at the prehospital system in Denver, Colorado. ALS scene times were found to average 9.9 minutes, during which one or more IV lines were placed and, if necessary, MAST applied and endotracheal intubation accomplished. Increases in blood pressure were noted in 55 percent of patients, whereas 32 percent experienced no blood pressure change and only 13 percent were found to have a blood pressure drop. Pons concluded that ALS interventions improve the hemodynamic status of these patients.

Finally, some insight as to the dynamics of one ALS intervention, IV therapy, was studied by Lewis [7]. In this study, computer modeling of the cardiovascular system was performed, with bleeding and IV inflow rates as variables. Patients with high bleeding rates (100 ml/min) benefitted from IV therapy if prehospital times were greater than 30 minutes. In modeled patients with slow (25 ml/min) bleeding rates, prehospital times of greater than 1 hour are necessary to accrue mild benefit from IV therapy. In patients with bleeding rates of 50 ml/min, significant benefit is obtained, but again only if prehospital times are greater than 50 to 60 minutes. Lewis concluded that IV infusions are of limited benefit in an urban EMS system, and advantages of IV therapy might be limited to rural systems.

Much of the scoop and run versus on-scene stabilization appears to be focused on the role

Table 5-1. Trauma Score

			Score
I. Respiratory rate	10–24	4	
	25–35	3	
	⩾36	2	
	1–9	1	
	none	0	I______
II. Respiratory expansion	normal	1	
	none/retractive	0	II______
III. Systolic blood pressure (mm Hg)	⩾90	4	
	70–89	3	
	50–69	2	
	0–49	1	
	no pulse	0	III______
IV. Capillary refill	normal	2	
	delayed	1	
	none	0	IV______
V. Glasgow Coma Score (see Table 4-1)	14–15	5	
	11–13	4	
	8–10	3	
	5–7	2	
	3–4	1	V______
Trauma score (sum I to V):			1–16

Note: The Trauma Score is a grading system for estimating the severity of injury. It is composed of physiologic parameters and the Glasgow Coma Scale.
Source: H. R. Champion et al., Trauma score. *Crit. Care Med.* 9:672, 1981.

of IV therapy, as noted in the articles by Lewis and Pons. IV therapy is only one stabilization technique that is used in the field. Other more critical physiologic derangements, such as airway obstruction and breathing abnormalities, may need attention in the field if the patient is to survive. Airway obstruction is poorly tolerated by a patient, even in the shortest transport distances. Time taken to intubate will be lifesaving. In the situation of intracranial injury, rapid and accurate endotracheal intubation, with subsequent oxygenation and hyperventilation, may indeed be life- and brain-saving.

Even in urban environments, prehospital times may be prolonged by extrication and problems attendant with prolonged transport times due to geography, traffic, and the like. Critical ALS procedures (intubation and external hemorrhage control) must be managed immediately. Less critical procedures, such as intravenous access, can be accomplished coincidental with extrication, skeletal stabilization, and transport. Limits can be placed on interventions (number of intubation or IV attempts) to ensure that time is not needlessly wasted.

Whether such interventions are indeed lifesaving depends on the skills maintained by the particular ALS system's personnel. Therefore, the quality of the ALS training is critical to what procedures paramedics are allowed to perform in the field as a part of on-scene stabilization. Summation of the data appears to point toward the fact that the proper management of the prehospital system can make a great deal of difference as far as the viability of the trauma patient delivered to the emergency department. It is imperative that the patient be delivered to the trauma center rapidly because excessive blood loss creates problems with hypothermia, clotting, and shock. Such conditions lead, in turn, to multiple organ failure, which the best surgeon cannot interdict once the blood loss has occurred. It is also clear that the maintenance of a proper airway and the administration of IV fluids, if done rapidly and accurately, can prevent progression of head injury, be lifesaving in terms of airway management, and prevent hypovolemic shock in certain cases. In this light, the role of the surgeon or emergency physician in prehospital care becomes quite clear. Without proper training and supervision, endotracheal intubation and IV fluid administration become life-threatening rather than lifesaving. The supervising physician must ensure that the training of the individuals to perform these critical ALS procedures is up to standards, otherwise continued use of these modalities in the field cannot be justified. Once the system has attained a capacity to perform such procedures accurately, it is the physician's task to make sure that these procedures do not prolong scene time, but are used judiciously and wisely with strict limitations on either time for procedure or time in the field. The judicious application of ALS stabilization techniques should not be criticized; however, excessive scene time to achieve these ALS interventions should not be condoned. The surgeon or emergency physician then has a role as an educator. If he is not the EMS medical director, he must maintain an active role to ensure that training of personnel in key ALS procedures takes place. In addition, the surgeon must either write or participate in writing protocols that deal with the prehospital treatment of trauma.

In our own system, we have allowed use of ALS procedures but have attempted to control scene time by placing limits on each individual procedure. Figure 5-1 shows the flow sheet for prehospital care of the trauma patient in the Jacksonville system and includes these limits as well as destination decisions.

In summary, the prehospital care of the trauma patient must again become the province of the physician through medical direction. The final outcome of the patient depends as much on his treatment in the prehospital areas as it does on the skill of the surgeon who finally stops the bleeding. If we abdicate this responsibility, we accept the fact that many patients will die unnecessarily, at the scene or in the emergency department, operating room, or intensive care unit, due to inadequate care at the scene.

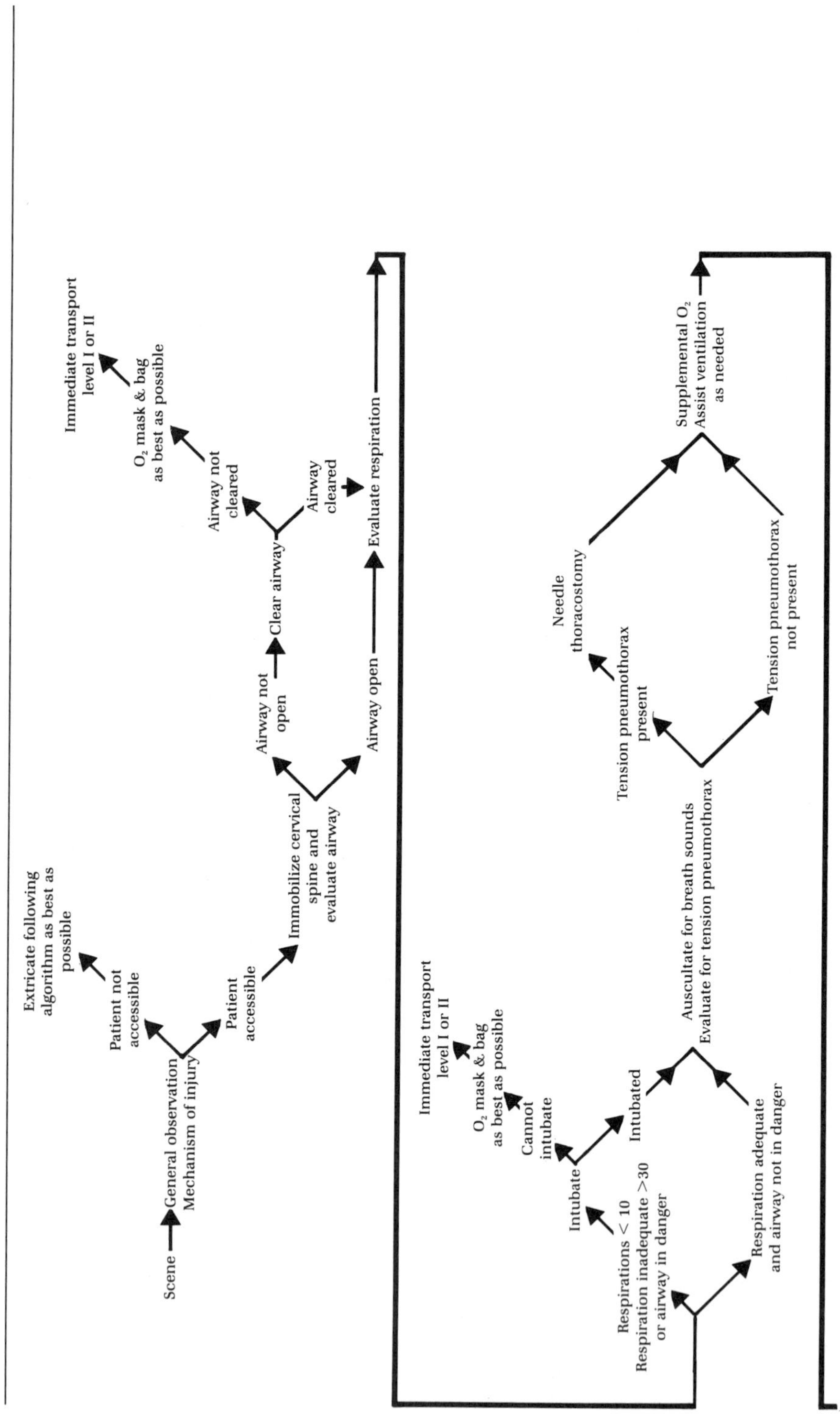
Scene
General observation
Mechanism of injury
Patient not accessible
Extricate following algorithm as best as possible
Patient accessible
Immobilize cervical spine and evaluate airway
Airway not open
Clear airway
Airway not cleared
O_2 mask & bag as best as possible
Immediate transport level I or II
Airway cleared
Airway open
Evaluate respiration
Respirations < 10
Respiration inadequate >30
or airway in danger
Intubate
Cannot intubate
O_2 mask & bag as best as possible
Immediate transport level I or II
Intubated
Respiration adequate and airway not in danger
Auscultate for breath sounds
Evaluate for tension pneumothorax
Tension pneumothorax present
Needle thoracostomy
Tension pneumothorax not present
Supplemental O_2
Assist ventilation as needed

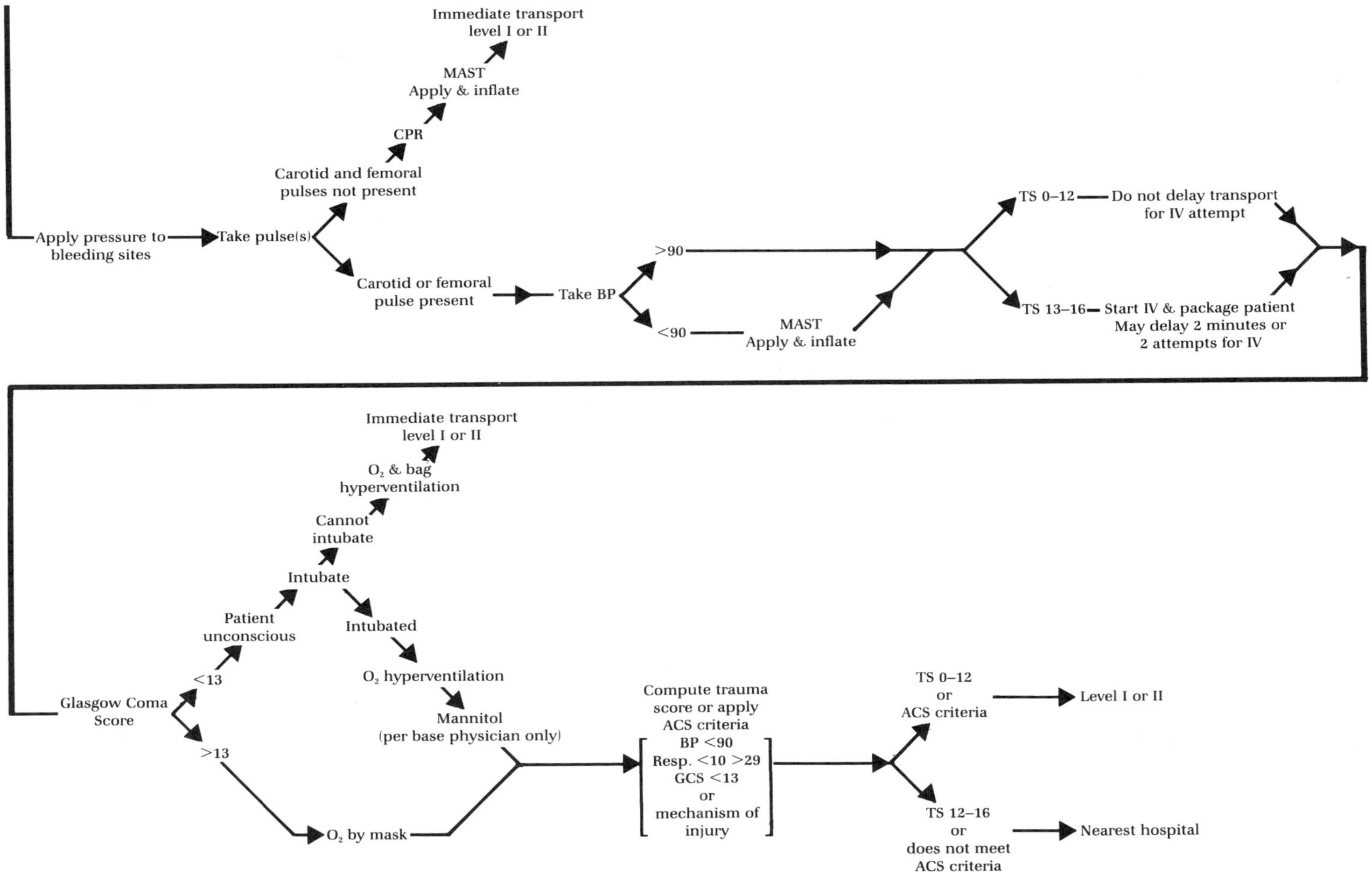

Fig. 5-1. Algorithm for prehospital treatment of trauma victims by Jacksonville, Florida fire rescue paramedics. TS = trauma score; ACS = American College of Surgeons; GCS = Glasgow Coma Score.

HELICOPTER PREHOSPITAL CARE

There are significant advances in military medicine associated with the use of rotorcraft transport from the front line to surgical units. At least part of the dramatic decrease in battlefield mortality must be attributable to the use of these aircraft in the Korean War and the Vietnam War (Table 5-2) [8]. Historically, the first dedicated use of rotorcraft for civilian transport was in Europe in the mid-1960s. St. Anthony's Hospital in Denver, Colorado, established the first rotorcraft EMS transport system in the United States in 1972 [9]. From that time to the present, there have been over 125 hospital-based helicopter programs begun in this country as well as countless other rotorcraft EMS transport programs associated with prehospital care systems, law enforcement, and other providers. It is well-established that the use of rotorcraft was lifesaving in military conflicts, and the capability of increasing the survivability of the trauma patient appears to be substantiated in civilian practice also. In West Germany, a system of level I trauma centers has been set up along the autobahns, or superhighways, of that country. Attached to each level I trauma center is a rotorcraft transport service, which has resulted in 90 percent of the West German population being within 15 minutes of a level I trauma center. This commitment to trauma care has decreased trauma mortality by 25 percent [10]. In the United States, several studies have been done that confirm the lifesaving capabilities of rotorcraft in EMS transport. In 1983, Baxt and Moody [11], compared ground transport to rotorcraft transport. Using the "Z statistic" (i.e., probability of survival index), they compared a ground transport system and an air transport system in terms of expected mortality for groups of patients. These patients were scored by the Severity Scoring System of Champion and associates [5]. Using this *Z* statistic, Baxt and Moody found that air transport increased survivability by 52 percent as compared to ground transport. Using the same technique, Baxt and colleagues [12], in 1985, studied seven rotorcraft programs spread throughout the United States. Rotorcraft-transported patients had a 21-percent lower mortality than that predicted by using trauma scores and the *Z* statistic to predict the probability of survival. In 1984, Urdaneta and coworkers [13] studied a rural population (Iowa) and found helicopter transport lifesaving in 27.4 percent of cases. It therefore becomes clear that a wealth of data reporting the lifesaving capacities of the EMS rotorcraft is emerging.

Table 5-2. Mortality per 100 Casualties During Major Wars Fought by the United States

War	Mortality per 100 serious injuries
World War II	8[a]
Korean War	2.5[b]
Vietnam War	1.3[b]

[a]Prior to the advent of rotorcraft transport.
[b]Rotorcraft transport used extensively.

It is notable that all the studies done were concerned with the transport of the trauma patient. A rotorcraft operating out of a trauma center has several distinct advantages. This aircraft increases the service area of the trauma center. Enlarged referral area makes a trauma center more cost-effective in terms of patient care. Additional patients also increase the expertise and experience of the trauma teams at the institution. In addition, rotorcraft transport ensures the rapid transportation of the traumatized patient to the facility, thereby saving precious moments that may be critical to the patient's survival. Helicopter transport also allows trauma centers to service rural areas. In Florida, the population is concentrated around the coastlines of the state. Central portions of the panhandle in Florida are sparsely populated and have few, if any, doctors or medical facilities. In such areas, even a level III trauma center becomes an impossibility. The study of vehicular mortality in the state shows the probability of dying in a motor vehicle accident in a rural county is some 200 times greater than that in a more urban area [14]. At least part of these mortality figures must be associated with an ability to obtain rapid trauma care. The use of rotorcraft transport in rural areas appears to be the only answer to providing quality trauma care to a population that cannot support even a level III trauma facility.

Since many helicopter programs associated with trauma centers are hospital-based, an effective interface between prehospital care and the trauma center is facilitated. The helicopter, under direct control of the hospital, can implement transport policies, facilitate training of prehospital personnel, and interface one-to-one with the existing prehospital organizations to a maximum degree. Since the established efficacy of the helicopter is mainly in the care of traumatized patients, it is imperative that a hospital seeking to be a high-volume trauma center have helicopter transportation available to it. In addition, direct influence and interaction by the trauma surgeons at the trauma center must take place to facilitate the optimum transport of the patient to the trauma center. In our own system, a surgeon is medical director of the helicopter program and is responsible for training of prehospital personnel as well as configuration of the helicopter. Mission design is directed toward the trauma patient. Helicopter transport is provided using a flight nurse and flight paramedic.

Baxt and Moody [15] have data that indicate the addition of a physician to the helicopter crew may be beneficial. Rhee and colleagues [16] and Carraway and associates [17] have presented data that indicate that 25 percent of patients may be benefitted by the presence of a physician on the helicopter. Although these data are convincing, it is also pertinent that much of the influence the physician has on the preservation of life in an aeromedical situation is that of providing judgmental skills. It is our thesis that the judgmental issues can be solved by prompt interface of the physician by radio contact with the trained flight crews on the helicopter. From a cost standpoint, this is a very important concept, in that use of physicians on an aeromedical transport unit costs approximately $85,000 per year [16]. In our own system, the helicopter is provided 24 hours of coverage by a physician known as the "medical control physician." These physicians are in contact with the helicopter, by cellular telephone, at all times. In this way, we feel that, in a majority of cases, the judgmental support, which appears to be the most important facet in the preservation of life in this situation, can be provided without the physician's actually having to be on board the aircraft.

The design of the aeromedical helicopter is critical as far as the trauma patient is concerned. First of all, we feel that safety is a primary consideration, since mortality involving EMS helicopters is the highest of any group of rotorcraft transport in the country by approximately five times. A twin-engine helicopter is preferable, and advanced navigational aids should be on board. We further stress a rigorous training program for our paramedics and flight nurses as well as a rigorous program of training for setting up landing zones and directing the helicopter on the part of the prehospital personnel with whom the program interacts. We follow a strict plan of localizing the helicopter at all times while in the air and, above all, maintain strict policies as to weather limitations and night flights.

The capabilities of the helicopter in terms of internal space are also critical. In our case, we have selected a BK-117, which facilitates the transport of two patients simultaneously, still giving total access to the patient from head to toe and ample access to perform any procedure necessary during flight. This space allows the capability of establishing IV lines, placing chest tubes or transthoracic needles, intubating, and performing other procedures during flight rather than at the scene. The BK-117 also has a rigid rotor system placed high off the ground. This allows safe "hot" loading (engines running) of patients. Normally, the helicopter turbines must be "warmed up" and "cooled down" for approximately 2 minutes before the helicopter lifts off or shuts down. This obviously delays the patient transport by at least 4 minutes should the helicopter need to be shut down because of low rotor height. Our "ideal standard" is to be on and off the ground at a scene within 2 minutes.

Internal configuration of the helicopter is extremely important, and various systems have been advocated for this. Many programs desire to design their own interior configurations. Some prefer a modular system made by Bucher in Switzerland. This is a standardized system that has the advantage of reaching from our primary helicopter to a backup with similar capabilities without reconfiguring equipment or losing crew familiarization with the internal medical systems.

Trauma surgeons in an institution must be acutely aware of the capabilities and limitations of a helicopter transport service if available at that institution. Used prudently, it is felt that the EMS helicopter provides a powerful tool for increasing the volume of trauma patients treated as well as their survivability.

EMERGENCY DEPARTMENT

The surgeon has responsibilities in the emergency department as the leader of the trauma team, a principle emphasized by the American College of Surgeons [18]. In the role of team leader, the surgeon is usually interacting with the emergency department physician. As modern trauma initiatives develop, it is apparent that the emergency physician–surgeon interface must be developed for smooth patient care. The marriage between emergency physicians and surgeons in trauma care can be a happy one once the initial "lovers' quarrels" are settled. The emergency physician is trained to stabilize the trauma patient and perform the initial resuscitation procedures. The surgeon, however, maintains control of the resuscitation as chief of the trauma team. The reason for this is quite simple. Whereas the emergency physician's role is rooted firmly in the present care of the patient, that is, stabilizing vital signs, assessing injuries, and caring for injuries that are treatable in that environment, the surgeon is looking at the patient as a preoperative or pre–intensive care unit patient. The surgeon's plan must be made for the future, to prepare the patient for the interventions that come later in the course of the illness. In that sense, the surgeon must have the latitude and authority to have ultimate control over the patient's management. The trauma surgeon must provide continuity of care from initial entry of the patient into the hospital until the moment the patient is discharged, and protocols must be written to reflect that type of relationship. To avoid conflictual relationships, these protocols assign not only what tasks are to be done in the emergency department but also who should be responsible for these tasks. The division of labor by protocol and assignment not only obviates the conflicts that might arise, but also positively benefits the patient, in that resuscitation is carried through smoothly and without anything "being forgotten." In addition, the emergency physician and the trauma surgeon must agree on critical resuscitation issues. As an example, a protocol decision must be made as to whether a urinary catheter should be placed in a patient with pelvic fractures before a cystogram is done. Protocol decisions "settle" arguable gray zones of medical knowledge to prevent confusion and dissension in the actual care of the patient. There is no time, in a trauma resuscitation, to debate the scientific merit of many procedures concerning when and on whom they should be done. In our own institution, we have various residents, by level and by specialty, assigned to a specific task within the protocol.

The other area of frequent conflict between emergency physicians and surgeons concerns the notification of the trauma team. Whether in a level I or level II institution, the surgeon must be called upon notification that a trauma patient is being transported to the institution. With the new triage standards set out by the American College of Surgeons [18], physiologic and "mechanism of injury" parameters can be used in the field easily to identify a patient who deserves a trauma center. It then makes perfect sense that those patients who need trauma centers need the trauma team and trauma surgeon. Upon notification that such a patient is en route to a trauma center, the trauma team or trauma surgeon should be immediately activated. Decisions as to the severity of injury are then placed back in the prehospital area, rather than in the emergency department, with the obvious advantage of saving many minutes of precious time. In our institution, the trauma team is alerted upon notification that a patient with a severity score of less than 12 or with a mechanism of injury indicative of a potential severe injury is being transported to us. We are currently in the process of changing from the old severity score in the prehospital system to that outlined by the American

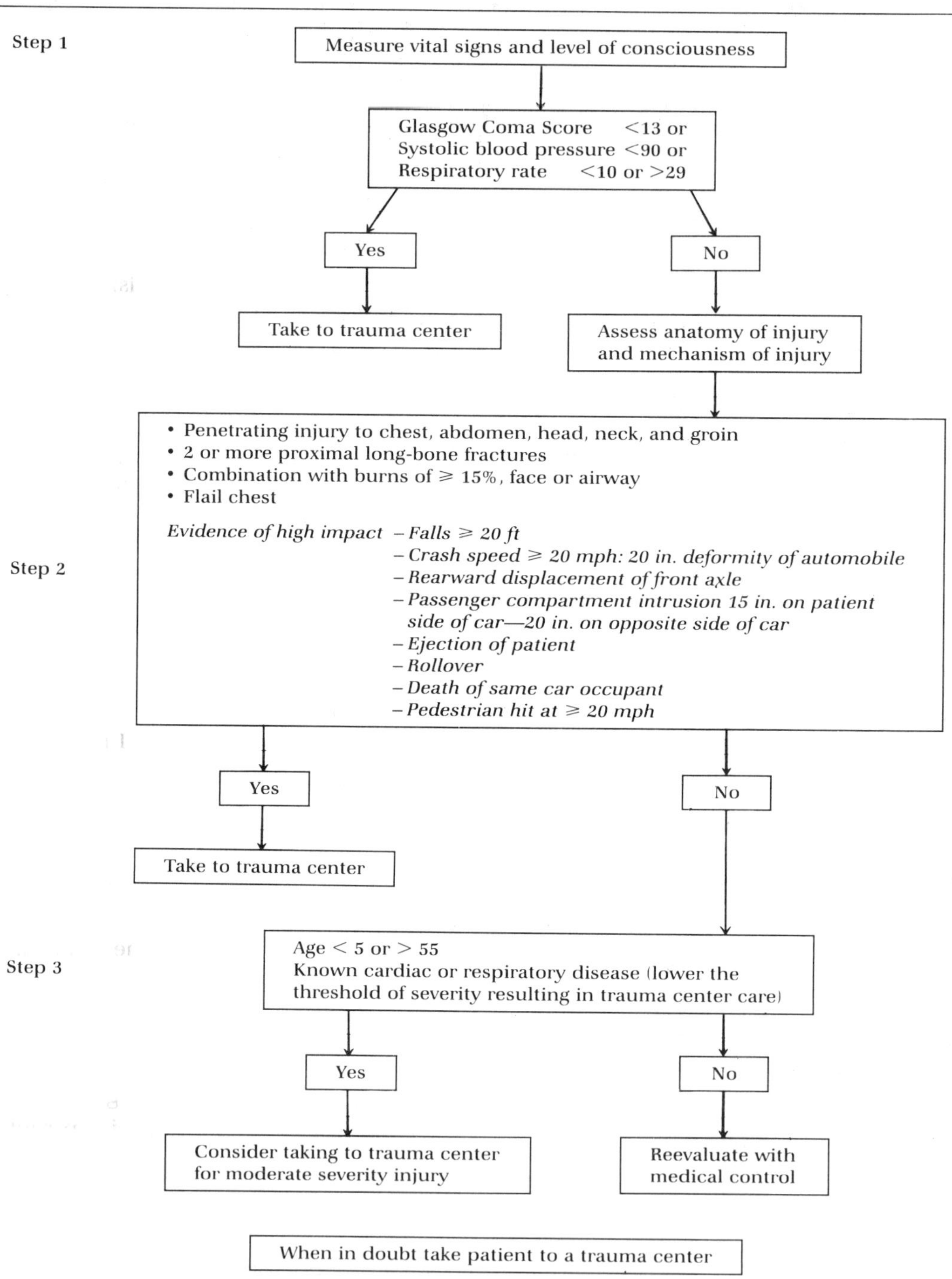

Fig. 5-2. Triage scheme for determining destination of trauma victims as published by the American College of Surgeons Committee on Trauma.

Table 5-3. Criteria for "Emergency Department Bypass" of Trauma Patients

Cardiac arrest
Hypovolemic shock unresponsive to volume infusion
Unstable vital signs secondary to blood loss due to
Penetrating injuries to neck, chest, and/or abdomen
Blunt trauma to chest and/or abdomen
Evisceration of abdominal contents
Major traumatic amputation or degloving injuries
Patients transferred from other hospitals known to need immediate surgery

College of Surgeons [18]. This triage scheme is depicted in Figure 5-2.

Of special mention in patient notification is that of the "emergency department bypass." Several authors have stated the wisdom of allowing a specific group of trauma patients to bypass the emergency department and go directly to the operating room [19,20]. Essential to such an effort is to have equipment in the operating room that would support a resuscitation ordinarily done in the emergency department. The specific indications for emergency department bypass are listed in Table 5-3.

When the patient arrives at the resuscitation area, members of the trauma team assume their assigned duties. Resuscitations are then carried out as per protocol. Protocols are broken down into a general overall protocol and an organ-specific protocol. The general protocol has both physician and nursing components, whereas the specific protocols mainly involve physician intervention.

CONFIGURATION OF THE TRAUMA RESUSCITATION AREA

The physical configuration of the trauma resuscitation area is very important for optimum care of the patient. The resuscitation area should be centrally located to both external support areas, that is, ambulance unloading area and helipad, and internal support systems, notably x-ray department, operating room, and computed tomography (CT) scanner. The space should be carefully planned, providing maximal support to a specific number of beds but having the capability of being an open area that could potentially expand greatly for a mass casualty situation. Primary resuscitation areas, ideally, should be reserved for trauma only. We dislike the "trauma room concept," as we typically deal with more than a solitary patient and sometimes as many as five patients simultaneously. Placing these patients in different areas spacially totally negates the ability of the trauma team to take care of multiple patients efficiently. Trauma resuscitation areas should be amply prepared with equipment necessary for the resuscitation of patients. Containers of intravenous fluids should be hung with tubing in place, and a set schedule for changing such containers established (Fig. 5-3). Intubation equipment and airway supplies should be available at the head of the table (Fig. 5-4). Also, special trays (e.g., peritoneal lavage, chest thoracostomy, thoracotomy, cutdown) should be available within seconds of the bedside (Fig. 5-5). A means of immediately and positively associating a trauma patient with his blood type and cross-matched samples, as well as an identifier until proper identification is established, is a necessity. We use a "type-

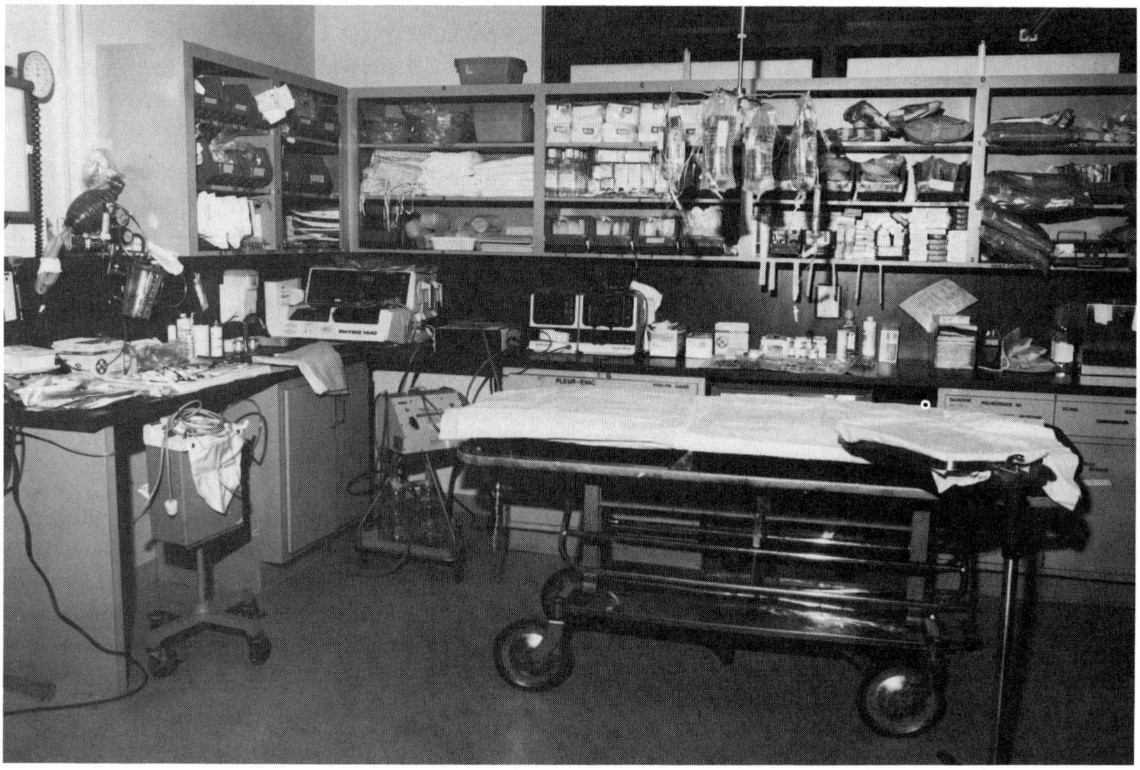

Fig. 5-3. Trauma resuscitation area. Note availability of supplies for immediate treatment of the patient.

nex" system in our center. The blood tubes, wrist band, and other identifiers are contained in a plastic bag, which is immediately opened on entrance of a patient into the trauma resuscitation area (Fig. 5-6). No effort is made to identify the patient by name until the patient has been stabilized. A special trauma resuscitation form is available at the bedside for the nurse to use immediately. When the trauma patient arrives, the nursing staff splits into two parts. The leader of the trauma nurse team and her assistants go immediately to the bedside, whereas one nurse will remain at a centrally located desk to be the "scribe." The resuscitation then proceeds as will be outlined in the next section. Within the next 2 years, we have planned to replace existing medical stretchers with a specially designed stretcher than can be put in use in the resuscitation area, double as an operating table, and be used as a recovery bed. Such a stretcher would obviate the need to transfer a patient with multiple lines and multiple support systems from stretcher, to operating ta-

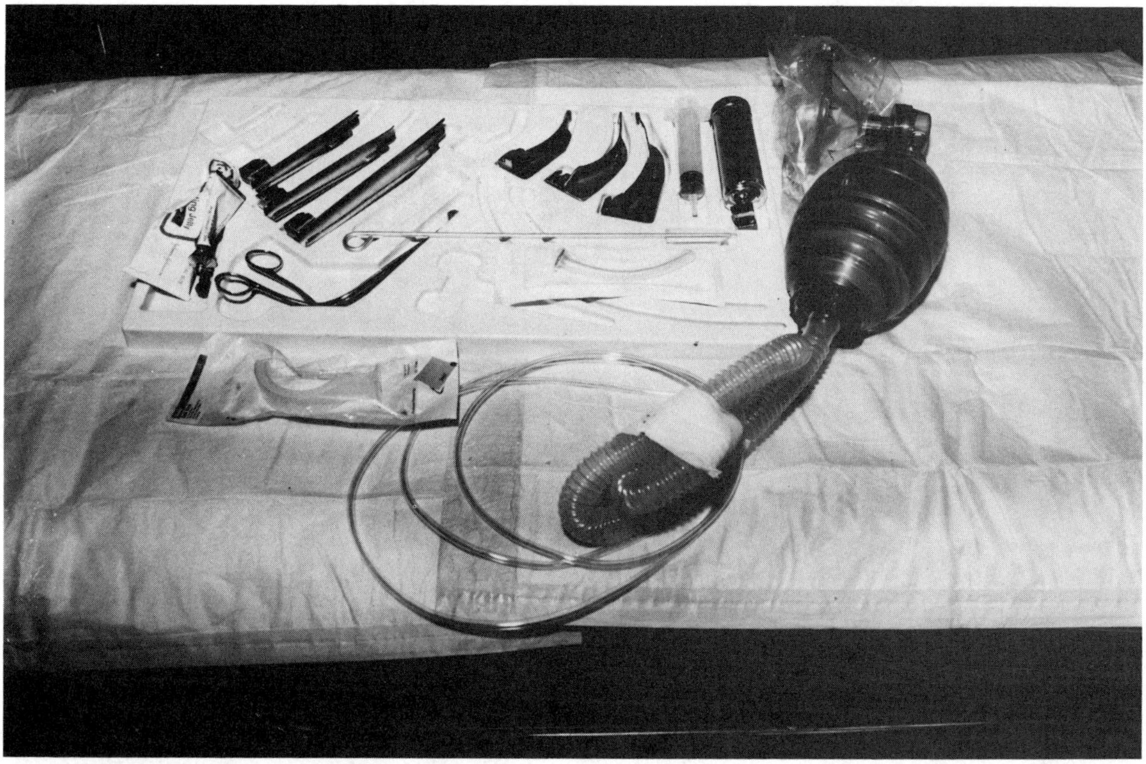

Fig. 5-4. Airway equipment (e.g., laryngoscopes, tubes, stylets) available at the head of the table. Equipment is continually checked to prevent a critical malfunction.

ble, to recovery bed. Such transfers, in our experience, endanger the patient's airway, intravenous lines, and other essential connections, such as chest tubes. Spinal cord stabilization is also compromised. The central monitoring of all trauma patients is greatly desirable.

Such physical capabilities can make an enormous impact on how rapidly the trauma patient is managed. While we have elected to build a special resuscitation area for the trauma patient similar to MedStar and other facilities, modifications of existing emergency facilities, reorganization of equipment and supplies, and minor expenditures for additional equipment, such as monitoring systems, will certainly suffice.

STAFFING OF THE TRAUMA RESUSCITATION AREA

In a few large cities, enough trauma is seen by a level I facility to justify the continuous staff-

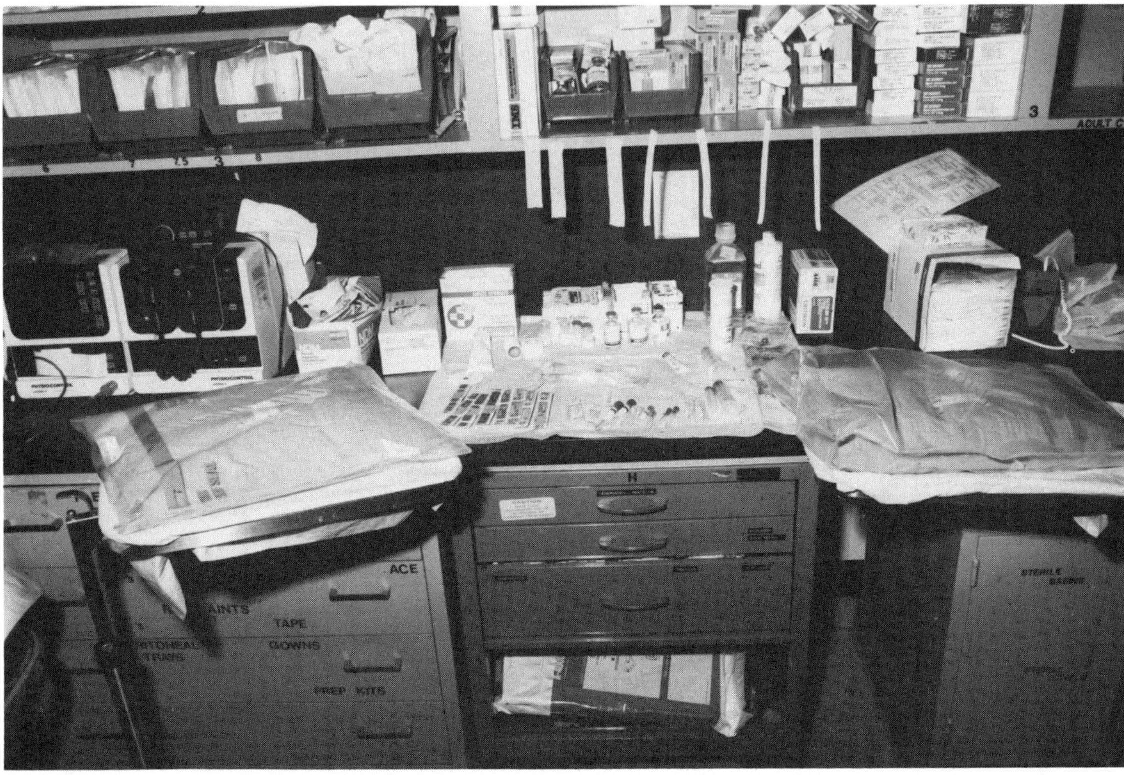

Fig. 5-5. Prepacked trays containing supplies for thoracotomy, peritoneal lavage, chest tube insertion, cutdown, and so on.

ing of the trauma resuscitation center or resuscitation area with a dedicated staff. Such is optimal for the treatment of the trauma patient, in that a dedicated staff is obviously more familiar with all the techniques and is a smoother functioning team. Unfortunately, financial constraints, as well as volume of trauma patients, would negate the use of such teams in many hospitals. In our own trauma center, we have been moving toward a model used by Dr. Howard Champion at MedStar. In such a model, there is a minimal staffing of the trauma center by dedicated personnel. This personnel is then augmented by various other groups when the trauma patient arrives. Other resources include paramedics and flight nurses aboard the helicopter, operating room personnel dedicated to the trauma operating room, and augmentation from personnel in other areas of the emergency department. Use of such personnel not only is cost-efficient but also builds a comradery among those individuals taking part in

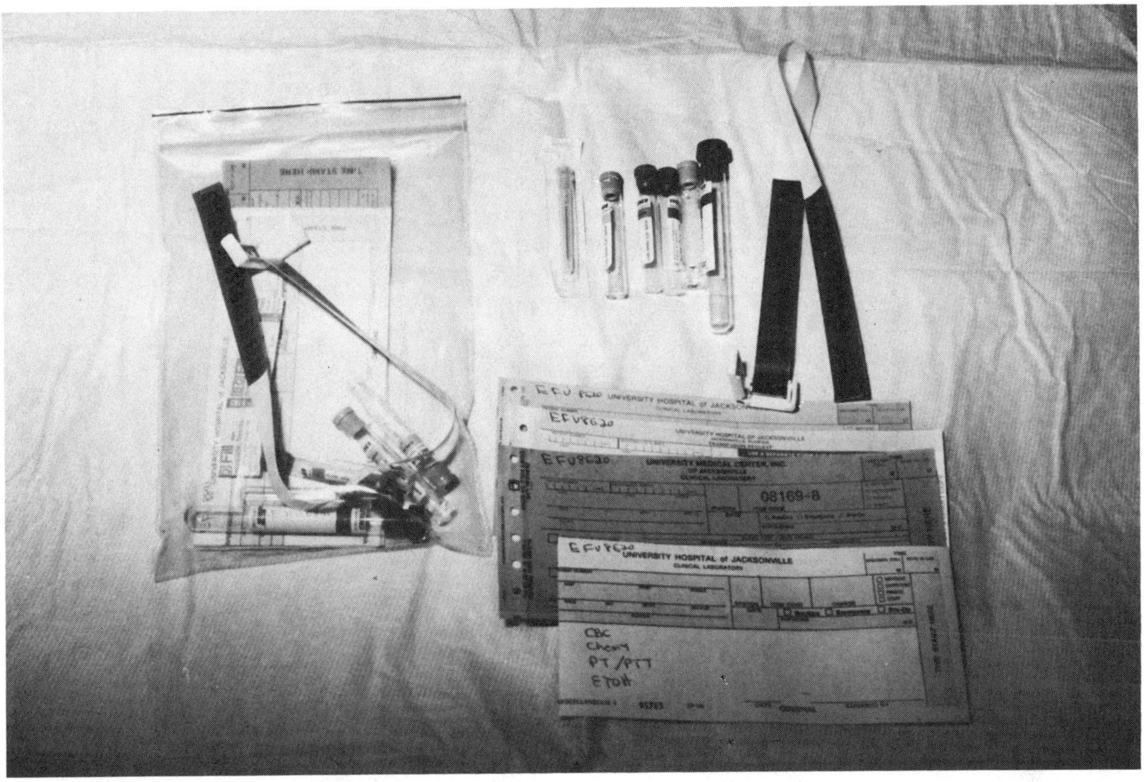

Fig. 5-6. "Typenex" system—sample tubes for protocolled blood work, numbers for charts, and x-rays—name band, all packaged in a plastic container.

trauma activities and blends together both the prehospital emergency department and in-hospital components of the trauma system. It is our feeling that one of the keys to good trauma care is the melding of all the prehospital emergency department and hospital areas into one coherent team rather than having the patient move, in a disjointed fashion, from one separate area of the hospital to another.

INITIAL RESUSCITATION OF THE TRAUMA PATIENT

As we have developed our trauma system at TraumaOne, we have found more and more need to protocol the initial resuscitation efforts, even down to assignment of different procedures to different team members. Even in a center that is not involved in residency training, assignment of specific procedures to different team members does prevent confusion or lessen the chance of some omitted procedure to the absolutely lowest level. Table 5-4 is the assignment that we use for active

Table 5-4. Assignment of Members of the Trauma Team at TraumaOne

Active team member I	Team leader
	Initial and comprehensive examination
Active team member II	Head of the patient
	Airway—respirations
	Cervical spine
	Head and neck
Active team member III	Right side venous access
	Central
	Peripheral
	Cutdown
	Nasogastric tube
	Right side chest tube
	Urinary catheter
Active team member IV	Left side venous access
	Central
	Peripheral
	Cutdown
	Left side chest tube
Supervisory team members	Assist and advise as needed

team members, in our trauma center a mixture of emergency physicians and surgeons.

Initial notification of the trauma team is of utmost importance. The decision whether to initiate a trauma team call is made by the dispatcher. This is done on the basis of mechanism of injury. The mechanism of injury parameters that we have used in the past have recently been modified according to guidelines of the American College of Surgeons [18] (see Fig. 5-2).

Initial resuscitation works in the following fashion. Upon notification that the helicopter or ground EMS vehicle is en route with a trauma patient, the trauma center dispatcher pages the trauma team on a "group pager." The trauma team immediately reports to the trauma resuscitation area. Team members take their places around the resuscitation bed and assume these positions according to their assigned job. All supplies needed for the resuscitation are at the bedside. As part of the trauma team notification, nursing team personnel, x-ray technician, and laboratory personnel come to the resuscitation area. The x-ray technician is ready to do cervical spine films, chest x-ray, and pelvic film immediately if needed. The laboratory technician assumes control of the blood sample and makes sure that the tubes are appropriately marked, that they contain adequate blood for the procedure, and that the blood therein is not hemolized. The blood is then delivered to the proper places within the laboratory for the various studies defined by protocol.

The model used for the trauma resuscitations is that described in the Advanced Trauma Life Support (ATLS) course [21]. First the patient receives a rapid initial assessment, which task is assigned to the team leader. Typically, in our program, the team leader is the person at the head of the table assigned to airway functions. The airway is then assessed. Foreign objects, facial fractures, intraoral bleeding, and inability to maintain an adequate airway due to a depressed level of consciousness are noted. Breathing is assessed by observing chest excursions and the presence of flail segments and open "sucking" chest wounds. The chest is next auscultated, noting dullness (blood) and hyperresonance (air). Percussion may reveal shift of the mediastinum. Circulation is evaluated by blood pressure, pulse, and capillary refill. Strong foot pulses and "warm feet" indicate near normal peripheral resistance. Carotid pulses alone indicate a pressure of approximately 60 mm Hg, carotid and femoral pulses indicate a pressure of 70 mm Hg, and a radial pulse indicates a pressure of above 80 mm Hg [21]. At this time, any external bleeding should be noted. Disability or neurologic status is best evaluated by the Glasgow Coma Scale (see Table 4-1). Pupillary size and sphincter tone are also important parameters. The presence of periorbital or mastoid hematomas and blood from the external meatus of the ear are important observations. The patient should always be exposed, that is, all clothes removed for proper observation.

After initial assessment, resuscitation is begun using ABCD prioritization. Initially, the airway is assured with cervical spine protection. The decision about how to manage the airway is made by the team leader. Simple means of controlling the airway without intubation are tried first. Intubation is felt to be indicated by the presence of upper airway obstruction, respiratory distress, profound shock, severe maxillofacial trauma, severe head or cervical spine injury, and significant hypoxemia or hypocarbia. If time permits, we will use blind endotracheal intubation. However, if this is not successful, either orotracheal or nasotracheal will be used, depending on the expertise of the person involved. Threading the tube over a fiberoptic bronchoscope, then placing the bronchoscope in the trachea under direct vision is a helpful technique. The head is stabilized by another member of the team while this procedure is taking place. Under situations of extreme instability of the neck, severe maxillofacial trauma, pharyngeal edema (particularly in burns), and difficulty in performing orotracheal intubation, we will move immediately to cricothyroidotomy. However, pediatric surgeons feel that this procedure is contraindicated in infants and in children up to approximately 10 years old. All patients, whether or not respiratory problems exist, are placed on oxygen.

Breathing is evaluated in terms of adequacy of respiration and the presence of life-threatening injuries, such as tension pneumothorax, open chest wounds, or flail chest. With pneumothorax and hemothorax, we prefer to place a thoracotomy tube directly rather than use needle thoracostomy. We can do this procedure rapidly and therefore feel comfortable that we are not compromising the patient by moving directly to the operative procedure. It is preferable to have a chest x-ray before such procedures are done, but in the case of very unstable patients, unilateral or bilateral chest tubes can be placed on clinical grounds. In extreme situations when the patient cannot be ventilated, we will do bilateral diagnostic tube thoracostomies. If there is a large hemothorax, we favor salvaging the blood for reinfusion if there are no contraindications.

Circulation is evaluated by blood pressure, pulse, and capillary refill. Treatment of circulatory problems involves the institution of intravenous lines. As in most centers, antecubital 14-gauge percutaneous catheters are our preferred route. The second preferred route of administration is saphenous cutdown or direct "stick" at the ankle. If the trauma team has the proper expertise, long catheters can be placed by a groin cut down at the saphenofemoral junction, feeding the long catheter through the saphenous vein well up into the vena cava. If there is a possibility of intra-abdominal caval injury, this catheter will then, hopefully, bypass the injury. Where there is a possibility of intra-abdominal interruption of the venous system, the use of lower extremity catheters is ill-advised.

Recently, we have found an advantage, in many patients, to insert the Swan-Ganz introducer, which typically is a 10-gauge plastic cannula. This can be easily performed with a needle guidewire technique, introducing a large cannula with one or more ports. This is most satisfactory for infusing large volumes of fluid in a very short length of time. These catheters do have the hazard of producing pneumothorax, and it is probably a good idea if the patient does have a pneumothorax to place the Swan-Ganz introducer on the ipsilateral side, which is controlled by the chest tube.

If the patient's pressure cannot be maintained despite rapid infusion of IV fluids, MAST trousers can be applied and inflated while the patient is transported to the operating room. This is particularly pertinent in patients who may have intra-abdominal injuries. In the operating room, the abdominal compartment can be carefully lowered after the patient is anesthetized. We will leave the legs inflated while the patient is prepared and draped, until the bleeding has been controlled. Patients with pelvic fractures can sometimes be temporarily controlled with the MAST until other means, such as embolization, embolization pelvic fixation, or direct operative intervention, can control this bleeding. One must remember to begin immediate monitoring of cardiac status by electrocardiogram (ECG) on admission to the emergency department.

Management of neurologic status is extremely important, and emphasis has to be placed, again and again, on a thorough neurologic examination, which includes all components of the Glasgow Coma Scale. Changes in pupillary status should be frequently assessed, and efforts should be made to assess the level of consciousness continually. One must remember the possibility of third-nerve palsy, causing unilateral pupillary dilation. The presence of a dilated pupil should not be automatically taken as a sign of impending neurologic catastrophe. Initial treatment for neurologic injuries should include the notification of the neurosurgeon, intubation with hyperventilation, ample oxygenation, and consideration of the use of mannitol.

As part of the trauma protocol, a nasogastric tube and urinary catheter are placed on all patients. One should observe the cautions given in the *ATLS Instructor Manual* [21] and not place a nasogastric tube in a patient with basilar skull fractures. We also do not place a urinary catheter if the patient has blood at the meatus, scrotal ecchymosis, or high-riding prostate. The protocol also calls for not placing urinary catheters in the presence of pelvic fractures. This is a very controversial issue in both the trauma and urologic literature. It is true that only a minuscule number of individuals with pelvic fractures and without the other cardinal signs mentioned above will have urethral transections [22]. Several cases, however, have been documented in the literature, and in general, the urologic community still adheres to the philosophy of withholding the urinary catheter in pelvic fractures. Further studies of the frequency of urethral disruption in various types of pelvic fractures should be done, as this constraint may be unnecessary.

The secondary assessment of the patient is a thorough physical examination. This includes repeat of the neurologic examination, as the neurologic status may change rapidly. Care should be taken to examine the back of the patient's head and torso, and the status of peripheral pulses should not be forgotten. Rectal examination is obviously an extremely important part of the examination. Sphincter tone, to indicate "sacral sparing," spinal cord injuries, presence of blood in the gastrointestinal tract, and the status of the prostatic urethra, can be evaluated.

After the secondary assessment, if the patient is stable, the abdomen is evaluated. Physical examination can be used in patients who are awake and have no evidence of alcohol consumption. If an equivocal examination exists, the patient has evidence of using alcohol or drugs, or the patient has an altered consciousness caused by the injury, peritoneal lavage is used. We prefer direct cutdown to the peritoneum, grasping the peritoneum between the forceps and making a small nick in this structure. This allows introduction of the peritoneal dialysis catheter without the use of a sharp stylet and the possibility of injuring bowel or mesentery.

Recently, the use of CT scanning has been reviewed in the literature as a method of assessing intra-abdominal injury. The advantage of the CT scan is that it is noninvasive and will accurately outline retroperitoneal hematomas. Its disadvantage is loss of control of the patient during the resuscitative period if the patient must go into the scanning room and his abdomen placed within the scanning ring.

Currently, in the literature, the accuracy of the CT scan is considered controversial [23, 24]. Excellent results are obtained if an experienced observer interprets the scan. In our own institution, we use traditional peritoneal lavage unless (1) the patient is to receive a head scan, (2) the patient refuses peritoneal lavage, or (3) lavage is contraindicated because of previous intra-abdominal procedures. Results with CT scanning have been excellent as far as the accuracy of the scan. However, there have been errors of interpretation by inexperienced radiology residents, which appear to confirm the tenor of the surgical literature.

When diagnostic peritoneal lavage is used, we adhere to the parameters described for this procedure and have found them to be accurate (Table 5-5) [25]. We also use diagnostic peritoneal lavage in selected stab wounds. In this situation, it is my own practice to lower the indications for a positive lavage to 10,000 red cells. Data on the use of peritoneal lavage in penetrating injuries are as yet unclear. However, several studies do suggest that 10,000 red cells result in the sensitivity one might desire [26].

The assessment of vascular injuries is of paramount importance. Obviously, the presence of a wide mediastinum indicates immediate angiogram for the possibility of a transected aorta [27]. Such a straightforward response to the wide mediastinum has to be modified when obvious intra-abdominal bleeding and instability exist. In such situations, the patient would go to the operating room for abdominal exploration followed by angiography. If such a procedure is contemplated prior to angiography, careful maintenance of a normal to slightly subnormal blood pressure is mandatory in the operating room.

It is our practice, at the present time, to treat all proximity injuries either by exploration or arteriography. A patient is explored without an arteriogram if lack of pulses, hemorrhage, or a large hematoma exists. In proximity injuries without these cardinal signs, it has been our practice to perform angiography. Freikberg and coworkers, at our institution, however, have studied nearly 100 consecutive proximity injuries with arteriography and have found four unsuspected injuries. These injuries were intimal flaps, which subsequently resolved without treatment. These results agree with the retrospective study by Gomez and associates [28], who found no operative arterial lesions in 72 patients with proximity injuries without clinical evidence of vascular injury. On this basis, we look forward to reassessing the policy of mandatory arteriography on all proximity injuries.

Table 5-5. Parameters Defining a Positive Peritoneal Lavage

Red blood cells	100,000/mm^3
White blood cells	500/mm^3
Amylase	175 μ/dl amylase/100 ml
Lavage positive for bile or bacteria	

Pelvic fractures are a troublesome entity to all trauma surgeons. Severe pelvic fractures can cause massive blood loss, requiring multiple transfusions, which in turn may lead to coagulopathies and more bleeding. Severe pelvic fractures are immediately assessed by the orthopedic surgeon or members of the trauma team. If the fractures appear to be responsible for appreciable blood loss, external fixation is considered based on the theory that reduction of the pelvic fractures will lead to cessation of the bleeding [29]. This procedure is occasionally indicated for posterior element fractures but is mostly required for unilateral or bilateral breaks in the pelvic ring or pelvic disruptions. Should external fixation fail, the patient is taken to the arteriography suite in an attempt to identify bleeding points. These bleeding areas are then embolized. We have had several patients recently who have had a combination of intra-abdominal and retroperitoneal hemorrhage. Therefore, the embolization of the retroperitoneal bleeding problems does not obviate the need to look for and operate on intra-abdominal pathology. Obviously, the individuals who have these types of injuries have very high mortalities, and exquisite timing, along with thorough cooperation between radiologist, orthopedic surgeon, and trauma surgeon, is absolutely essential.

Once the initial assessment, resuscitation, and secondary survey are done, the patient is ready for continued care in the intensive care unit or operating room.

The trauma patient, after leaving the emergency department, usually goes to one of three areas: the operating room, the CT scan facility, or the angiography suite. The operating room option will be discussed in detail in a later section. Emergence of CT scanning and arteriography as primary diagnostic and treatment modalities for the trauma patient offers new challenges and problems for the trauma team. Traditionally, these have been diagnostic tools for predominantly stable patients and have been staffed, configured, and equipped accordingly. Computed tomography has become the mainstay in the diagnosis of head injury. In addition, an increasing number of centers are using the CT scan for diagnosis of intra-abdominal injury. It is also frequently used in patients with pelvic fractures to assess the extent of pelvic injury as well as the magnitude of a retroperitoneal hematoma. It then becomes mandatory that appropriate monitoring equipment, IV fluids, drugs, airway equipment, and other modalities be instantly available. Provisions must be made to maintain the patient on respiratory support while being scanned. Appropriate nursing care and physician interaction must be provided in this facility.

The special location of such a facility is also of great importance. In our institution, we have followed the lead of Dr. Donald Trunkey who, while at San Francisco General Hospital, was instrumental in installing the CT unit adjacent to the emergency department. Our old unit was quite a distance away from the resuscitation area, thereby presenting a transportation and logistics problem. We have now moved the CT scanner adjacent to the emergency department, where these problems can be minimized.

Angiography, like the CT scanner, has become more important as a diagnostic and treatment modality for the acute trauma patient. Diagnosis of arterial injuries now rests heavily on the use of angiography in the absence of the cardinal signs of arterial injury (pulse deficit, active hemorrhage, or expanding hematoma). Acceleration injuries producing aortic tears can be ruled out only by angiography. The use of embolic therapy in severe pelvic hemorrhage is becoming one of the primary therapeutic maneuvers in controlling this devastating traumatic event. Again, the angiography suite area has seldom been configured as a primary treatment area, and it needs to be reassessed in terms of the supplies, staffing, and support systems for resuscitation and respiratory care that must be provided to a trauma patient. Surveillance may be extremely difficult in a dark and cluttered angiography suite, and such physical problems must be solved in some way. In both the CT and angiography suites, direct physician interaction with the patient, by members of the trauma team, is mandatory.

OPERATING ROOM

Trauma care is focused on the ability to deliver rapid operative therapy for those patients who require such therapy. Components necessary to make this area rapidly responsive to the trauma patient are immediate availability of the surgeon, operating room, operating room staff, and anesthesia. Although the trauma surgeon may be immediately available or in-house, the availability of operating room support is the critical issue of survivability of many patients. The American College of Surgeons guidelines require a certified registered nurse anesthetist in-house 24 hours a day in level II trauma centers and in-house anesthesia coverage by board-certified anesthesiologists in level I and, preferably, level II trauma centers [18]. Anesthesia support should be attuned to the particular needs of the trauma patient. Rapid induction of anesthesia, coupled with the possible needs for large volumes of fluid and for management and monitoring of a large number of lines, would suggest that one anesthesiologist or nurse anesthetist in the operating room is certainly not adequate. An additional person and, in many cases, an additional two to three people are essential to perform the tasks required to maintain the patient during the induction of anesthesia and continued resuscitation of the patient. There are various ways of providing this manpower, such as additional nurse anesthetists, anesthesia residents, additional anesthesia staff, or perhaps members of the trauma team. It is important, however, to take this matter into consideration, as the large multidisciplinary trauma team, consisting of emergency physicians, emergency nurses, and surgeons, quickly disappears as the emergency physicians and nurses file back to the emergency department and the surgeon disappears into the scrub room. This situation often leaves a solitary anesthesiologist or nurse anesthetist to attend a desperately ill individual without adequate supporting staff.

Availability of operating room staff and an open operating room is critical. In most institutions, a dedicated operating room cannot be spared, particularly during the busy daytime hours. It is then the responsibility of the operating room supervisor to maintain an open room at all times and provide equipment in the room such that the facility can rapidly respond to an unstable trauma patient. In our own institution, we have solved this problem by attempting to maintain a room as a primary trauma room. Other hospitals find that their operating facilities lend themselves best to availability of different rooms during the day.

Integral and important to the maintenance of a trauma operating room is the movement of equipment needed for resuscitation of the trauma patient from room to room as that "open room" is maintained. In most institutions, the trauma room is outfitted with the basic instruments (e.g., lap packs, drapes) needed to start a trauma case, with immediate availability of specialty instruments such as vascular instruments in separate sterile packs. In addition, the important features of continued resuscitation of the patient (i.e., blood pumps, blood warmers, monitors, oxymetric computers, pressure transducers) should always be in the designated operating room (Fig. 5-7).

In addition to a designated operating room, a dedicated operating room staff for trauma

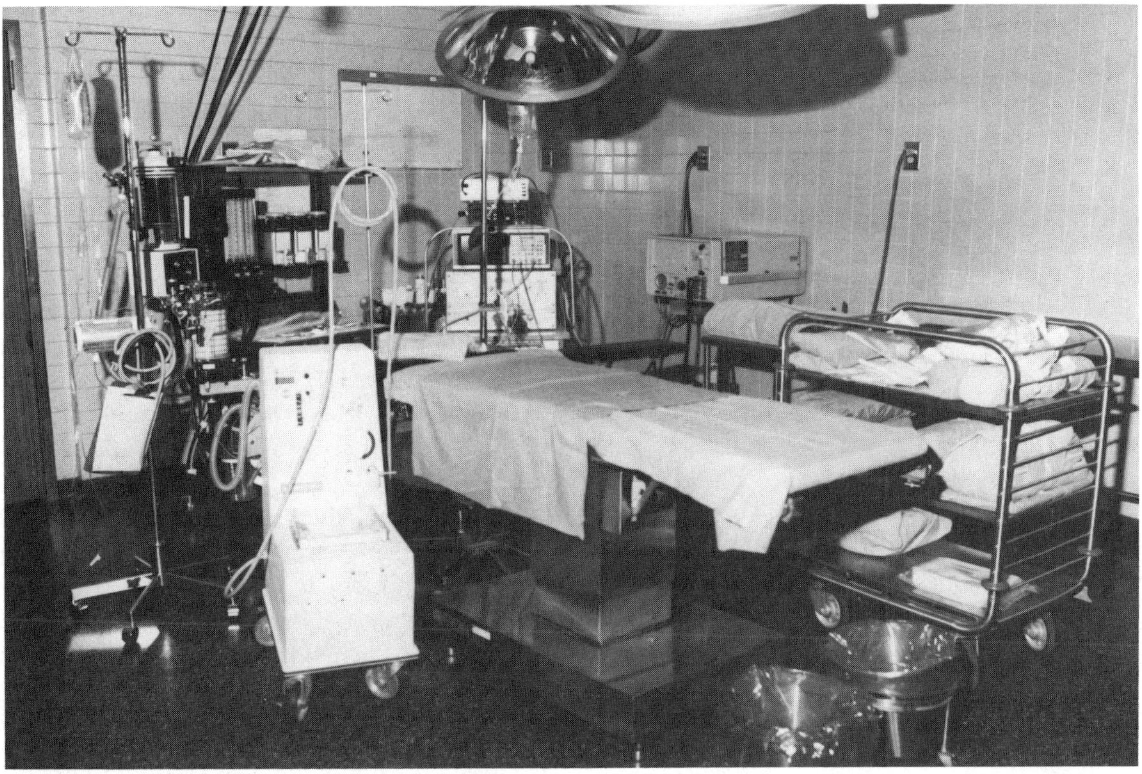

Fig. 5-7. Operating room configured and equipped for the rapid operative management of the trauma patient. Note patient warming device and arterial, venous, ECG, and oxymetry monitoring capabilities; "Cell Saver" is readily available.

should be maintained night and day. During busy daytime hours, an operating room team should be reserved and available at all times to respond to the trauma patient. At night, at least one operating room crew should be available in-house for the treatment of the trauma patient. This requires several tiers of backup in most cases. If one in-house operating room crew becomes occupied with a patient, a second team must be available in the operating room, ideally, before the first team starts the case in question. In our own situation, we start an evening shift with two operating room teams available; one can respond to the trauma patient or may become involved in another surgical case. The other team will then be instantly available for another trauma patient. We also have an additional tier on call so that, if the two teams become occupied, a third team is in-house. Upon the scheduling or anticipation of the second case in the evening, the third team is immediately called in. Obviously, at some point in time, the resources of a hospital to provide an "infinite number" of operating room teams, as rooms fill, become limited. Each hospital must decide, on the basis of volume, how much backup of operating room staff is needed for that trauma center. However, at least one tier of backup should be provided.

When the critical trauma patient is brought to the operating room, the entire staff must function rapidly to facilitate the immediate start of the procedure. The scrub nurse should immediately prepare routine instruments. Ideally, a member of the operating room staff should respond to the emergency department as a member of the trauma team. This person not only can offer help there but will also be able to predict special needs of the operating surgeons when they later arrive in the operating room. The scrub nurse can prepare specialized instruments while the anesthetist, anesthesiologist, and assistants are stabilizing and anesthetizing the patient for the operation.

In most hospitals, the trauma operating room is not contained within the boundaries of the resuscitation area. Therefore, the patient must undergo some short periods of transport. In the unstable patient, however, this transport will necessitate a reevaluation of the patient's status, that is, a repeat of the "initial assessment" on arrival in the operating room. Tube placement, chest excursion, and evaluation for pneumothorax must be rapidly accomplished. Usually some alterations in the patient's cardiovascular status have occurred, and additional fluid and blood resuscitation must be accomplished. The fact is particularly true after anesthetic induction, in that most anesthetic gases result in vasodilatation. This physiologic alteration must be anticipated. If the patient arrives in the MAST, all compartments should remain inflated until the anesthesiologist is content that the volume status and overall status of the patient is satisfactory. Only the abdominal compartment should be deflated to allow the patient to be prepared. In our own institution, we leave the leg compartments inflated until the patient's blood loss has been operatively controlled.

In the critically ill patient whose blood pressure is extremely unstable, one must consider modes of temporarily controlling bleeding while definitive operative control is facilitated. Many surgeons prefer to control massive intra-abdominal bleeding by aortic occlusion in the chest. In the extremely unstable patient who might not survive the lack of tamponade when the peritoneal cavity is opened, we will use this approach. A separate left chest incision with cross-clamping of the aorta is accomplished by part of the operative team. Meanwhile, the other half of the team begins the abdominal incision but does not open the peritoneum. In most situations, however, we are comfortable with controlling intra-abdominal hemorrhage upon opening the abdominal cavity. This is greatly facilitated by the use of an "aortic occluder," an instrument designed to fit over the aorta (Fig. 5-8), compressing it against the vertebral bodies. In the absence of such an instrument, a Richardson retractor can be used in a similar fashion. The occluder is placed, ideally, above the left

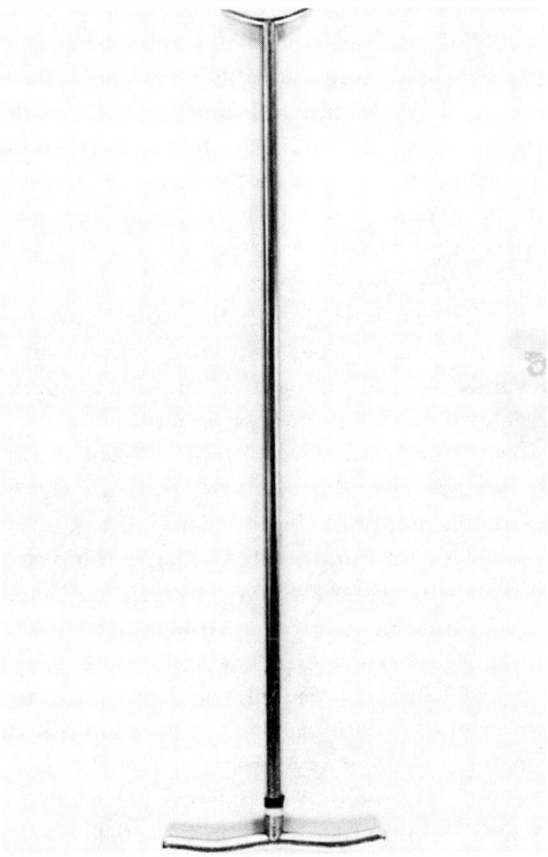

Fig. 5-8. Aortic occluder. This device can be used at any level but is usually placed above the left lobe of the liver to compress the aorta against the anterior vertebral body.

lobe of the liver, compressing the abdominal aorta at this point. This device can effectively control the proximal inflow even in the most catastrophic abdominal events.

Having entered the abdomen, we immediately use large laparotomy packs to pack all four quadrants of the abdomen. The other areas of the abdomen are then quickly scrutinized. Midline bleeding that may come from the vena cava or aorta is controlled by direct pressure, by laparotomy pads, or by hand or finger compression. Caval bleeding can often be controlled by sponge sticks proximal and distal to the lesion. In the absence of large-vessel bleeding, blood is aspirated from the abdomen with four quadrant packs in place. One by one, the packs are then removed to identify the source of bleeding. Control of caval bleeding is facilitated by doing a "Kocher" maneuver and bringing the duodenum far left of the aorta. The approach used for possible aortic injuries is that described by Mattox and colleagues [30], in which the left colon is taken down from its peritoneal attachments and kidney, spleen, pancreas, and other intra-abdominal structures swept to the right of the aorta. Liver injuries are tamponaded by laparotomy sponges until a definitive approach can be planned; bleeding from the spleen is handled in the same fashion. Systematically, after large bleeding areas have been controlled, the abdomen is explored. The exploration is usually begun retrograde, inspecting the area of the bladder and rectal area in the depths of the pelvis and then exploring the remainder of the colon. The small bowel is carefully inspected, as is its mesentery. Special attention is placed at the ligament of Treitz, and if doubt exists as to the integrity of the duodenojejunal junction, this area is dissected out. The duodenum, gallbladder, stomach, and esophageal gastric junction are then inspected carefully. The liver and spleen are examined in every aspect. In blunt trauma, the lesser sac is usually opened, and direct inspection of the pancreas is carried out.

Operating room equipment needed for the

trauma patient should be somewhat different than for the ordinary surgical patient. The operating room should be quite large, so that two or more teams of surgeons could simultaneously operate on the patient. The operating table should be fitted with a warming blanket ready to be used. In addition to transducers and monitors, automatic blood pressure cuffs and a pulse oximeter should be available. Blood warmers should be available in the room, as should a chest suction apparatus. These should be assembled and stored in the trauma room. An autotransfusion device should be available. Some method for rapidly utilizing this apparatus must be developed, since special technical help is usually required for use of this device. A microwave oven in the room for rapidly warming crystalloid IV fluids to body temperature is a useful adjunct to therapy. Separate temperature control of the trauma operating room is desirable because hypothermia is a significant problem in patients who require multiple transfusions and large volumes of crystalloid and who lose heat through large abdominal incisions. The temperature of the operating room must be uncomfortably warm to the surgeon to prevent significant hypothermia problems in the patient.

SURGICAL/TRAUMA INTENSIVE CARE UNIT

The multiply injured patient is probably one of the most challenging seen by surgical intensivists. The involvement of multiple organs, a result of the injury added to the frequent failure of other organ systems, places an incredible demand on the intensive care facility. In general, this facility must be configured to accommodate this level and intensity of effort. Ideally, around-the-clock staffing by residency staff or intensivists should be provided. More importantly, well-trained nurses experienced in trauma need to be provided in adequate numbers. Usual guidelines called for a ratio of two patients for one nurse; however, we have found this totally inadequate in many cases. For the acutely and severely injured patient, a nursing staff of greater than one nurse per patient may be required. In our own institution, we have found it necessary to adopt a measurement system to match acuity of nursing care with patient needs. We have found the Nursing Intervention Scoring System (NISS) to be quite satisfactory in this respect [31]. In this system, each nursing task has been related to a certain numerical value representative of the minutes required to do the task. Normally, each nurse can provide the equivalency of 60 NISS points per shift. Therefore, two patients requiring 30 or less NISS points each can be satisfactorily managed by one nurse. On the other hand, a patient requiring 90 NISS points per shift can only be adequately managed if one nurse is entirely devoted to that patient's care and one-half of another nurse's time is also available. Without such a system, the surgical intensive care unit cannot be responsive to the needs of the patients or the physical capacities of the nurses.

The surgical intensive care unit must also be equipped with modalities routinely needed for the multiply injured patient. Respirators capable of delivering wide ranges of volumes and high pressures must be provided. Traditionally, the availability of full support for hyperalimentation both parenteral and enteral is necessary. Facilities to monitor arterial lines and Swan-Ganz catheters are absolutely essential, as is the ability to perform cardiac outputs. Recently, we have found the use of catheters to measure saturation of mixed venous oxygen in addition to cardiac output to be very advantageous. Instantaneously, changes in the patient's respiratory or cardiac status can be detected by such "on-line" continuous measurements.

The addition of a trauma unit to the intensive care facilities of a hospital or the introduction of a large volume of trauma patients in existing surgical intensive care units presents particular problems in infectious disease management. As all these patients are being severely compromised, they are continuously subject to infections from opportunistic organisms. Frequently, the unit is beset by problems with resistant *Klebsiella* or *Serratia,* which can be devastating to an otherwise viable patient. Recently, more and more hospitals, particularly those managing large volumes of trauma patients, have been beset by methicillin-resistant *Staphylococcus aureus.* A key to minimizing the problems with such infectious agents is continuous, meticulous surveillance not only of patients residing in the intensive care areas, but also of those who have passed through the unit and gone to ward facilities. Great emphasis must be placed on hand washing within the unit itself. Particular offenders in this regard are physicians. However, an overburdened nursing staff can easily lapse into the habit of carrying organisms from room to room because of inadequate time to practice the hygienic principles necessary to control the organisms.

WARD CARE

The ideal situation of a trauma patient would be the transfer from the intensive care unit to a ward specialized in trauma care. Such a ward is unique in several respects. First, the nurses are trained to take care of both operative wounds and wounds resulting from the injury process. Many of these require special treatment, in that large areas of tissue loss are incurred during the accident. Patients are often immobile due to spinal cord injuries and fractures and may be debilitated and nutritionally devastated. Such patients will easily develop decubitus ulcers if not meticulously cared for, sometimes in a special bed such as a rotorbed or Ken-Air bed. Motivated, well-trained nurses of adequate numbers must be provided if these special areas of care for the trauma patient are to be provided.

Additionally, parenteral or enteral hyperalimentation may continue in the ward setting. Patients with chest tubes, nasogastric tubes, and various drains may also be present in large numbers on the trauma ward. Again, the nursing staff must be thoroughly familiar and comfortable with managing these adjuncts to therapy. Because these devices require greater acuity in nursing services, the trauma ward should obviously be staffed at a greater level than an ordinary postsurgical ward.

The trauma ward should also have adequate provisions for performing the first steps of rehabilitation. Physical and occupational therapy should be available in such a facility.

REHABILITATION

Trauma is a disease of young individuals and, as so often stated, the most common cause of death and disability between the ages of 1 and 44. Because of its relation to younger individuals, it is incumbent on trauma centers to return those patients back to society as functional as possible. Such a commitment requires great resources in rehabilitation. Needs of the trauma patient for rehabilitative therapy are legion. These include the obvious problems of head injuries, cervical spine problems, paralysis problems due to spinal cord injury, and problems of muscle loss and contracture as a result of fractures and immobility. Ideally, a physiatrist to direct such activities would be present at every level I trauma center. Rehabilitation, beginning as soon as feasible after injury, is mandatory. An adequately staffed and fully equipped physical therapy unit is, again, essential.

AFTERCARE

As the trauma patient often has injuries that require a prolonged amount of time for that individual to reach maximum medical benefit, and since greater and greater emphasis is being placed on home care or care outside the hospital setting, a planned program of outpatient reassessment and rehabilitation must be set up. Again, ideally, this would be a multidisciplinary clinical setting in which the orthopedic surgeon, trauma surgeon, neurosurgeon, and physiatrist could interact in the same area at the same time for the maximum benefit of the trauma patient. Integral to such a program would be the presence of visiting nurses who would also be physically present at the clinic at the time the patient was reassessed. Convalescent care facilities of an advanced level are necessary if the mission of the trauma center is to be carried out to its maximum extent. Ideally, the presence of physical and occupational therapy in these facilities should be not only desirable but mandatory. Commitment on the part of the convalescent facility is just as important as commitment on the part of the trauma center. That commitment should be pointed toward returning the patient to as near his normal state as possible in the shortest length of time possible. In spite of its importance, this component of the care of the trauma patient has probably received the least amount of attention.

QUALITY ASSURANCE

Quality assurance in trauma care must transcend the artificial boundaries set up within the usual health care system. Such a quality assurance plan must take into consideration all aspects of patient care from the time of injury until the time maximum medical benefit is received. This would necessitate the "erasure" of boundaries between prehospital and emergency department care, between emergency department care and in-hospital care, and finally, between inpatient care and posthospital care. The most important component of such a quality assurance program would be the trauma registry. This registry would ideally track the patient throughout the illness. Necessarily, the trauma register must transcend not only the boundaries previously mentioned but also the boundaries of a particular hospital or agency. In the ideal situation, quality assurance should be maintained for the entire trauma system by the system's trauma council or other public agency. Perhaps the most far-reaching and functional program in existence today is present in San Diego, where such a council includes representatives of the trauma service of all hospitals in the system [32]. In this way, all components can be brought together and the entire system made to function harmoniously and efficiently. Although the quality assurance plan should be systemwide, feedback should include the individuals involved in the care. This would include individual paramedics, surgeons, and visiting nurses.

OUTREACH

It is the responsibility of a trauma center to provide support and help to outlying hospitals and physicians in every aspect of trauma care. This would necessarily require a close liaison between those hospitals and the trauma center. An attempt to establish transfer agreements and transfer protocols from a nontrauma center to the trauma center is an excellent first step in the outreach process. Additionally, physicians in outlying hospitals should be invited to trauma grand rounds. If possible, physicians from the trauma center should be made available to the outlying hospitals for lectures on topics in which they are interested. In our own center, we couple these physician lectures with "marketing" flights by the helicopter. In this way, we can minimize the amount of travel time for the physician, provide the continuing education, and acquaint the hospitals with our transport system. The sponsorship or actual administration of ATLS courses and other courses, such as Pre-Hospital Training Life Support (PHTLS) and nurse trauma life support, is another excellent way that the trauma center can reach out to both prehospital and hospital personnel. Nursing trauma rounds for the continuing education of nurses within the trauma center can also be made available to nurses in outlying hospitals as part of the outreach program. Finally, the availability of an on-call trauma team to physicians in outlying areas, through the use of a toll-free line, is also helpful in providing support and education to referring hospitals.

PUBLIC EDUCATION

The responsibility of the trauma center is not only to treat the victims of trauma but also to educate the public as to trauma prevention. Most experts agree that many accidents can be prevented if effective measures are instituted both on a societal and individual level. Hospital sponsorship of programs to promote prevention of teenage drinking and driving and control of the drunk driver are examples. Programs, in conjunction with civic clubs, law enforcement, and the media, can facilitate the education of the public in accident prevention. Funding alternate modes of transportation to drinkers during holidays, proms, and other large social events keeps such individuals off the highways and focuses attention on drinking problems. Programs such as "feet first, first time" for prevention of spinal cord injuries due to diving accidents are extremely effective. Campaigns for laws to require seat belts, child restraints, and air bags should be led by physicians in the trauma center. We have found a very cooperative attitude in public safety officials, media, and government leaders. A catalyst for such functions, however, must be the trauma center, in that the trauma physicians, armed with data from the trauma registry, can focus attention to the important problems in a community. More and more attention is being paid to trauma prevention, and more resources are available within the medical community for public education. The Committee on Trauma of the American College of Surgeons and the American Trauma Society are excellent resources for such programs.

In conclusion, the trauma system is extraordinarily complex and requires an immense amount of resources. The financial commitment required for the ideal system is immense. Realistically, certain compromises may need to be made at the start of the system to facilitate better trauma care. Better an imperfect system be instituted than a nonsystem resulting in the usual 30-percent unnecessary death rate. Unfortunately, however, many of the shortcomings of a system can be overcome with a component that the American College of Surgeons feels is the most important aspect of quality trauma care. That component is commitment. Commitment of paramedics, emergency physicians, surgeons, physical therapists, visiting nurses, and convalescent centers can overcome many of the problems involved in this complex system. In spite of the amount of money available for trauma care, without the component of commitment, the system will ultimately fail.

REFERENCES

1. *Emergency Medical Technician–Ambulance: National Standard Curriculum* (3rd ed.). Washington, D.C.: U.S. Department of Transportation, National Highway Traffic Safety Administration, 1984.
2. Gervin, A. S., and Fischer, R. P. The importance of prompt transport in salvage of patients with penetrating heart wounds. *J. Trauma* 22:443, 1982.
3. Aprahamian, C., Thompson, B. M., Towne, J. B., et al. The effect of a paramedic system on mortality of major open intra-abdominal vascular trauma. *J. Trauma* 23:687, 1983.
4. Jacobs, L. M., Sinclair, A., Beiser, A., et al. Prehospital advanced life support: Benefits in trauma. *J. Trauma* 24:8, 1984.
5. Champion, H. R., Sacco, W. J., Carnazzo, A. J., et al. Trauma score. *Crit. Care Med.* 9:672, 1981.
6. Pons, P. T., Honigman, B., Moore, E. E., et al. Prehospital advanced trauma life support for critical penetrating wounds to the thorax and abdomen. *J. Trauma* 25:828, 1985.
7. Lewis, F. R. Prehospital intravenous fluid therapy: Physiological computer modelling. *J. Trauma* 26:804, 1986.
8. Uhlhorn, R. W., and Jacobs, L. M. Helicopters: Extending the prehospital transportation system. *Med. Instrum.* 16:202, 1982.
9. Cleveland, H. C., Bigelow, D. B., Dracon, D., et al. A civilian air emergency service: A report of its development, technical aspects, and experience. *J. Trauma* 16:452, 1976.
10. Trunkey, D. D. Trauma. *Sci. Am.* 249:28, 1983.
11. Baxt, W. G., and Moody, P. The impact of rotorcraft aeromedical emergency care service on trauma mortality. *J.A.M.A.* 249:3047, 1983.
12. Baxt, W. G., Moody, P., Cleveland, H. C., et al. Hospital-based rotorcraft aeromedical emergency care services and trauma mortality: A multicenter study. *Ann. Emerg. Med.* 14:859, 1985.
13. Urdaneta, L. F., Sandberg, M. K., Cram, A. E., et al. Evaluation of an emergency air transport ser-

vice as a component of a rural EMS system. *Am. Surg.* 50:183, 1984.
14. Alexander, R. H., Pons, P. T., Krischer, J., et al. The effect of advanced life support in sophisticated hospital systems on motor vehicle mortality. *J. Trauma* 24:486, 1984.
15. Baxt, W. G., and Moody, P. Differential impact on the mortality of major trauma victims of a physician staffed and non-physician staffed aeromedical emergency care service. Presented at the Sixth Annual American Society of Hospital Based Emergency Aeromedical Services/National Flight Nurses Association Conference, Reno, Nev., December 4, 1985.
16. Rhee, K. J., Strozeski, M., Burney, R. E., et al. Is the flight physician needed for helicopter emergency medical services? Presented at the Sixth Annual American Society of Hospital Based Emergency Aeromedical Services/National Flight Nurses Association Conference, Reno, Nev., December 4, 1985.
17. Carraway, R. P., Brewer, M. E., Lewis, B. R., et al. A true American rarity—E.D. physician/flight nurse on every flight: A critical part of Life Saver (Alabama's Airborn Emergency Service). Presented at the International Aeromedical Evacuation Congress, Zurich, Switzerland, September 10–13, 1985.
18. Committee on Trauma of the American College of Surgeons. Hospital and prehospital resources for optimal care of the injured patient. *Bull. Am. Coll. Surg.* 71:4, 1986.
19. Law, D. K., Law, J. K., Brennan, R., et al. Trauma operating room in conjunction with an air ambulance system: Indications, interventions, and outcomes. *J. Trauma* 22:759, 1982.
20. Hoyt, D. B., McGill, T., Shackford, S. R., et al. Operating room resuscitation. Presented at the Sixth Annual American Society of Hospital Based Emergency Aeromedical Services/National Flight Nurses Association Conference, Reno, Nev., December 4, 1985.
21. Committee on Trauma. *Advanced Trauma Life Support Instructor Manual.* Chicago: American College of Surgeons, 1984.
22. Guerriero, W. G. *Urologic Injuries.* Norwalk, Conn.: Appleton-Century-Crofts, 1984.
23. Marx, J. A., Moore, E. E., Jorden, R. C., et al. Limitations of computed tomography in the evaluation of acute abdominal trauma: A prospective comparison with diagnostic peritoneal lavage. *J. Trauma* 25:933, 1985.
24. Peitzman, A. B., Makaroun, M. S., Slasky, B. S., et al. Prospective study of computed tomography and initial management of blunt abdominal trauma. *J. Trauma* 26:585, 1986.
25. McLellan, B. A., Hanna, S. S., Montoya, D. R., et al. Analysis of peritoneal lavage parameters in blunt abdominal trauma. *J. Trauma* 25(5):393, 1985.
26. Merlotti, G. J., Marcet, E., Sheaff, C. M., et al. Use of peritoneal lavage to evaluate abdominal penetration. *J. Trauma* 25:228, 1985.
27. Moore, E. E. Resuscitation and Evaluation of the Injured Patient. In G. Zuidema, R. Rutherford, and W. Ballinger (eds.), *The Management of Trauma* (4th ed.). Philadelphia: Saunders, 1985. P 18.
28. Gomez, G. A., Kreis, D. J., Ratner, L., et al. Suspected vascular trauma of the extremities: The role of arteriography in proximity injuries. *J. Trauma* 26:1005, 1986.
29. Moreno, C., Moore, E. E., Rosenberger, A., et al. Hemorrhage associated with major pelvic fractures: A multispecialty challenge. *J. Trauma* 26(11):987, 1986.
30. Mattox, K. L., McCollum, W. B., Jordan, G. L., et al. Management of upper abdominal vascular trauma. *Am. J. Surg.* 128:823, 1974.
31. Alexander, R. H., Rumley, T. O., and Blikken, W. Use of the Nursing Intervention Scoring System in management of a surgical intensive care unit. *South. Med. J.* 77:1248, 1984.
32. Shackford, S. R., Eastman, A. B., and Virgilio, R. W. Assuring quality of care within a trauma system: The Medical Audit Committee. Composition, function, cost, and first year's experience. Presented at the American Association for the Surgery of Trauma, Honolulu, Hawaii, September 19, 1986.

6

Central Nervous System Trauma: Brain

Philip A. Villanueva

Injury to the brain poses a number of special problems in trauma management. Head injury may result in an alteration of consciousness, ranging from mild confusion to frank coma. Also, depending on the area of brain involved, there may be derangements of sensory, motor, and autonomic function. These factors, alteration of consciousness and sensorimotor deficits, may alone or in combination mask certain findings (e.g., abdominal tenderness) that would otherwise alert the treating physician to the presence of a traumatic injury. However, perhaps the single most important factor in terms of brain injury is the injury itself and the resultant immediate and potential neurologic deficit. In addition to causing a purely neurologic deficit, these injuries, by virtue of the brain's role in regulating autonomic and vegetative function, may create significant systemic problems as well. This feature gains added importance when the concepts of primary and secondary brain injury are considered.

This chapter will not provide an in-depth review of pathologic anatomy and physiology; rather, it will concentrate on the clinical aspects of craniocerebral trauma and its management. However, a basic understanding of normal neuroanatomy and physiology is necessary to treat the pathologic state effectively.

ANATOMY

The brain is housed in a rigid container, the skull. Externally, it is relatively smooth and rounded and covered with the scalp, which acts as a "shock absorber." On the other hand, the inner surface of the skull is very irregularly shaped, with numerous ridges and depressions that serve to hold the brain loosely in place. However, a blow to the head may cause the brain to move rapidly over these irregularities, leading to damage to its surface. In addition to the irregularities of the inner surface or table of the skull, there are multiple foramina that provide entry and exit sites for the cranial nerves, as well as the arterial supply and venous drainage of the brain. All but one of these foramina are relatively quite small. Only the foramen magnum at the posterior base of the skull is large enough to permit significant egress of neural tissue. The thickness of the skull varies from extremely thick at the base and posterior (occipital) regions to quite thin in the temporal or anteroinferolateral areas.

Between the inner table of the skull and the surface of the brain lie three membranes, or meninges. Working from the outermost inward, they are the tough, fibrous dura mater, which is supplied by several nutrient arteries (the chief being the middle meningeal) and also carries the large draining veins of the brain or venous sinuses and folds upon itself to form partitions between the right and left sides of the cerebral hemispheres (falx cerebri) and upper and lower portions of the intracranial cavity (tentorium). Encountered next is the bilayered arachnoid, thin and weblike, through whose interstices course the arterial supply and tributary venous drainage of the brain as well as cerebrospinal fluid (CSF). Between the arachnoid and dural sinuses run the bridging veins, which funnel the blood from the tributary veins into the sinuses. Innermost is pia mater, which is closely applied to the brain's surface.

The brain itself is composed of three main divisions: the cerebrum, the cerebellum, and the brain stem. Roughly speaking, the cerebrum controls higher functions such as memory, speech, volitional movement, sensory perception, and cognitive function; the cerebellum controls balance and coordination; and the brain stem controls (or at least regulates) consciousness and vegetative functions such as respirations, blood pressure, and pulse. Deep within the brain stem also lies the ascending reticular activating system (ARAS), a loosely organized network of nerve cells and projections that acts as the "switching" center of the brain; essentially all incoming and outgoing pathways either pass through or send branches to the ARAS. The ARAS must be functioning properly for the patient to maintain consciousness. Lesions to this area may result in permanent loss of consciousness (coma).

Within the brain are cavities (ventricles) in which the CSF is manufactured and stored. There are two lateral ventricles, one in either hemisphere of the cerebrum. They connect through the foramen of Monro to the midline third ventricle located in the midbrain (at the junction of the upper brain stem and cerebrum). This third ventricle is in turn connected to a midline fourth ventricle in the lower brain stem through the relatively narrow aqueduct of Sylvius. The ventricular system connects in turn to the subarachnoid space through three foramina at the brain stem level. CSF is being produced constantly at the rate of 0.3 to 0.5 ml/min. To prevent a net increase in CSF, the CSF must pass from the ventricles into the subarachnoid space, over the surface of the brain and be absorbed into the dural venous sinuses through arachnoid villi, which are projections of the arachnoid into the venous sinuses. If there is obstruction to flow at any point, there occurs a buildup of CSF with resultant pressure on the brain. The total pressure exerted by all of the intracranial contents, that is, brain tissue (including brain water), blood (arterial, venous, and capillary), CSF, and any other intracranial entity, equals the intracranial pressure. This important term will be examined in a later section.

PHYSIOLOGY

The brain demands an adequate supply of glucose and oxygen to function. Inadequate oxygenation leads to a shift to anaerobic pathways, which do not provide for an adequate production of adenosine triphosphate (ATP) to allow proper neural function. Therefore, there is an attempt by the body to maintain cerebral blood flow within a certain range (approximately 55 ml/gm brain/min). This is maintained over a relatively wide range of mean arterial blood pressures through the process of autoregulation, which allows the resistance of the cerebral arteries to change in order to maintain an adequate cerebral blood flow. This autoregulatory function may be influenced by arterial tensions of oxygen (PO_2) and carbon dioxide (PCO_2). At low PO_2, there is dilatation of the cerebral arteries with an increase in cerebral blood flow; at low PCO_2 (and high pH), there is vasoconstriction, while high PCO_2 (with low pH) leads to dilatation. In general, the PCO_2 response is seen most markedly in the range of 25 to 30 torr.

Cerebral blood flow may be considered from another, analogous view, that of cerebral perfusion pressure (CPP). This is the pressure at which blood enters the brain and may be derived by subtracting the intracranial pressure (ICP) from the mean arterial pressure (MAP):

$$CPP = MAP - ICP$$

As a rule, a minimum cerebral perfusion pressure of 60 torr must be maintained to allow for adequate cerebral blood flow. Below 60 torr, and in certain individuals even at that level, neurologic dysfunction may occur. Much of the management of head injury is directed toward maintaining cerebral perfusion pressure at or above 60 torr, by adjusting either the mean arterial pressure or intracranial pressure, or both.

TRAUMATIC INJURIES

Scalp

Most scalp injuries are due to bleeding from the highly vascular galeal layer. If no overyling laceration exists, the blood will collect in the subgaleal or subperiosteal space and form a cephalohematoma. This collection usually resorbs without complication, but in the pediatric age group, a significant amount of blood may be sequestered so as to result in anemia. Open injuries may range from simple laceration to frank scalp avulsion. Because of the significant vascularity of the scalp, a relatively large volume of blood may be lost, causing hemodynamic instability.

Skull Fractures

Skull fractures can be classified in several ways: linear versus comminuted, closed versus open, calvarial versus basilar, or combinations of these. Linear or nondisplaced fractures may be identified on x-ray as straight, unbranched lines and are of significance when they cross dural vascular channels embedded within the skull. In these cases, the channel may be torn by the fracture and result in bleeding. In children, the dura alone may be torn, and consequently, the CSF-filled arachnoid may bulge between the fractured bony plates. With time, given the normal pulsations of CSF and brain growth, this outpouching may enlarge, further splitting the bony plates and forming a "growing" fracture. This is not seen in adults. Comminuted fractures are those resulting in multiple fragments of bone and are said to be "depressed" if any fragments are pushed inward toward the dura and brain. Meningeal and brain injury may result from these fractures.

Closed fractures have no communication to the external environment, while open fractures may communicate through an overlying scalp laceration, air sinuses, or middle or external ear spaces. These are of special clinical significance because of the infective risk created by the continuity between the intracranial space and the external environment. If the dura and arachnoid have been torn by the fracture, there may be leakage of CSF through the nose (rhinorrhea) or ear (otorrhea).

Calvarial or vault fractures involve those bones that compose the sides and top of the skull, while basilar refers to fractures of the skull floor or base. The key feature of basilar fractures is the frequent association of a dural/arachnoid tear and CSF leak as noted above. These injuries are often difficult to identify on standard skull x-rays but may be seen by computed tomography (CT) or polytomography. The diagnosis of basilar skull fracture is usually made on clinical grounds.

Concussion

Concussion, one of the most commonly occurring types of head injury, is a frequently employed term but is poorly understood as an entity. It is characterized by a transient loss of consciousness with a variable amnesia for events preceding and following the trauma. No focal neurologic deficits are seen, but there may be complaints of headache, dizziness, nausea, and subsequent alterations of cognitive and/or emotional functions. No lesion is identifiable on CT scan, and magnetic resonance imaging (MRI) findings to date have been inconclusive [1]. At autopsy of known concussed patients who have died from other causes, brain stem changes have been noted, but again these are not universally recognized. A popularly accepted mechanism for concussion proposes that there is mechanical stretching of the fibers in the ARAS, with temporary disruption of neural transmission resulting in transient loss of consciousness.

Intracranial Lesions

Traumatic intracranial lesions are all secondary to bleeding, either from the dura or from the brain itself. Dural bleeding may be either extradural (epidural) or intradural in nature. The key principle to remember is that none of these have an immutable clinical picture, although some findings may be seen more frequently. The hallmark of intracranial bleeding is that symptomatology depends mainly on the portion(s) of brain being affected by the bleed, or brain shift, and not the type of bleed. The principal types of bleeds will be discussed, again proceeding from the outermost to innermost.

Epidural Hematoma

Epidural hematomas arise from a tearing of either a meningeal artery or a dural venous sinus by an overlying fracture, with bleeding into the epidural space (Fig. 6-1). It is relatively uncommon in the very young or elderly, due to the tight apposition of the dura to the inner surface of the skull, which tends to limit the amount of dural dissection the clot can create. If an artery (usually the middle meningeal, which underlies the thin temporal bone) is involved, the bleeding may be quite brisk, and symptoms may develop within minutes to hours. If a venous sinus is involved, the bleeding is usually slower and may not manifest itself for days. The classic picture of an epidural hematoma due to a tear in the middle meningeal artery is that of unconsciousness followed by a lucent period, then progressive diminution of consciousness with an ipsilateral dilated and nonreactive ("blown") pupil on the side of the lesions and a contralateral motor weakness. This pattern is due to the pressure exerted by the hematoma on the underlying temporal lobe, which in turn compresses the third cranial nerve (causing the pupillary change) and the motor pathways that supply the opposite body side. In a minority of patients, the motor deficit is on the *same* side as the mass lesion and the pupillary change (Kernohan's notch phenomenon)

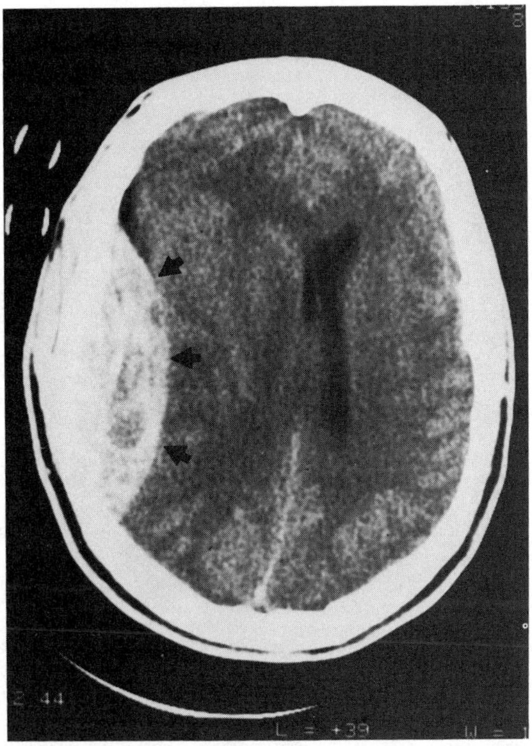

Fig. 6-1. Epidural hematoma (*arrows*).

[2]. In such a situation, it must be remembered that the lesion is almost invariably (>90 percent of the time or more) on the same side as the "blown" pupil [3].

Subdural Hematoma

Subdural hematomas usually result from a tearing of the veins that bridge the subdural space between the surface of the brain and the large dural venous sinuses (Fig. 6-2). They are found in infancy, in old age, and in alcoholics, all situations where the subdural

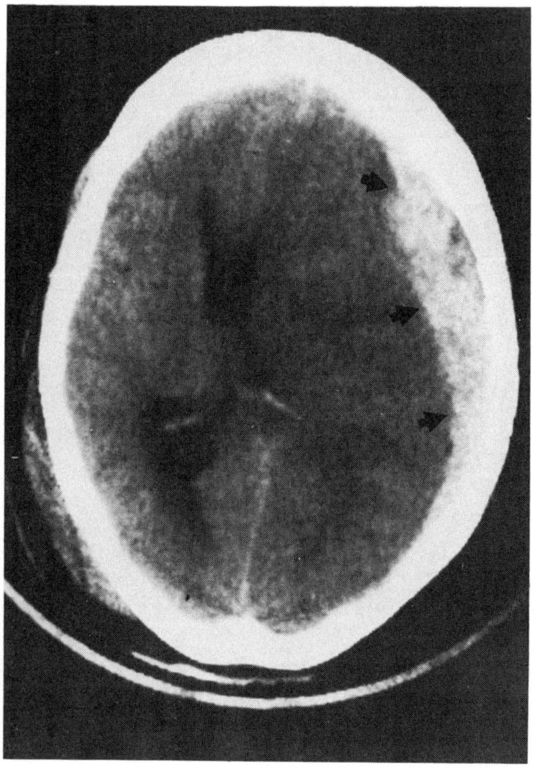

Fig. 6-2. Subdural hematoma (*arrows*).

space is increased, either due to immaturity of the brain, as in the former case, or to atrophy, as in the latter two. In these situations, the bridging veins are under relatively increased tension and may be torn by relatively mild trauma. It is also a frequent site for bleeding in patients with coagulopathies. Blood may also collect in the subdural space when there is actual brain laceration or rupture of an intracerebral clot through the brain's surface. As these lesions are usually venous in nature, the rapidity of bleeding may vary, as may the time of onset of clinical symptoms, and subdural hematomas can be classified as acute, subacute, and chronic. There are no universal criteria for these categories, but generally collections less than 3 days old are considered acute, those over 14 days chronic, and subacute those in between [4]. By the third day, organization of the clot has begun along with the formation of an enveloping membrane. Eventually, the clot may liquefy and even be resorbed. However, the membrane itself is frequently quite vascular, and subsequent trauma may trigger rebleeding, resulting in areas of varying chronicity within the same collection. Again, as with the epidural clot, the clinical picture is dependent on the area of brain involved and may range from headache or mild confusional/personality changes to frank coma with focal findings.

Subarachnoid Hemorrhage

The subarachnoid hemorrhage of trauma is different from that resulting from the rupture of a berry aneurysm or vascular malformation. It is due to the tearing of small vessels on the brain's surface and resultant leakage of blood into the CSF-containing subarachnoid space. Frequently, there is associated contusion of the brain surface. Blood in the subarachnoid space can be extremely irritating, resulting in headache, nausea, photophobia, and neck stiffness. However, no focal findings are usually attributable to this condition, and it tends to be self-limiting in its course. In some patients, the symptoms attributable to "concussion" may be at least partially due to subarachnoid blood.

Intracerebral Contusion and Hematoma

Contusion and hematoma may be said to lie along the same spectrum of brain tissue injury. Contusions are areas of hemorrhage within necrotic, swollen, brain tissue, while hematomas are essentially homogenous areas of blood (Fig. 6-3). Frequently, contiguous contused areas may coalesce into a hematoma, or there may be a gradation from mild to severe contusion to frank hematoma within the same general area. These lesions may arise from several different causes. Brain surface contusions are usually caused by a blow to the head that imparts its energy to the brain subadjacent to where the blow is struck (coup lesion). The brain, in response to the blow, may be shifted so as to strike a portion of the inner table of the skull almost diametrically across from where the original insult occurred. This secondary injury, caused by the "ricochet" effect, may also lead to a contusion (contrecoup). Coup/contrecoup lesions may show a range of severity, that is, the coup lesion may be more, equal to, or less severe than the contrecoup. Differentiation between the two types may be difficult. Usually scalp/skull trauma marks the site of the coup lesion, although when there are multiple blows to the head, the value of this criterion is diminished. Contusions and hematomas may occur at sites away from the primary blow or the opposite pole of the brain. As the brain is shifted within the skull from the force imparted to it, there is contact with the rough, irregular floor of the skull and the dural partitions. Because of the surrounding bony anatomy, the tips of the frontal, temporal, and occipital lobes (especially their inferior surfaces) are most frequently affected, even to the point of actual laceration. Occasionally, contusions/hematomas may occur deep within the brain structure, without any apparent lesions on the surface. These are usually due to shearing forces within the brain that occur during rapid acceleration/deceleration events [5]. The deep white matter structures are affected, and the prognosis is extremely poor. Discrete intracerebral clots may also be due to penetrating injuries, be they caused by mis-

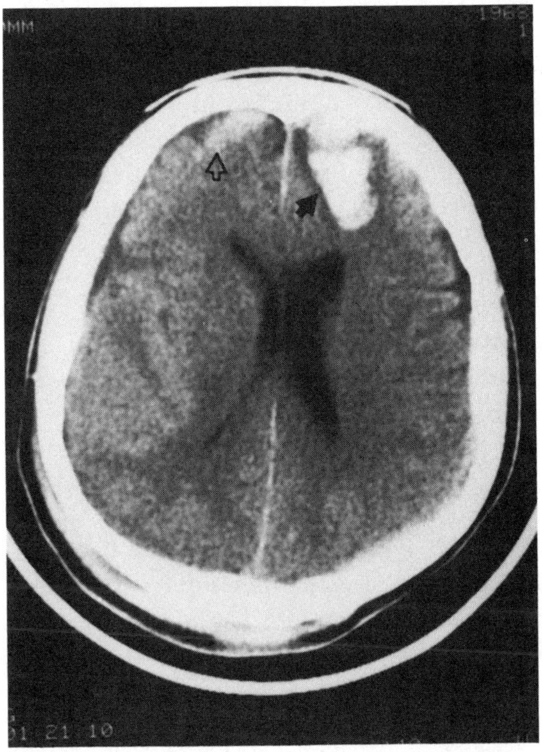

Fig. 6-3. Intracerebral hematoma (*solid arrow*) and cerebral contusion (*open arrow*).

siles or indriven fragments of bone and other tissue. Because of the penetration of the brain surface, blood may be extravasated into the subarachnoid, subdural, epidural, or ventricular spaces. Depending on the nature of the foreign body as well as the location, neurologic deficit may vary from minimal to severe.

DIAGNOSIS AND MANAGEMENT OF HEAD TRAUMA

Evaluation of the Patient

As with any trauma patient, the ABC approach is utilized: *a*irway, *b*reathing, *c*irculation. In neurologically injured patients, especially those whose level of consciousness is decreased, it *must* be assumed that there is a concomitant cervical spine injury until ruled otherwise [6]. Therefore, the airway must be secured *without* neck manipulation. (It would be hoped that the patient has been transferred from the scene on a "spine board" with the head and neck secured by sandbags in a neutral position.) If an emergency airway is needed, then intubation should be attempted. If this is not feasible, then a cricothyroidotomy should be initiated. Once the airway has been secured, breathing patterns should be noted, although with the exception of grossly irregular (ataxic) breathing (which indicates brain stem involvement), one cannot reliably attribute a specific pattern to a specific area of injury.

Circulatory function is critical. Hypertension with concomitant bradycardia may indicate increasing intracranial pressure, while hypertension with tachycardia may indicate a response to pain and discomfort. Hypotension with tachycardia usually indicates blood loss from a *nonintracranial* source, while hypotension with bradycardia may point to a concomitant spinal cord injury. It should be remembered that "shock" is very rarely associated with a primary neurologic injury, and systemic sources of blood loss should be investigated carefully.

Assessment of the patient's level of consciousness should be performed next, unless intervention to remedy a derangement of the ABCs is needed. The best means of assessing consciousness is the Glasgow Coma Scale [7] (Table 6-1). This system allows a rapid, concise means of determining level of consciousness and one that may be reproduced by various examiners without the use of subjective terminology such as "lethargic," "stuporous,"

Table 6-1. Glasgow Coma Scale

Test	Score
Verbal response	
None	1
Incomprehensible sounds	2
Inappropriate words	3
Confused	4
Oriented	5
Eye opening	
None	1
To pain	2
To speech	3
Spontaneously	4
Motor response	
None	1
Abnormal extensor	2
Abnormal flexion	3
Withdraws	4
Localizes	5
Obeys	6
Total score	

or "somnolent." The score for each category should be recorded, as well as the total score, and the procedure repeated every 5 to 15 minutes as needed.

Pupillary function should also be checked. As noted, raised intracranial pressure may cause a shift of the brain that compresses the oculomotor (third cranial) nerve and interferes with pupillary function, and this must always be considered when pupillary dysfunction or irregularity follows trauma. However, direct ocular injury may cause a pupil to dilate and react sluggishly or not at all (traumatic mydriasis). This is far more common in the patient who is otherwise neurologically intact or who has evidence of orbital/ocular injury. Another cause, though less frequent, is the presence of an ocular prosthesis. Small pupils (2 mm or less) are rarely caused by trauma, unless the pons (part of the brain stem) is affected, and other neurologic signs would be expected to be present. Frequently, small pupils are associated with illegal drug usage, usually narcotics or cocaine.

Eye motility or extraocular movement should also be evaluated. Normally, the patient should be able to look in all directions without double vision (diplopia). If impairment of extraocular movement exists, there may be injury to the controlling neural pathway. However, in the case of orbital or direct ocular trauma, entrapment of one or more extraocular muscles may be the cause ("blowout" orbital fracture). Double vision may result from any impairment of extraocular movement, but when it occurs during testing of each eye separately (monocular diplopia), the cause is almost invariably hysteria. Synchronous eye movement in the comatose patient may be assessed by passively turning the head from side to side (doll's-head maneuvering) or injecting ice water in the external ear canal (cold caloric testing). However, the former should never be performed until an adequate lateral cervical spine x-ray has been obtained, and the latter is contraindicated when basilar skull fracture is suspected. These tests are best performed by the neurologic or neurosurgical consultant.

The sensory examination may be variable and indeed quite confusing. In general, response withdrawal to nail bed pressure should be evaluated, especially if spinal trauma is suspected. A more detailed examination would be performed by the neurosurgical consultant.

The extremity examination would, in part, have been conducted while determining the Glasgow Coma Score. Of special concern is posturing, or nonpurposeful movement to stimulus. Two major types may be seen: flexor (decorticate), where the arms are flexed upward on the chest/abdomen, with flexion of the wrists and fingers, but without an attempt to localize the site of stimulation; and extensor (decerebrate), in which there is extension of the arms, hands, and fingers, with outward rotation of the hands. In both cases, the lower extremities are extended. A severely head-injured patient may exhibit either posture unilaterally and may show a combination of both. When testing for the ability to localize pain, it may be helpful to stimulate above (supraorbital ridge pressure) and below (anterior iliac crest pressure) the waist. Response only to the former may indicate a cervical spinal cord injury.

The remainder of the neurologic examination would normally be performed by the consulting neurosurgeon or neurologist.

Diagnostic Tests

There is some degree of controversy regarding the use of skull films [8]. Certainly, they are indicated in the patient who is unconscious or has an altered mental status, focal neurologic findings, or open injury. The argument arises in the case of the patient who has had a concussion and/or a scalp laceration. Our policy has been to obtain a skull series (anteroposterior and lateral views) in patients who have suffered a full-thickness laceration (galeal involvement) or who have suffered a loss of consciousness (documented or suspected due to post-traumatic amnesia/confusion). Unquestionably, this may represent an "overkill" policy, and several factors must be considered when establishing radiographic guidelines for "minor" head trauma, such as documentation of unconsciousness (including reliability of patient/witnesses), the potential postdischarge situation of the patient, and unfortunately, the medical-legal climate of the community. It should be reiterated that the most important initial x-ray in a patient with altered mental status is a lateral cervical spine view, with visualization of C7. Associated cervical spine trauma occurs in 5 to 10 percent of head injury, and proper radiographic evaluation of the entire cervical spine must be performed as quickly as possible to prevent spinal cord trauma. If necessary, the shoulders may need to be pulled downward or the patient positioned for a lateral "swimmer's" view to enable exposure at C7.

Tests such as blood chemistry, complete blood count, urinalysis, arterial blood gases, and clotting studies should also be drawn at the time of initial evaluation. It may not be necessary to obtain all of these studies, depending on the status of the patient. If there is an alteration of consciousness associated with the odor of alcohol, blood alcohol level may be drawn, as well as other toxicology screening tests, depending on the individual policy of the institution. Because of the potential legal implication of these tests, there may be certain restrictions on obtaining them. However, if this information is deemed necessary for adequate diagnosis and therapy, there is usually little difficulty encountered. Other tests evaluating the remaining body systems are dealt with in other chapters of this text.

Perhaps the most definitive test is the CT scan. While it is of tremendous aid in determining the presence or absence of an intracranial mass, it is not entirely foolproof in certain situations, nor is it a low-cost test. There are no universally accepted criteria for CT scan usage in head trauma; however, the following guidelines may assist the clinician in deciding to scan the head-injured patient. They are evidence of penetrating injury by clinical examination or skull x-ray; focal neurologic deficit; depressed skull fracture by clinical examination or x-ray; Glasgow Coma Score of 12 or less in a patient who will require general anesthesia for a non-neurosurgical procedure or controlled ventilation; and coma (Glasgow Coma Score of 8 or less) with clinical evidence of head injury or no metabolic explanation. These are not intended to be absolute indications but are simply guidelines. The clinician should always follow his acumen in the individual circumstance. Other tests such as lumbar puncture, radionuclide scan, MRI scan or positron emission transaxial (PET) scan, or electroencephalogram (EEG) are of little to no value in the acute diagnostic and management stage. In the absence of CT scan, two other tests may be performed. If the patient is stable systemically and neurologically, cerebral angiography may reveal a displacement of the intracranial vessels, indicating a mass lesion. If there is rapid neurologic deterioration, burr holes or smaller twist drill holes may be placed. These are placed initially ipsilateral to an enlarged pupil (if any) or opposite to the side of worse motor function. They are placed over the temporal, frontal, and parietal areas. The epidural space is examined for clot, and if negative, the dura is opened. If such exploration is negative, the procedure is repeated on the opposite side. If these are negative, then bilateral holes are placed over the posterior fossa. It must be stressed that this procedure is performed only when a definitive study (CT scan or angiogram) is unavailable or cannot be performed due to patient instability. Likewise, it should be performed only by a neurosurgeon or one specifically trained in the technique.

Diagnosis and Treatment of Specific Lesions

Scalp Injuries

Closed scalp injuries (cephalohematomas) are diagnosed clinically, although if there is concern about an underlying fracture, skull x-rays, especially tangential views, may help to define the soft tissue swelling and rule out a bony injury. Usually these injuries resolve spontaneously, but in a minority of patients, bleeding may continue and so require a compression dressing to tamponade the bleeding. In rare cases (usually very young children), the bleeding may be enough to require transfusion and/or surgical intervention.

Scalp lacerations require treatment depending on their degree of severity. Simple abrasions require only local cleansing and topical antibiotics. Lacerations, regardless of thickness, should have the surrounding area shaved, irrigated with antibiotic solution (usually a povidone/hydrogen peroxide mixture), and closed. Necrotic edges should be debrided and, if the galea is not penetrated, the wound closed in a single layer. If galeal penetration has occurred, then the galea must be included in the closure, either as part of a single-layer technique or with its individual layer. If there is question of contamination or the injury is over 12 hours old, then a single-layer closure, using nonreactive suture and incorporating the galea, may be advisable. It must be remembered that because of the vascularity of the scalp, significant blood loss may occur from scalp injuries, even to the extent of causing hypovolemic shock.

Skull Fractures

The diagnosis of a skull fracture may be straightforward, as in an open, comminuted injury, or may be more difficult, as in certain basilar fractures. The basic diagnostic test is the skull series of plain radiographs. This would include lateral, Waters' and Towne's views. Linear fractures of the vault will appear as lucencies not in the distribution of normal vascular markings. As a rule, linear fractures usually do not cross bony suture lines but may cause a splitting of the suture. Basilar skull fractures usually involve the petrous bone posteriorly or the frontal bone anteriorly. Frequently, they may also involve an air sinus, resulting in bleeding into that space. Although the fracture itself may be seen on as little as 30 percent of plain radiographs, secondary evidence of such a fracture may be manifested by "clouding" of a contiguous air sinus, an air-fluid level in such a sinus (both due to bleeding), or the presence of intracranial air. This last condition indicates a concomitant dural tear, allowing ingress of air. A CT scan will frequently demonstrate the fracture if "bone" windows are used. Externally, both linear and basilar fractures may show little evidence of their presence. There is usually pain and tenderness and scalp swelling. A fracture line is rarely palpable. Basilar fractures, by virtue of an associated tear, may manifest leakage of CSF otorrhea or rhinorrhea. In the former case, there is often an ecchymosis and bogginess in the postauricular area (Battle's sign), while in the latter, periorbital ecchymosis without conjunctival bleeding (panda-bear or raccoon eyes) may be seen. Posterior basilar fractures may also exhibit a tear of the external auditory canal or trapping of extravasated blood behind the eardrum (hemotympanum). The petrous bone may be fractured, causing trauma to the fifth, seventh, and/or eighth cranial nerves.

When fractures are closed (i.e., there is no violation of the skin or at least the galea) and linear with no focal neurologic findings, then no surgical therapy is needed. The patient is to be admitted for 24 hours and observed closely with neurologic checks. If the fracture site crosses a major vessel, 48-hour observation should be carried out. In pediatric linear fractures, skull x-rays should be repeated in approximately 1 month to check for a "growing fracture." In the very young, serial daily hematocrits should be performed to rule out significant bone bleeding (which would manifest as a cephalohematoma). Basilar fractures are treated similarly in terms of admission and observation. A CT scan may be performed to determine the fracture site. If there is leakage of CSF, then the patient should be nursed in the upright position, with the head of the bed as close to 90 degrees as possible at all times. This will allow the brain to "settle" over the dural tear site and hopefully "plug" the leak. If the leakage has not ceased over a 7-day course, then a lumbar subarachnoid drain may be placed to divert CSF away from the dural tear and allow the brain to tamponade the leakage site. Failure to achieve closure of the leak after a week's lumbar drainage has usually been seen as an indication for positive-contrast CT cisternography to identify clearly the site(s) of leakage prior to craniotomy for dural repair. There is some variation of opinion regarding the use of prophylactic antibiotics in the case of CSF leaks [9]. As a rule, we have not utilized this approach because of concern for the selecting out of resistant organisms. However, other authors have advocated it with little or no complications. A special case arises when there is CSF leakage in patients who have an associated endo- or nasotracheal tube in place. In our experience, we have found an increased incidence of meningitis when the airway is kept in place for over 72 hours. The organism involved has usually been part of the respiratory flora, implying retrograde spread from the tracheobronchial tree, along the airway, through the CSF leakage pathway, and across the torn meninges. Prophylactic antibiotics have not, again in our experience, been of significant help. Rather, if intubation is required beyond 72 hours, then we have adopted a policy of tracheostomy and removal of as many oro- and nasopharyngeal tubes as necessary. Although the creation of a surgical airway is not without risk, we have found a significant decrease in the incidence of CSF infection in this patient group.

Depressed and comminuted fractures require operative therapy if the depression is equal to or greater than the thickness of the skull or if the fracture is open. CT scanning is of significant value in the former case. If this is not available, then tangential view of the skull may help to determine the extent of depression. CT scan is also important to help identify any underlying contusion/hematoma or whether the fragment of bone overlies a major vascular structure. Operative therapy is aimed at evaluating the bone fragments, removal of any underlying clots, and dural repair, primarily or with pericranium or allograft, if necessary. If the fracture is closed, the bone may be sutured in place or a primary cranioplasty performed. In patients with open depressed fractures, we have left the contaminated bone out and then performed a cranioplasty after waiting 6 months to a year. In the immediate postoperative period, patients with open depressed fractures are treated with at least 1 week of intravenous antibiotics. Open linear fractures, if the wound is adequately debrided and there is no underlying increased infective risk, are usually treated with 3 days of intravenous, then 7 days of oral antibiotics.

Concussion

The hallmark of a concussion is its lack of focal deficit following a brief loss of consciousness. External signs of head injury (including skull fracture) may or may not be present. CT scanning is negative. For most concussions, a skull series is adequate, with cervical x-rays performed only if neck pain is present. There is no absolute criterion for admission of these injuries. As a rule, patients with a loss of consciousness are admitted for 24-hour observation. In some centers, if the loss of consciousness has been less than 5 minutes, and if the patient has a normal Glasgow Coma Scale and will have a friend or relative in attendance for the following 24 hours, the patient may be discharged home with a "head sheet" or checklist for the observer. This is a listing of signs and symptoms to observe for (e.g., persistent nausea/vomiting, lethargy, seizures, weakness, and visual changes) and instructs that the patient be returned to the hospital immediately if any of the listed changes occur. Following concussion, it is common for the patient to have a period of post- as well as pretraumatic amnesia, with some headache and dizziness. There may also be some transient nausea and vomiting. As a rule, these findings subside to a great extent over several days. In the case of persistent symptoms, a CT scan may be performed with attention to the petrous area to look for an occult basilar skull fracture with concomitant disruption of the vestibular system.

Epidural Hematoma

The hallmark of the arterial epidural hematoma is rapidity of presentation. Although a lucent period is described in the classic cases, frequently there is no such interval and the patient remains unconscious from the time of the initial trauma and exhibits the clinical findings described previously. Venous epidural bleeds may be slower in presentation. In either case, the diagnosis is to be suspected when a fracture line is seen to overlie a major dural vessel or x-ray. The definitive diagnosis is made by CT scan, which reveals a lenticular-shaped hyperdense collection. Most epidural hematomas require evacuation. In the case of rapid neurologic deterioration, a temporal burr hole may be placed on the side of the dilated pupil for immediate decompression. This hole may then be included in a formal craniotomy incision and bone flap, which will allow the entire clot to be evacuated and the source of the bleeding controlled. An arterial bleed may necessitate the rongeuring of bone at the base of the middle fossa to allow control of the middle meningeal artery at its entry point in the foramen spinosum. With venous sinus tears, the sinus may require pericranial or dural allograft patching if primary repair does not suffice. The bone flap is usually replaced and an epidural drain left in place for 24 to 48 hours postoperatively. The intracranial pressure is likewise usually monitored due to the compression injury to the underlying brain. A small number of epidural hematomas with CT scan shifts of less than 15 mm may be treated conservatively with close neurologic observation and repeated CT scanning to detect any expansion of the clot that may cause neurologic deterioration. It must be stressed that these lesions are a minority, and deterioration is a definite risk. Observation should be carried out for at least a week.

Subdural Hematoma

An acute subdural hematoma often carries a more serious prognosis than an epidural clot, since the forces that lead to a tear of bridging veins frequently cause significant movement of the brain with resultant contusions to the brain's surface. Likewise, intracerebral clots may rupture into the subdural space and present with a combined picture. Clinically relevant subacute or chronic subdural hematomas may present more slowly, becoming symptomatic only when they have reached a relatively large size. There is no standard clinical picture, the findings being dependent on the area of the brain involved. (There is a tendency for subacute and chronic collections to localize beneath the parietal bone, where the distance between the brain surface and the inner aspect of the dura is potentially greatest.) CT scan reveals a crescent-shaped mass lesion over the cortex. Depending on the acuity, the density may be high (acute) or low to isodense with brain (subacute and chronic). The patient with an acute subdural clot will frequently be "sicker" due to the rapidly expanding mass lesions, while in the subacute and chronic states, there may be some compensation by the brain for the more slowly expanding mass. The acute subdural hematoma, because of its acute mass effect, is a surgical emergency, requiring a craniotomy for evacuation of the coagulated mass and occlusion of the torn veins. Studies have shown the best results in patients operated on within 4 hours of their injury [10]. On the other hand, the subacute and chronic lesions will have undergone varying degrees of liquefaction, and evacuation may be accomplished through burr or twist drill holes. An exception is the situation where there exists a vascular membrane (contrast enhancing on CT scan), which must be coagulated or removed to minimize the risk of recurrent bleeding. Usually the acute lesion will be accompanied by a significant degree of brain swelling, and postoperative intracranial pressure monitoring and control is carried out, while in the nonacute lesions, the degree of brain swelling is considerably less.

Cerebral Contusion/Intracerebral Hematoma

These lesions, as noted previously, represent a spectrum. They represent a twofold problem, that of an acute mass lesion plus a surrounding zone of edema. The clinical picture is dependent on the size of the lesion, its location, and the surrounding edema. The resultant mass effect increases intracranial pressure and may impair cerebral perfusion pressure. As a rule, contusions are treated without surgical intervention, and intracranial pressure monitoring and management may be of great value. Control of systemic factors is also important in preventing further bleeding or edema formation. Intracerebral hematomas require surgical therapy depending on size and location as well as degree of CT shift (usually 15 mm or greater). Hematomas associated with open injuries, however, almost invariably require removal and debridement of devitalized brain along the track. An important subset of penetrating injuries is the impalement injury. The key point here is to leave the foreign body in place until it can be removed under controlled circumstances in the operating room. If the object hinders a diagnostic CT scan (which is the test of choice for contusions/intracerebral hematomas), then it may be trimmed off close to the entry point to allow the study to be performed. Following the removal of an intracerebral clot, intracranial pressure monitoring and management are again performed, with attention given to managing edema associated with the excised lesion.

Traumatic subarachnoid hemorrhage may also be seen as an entity related to contusion in that it is usually seen with a concomitant contusional injury to the inferior surface of the brain due to movement of cerebral tissue over the irregular skull base. Focality depends on the contusional component. The major sequela of the hemorrhage, which appears on CT as high-density collections within the subarachnoid space, is obstruction of the CSF pathways resulting in hydrocephalus. This may be acute or even after lysis of the blood.

STEROIDS AND HEAD INJURY

At the present time, there is little evidence to support the use of steroids in head trauma. While some studies have shown an increased survival with the use of very high doses of these drugs [11], the overall quality of survival has not shown a similar improvement [12]. In addition, the potential risks of steroids, such as infection, hyperglycemia, electrolyte imbalance, and impairment of wound healing, would not appear to justify their inclusion in the therapeutic armamentarium. We therefore do not, as a rule, utilize them in our treatment of head trauma.

ANTICONVULSANTS AND HEAD INJURY

There exists some difference of opinion as to the use of anticonvulsants in head injury. There is a significantly increased risk of seizures in open or penetrating head trauma. In closed trauma, however, the incidence of postinjury epilepsy varies according to a number of factors, such as the presence of a hematoma or fracture, duration of post-traumatic amnesia, and unconsciousness. Based on our experience, as well as literature studies [13], it has been our practice to place the following groups of patients on anticonvulsants: patients with open injuries with violation of the dura, patients with closed injuries who exhibit seizure activity at the time of the trauma, and patients with closed trauma with CT-demonstrated or grossly visible cerebral contusion or intradural hematoma (this includes the group with traumatic subarachnoid hemorrhage). All patients in these groups are given a baseline EEG and continued on a regimen of phenytoin or phenobarbital until they are seizure-free for at least 1 year, at which time the EEG is repeated. If no obvious epileptic focus is noted, then the anticonvulsants are weaned over a 6- to 12-month period. Seizure recurrence dictates a return to the anticonvulsant medication.

INTRACRANIAL PRESSURE MONITORING

Intracranial pressure monitoring is of value in the management of the brain swelling that accompanies significant head injury, either isolated or in the multitrauma patient. Because multiple systemic factors may influence intracranial pressure, it is of special value in the latter group, especially in the anesthetic management of extracranial surgery. Also, intracranial pressure monitoring may be of value in the intensive care management of the multitrauma patient [14]. The goal of this monitoring is the determination of the intracranial pressure (ICP) in the equation:

$$CPP = MAP - ICP$$

In this manner, it becomes possible for the clinician to maintain the cerebral perfusion pressure at a level to provide adequate cerebral blood flow. The monitor of choice in our experience has been the ventricular catheter, as this allows both monitoring as well as drainage of CSF to reduce elevated intracranial pressure. When the ventricular size prohibits the placement of such a monitor, a subdural or subarachnoid bolt or catheter is placed.

BRAIN DEATH

Brain death defines the state of irreversible and complete cessation of all brain function. This includes the neurovegetative centers in the brain stem. The concept is based on two characteristics of the brain: its need for a constant supply of glucose and oxygen and its inability to regenerate nerve cells (neurons). This state may occur as a result of a number of factors: hypoxia, hypoperfusion, and raised intracranial pressure. The determination of brain death is based on the clinical examination, that is, there must be no brain function, including that of the brain stem. Therefore, the patient must be apneic, areflexic (including cranial reflexes), and comatose. Spinal reflexes may be preserved and can exist independent of brain death. Because certain toxic-metabolic states may block the neurologic examination to the above extent, it becomes mandatory for the clinician to rule them out prior to declaring brain death. Because this frequently cannot be done (especially in the trauma patient where the pretrauma metabolic state is unknown or where the central nervous system injury has required the use of medications to control the intracranial pressure but also block the examination [e.g., barbiturates]), most criteria for declaring brain death include the use of a confirmatory test that may be independent of the toxic-metabolic state. This test may either demonstrate lack of neural function (EEG, evoked potentials) or lack of brain blood flow (cerebral angiogram, radionuclide scan, dynamic CT scan). In the former case, it must be determined that no blocking medications or drugs are on board, and in the latter, the lack of flow must be shown to exist over such a time as to cause "irreversible and complete" loss of function (usually 15–30 minutes). In our experience, the radionuclide scan has proved to be the optimal test, as it is portable, provides documentation over 30 minutes, and has been proven an effective determinant of brain death [15]. The choice of test, however, must be dictated by the facilities available at the particular institution.

REFERENCES

1. Jane, J. A., Rimel, R., Pobereskin, L., et al. Outcome and Pathology of Minor Head Injury. In R. Grossman (ed.), *Seminars in Neurological Surgery.* New York: Raven Press, 1982.
2. Kernohan, J. W., and Woltman, H. W. Incisura of the crus due to contralateral brain tumor. *Arch. Neurol. Psych.* 21:274, 1929.
3. Byrnes, D. P. Head injury and the dilated pupil. *Am. Surg.* 45:139, 1979.
4. Cooper, P. R. Post-Traumatic Intracranial Mass Lesions. In P. R. Cooper (ed.), *Head Injury* (2nd ed.). Baltimore: Williams & Wilkins, 1987.
5. Adams, J. H., Graham, D. I., and Gennarelli, T. A. Contemporary Neuropathological Considerations Regarding Brain Damage in Head Injury. In D. P. Becker and J. T. Povilshock (eds.), *Central Nervous System Trauma Status Report.* Bethesda: NINCDS, 1985.
6. Alker, G. J., Young, S., and Leslie E. V. High cervical spine and cranio-cervical junction injuries in fatal traffic accidents: A radiologic study. *Orthop. Clin. North Am.* 9:1003, 1978.
7. Teasdale, G., and Jennett, B. Assessment of coma and impaired consciousness: A practical scale. *Lancet* 2:81, 1974.
8. Cooper, P. R., and Ho, V. Role of emergency skull x-ray films in the evaluation of the head-injured patient: A retrospective study. *Neurosurgery* 13:136, 1979.
9. Ommaya, A. K. Spinal fluid fistula. *Clin. Neurosurg.* 23:363, 1976.
10. Seelig, J. M., Greenberg, Greenberg, R. P., Becker, D. P., et al. Traumatic acute subdural hematoma: Major mortality reduction in comatose patients treated within four hours. *N. Engl. J. Med.* 304:516, 1981.
11. Gobiet, W. The Influence of Various Doses of Dexamethasone on Intracranial Pressure in Patients With Severe Head Injury. In H. M. Pappius and W. Feindel (eds.), *Dynamics of Brain Edema.* Berlin: Springer-Verlag, 1976. Pp. 351–355.
12. Braakman, R. Schouten, H. J. A., Blaauw-Van-Dishoeck, M., et al. Megadose steroids in severe head injury: Results of a prospective double-blind clinical trial. *J. Neurosurg.* 58:326, 1983.
13. Jennett, B. *Epilepsy After Non-missile Head Injury* (2nd ed.). Chicago: Year Book, 1975.
14. Villanueva, P. A. Intracranial pressure monitoring in the postinjury patient. *Trauma Q.* 2:56, 1985.
15. Schwartz, J. A., Baxter, J., Brill, D., et al. Radionuclide cerebral imaging confirming brain death. *J.A.M.A.* 249:246, 1983.

7

Central Nervous System Trauma: Spine and Spinal Cord

Scott H. Kitchel
Barth A. Green
Frank J. Eismont

Spinal cord injury represents a multibillion dollar health care problem in the United States and around the world. In this country there are between 250,000 and 500,000 living spinal cord–injured patients, with an estimated 10,000 new injuries occurring every year [1]. Because of the high morbidity, mortality, and economic impact associated with these paralyzing injuries, they represent a catastrophic problem.

Spinal cord injury continues to be a disease of young people, the highest incidence being among males in their second and third decades. The most common etiology is motor vehicle accidents, followed by falls, industrial accidents, gunshot wounds, and sporting injuries. The majority of the patients suffer multisystem trauma, with associated long-bone injuries, visceral injuries, and head injuries [2].

Quadriplegia and paraplegia victims are approximately equally distributed [3,4]. The most common injury site is the lower cervical spine, followed by the thoracolumbar junction [3,4]. The predilection for injury at these levels is explained by their relative mobility as compared to the other spinal segments. In past years, the distribution of complete versus incomplete spinal cord injuries has been roughly equal [3,4]. However, in recent years, there has been a trend toward more patients having incomplete lesions on presentation [3].

Presently, there is little worldwide consensus on management of these trauma victims. The European standards were established through work at Stoke Mandeville Spinal Injury Center in England 40 years ago. Sir Ludwig Gutman established a protocol of nonsurgical immobilization and stabilization followed by a prolonged period of bedrest [5]. In North America, there is emphasis on early stabilization and mobilization. Most patients undergo some type of surgical procedure or have an external orthosis applied to allow rapid mobilization and institution of rehabilitation. At the present time, there are no good data available to prove either treatment strategy superior. Until these data are available, with long-term follow-up, treatment will remain variable.

PREHOSPITAL MANAGEMENT

The recent improved prognosis in spinal cord injury is directly attributable to advances and refinement in the prehospital management of the patients. The modern paramedic has training and equipment to provide optimal prehospital care and ensure expeditious transport to a hospital with preservation of maximal neurologic function. This is a vast improvement over the traditional first responder at an accident scene with no spinal cord injury training.

At the scene of the accident, the initial consideration is the recognition of the patient with a spinal cord injury. Any unconscious patient must be considered to have a spinal cord injury until proved otherwise. The most significant signs and symptoms found in patients with spinal cord injuries are

1. Motor signs: weakness or paralysis of extremities and/or the trunk
2. Sensory signs: alteration of sensation over trunk or extremities
3. Incontinence: loss of control of bowel or bladder
4. Superficial signs: abrasions, lacerations, or deformities of the spine, neck, trunk, or head
5. Pain: tenderness on palpation of the spine

Once the trauma victim has been identified as potentially having a spinal cord injury, then the priorities are established. First comes respiratory and cardiovascular stabilization, followed by immobilization of the individual in a neutral supine position. The entire spine must be immobilized because of the incidence of spinal injuries occurring at multiple levels [3]. The simplest and most effective method of immobilization remains the combination of a spine board, sandbags, and adhesive tape. We do not recommend the use of cervical collars at the accident because they do not provide adequate immobilization and may give a false sense of security. Similarly, the use of cervical traction at the accident scene is inappropriate. This may exacerbate the deformity and increase the neurologic deficit if not done with radiographic control.

If extrication or movement of the patient is required, the most important factor is common sense [6]. Victims should never be moved or lifted until splinted to minimize the chance of neurologic injury. Once the patient is splinted in the neutral supine position, the movement may be safely accomplished.

The emergency medical system coordinator can implement an optimal transport plan. Transportation may be accomplished in standard ground ambulances, helicopters, or fixed-wing aircraft. Considerations in determining the means of transport and the receiving center include distance, available resources, patient condition, and weather.

A prehospital standard neurologic assessment for use by paramedics at the accident scene has been developed (Fig. 7-1). It can be performed in less than 2 minutes [7]. This does not significantly delay implementation of the accident scene protocol or transport time. Invaluable information regarding the baseline neurologic examination can be forwarded to the receiving center that, if changed, could result in a change in the therapeutic direction.

EMERGENCY DEPARTMENT MANAGEMENT

The emergency department management of the spinal cord–injured patient requires a well-organized, multidisciplinary team approach. The trauma surgeon or emergency department physician is the key to appropriate triage and implementation of care. Close communication between all evaluating physicians is crucial in treating these patients with multisystem injuries.

The same priorities established at the accident scene must be reassessed. Respiratory and cardiovascular stabilization comes first, then spinal column immobilization. In our center, two large-gauge IV catheters, a Foley catheter, and a nasogastric tube are inserted. Baseline blood and urine samples are analyzed. The vital signs are checked, and the emergency department physician or trauma surgeon performs a careful, detailed history and physical examination. Arterial blood gases and vital signs are maintained within normal ranges. The treatment of multisystem injuries must be prioritized based on lifesaving measures. Spinal column and spinal cord injuries must be considered as preserving neurologic function and not lifesaving.

When the respiratory and cardiovascular systems have been stabilized, it is time to assess the spinal injury. The initial neurologic assessment is of paramount importance for management of these patients. A systematic approach of history taking, physical examination, radiographic assessment, and data recording is essential.

A patient who is responsive may provide a history with critical information. This should include the mechanism of the injury, the velocity with which the injury occurred, the patient's perception of neurologic function immediately following the injury, and any changes that have occurred since that time. Any history of prior neurologic dysfunction or spine injury in the patient should be obtained. If the patient is unresponsive, then much of this information can be obtained from paramedics, accident witnesses, and family members or friends.

Once the history has been obtained, a thorough physical examination should be carried out. General inspection of the patient may reveal helpful information. The alignment of the trunk and neck should be observed. Any abrasions about the thorax or head and neck may give clues as to the mechanism of injury.

A careful neurologic assessment is required. This must include a thorough sensory evaluation, motor examination, evaluation of reflexes, and a rectal exam. The sensory examination is best documented with sharp/dull discrimination checked in all dermatomes. It is critical that perianal sensation be documented, as well as sensation over the trunk and extremities.

Voluntary motor function must be assessed in the extremities. Inexperienced examiners are often deceived by reflex withdrawal of an extremity to a painful stimulus. Only voluntary motor function can be considered in defining the completeness of injury. A system-

Fig. 7-1. A standardized two-part form to record the spinal cord–injured patient's neurologic examination at the scene of injury. The same form or a similar one may be used by the emergency department physician.

University of Miami
Department of Neurological Surgery
CNS Trauma Research

Site of Injury Motor Assessment

Name ____________________
Examiner ____________________
Date of assessment ____________________

Code: Present = 3 Normal strength & range of motion
Abnormal = 2 Weak strength, flicker of muscle or loss of range of motion
Absent = 1 No motion

This exam is to be done only with the patient in a neutral supine position.

		L	R	
Shoulder elevation	(Shrug shoulders)			(10–11)
Elbow flexors	(Bend elbow)			(12–13)
Elbow extensors	(Straighten elbow)			(14–15)
Wrist extensors	(As though raising hand to stop traffic)			(16–17)
Interossei	(With hand & fingers flat spread and close fingers)			(18–19)
Upper abdominals	(Ask patient to tighten stomach muscles, then feel)			(20–21)
Lower abdominals	(Ask patient to tighten stomach muscles, then feel)			(22–23)
Hip flexors	(Raise knee to chest)			(24–25)
Knee flexors	(Tester raise thigh, ask patient to bend knee)			(26–27)
Knee extensors	(Tester raise thigh, ask patient to straighten knee)			(28–29)
Foot flexors	(Point toe as in stepping on gas)			(30–31)
Foot dorsiflexors	(Opposite of above; ankle up)			(32–33)

Code: 0 = Absent
1 = Present

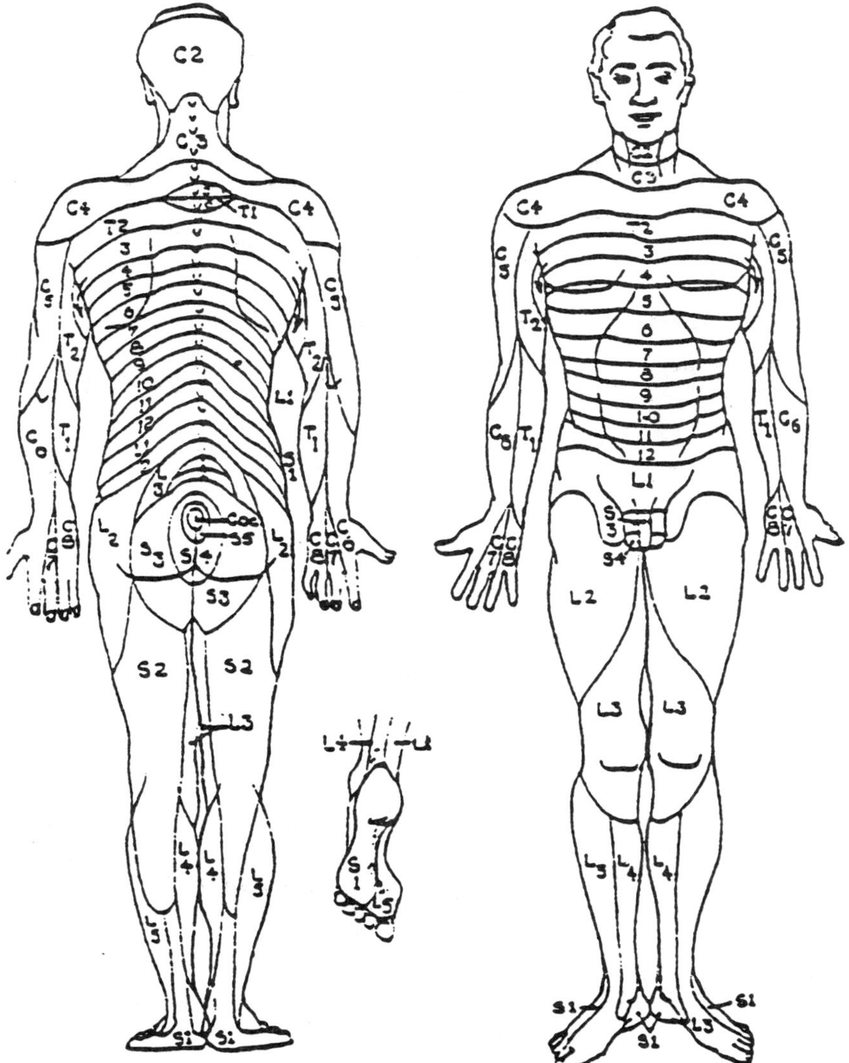

Left	Right
-C2	(16–17)
-C3	(18–19)
-C4	(20–21)
-C5	(22–23)
-C6	(24–25)
-C7	(26–27)
-C8	(28–29)
-T1	(30–31)
-T2	(32–33)
-T3	(34–35)
-T4	(36–37)
-T5	(38–39)
-T6	(40–41)
-T7	(42–43)
-T8	(44–45)
-T9	(46–47)
-T10	(48–49)
-T11	(50–51)
-T12	(52–53)
-L1	(54–55)
-L2	(56–57)
-L3	(58–59)
-L4	(60–61)
-L5	(62–63)
-S1	(64–65)
-S2	(66–67)
-S3	(68–69)
-S4	(70–71)
-S5	(72–73)
-C01	(74–75)

atic approach is necessary to evaluate motor function at each spinal level and to grade the strength. We advocate the system adopted by the American Spinal Injury Association. This grades muscle strength on a scale of 0 to 5:

5: Normal strength
4: Less than normal strength but the ability to move the joint through a full range of motion against resistance
3: Ability to move the joint through a full range of motion against gravity, but not against resistance
2: Ability to move the joint through a full range of motion with gravity removed
1: Palpable or visible contraction of the muscle with no motion at the joint
0: No palpable or visible muscle contraction

Each muscle group tested should be recorded for both right and left. Testing must be done on a muscle group representative of each motor root segment.

Reflex function should be checked in the extremities as well as the spinal cord–mediated reflexes. Deep tendon reflexes may be obtained for the biceps brachii, triceps, and brachioradialis in the upper extremity. The quadriceps (knee jerk) and gastrocnemius-soleus (ankle jerk) reflexes are readily checked in the lower extremities. These may be recorded by the standard 0 to 4 scale. The bulbocavernosus, cremasteric, and anal wink reflexes should also be recorded. The presence or absence of reflexes has not been as reliable a predictor of prognosis or diagnosis in spinal cord injuries as the motor and sensory levels.

A rectal examination is very important in the acute phase of assessment. It will give information about perianal sensation and motor function and allow assessment of anal wink and bulbocavernosus reflexes. Careful rectal examination with detection of tone or of perianal sensory sparing may change the classification of the patient and his immediate management.

All the data obtained in the history and physical need to be recorded in an organized, reproducible fashion so that it can be checked against follow-up examinations to determine the patient's course. We recommend the use of a spinal cord worksheet.

Once the history and physical examination have been completed, the patient can be classified according to the conventions of the American Spinal Injury Association. First, a functional level is described. This is defined as the lowest neurologic level with completely normal function. For instance, a patient with normal sensation in the C6 dermatome and 5/5 muscle strength in the biceps brachii and radial wrist extensors but deficits at the C7 level is termed a C6 quadriplegic. However, if adjacent levels have partial innervation, motor or sensory, then the patient may be termed a complete C6 with an incomplete C7. This is in contrast to the classic definition of complete or incomplete lesions. A complete lesion is defined as a total loss of motor and sensory function below the level of injury. Any residual function, either sensory or motor, distal to the level of injury makes the injury incomplete. As a general rule, patients with incomplete lesions will show some degree of neurologic recovery, while those with complete lesions rarely show any significant neurologic recovery beyond adjacent root recovery.

Once a careful history and physical examination have been completed and the patient is determined to be stable, radiographic procedures may be carried out. Anteroposterior and lateral projection radiographs should be obtained of the entire spine. These can be performed without jeopardizing the immobilization of the patient in the neutral supine position. Once the routine radiographs have been evaluated, then further specialized studies such as oblique radiographs or cone-down views may be obtained in the emergency room as indicated.

Postassessment Management

Once the patient is identified as having a spinal cord injury and has been assessed neurologically, then management should be instituted. The administration of systemic steroids or any other pharmacologic agents in the acute injury setting presently has no justification in the literature. There is good evidence that steroid administration is associated with increased morbidity [8]. For these reasons, we do not advocate the use of systemic corticosteroids in the acute injury setting. There are currently ongoing clinical studies to evaluate the use of the neuropeptides, thyrotropin releasing hormone (TRH), and naloxone (Narcan) in acute spinal cord–injured patients. None of these studies has been completed at the time of this publication.

Reviewing the patient's history, physical examination, and radiographs will dictate the immediate management. The hallmark of treatment in these patients is realignment of the spinal column, with resultant decompression of the spinal canal. When patients have neurologic deficit but no apparent spinal column disruption, they should be treated as if a spinal injury does exist at the clinically indicated level in spite of plain radiographs.

In the cervical spine, this translates into applying cervical traction to all patients who have any evidence of spinal cord injury. Gardner-Wells tongs are used for applying primary cervical traction in the emergency department. A small area is shaved above both ears, two fingerbreadths above the anterior tragus. The area is sterilely prepared and infiltrated with 1% lidocaine. The tongs knobs are tightened simultaneously until the pressure gauge protrudes several millimeters. The bolts on both sides are then wrench-tightened to assure no migration of the tongs.

In cervical spinal cord injury without obvious spinal disruption, traction with 10 pounds is applied until further evaluation is completed. If spinal column injury is apparent on the plain films, then 5 pounds of weight are added per level from C1 to the level of injury. When severe spinal disruption is present on the plain radiographs, then 5 pounds should be used initially and further radiographs obtained to be sure there is no overdistraction at the level of injury. Weight may then be added in 5-pound increments with serial radiographs being obtained. If there is difficulty in realigning the spine because of severe disruption, a halo apparatus should be applied while traction is maintained in a horizontal plane.

In attempting realignment of the cervical

spine, it is not indicated to apply greater than 10 pounds of traction per interspace. Any further weight will increase neck pain and spasms. If this amount of traction does not realign the spine within 1 hour, then a nasotracheal intubation is performed and the patient is paralyzed with an intravenous dose of *d*-tubocurarine. The patient must be manually respirated while the agent is working. The muscle paralysis allows spinal column realignment requiring less traction. Once realignment has been attained and the paralysis reversed, then the patient is extubated unless there is any question of respiratory status. Often, high-level quadriplegics are left intubated to prevent catastrophic respiratory complications.

The goal of realignment of the spinal canal is to decompress the spinal cord and nerve roots. Perfect alignment does not have to be achieved as long as the spinal cord is decompressed. If this is achieved, then a 1- or 2-mm subluxation may be accepted. Spinal cord decompression can be judged by measuring the spinal canal diameter on a lateral radiograph. The distance from the posterior aspect of the body to the spinolaminar line in an adult should be at least 15 mm (Fig. 7-2).

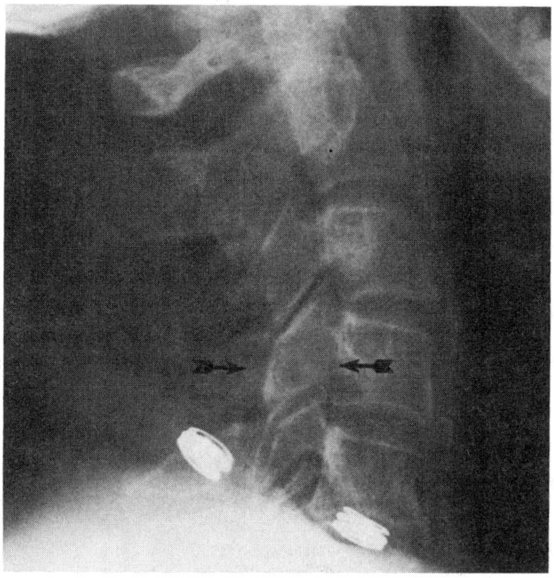

Fig. 7-2. The sagittal diameter of the spinal canal can be measured on a lateral radiograph. This is done by measuring from the posterior aspect of the vertebral body to the spinolaminar line (*arrows*). The spinolaminar line represents the anterior aspect of the lamina.

Once realignment has been achieved, the amount of weight may be reduced as long as the alignment is maintained. This will enhance the patient's comfort and prevent delayed overdistraction.

Attempts at closed postural reduction of thoracolumbar fractures have not proved successful. This may result in increased pain and neurologic deficit. In general, once these fractures are evaluated and the patient physiologically stabilized, the patient should be taken to the operating room for open reduction if indicated or treated conservatively with an appropriate orthosis.

Neuroradiographic Evaluation

Neuroimaging is performed once the spinal column is realigned in cervical injuries. Since this is rarely achievable in thoracolumbar injuries, the imaging is performed after emergency department triage. There still exists some controversy as to what is the most appropriate radiographic study to obtain.

In our center, the combination of plain radiographs and high-resolution computed tomography (CT) scans with 3-mm cuts and sagittal reconstruction permits us to evaluate the factors necessary to make a therapeutic decision. Based on these two studies, we can evaluate extrinsic compression of the spinal cord and spinal column stability. We have discarded the use of metrizamide myelography in the acute setting after reviewing a series of 250 cases where the myelogram information influenced the therapeutic decision in less than 1 percent. In settings where high-resolution CT is unavailable, metrizamide myelography is an acceptable alternative.

The advent of magnetic resonance imaging (MRI) presents the potential for a single study to provide more information than a myelogram and CT scan. Several centers are currently studying this question and the technical difficulties of utilizing MRI in the acute trauma setting. Until these results are available, one cannot recommend MRI for acute spinal cord–injured patients.

Optimally, the time required for neuroradiologic assessment should be 1 hour. In uncomplicated cases, the triage and assessment time in the emergency department should also be approximately 1 hour. This allows initiation of definitive medical and/or surgical treatment within 2 hours of arrival. Of course, this time may be significantly prolonged in the complicated multisystem trauma patient.

Therapeutic Pathways

After the baseline assessment including history, physical examination, and complete radiologic evaluation, then the patients with neurologic deficit are placed into one of five categories. Realignment of the spinal column is attempted on all cervical injuries as described previously.

1. Patients with no extrinsic compression on the spinal cord or nerve roots and a stable spinal column. These patients are transferred to the intensive care unit or ward as appropriate, with no indication for surgery.
2. Patients with no extrinsic pressure on the spinal cord but with spinal column instability. These patients are transferred to the intensive care unit or ward and plans made for spinal stabilization by surgery, orthoses, or both.
3. Patients with extrinsic spinal cord and/or nerve root compression. These patients are taken immediately to the operating room for decompression if they arrive within 24 hours of injury. The exception to this is the patient with a complete [1] injury below T1 but above T12. This patient is considered to have an irreversible lesion, and surgical stabilization is performed electively.
4. Patients with penetrating low-velocity wounds of the spinal column. Patients with complete neurologic lesions are not explored. Incomplete lesions are considered for exploration on a case-by-case basis depending on the level of injury, mechanism of injury, and neurologic function. Life-threatening multisystem injuries take priority over the spinal cord injury.
5. Patients with life-threatening multisystem injuries that take priority over closed neurologic injuries. Once these patients are stabilized by the trauma team, they are recategorized into one of the above groups.

SPINAL COLUMN INJURIES WITHOUT NEUROLOGIC INJURY

The principles of early treatment for spinal column injuries without neurologic deficit are fundamentally the same as those for spinal cord injuries. First, the patient with a spinal column injury must be identified and precautions taken to avoid further injury or creation of a neurologic injury. Then the patient must be triaged and assessed by the trauma surgeon or emergency department physician for priorities in care. Spinal column injuries without neurologic deficit are not a life-threatening priority. However, they must be properly immobilized to prevent catastrophic neurologic complications. Once the respiratory and cardiovascular systems have been stabilized, attention may be turned to the spinal column.

Identification of the patient with a spine injury will most often be accomplished by the history. The patient will complain of localized pain about the region of injury. Once this patient has been identified, then he should be aggressively evaluated and immobilized as if he had an impending spinal cord injury. When a complete history and neurologic evaluation have been completed and found to be negative for any neurologic deficit, then the patient is ready for radiographic evaluation of the entire spine. This should be completed while the patient is still immobilized in the neutral supine position. Further emergency department management will be based on careful evaluation of these initial radiographs and correlation with the history and physical examination.

Initial radiographic evaluation should include anteroposterior and lateral radiographs of the entire spine. The physician should not be misled by the negative appearance of these radiographs. It is critical that they be evaluated carefully and systematically for overall spinal alignment, soft tissue swelling, and any bony abnormalities. Once this has been determined, consultation with an orthopedic surgeon and/or neurosurgeon familiar with spinal column injuries is indicated.

If after careful review of the plain radiographs no abnormality is detected, stress views of the symptomatic region are indicated. This is particularly important in the cervical and lumbar spine, where there is relatively more mobility than in the rigid thoracic spine. Prerequisites for flexion-extension views of the spine are a cooperative, fully awake, neurologically intact patient with radiographs that show no gross malalignment of the spinal column. The patient is returned to the x-ray suite, where lateral flexion-extension radiographs are obtained with physician supervision. The flexion and extension should be completely volitional by the patient and not forced.

Special attention must be paid to changes in spinal column alignment with flexion and extension. Criteria have been established to determine evidence of cervical spine instability on these radiographs [9]. Any subluxation of greater than 3.5 mm, angulation of greater than 11 degrees as compared to adjacent vertebrae, or severe disruption of anterior or posterior elements is absolute evidence of instability. Such strict criteria are not available in the thoracic or lumbar spine. In practical terms, for emergency department management, any subluxation or angulation across one level should alert the physician to the possibility of a significant injury. This patient should then be seen in consultation by an orthopedic surgeon and/or neurosurgeon familiar with spinal column injuries.

If flexion-extension radiographs are negative, a conservative course of treatment may be elected. In the cervical spine, this includes immobilization in a rigid collar and appropriate analgesia. The patient should then be followed up with repeat evaluation in 1 to 2 weeks with repeat radiographs if symptoms persist. In the thoracic and lumbar spine, if all radiographs prove negative, the patient is managed with immobilization and analgesia as required by the pain.

REFERENCES

1. Thomas, J. P. Rehabilitation of the spinal cord injured. *Spinal Cord Injury Dig.* 1:3, 1979.
2. Green, B. A., and Eismont, F. J. Acute spinal cord injury: A systems approach. *Cent. Nerv. Syst. Trauma* 1:2, 1984.
3. Young, J. S., Burns, P. E., Bowen, A. M., et al. *Spinal Cord Injury Statistics. Experience of the Regional Spinal Cord Injury Systems.* Phoenix: Good Samaritan Hospital, 1982.
4. Ducker, T. B., and Perot, P. L. National Spinal Cord Injury Registry, Division of Neurosurgery, Medical University of South Carolina, Charleston, 1984.
5. Guttman, L. *Spinal Cord Injuries: Comprehensive Management and Research* (2nd ed.). Edinburgh: Blackwell, 1979.
6. Green, B. A., Eismont, F. J., and O'Heir, J. T. Prehospital management of spinal cord injuries. *Paraplegia* 25:3, 1987.
7. Hall, W. J., Green, B. A., and Colodonato, J. P. Spinal cord injury: Emergency management. *Emerg. Med. Serv.* 5:3, 1976.
8. Bracken, N., Collins, W. F., and Freeman, D. F. Efficacy of methylprednisolone in acute experimental spinal cord injury. *J.A.M.A.* 251, 1984.
9. White, A. A., Southwick, W. O., and Panjabi, M. M. Clinical instability in the lower cervical spine. *Spine* 1:15, 1976.

8

Maxillofacial Trauma

Stuart N. Kline

High-speed transport accidents, community violence, and the use of firearms explosively disrupt the facial skeleton and its overlying tissues.

Each year there are over 625,000 hospital-treated facial injuries from vehicular accidents. Within this group, there are a reported 29,000 patients who have suffered severe facial fractures [1] (Fig. 8-1). The loss of sight, smell, hearing, jaw function, and facial form is part of the injury potential.

Facial injuries do not usually pose a threat to life. Asphyxiation from the aspiration of blood, occlusion of the airway from displaced bone, and the traumatically induced loss of laryngeal architecture are the primary causes of death secondary to maxillofacial injuries [2]. Hypoxia associated with the obliteration of anterior tongue support in a patient with closed head trauma can prove to be disastrous. Thus, airway management, from the time of initial injury to the period of definitive care, is assigned the highest priority in the management of patients with maxillofacial trauma.

AIRWAY MANAGEMENT

Initial Care

Assessment of the airway at the scene of the accident will establish the patient's transport position. If the airway is not embarrassed, a semiprone position protects the airway by providing an escape for blood, vomitus, and oral secretions (Fig. 8-2). The semiprone position also prevents shredded soft tissues of the tongue, cheeks, and lips from collapsing into the oral cavity.

Acceleration-deceleration accidents resulting in acute maxillofacial injuries require transport of the patient in a supine position with the head immobilized, since injury to the cervical spine is assumed until proved

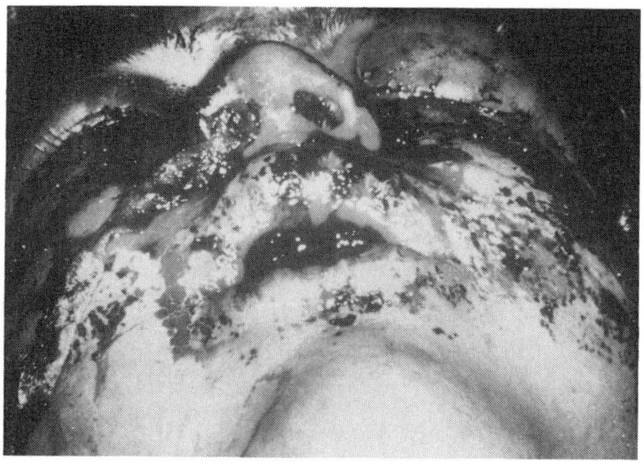

Fig. 8-1. Acute mid-third facial fractures in which the passenger struck the dashboard.

otherwise (Fig. 8-3). The supine position may further compromise the airway, and if intubation is not feasible in the field, then advancing the jaw with a forefinger and thumb will effectively support the airway until the patient is received at the hospital.

Definitive Airway Control

Adequate light and suction are essential in definitive airway control. The mouth and pharynx are suctioned well and inspected. Missing teeth, portions of teeth, dentures, and bridgework are frequently displaced and pose the threat of aspiration (Figs. 8-4 and 8-5). A

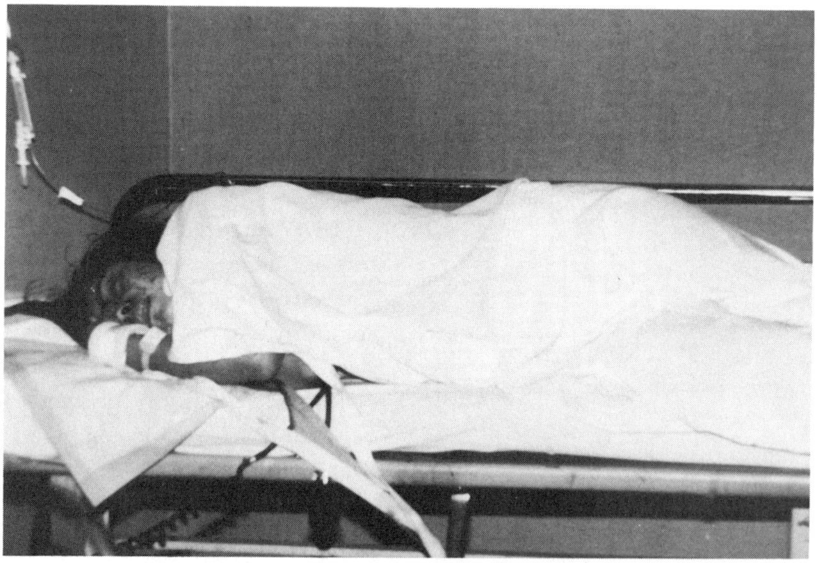

Fig. 8-2. Transport and maintenance of patient in semiprone position supports the airway.

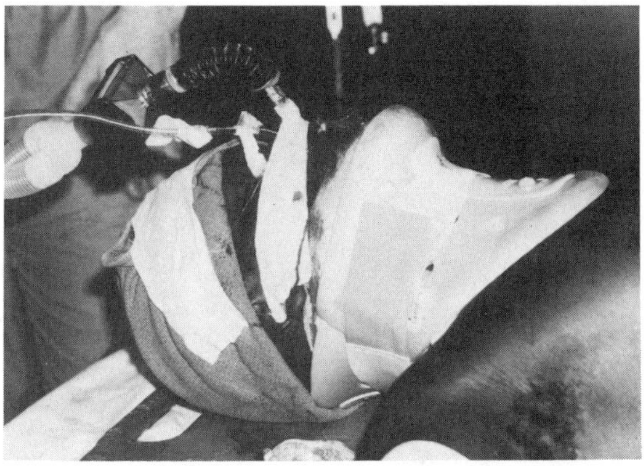

Fig. 8-3. If the cervical spine has not been cleared, minimal manipulation of facial injuries is possible.

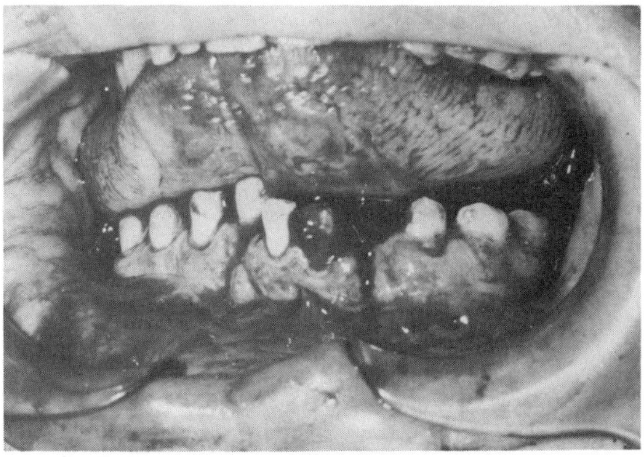

Fig. 8-4. Multiple mandibular fractures with disruption of the floor of the mouth and the loss of a tooth.

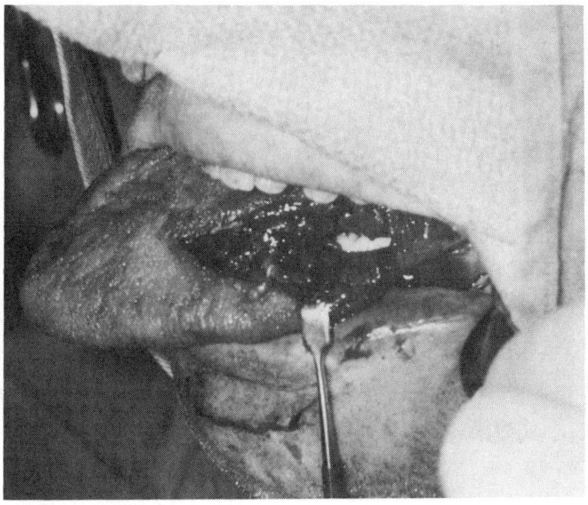

Fig. 8-5. Tooth found during debridement of tongue laceration.

gloved finger, sweeping the pharynx and mouth will dislodge foreign bodies, clots and debris which can be evacuated. Rapid pharyngoscopy and review of chest and abdominal films must be performed if missing teeth and other suspected foreign bodies are not located (Fig. 8-6).

An oral airway will support the tongue and mandible in the unconscious patient, but in the conscious patient, the airway is usually rejected. An alternative is the placement of a large suture through the dorsum of the tongue as far back as feasible (Fig. 8-7). Tension on the suture will bring the tongue forward and improve the volume of the airway. A well-lubricated nasopharyngeal tube will aid in achieving airway competence. However, the tube can become a liability, since it easily becomes plugged with secretions and clots. Frequent suctioning is needed to guarantee its continued patency (Fig. 8-8).

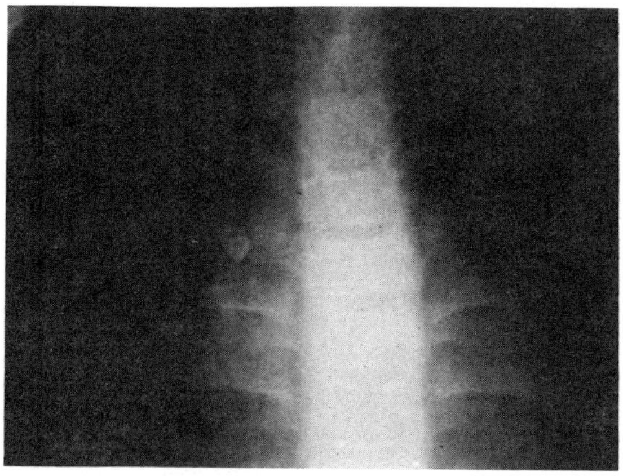

Fig. 8-6. A missing tooth was found on the chest film. It was removed by bronchoscopy at the time of maxillofacial repair.

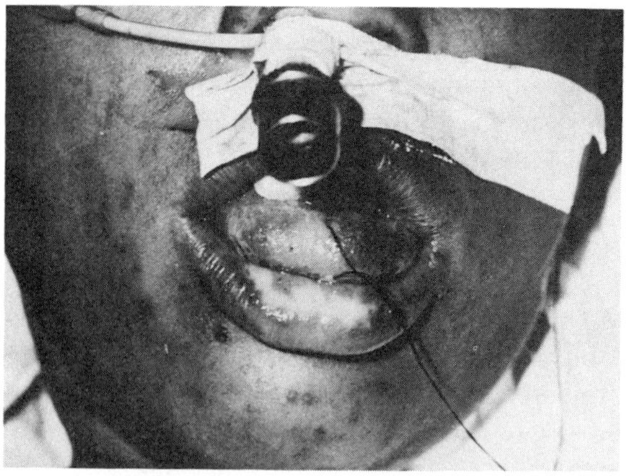

Fig. 8-7. Suture placed in tongue to maintain airway until definitive intubation.

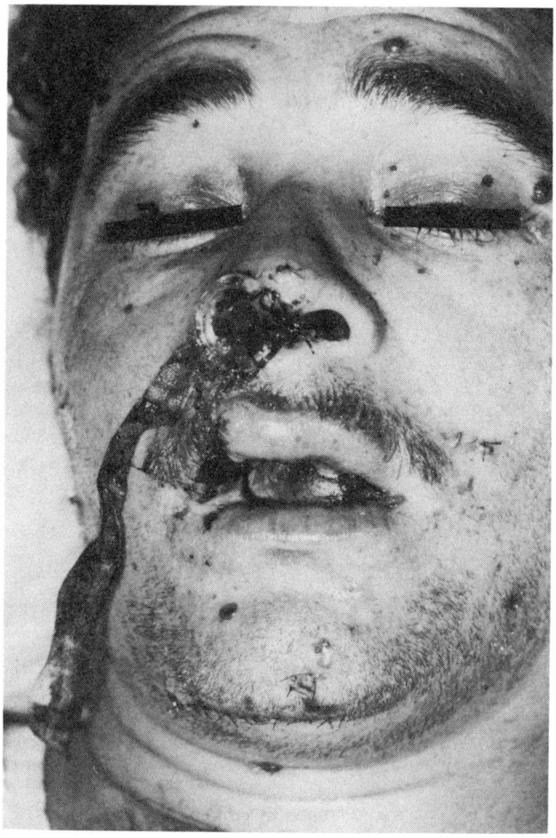

Fig. 8-8. Airway distress will become more acute if the nasopharyngeal tube is allowed to become plugged.

Endotracheal Intubation

The continued presence of persistent and copious hemorrhage, the displacement of the bony architecture of the maxillofacial area, and the potential for massive edema with the loss of compliant tissues require intubation for positive airway management (Fig. 8-9).

Oral intubation is preferred, especially in patients with nasomaxillary-ethmoid fractures.

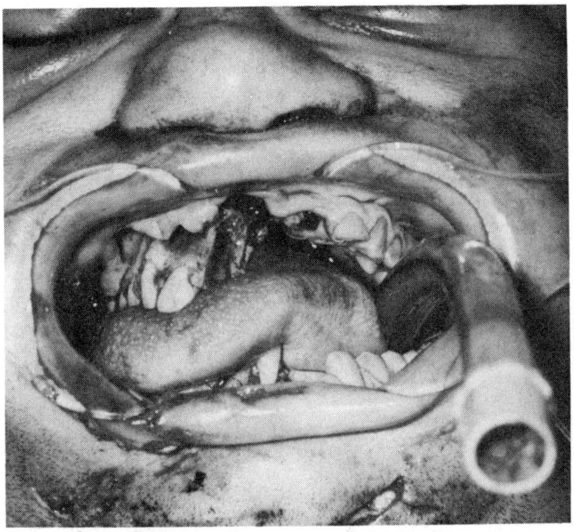

Fig. 8-9. Massive maxillofacial injury with intubation to preserve the airway. Patient expired secondary to ruptured thoracic aorta.

Insertion of nasal endotracheal tubes in patients with midface fractures can inadvertently be passed submucosally. Furthermore, endotracheal tubes in close proximity to fractures of the ethmoid cells that are associated with dural tears can provide the environment for a bacterial population consistent with the development of meningitis. Reintubation of patients with maxillofacial injuries is extremely difficult. As time progresses, the traumatized tissues become immobile secondary to edema and interstitial hemorrhage. Once placed, the endotracheal tube must be well attached to the skin with tape, sewn to the skin, or wired to the patient's teeth.

For whatever reason, if the airway cannot be maintained, then cricothyroidotomy is indicated.

Cricothyroidotomy

Cricothyroidotomy is an acceptable procedure for airway control when intubation has failed in the management of airway obstruction related to maxillofacial injuries [3].

In 1921 in a classic paper, Jackson [4] identified that subepiglottic stenosis was the end product of laryngotomy, cricothyroidotomy, and stabbing procedures when used as emergency measures to obviate airway obstruction. His dictum was accepted for over 50 years until Brantigan and Grow [5] reported their findings in 655 cricothyroidotomy procedures in which patients had tubes in place from hours to months. Their complication rate of 6.1 percent included only eight cases of airway obstruction following extubation. Morain [6] and others [7–9] have supported the fact that cricothyroidotomy appears to be a safe and effective procedure.

The emergency control of airway obstruction due to maxillofacial injuries, foreign body obstruction of the upper airway secondary to trauma, cervical spine injuries that preclude the movement of the head, and clenched teeth are the prime indications for emergency cricothyroidotomy [3]. Injuries to the larynx that pose a threat to airway patency are best managed by tracheostomy [10] (Fig. 8-10).

Surgically, the cricothyroid membrane can be palpated between the lower border of the thyroid cartilage and the superior aspect of the cricoid cartilage. The cricoid membrane is very superficial and quite easily exposed. The larynx is stabilized, and a vertical incision is made through the skin. The area is not free of potential hemorrhage, since bleeding is one of the frequent complications of emergency cricothyroidotomy [11]. The cricoid artery

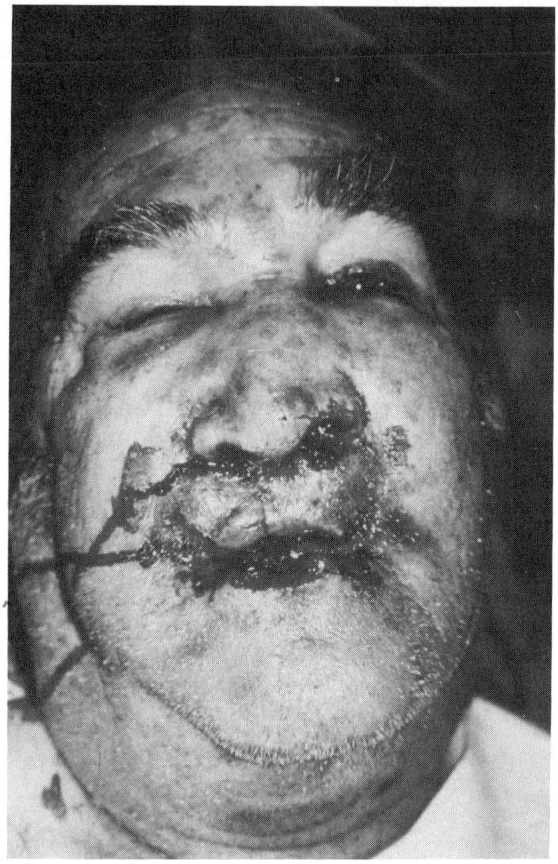

Fig. 8-10. Ecchymosis suggested fractured larynx, which collapsed during intubation. Immediate tracheostomy would have been a better choice.

runs transversely at the level of the inferior surface of the thyroid cartilage and gives off small branches that course down the face of the cricothyroid membrane. The dissection can be performed without hemorrhage if the incision through the membrane is made just above the cricoid cartilage and if the smaller vessels are ligated. The membrane is opened with a transverse incision in a stablike manner. The opening is dilated, and either an endotracheal tube or a No. 4 Shiley tube is inserted. The cricothyroidotomy when indicated can be replaced with a traditional tracheostomy in the controlled atmosphere of an operating room, or it can be retained and removed within 5 days following definitive maxillofacial repair.

BLUNT LARYNGEAL TRAUMA

Nonpenetrating laryngeal injuries are occasionally associated with maxillofacial trauma. The low incidence of laryngeal trauma is related to the mechanism of injury as well as to the anatomy of the area.

In vehicular accidents, when the head is hypoflexed, the mandible covers and protects the larynx. The larynx is further protected by its resiliency and mobility, which resist disruption. However, when the head is hyperflexed, the unprotected neck strikes the steering wheel with devastating effect [12].

Symptoms related to laryngeal injuries vary but may include pain to palpation, pain on swallowing, ecchymosis, edema of the neck, dysphagia, hoarseness, progressive respiratory distress, and stridor. The presence of subcutaneous emphysema and crepitus suggests separation of the larynx or trachea [13].

Indirect laryngoscopy is often diagnostic [14]. In the conscious patient, indirect laryngoscopy can identify mucosal tears, exposed cartilage, edema, hematoma, and vocal cord movement.

Tracheostomy is indicated in acute laryngeal injuries rather than intubation. Premature intubation can obscure important diagnostic considerations as well as precipitate life-threatening airway decompensation if the trachea is completely transected or if the larynx is fractured or distorted [15]. Direct laryngoscopy should be deferred until all resuscitative measures have been accomplished and the airway is maintained by tracheostomy.

Lateral x-rays of the neck, tomography, and especially a computed tomography (CT) scan will reveal the site of injury to the larynx as well as dislocation of the epiglottis and arytenoids.

Nonoperative treatment is indicated in edema, hematoma without mucosal disruption, single nondisplaced thyroid cartilage fractures in the otherwise stable larynx, and small lacerations not involving the anterior commissure.

Open exploration is indicated, if after tracheostomy and laryngoscopic examination, mucosal tears, cartilage exposure, vocal cord immobility, and comminuted fractures are recognized [16]. Early surgical intervention is indicated, as it provides the best opportunity for primary repair of all involved tissues [10].

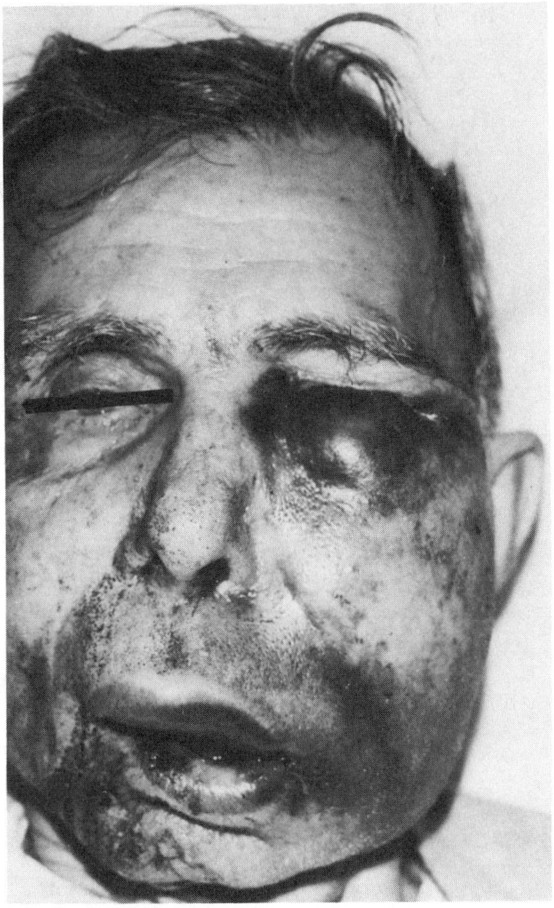

Fig. 8-11. Facial fractures with minimal dislocation result in contained hemorrhage.

MAXILLOFACIAL HEMORRHAGE

Soft tissue injuries associated with maxillofacial trauma can be managed by direct pressure. Once the hemorrhage has ceased, the wounds are lavaged with saline, and an occlusive pressure is placed until the lacerations are ready for definitive closure. Too often interested parties lift the dressing to view the extent of the injury. This practice should be discouraged, as it can only lead to contamination and infection.

Mid-third facial fractures that are minimally displaced usually do not provoke extensive hemorrhage. The tissues fill with blood, become distended, and tamponade the bleeding (Fig. 8-11). When gross separation of fractured

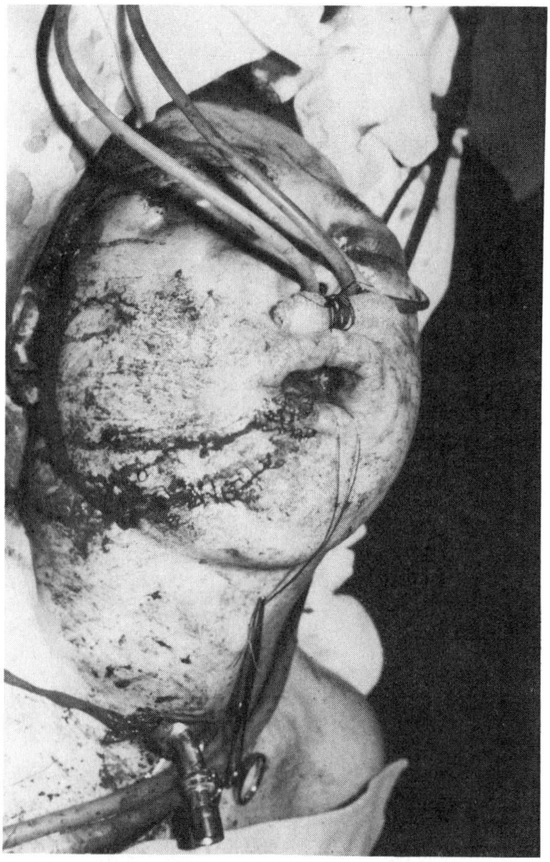

Fig. 8-12. Foley catheters and posterior nasal plugs controlling acute maxillofacial hemorrhage.

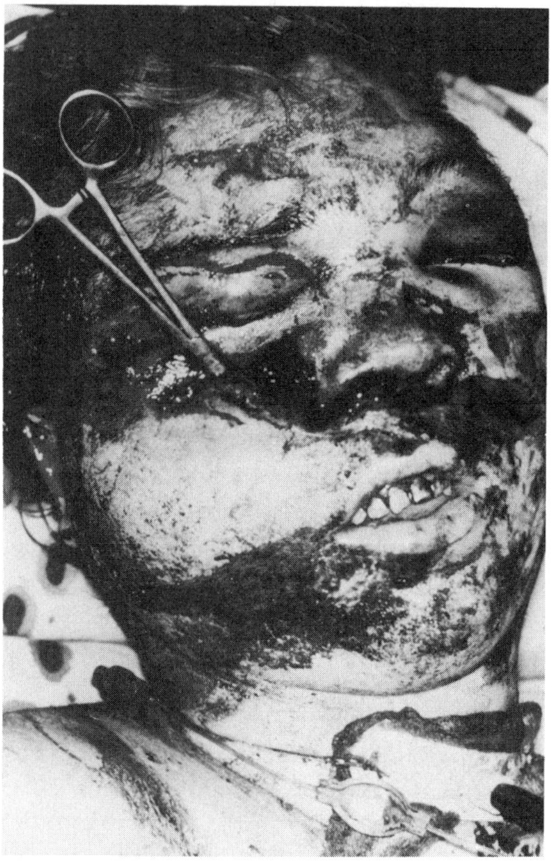

Fig. 8-13. Definitive ligation of a major vessel should take place in an operating room.

segments occurs, local vessels and mucosa are lacerated. This results in profuse hemorrhage with volume depletion. Digital repositioning of the fractured bone, occlusion of the nasopharynx with posterior nasal plugs, the use of inflated Foley catheters, and packing open wounds will effectively control the hemorrhage. It is rare to have to resort to ligating the external carotid system to control maxillofacial hemorrhage (Fig. 8-12).

Nasal packing in the presence of cribriform plate fractures associated with rhinorrhea is a liability due to its potential for becoming saturated with bacteria and the possibility of producing a meningitis. Obviously if the packing is necessary, it should be used, but the packing should be removed as early as possible.

The use of hemostats to control peripheral bleeders in the maxillofacial area is to be avoided, since injury to branches of the seventh nerve is a possibility. Clamping a major vessel to control extensive bleeding can be accomplished, but once done, any further dissection or ligation should be performed in the operating room (Fig. 8-13).

Maxillofacial hemorrhage can produce a significant hypovolemic state resulting in shock. Once resuscitated, if the patient continues to demonstrate a continuation of lost volume, a search should be made for an occult source of hemorrhage.

RECOGNITION OF MID FACE FRACTURES

Early recognition of mid face fractures is essential since many facial fractures can be brought to a successful conclusion during, or immediately following, an exploratory laparotomy, neurosurgical intervention, or an orthopedic procedure.

Definitive maxillofacial repair should be accomplished, if possible, before the patient's tissues become edematous. The use of computed axial tomography (CAT) for the evaluation of head injuries has made this premise feasible. One does not have to wait 4 or 5 days or longer until all the edema has receded. Everything being equal, the patient with maxillofacial injuries should undergo surgery as soon as possible.

Fracture separations of the maxillae and associated osseous structures are referred to as middle third facial fractures. They are classified as LeFort I, II, and III fractures. The classification stems from the research of French anatomist Rene LeFort [17]. Dropping cannon balls at various levels on the face of cadavers, LeFort was able to demonstrate predictable fracture lines. In LeFort I injuries (Fig. 8-14A) the lines of fracture involve the maxillae at a low level. The fracture lines extend from the pterygoid plates to below the zygomatic butress and continue forward to the pyriform aperture. A fracture at this level will produce a malocclusion as its most distinctive feature (Fig. 8-15).

LeFort II fractures (see Fig. 14B) are more extensive and usually require more applied force in their development. The fracture lines run in a manner similar to the LeFort I fracture except that the fracture line turns upward on the anterior maxillary surface to involve the infraorbital rim, the medial portion of the orbit, and the nasomaxillary process. The line of fracture stops short of the nasofrontal suture. The fracture may or may not produce anesthesia over the distribution of the infraorbital nerve. The fracture is associated with a disturbance of occlusion and if severely displaced an anterior open bite results (Fig. 8-16). Bilateral ecchymosis of the lower eyelids is consistent with a LeFort II fracture (Fig. 8-17).

It takes significant trauma to produce a LeFort III injury. The impact of a patient's face against the dashboard, or a base ball bat repeatedly striking the mid face results in a craniofacial dysfunction (see Fig. 8-14C). This form of fracture includes total separation of

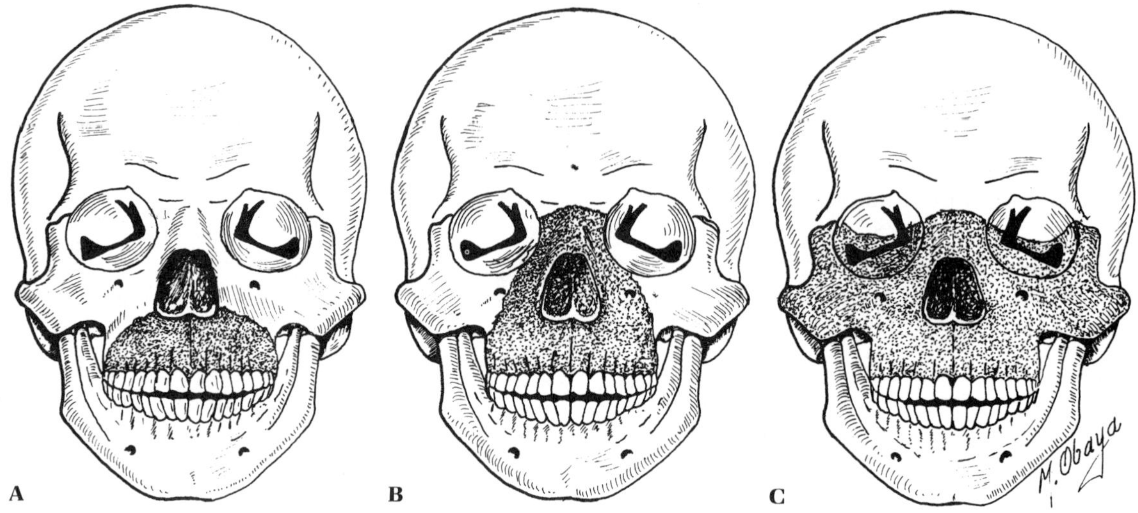

Fig. 8-14. LeFort areas of fracture. *A.* LeFort I fracture. *B.* LeFort II fracture. *C.* LeFort III fracture.

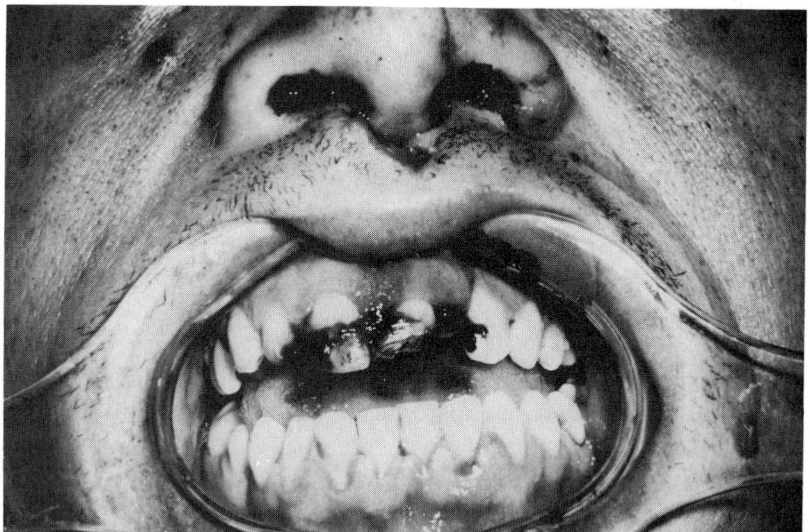

Fig. 8-15. Malocclusion related to a LeFort I fracture.

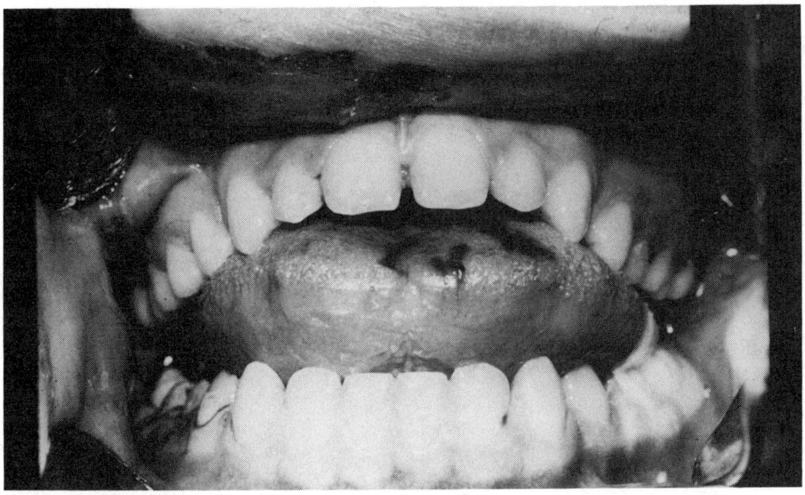

Fig. 8-16. Superiorly and posteriorly displaced LeFort II fracture resulting in an open bite deformity.

both zygomas, orbits, maxillae, nasal bones, ethmoids, and vomer. In effect, the mid face is taken off the cranial base. The fracture lines involve the nasofrontal and nasomaxillary junctions, transcend the nasolacrimal groove, and extend posteriorly along the ethmoids to the optic foramen. Fortunately, the dense optic foramen does not readily fracture. Thus, sight is preserved in most LeFort III fractures. The fracture continues on to involve the orbital floor, the sphenopalatine fossae, and the pterygoid plates. Other fracture lines develop within the orbits and involve the inferior orbital fissure, the junction of the zygoma and the greater wing of the sphenoid, and the zygomaticofrontal suture. After the edema has subsided the changes in the patient's facial form can be appreciated. The LeFort III fracture increases the vertical dimension of the face (Fig. 8-18). If there has been disruption of the nasal bones, as well as posterior impaction of the nasoethmoidal complex, the middle third of the face from a lateral view becomes concave or "dishpan" in appearance (Fig. 8-19).

Clinical examination of mid face fractures requires observation and palpation. A radiologic review serves to confirm a clinical impression. Frequently the patient's general condition will not allow routine facial bone films, however, a CAT scan can be performed at the same time that potential injuries to the brain are being scanned. Taken at 3-mm sections, the CAT scan increases the time in x-ray but the information gained is worth the minor delay.

Mid facial fractures are more often than not masked by edema, hemorrhage, emphysema, ecchymosis, and hematoma formation. How-

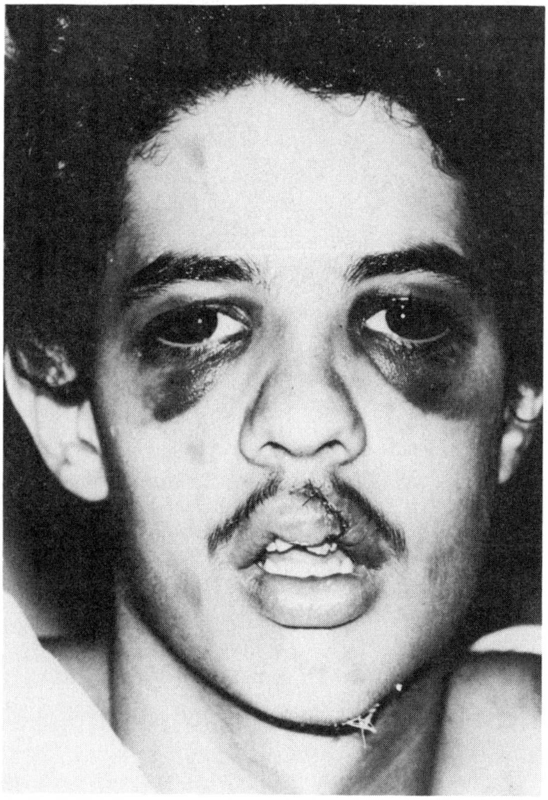

Fig. 8-17. Lower eyelid ecchymosis related to a LeFort II fracture.

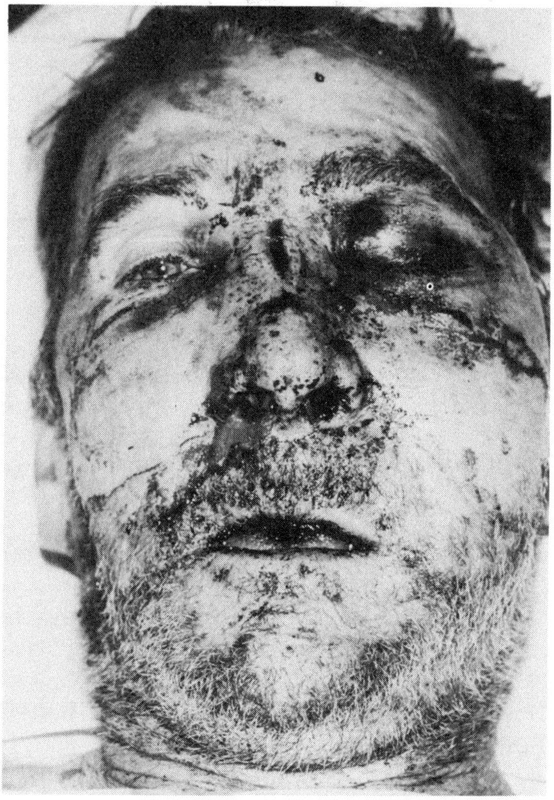

Fig. 8-18. Increased vertical dimension of the face following a LeFort III fracture.

ever, depressions of the zygoma, nasoethmoidal area, and orbits can still be defined by observation.

Characteristic of LeFort III fractures when there is involvement of the cribriform plate of the ethmoids is the presence of cerebrospinal rhinorrhea. It is assumed that following a LeFort III fracture, any clear discharge from the nose is cerebrospinal fluid until proven otherwise.

Orbital floor and wall fractures are associated with LeFort II and III injuries. A cursory examination to determine visual acuity, pupillary size and response, the presence of foreign bodies, corneal abrasions, hyphema, diplopia, and ocular mobility is necessary. Gross disruption of the orbital floor will allow the orbital fat to prolapse into the underlying maxillary sinus. Loss of volume support to the globe occasionally results in enophthalmos.

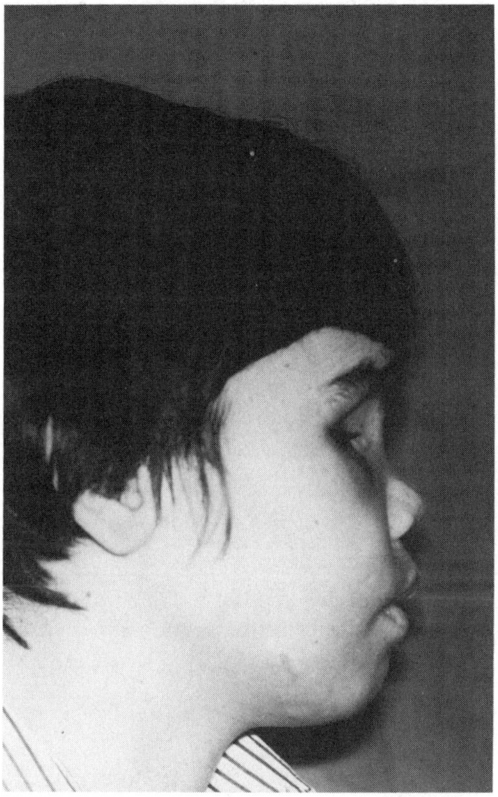

Fig. 8-19. Residual concave deformity following the repair of a chronic facial dysfunction.

The inferior oblique and inferior rectus muscle fibers can become trapped in the bone spicules of the orbital floor. Tethering of extra ocular movements follows the muscle entrapment.

The oral cavity should be inspected and palpated in LeFort injuries. Mobility of segments must be determined in order to clarify the extent of involvement. A fractured palate can be identified by mucosal tears and independent movement of the respective alveolar segments. Displaced maxillary fractures produce a malocclusion. The usual dislocation of the maxillae is posteriorly and inferiorly. Ecchymosis in the vestibule and a palpable defect between the zygoma and alveolar ridge point toward an underlying fracture.

Bimanual palpation of the mid third facial skeleton is used to identify fractured segments. While someone else holds the head, one hand grasps the dentition while the other palpates suspected areas of fracture. In fractures at the level of the dentition, movement can be detected in the dentoalveolar component. In LeFort II fractures, movement at the inferior orbital rims can be palpated when the maxillary arches are moved with finger pressure. In LeFort III dislocations, movement is discernible at the nasofrontal suture, as well as at the zygomaticofrontal suture when pressure is applied to the maxillary teeth.

LeFort II and LeFort III fractures frequently involve the medial canthal ligament. Crepitus and movement in the medial canthal area suggests a loss of continuity and ligament detachment; when the ligament is displaced, the development of a traumatic telecanthus is possible. The intercanthal distance should be measured. The normal measurement is 33 to 35 mm. An increase in the width of the intercanthal distance requires an open surgical exploration and the reattachment of the ligament.

In LeFort III fractures, the lateral canthal ligament, which is attached immediately below the zygomaticofrontal suture, is frequently displaced and will result in a narrowing and inferior positioning of the lateral palpebral fissure.

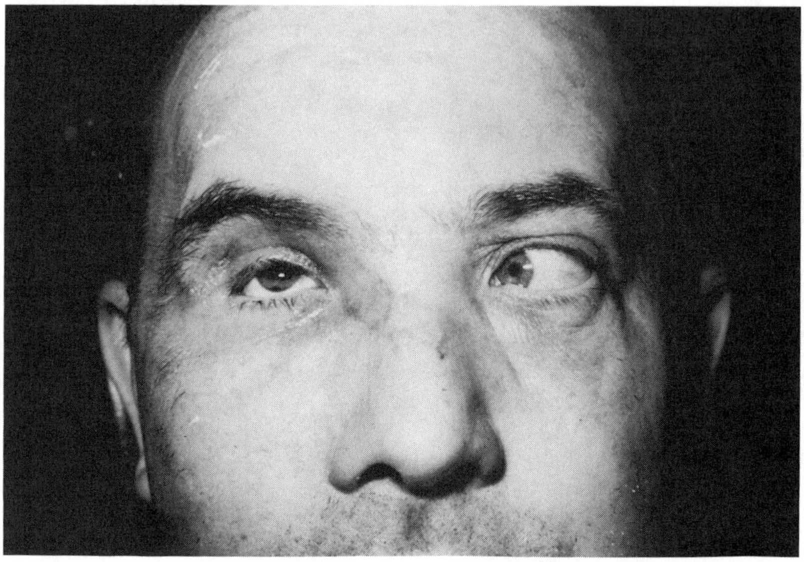

Fig. 8-20. Superior orbital fissure syndrome. The patient is attempting right lateral gaze.

Gross hemorrhage or edema within the superior orbital fissure can be recognized by ophthalmoplegia, a fixed dilated pupil, ptosis, and anesthesia over the distribution of V_1. Cranial nerves III, IV, and VI are compressed, as well as the ophthalmic division of the trigeminal nerve and the sympathetic plexus from the cavernous sinus [18]. This condition is appropriately termed the superior orbital fissure syndrome (Fig. 8-20).

Nasal-orbital-ethmoidal injuries are usually the result of high velocity trauma. The nasal structures are shelved from the frontal bone. The osseous anatomy of the area comprises thin bony structures that lend themselves to comminution and displacement. The fractured segments are driven posteriorly to involve the ethmoid cells and the medial walls of the orbits. Depending on the violence, the entire nasal bridge can be telescoped posteriorly (Fig. 8-21). The medial palpebral canthus widens and becomes round in appearance. Beneath the canthus, the medial canthal ligaments are at risk. The tissues rapidly become ecchymotic and edematous. Cerebrospinal rhinorrhea and occasionally permanent anisomia develop with involvement of the ethmoid cells and the cribriform plate. Ocular injuries are frequently associated with a naso-orbital ethmoidal crunch injury. Opthalmologic consultation is always indicated.

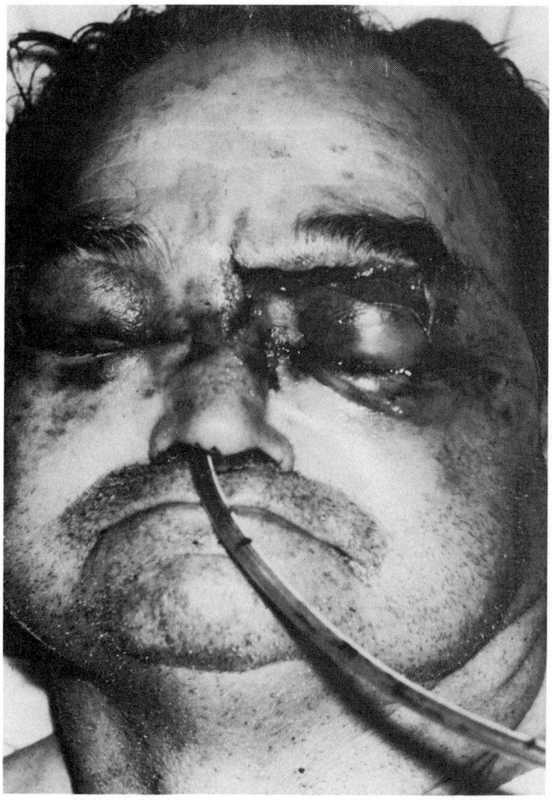

Fig. 8-21. Nasoethmoidal complex fracture with telescoping of the nasal bridge into the frontal sinus.

REFERENCES

1. Karlson, T. A. Incidence of hospital treated facial injuries from vehicles. *J. Trauma* 22:303, 1982.
2. Edgerton, M. T. Emergency Care of Maxillofacial Injuries. In: G. D. Zuidema, R. B. Rutherford, and W. F. Ballinger (eds.), *The Management of Trauma* (3rd ed.). Philadelphia: Saunders, 1979.
3. McGill, J., Clinton, J. E., and Ruiz, E. Cricothyrotomy in the emergency department. *Ann. Emerg. Med.* 11:361, 1982.
4. Jackson, C. High tracheotomy and other errors: The chief causes of chronic laryngeal stenosis. *Surg. Gynecol. Obstet.* 32:392, 1921.
5. Brantigan, C. O., and Grow, J. B. Cricothyroidotomy: Elective use in respiratory problems requiring tracheotomy. *J. Thorac. Cardiovasc. Surg.* 71:72, 1976.
6. Morain, W. D. Cricothyroidostomy in head and neck surgery. *Plast. Reconstr. Surg.* 65:424, 1980.
7. Gleeson, M. J. Cricothyroidostomy: A satisfactory alternative to tracheostomy (Editorial). *Clin. Otolaryngol.* 1:2, 1984.
8. Van Hasselt, E. G., Bruining, H. A., and Hoeve, L. J. Elective cricothyroidotomy. *Intens. Care Med.* 11:207, 1985.
9. Holst, M., Hedenstierna, G., and Kumlien, J. A., et al. Five years experience of coniotomy. *Intens. Care Med.* 11:202, 1985.
10. Trone, T. H., Schaefer, S. D., and Carder, H. M. Blunt and penetrating laryngeal trauma: A 13-year review. *Otolaryngol. Head Neck Surg.* 88:257, 1980.
11. Little, C. M., Parker, M. G., and Tarnopolsky, R. The incidence of vasculature at risk during cricothyroidostomy. *Ann. Emerg. Med.* 15:805, 1986.
12. Nahum, A. M., and Siegal, A. N. Biodynamics of injury to the larynx in automobile collisions. *Ann. Otol. Rhinol. Laryngol.* 76:781, 1967.
13. Sofferman, R. A. Management of laryngotracheal trauma. *Am. J. Surg.* 141:412, 1981.
14. Lucente, F. E., Mitrani, M., Sacks, S. H., and Billen, H. F. Penetrating injuries of the larynx. *Ear Nose Throat J.* 64:406, 1985.
15. Fitz-Hugh, G. S., and Powell, J. B., III. Management of laryngotracheal injuries. *V. Med.* 97:490, 1970.
16. Schaefer, S. D. Primary management of laryngeal trauma. *Ann. Otol. Rhinol. Laryngol.* 91:1982.
17. LeFort, R. Étude expérimental sur les fractures de la mâchoire supérieure. Parts I, II, III. *Rev. Chir. Paris* 23:201, 1901.
18. Pogrel, M. A. The superior orbital fissure syndrome. *J. Oral Surg.* 38:215, 1980.

9

Chest Trauma

John A. Elefteriades

It has been estimated that chest injury accounts directly or indirectly for one of every two deaths due to trauma [1]. This underscores the importance of understanding chest injuries to the physician caring for injured patients.

The early physiologic management of abdominal and extremity injuries is usually straightforward. The acute derangement that threatens life is hypovolemia from hemorrhage. Later, sepsis may supervene. Cardiac and thoracic injuries, however, do not present such a clear physiologic picture; a number of other catastrophic conditions besides hemorrhage can occur. Trauma to the heart and lungs can pose an immediate threat to life by interfering *mechanically* with the processes of *circulation* and *ventilation*. The physiology of these injuries can be complex and, in some cases, remains to this day incompletely understood. A working understanding of these injuries is essential in the care of traumatized patients.

The current discussion will be divided into two parts. The first will deal with the general management of thoracic injuries. The emphasis will be on what needs to be known to keep patients with thoracic injuries alive during the early minutes in the emergency room. Physiologic principles will be carried to their therapeutic implications. It has been estimated that fully 85 percent of chest injuries can be handled without surgery by straightforward emergency room procedures.

The second phase of discussion will deal with the particular management of specific injuries. This will include discussion of surgical procedures required for definitive management. Chest wall, lung, heart, and esophageal injuries will be discussed. Great vessel injuries are covered in Chapter 12.

GENERAL MANAGEMENT

There are six general categories of physiologic abnormality following chest trauma that are acutely life-threatening [2,3]:

Airway obstruction
Flail chest
Sucking chest wound
Massive hemothorax
Tension pneumothorax
Cardiac tamponade

These are the conditions that can take a patient's life within minutes of arrival in the emergency room (Fig. 9-1). Note that these are categories of physiologic abnormality, not specific injuries. Each category may follow any of a number of specific injuries, and a given injury may bring about several of these abnormalities. For example, massive hemothorax may be the result of an aortic transection from a motor vehicle accident, a gunshot wound of the lung parenchyma, or a knife wound of an intercostal blood vessel. Likewise, a gunshot to the chest may cause both massive hemothorax and cardiac tamponade.

Because each of these conditions can take the patient's life within minutes, only minutes are available for diagnosis and treatment. With knowledge and experience, diagnosis is usually straightforward. It depends on vital signs, physical examination, and only a single laboratory test—the *chest x-ray.* The vital signs can be assessed, the examination done, and the x-ray obtained within minutes. While other diagnostic procedures (e.g., hematocrit, blood gases, electrocardiogram [ECG], angiogram) may well prove useful, only the chest x-ray is absolutely essential in the crucial first minutes for preservation of life. As will be seen, the immediate treatment for these conditions—to the extent required to preserve life—can usually be administered within several minutes.

Airway Obstruction

The term *airway obstruction* (Fig. 9-1A) is self-explanatory: The flow of air into and out of the tracheobronchial tree is impaired or eliminated. The trachea can be injured in its cervical portion; these injuries are discussed in Chapter 8. Of concern in this chapter are injuries to the trachea in its thoracic extent. The lumen of the thoracic trachea can be obstructed or the trachea may in fact be transected by blunt trauma, with resultant loss of continuity. These can be devastating injuries, and in fact, it is thought that most serious injuries to the intrathoracic trachea are fatal in the field [2,4].

The patient with an obstructed intrathoracic trachea suffocates. If the airway is only partially obstructed, the patient suffers from hypoventilation; that is, the minute volume (the product of tidal volume times number of breaths per minute) of ventilation falls. As minute volume falls, PCO_2 rises; PO_2 is often preserved until minute volume falls very low [3]. Thus, the patient with traumatic partial airway obstruction will be hypoventilated; in the late stages, he may be hypo-oxygenated as well.

Airway obstruction is an obvious clinical diagnosis. The patient tries to move air but cannot. The respiratory muscles act, but the chest does not expand. Good air movement cannot be felt or heard at the nose and mouth. Experience on an anesthesia service

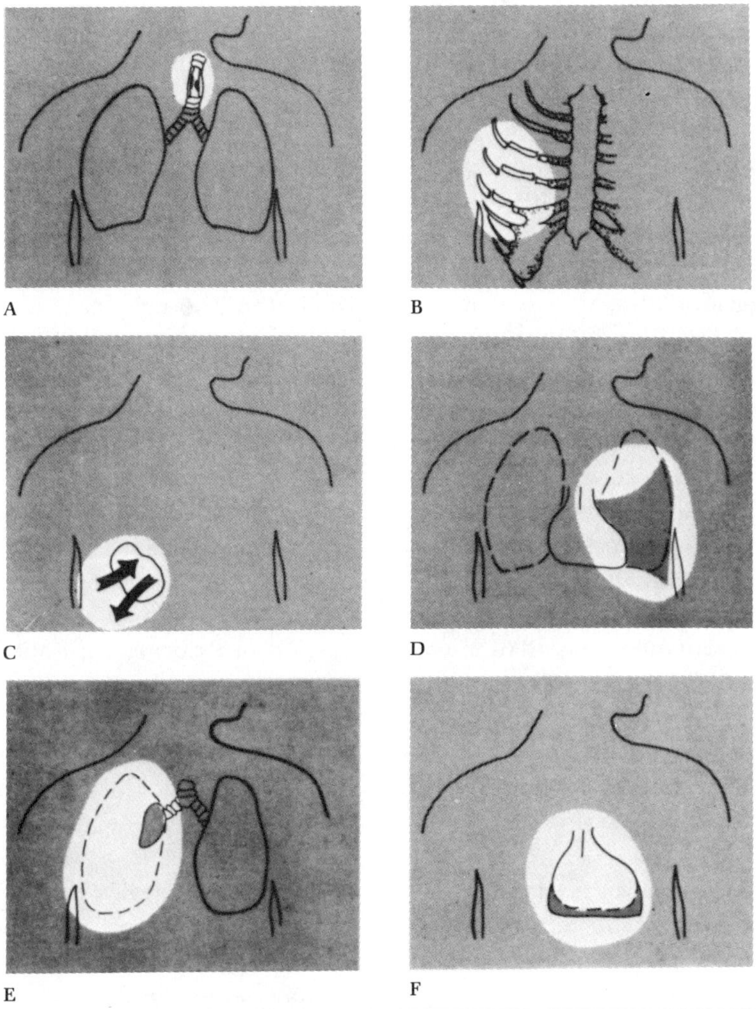

Fig. 9-1. **Schematic representation of the six major physiologic categories of injury that can take a patient's life within the first few minutes of chest trauma. *A.* Airway obstruction. *B.* Flail chest. *C.* Sucking chest wound. *D.* Massive hemothorax. *E.* Tension pneumothorax. *F.* Cardiac tamponade. (From J. A. Elefteriades and A. S. Geha, *House Officer Guide to ICU Care.* Rockville, Md.: Aspen Systems, 1985.)**

confers to the physician responsible for emergency care an excellent appreciation of the airway and states of obstruction, for airway obstruction is part of standard general anesthetic induction.

As mentioned, injuries of the intrathoracic

great airways can be devastating. Unlike the situation with neck injuries to the larynx or upper trachea, where tracheostomy provides access to the airway beyond the injury, tracheostomy is not useful with injuries to the intrathoracic trachea. Judgment and experience are key. Sometimes, even with transection of the trachea, partial airway continuity may be maintained, as the pleural and connective tissues around the airway conduct the tidal volume, allowing some effective spontaneous ventilation.

In this situation, it may be most prudent to allow spontaneous ventilation to continue until expert assistance is available. At times, in such circumstances, intubation may exacerbate the injury or positive pressure ventilation may disrupt the connective tissues, leading to tension pneumothorax.

At other times, spontaneous ventilation will clearly be inadequate, and intubation and positive pressure ventilation will be necessary. Flexible bronchoscopy through the endotracheal tube can assess the injury and clarify optimal tube positioning if air exchange is still inadequate.

The rigid bronchoscope is the thoracic surgeon's cardinal instrument in airway injury. This scope provides excellent visualization of the airway and its injury (as blood is suctioned easily and fully); further, it can be negotiated through a partially obstructed area of tracheal injury to provide access to the normal trachea beyond. Positive pressure ventilation can be provided through the scope, which is left in place until operative repair can be effected.

Rigid bronchoscopy is a specialized technique; the emergency physician on the scene may serve the patient best by recognizing airway obstruction early and obtaining early specialized assistance.

Flail Chest

Flail chest (Fig. 9-1B) is a disruption of the continuity of the rigid thoracic cage, with paradoxical movement of the disrupted segment. Since the thoracic cage in the transverse plane is a rigid oval, with ribs attached posteriorly at the spine and anteriorly at the sternum, flailing requires that at least one rib be broken in at least two places. If one rib were broken in one place only, it would still be attached anteriorly and posteriorly. Usually, a number of adjacent ribs are broken in multiple spots, so that a segment of chest wall is free to be sucked in during inspiration and pushed out during expiration, while the intact chest cage moves oppositely during each phase.

The physiology of flail chest is complex. A colorful theory is the old German concept of "Pendelluft," or ineffectual to-fro movement of end-expired air between the flail and normal lung. Modern studies cast serious doubt on this concept [5]. It is safe to say that the pathophysiology of flail chest is currently inadequately understood. A certainly oversimplified view, but one that leads to appropriate therapy, is that tidal volume is wasted in moving the flail segment in and out. The movement of the flailed chest wall represents a wasted tidal volume equal to the area in square centimeters of the defect multiplied by the length of its to-and-fro travel (similar to the volume of displacement in a cylinder in an automobile engine, equal to bore times stroke). This volume is lost from each breath, and the patient is overwhelmed by the work of breathing and may die.

Flail chest is a diagnosis of inspection. Many times, flails are missed because concentrated inspection of chest wall motion is omitted.

It is important that severely traumatized patients have all clothing removed. With attention to the chest, a flail will be apparent as a segment of chest wall that moves in with inspiration and out with expiration—out of synchrony with the remainder of the chest. This paradoxical movement can be appreciated also on palpation, and rib fractures and tenderness can also be found. Flail chest is not a sophisticated diagnosis; rather, with good observation, it is an obvious one.

Flail chest has historically been treated by immobilization of the flail segment. This has been done by immobilizing in the "in" position (by sandbags or bricks) or in the "out" position (by grasping a rib with a towel clip attached to a weight hanging over a pulley). On occasion, internal fixation of rib fractures has been carried out surgically. This is fraught with difficulties and is usually unnecessary.

The modern treatment for flail chest is intubation and positive pressure ventilation. When the lungs are expanded by positive pressure within the tracheobronchial tree, it makes no difference, physiologically, what the flail segment does. After 10 days to 2 weeks of ventilation, the chest wall begins to solidify, flailing diminishes, and the patient can be weaned to spontaneous ventilation and extubated.

Not every patient with flail chest requires intubation and positive pressure ventilation. Flails have different degrees of severity, and patients differ in the degree of embarrassment they can tolerate (i.e., the amount of ineffective tidal volume they can afford to lose). If a particular flail is well tolerated in a given patient without distress and without hypoventilation, no specific treatment is required. It is important to remember that elderly patients, especially, may initially tolerate the flail but tire progressively from the respiratory embarrassment. It is important that such patients be watched carefully over the first several days, both by clinical observation and by arterial blood gas measurements.

In recent years, increasing attention has been drawn to the fact that in flail chest significant pulmonary contusion, more often than not, accompanies the mechanical chest wall defect [6,7]. It has been learned that the underlying contusion may be equally as important as the chest wall defect and perhaps more so in certain cases. It has been shown that the contused lung is very sensistive to fluid administration; vigorous fluid and crystalloid administration by the trauma team can lead to pulmonary edema in the contused lung segments, with resultant hypoxia. While avoidance of overtransfusion and "running the patient dry" are now accepted as important aspects of the care of patients with flail chest, most authorities would still agree that severe flails with respiratory embarrassment continue to require intubation and mechanical ventilation.

One recent report [8] shows a beneficial effect, in avoiding intubation in some patients with flail, from performing epidural analgesia by an indwelling catheter to relieve the pain of flail and permit better breathing and coughing; there were, however, several very serious complications from the catheter itself.

Sucking Chest Wound

A sucking chest wound (Fig. 9-1C) results from loss of integrity of the chest wall, so that air is free to move in and out of the pleural space to the atmsophere. (A chest tube, before it is hooked to the suction device, represents a sucking chest wound. The to-and-fro rush of air with breathing is one sign that the surgeon looks for to confirm that the tube is well situated in the pleural space.)

Many mechanisms have been proposed to explain the distress seen with sucking chest wounds; none is totally satisfactory. It is safe to say that distress can occur even without development of tension pneumothorax, that simple loss of function of the ipsilateral lung is not the critical defect, and that some disturbance of the thoracic bellows appears likely [9]. With large wounds, as the chest expands, air moves through the chest opening into the pleural space, rather than through the trachea into the tracheobronchial tree [10]; this represents, of course, wasted tidal volume and wasted ventilation. The bigger the defect, the greater the ventilatory burden. Even a young, robust patient can succumb if the defect is large. The patient who succumbs to a sucking chest wound dies hypoventilated, with a high PCO_2.

Sucking chest wound is a diagnosis made by listening—not through a stethoscope, but with one's ear. Once heard, the sound of air rushing in and out of the pleural space with each breath is unmistakable. It is the same sound that is made through a chest tube before the tube is connected. Again, this is not a sophisticated diagnosis. Usually it is obvious the moment the patient is brought into the trauma room that he has a sucking chest wound—from the sound of the air rushing to-and-fro. From that point on, it is just a matter of removing the patient's clothing to identify the site of the chest wall defect.

The immediate treatment for a sucking chest wound is placement of an occlusive dressing. Vaseline gauze covered by sponges and tape works well. The occlusive dressing prevents the loss of tidal volume through the defect (the wasted ventilation of the pleural space). Usually a closed (nontension) pneumothorax remains after placement of the occlusive dressing, but this does not represent a life-threatening condition. Astute medical technicians in battlefield circumstances have learned to have the injured patient with a sucking chest wound exhale fully immediately before placement of the occlusive dressing. This maneuver serves to minimize or eliminate residual pneumothorax. In the emergency room setting, a chest tube can be placed after application of the occlusive dressing to eliminate a residual pneumothorax.

Major chest wall defects will need eventually to be debrided and closed formally in the operating room. The treatment outlined above will prevent respiratory demise until formal treatment is undertaken.

Massive Hemothorax

Hemothorax is the presence of blood in the pleural space, and massive hemothorax (Fig. 9-1D) is the presence of large amounts of blood in the pleural space. Massive hemothorax is distinguished from simple hemothorax because a small hemothorax is not acutely life-threatening.

The physiology of massive hemothorax is important. It is not the case that the patient succumbs because the blood impinges on the lung, impairing its respiratory function. This is not the mechanism. A young, otherwise healthy patient will usually not even be symptomatic if one entire pleural space is filled with fluid. Such a patient manages to ventilate adequately with the opposite lung. Pneumonectomy can be done even in elderly patients with poor lung function, and they are not rendered dyspneic at rest. (This situation is not entirely analogous, for in pneumonectomy, the pulmonary artery is interrupted as well, preventing the shunting of blood through a collapsed lung.) In any case, the patient with a massive hemothorax dies by exsanguination into the pleural space, not by restriction of pulmonary function. Nearly an entire blood volume can be lost into one hemithorax.

Massive hemothorax and tension pneumothorax share one physical finding and are disparate in another. The physical finding they share is decreased breath sounds. The physical finding in which they are disparate is resonance to percussion: hemothorax is dull, and pneumothorax is hyperresonant. The dullness of hemothorax may not be easy to appreciate in a noisy, hectic trauma room. The severely injured patient will be supine; the dullness of the hemothorax will be, accordingly, posterior only.

The diagnosis of massive hemothorax or tension pneumothorax will be confirmed by chest x-ray, which is available within minutes in emergency wards. Hemothorax, even massive hemothorax, may be a subtle chest x-ray diagnosis. Most house officers are accustomed to interpreting upright chest x-rays. On an upright chest x-ray, a pleural effusion shows its characteristic meniscus-type layering shadow on posteroanterior and lateral views. On upright studies, a massive hemothorax would appear just like a large pleural effusion. In severely traumatized patients, however, the chest x-ray will likely need to be obtained supine.

On a supine chest x-ray, a massive hemothorax will show only as a diffuse increase in density of the affected hemithorax. A liter of fluid may be just detectable to the astute observer. Two liters of fluid may be subtle. It is important to be alert that in the traumatized patient a homogeneous increase in density of a hemithorax likely represents major hemothorax. If the patient stabilizes before treatment is required, upright and lateral chest x-rays may clarify the diagnosis.

Treatment of massive hemothorax requires more than just placement of a chest tube. While a chest tube is certainly helpful, the loss of ipsilateral lung function is not the key physiologic element in massive hemothorax. Rather, the key feature is hypovolemia—the patient exsanguinates. Thus, the treatment of massive hemothorax is volume replacement—specifically, administration of blood. While not usually critical, restoration of ipsilateral lung function by emptying the pleural space is also beneficial. Placement of a chest tube is therefore helpful and allows evaluation of the amount of blood lost and the ongoing rate of bleeding.

The house officer should not be shocked if

large amounts of blood are evacuated immediately. It is not uncommon for one drainage device to fill immediately. This volume usually represents blood already shed. The key criterion in further management is the ongoing rate of bleeding. If bleeding continues at more than 200 ml/hr for 3 hours, operative intervention should be considered. The specialist can address this question. The critical aspect of initial care is volume replacement.

It is important to note that the overwhelming majority of knife wounds of the lung and large majority of gunshot wounds of the lung do not require surgical treatment. The pulmonary arterial circuit is a low-pressure system. When the lung is expanded to the chest wall after tube placement, the irritated visceral and parietal pleural surfaces appose and adhere. Between the low pressures involved and the tamponading by apposed tissues, most pulmonary parenchymal injuries stop bleeding without exploration.

Tension Pneumothorax

Pneumothorax is the presence of air in the pleural space; tension pneumothorax (Fig. 9-1E) is the presence of air under pressure. An ordinary pneumothorax is not acutely life-threatening, whereas tension pneumothorax may be so.

As with massive hemothorax, tension pneumothorax does not kill the patient simply by eliminating function of the affected lung. Again, the patient could survive well with just the opposite lung functioning. Rather, the patient with tension pneumothorax dies from circulatory embarrassment. The superior vena cava (SVC) is relatively fixed to the adjacent organs. The inferior vena cava (IVC) is fixed to the liver. When pressure develops in one chest, the heart is displaced toward the opposite side. If displacement is great enough, it is thought, the venous return through the SVC and IVC can be impaired. Stroke volume and cardiac output suffer because of inadequate blood return to the heart. Shock may supervene. (This commonly accepted pathophysiology is oversimplified; experimental study in the animal model [11] has shown that the actual physiology may be much more complex.)

The clinical signs in tension pneumothorax are decreased breath sounds and hyperresonance to percussion on the affected side. The trachea may be shifted to the opposite side. The chest may be visibly overexpanded on the affected side. Subcutaneous emphysema may be present if the air under pressure has found a route into the soft tissues.

The treatment for tension pneumothorax is chest tube placement. This is fairly straightforward. Occasionally, a physician will instrument the chest with a needle or plastic intravenous cannula. While these maneuvers may occasionally be helpful, placement of a chest tube takes little more time and is far superior. Most physicians should know how to place a chest tube, as many will perform procedures that can be complicated by tension pneumothorax (especially thoracentesis and placement of central venous lines).

Cardiac Tamponade

Cardiac tamponade (Fig. 9-1F) refers to impairment of cardiac function by fluid under pressure in the pericardial space. In the context of trauma, the offending fluid is blood. In nontraumatic conditions, transudates, exudates, purulent fluids, and chyle can cause tamponade.

The physiology of tamponade is of importance, as it dictates early treatment. Studies [12,13] have demonstrated that, because the pericardial sac is relatively inelastic, accumulation of fluid in the pericardium causes positive pressure around the heart, compresses the cardiac chambers, prevents filling of the heart, and thus impairs stroke volume. Basically, in cardiac tamponade, the heart cannot pump because the heart cannot fill. The untreated patient dies hypotensive, in cardiogenic shock.

Beck's classic triad of diagnostic findings in cardiac tamponade includes decreased pulse pressure (difference between systolic and diastolic pressure), distant heart sounds, and jugular venous distention (indicative of high central venous pressure [CVP]). Pulsus paradoxus (>15 mm Hg inspiratory decrease in blood pressure) and widened cardiac silhouette on chest x-ray are other classic features.

These classic findings are more typical of subacute or chronic tamponade (e.g., from uremic pericarditis). In traumatic tamponade, the classic findings are often *not* present. Heart tones may be difficult to evaluate in the noisy trauma room where many staff are doing many things all at once to a critically injured patient. Pulsus paradoxus is often not present in traumatic tamponade [12]. The cardiac silhouette is usually *normal* in traumatic tamponade; it is precisely because the pericardium is inelastic and cannot stretch that acute tamponade occurs. Only with chronic tamponade, over time, does the classic widened heart shadow occur.

The most important diagnostic principle regarding traumatic tamponade is to suspect this diagnosis in any patient with circulatory embarrassment and a penetrating wound that may have injured the heart. Confirmation of diagnosis goes hand in hand with treatment.

It is useful first to consider the medical (i.e., the nonsurgical) treatment of tamponade. This emerges as a therapeutic correlate of the pathophysiology. In tamponade, the heart cannot pump because the heart cannot fill. To get the heart to fill, one must provide a gradient from the cavae (superior and inferior) to the right ventricle. As the right ventricular pressures are high due to pressure transmitted from the pericardial space, the CVP must be raised quite high to achieve a gradient. Thus, the medical treatment of tamponade is *volume* [14].

The trauma surgeon should be cautioned that nurses and inexperienced physicians may look skeptically on giving volume to a patient whose CVP is already high. Nonetheless, when blood pressure is failing in tamponade, one must drive the CVP as high as possible to fill the heart and get the heart to pump. Pulmonary edema is not an issue. Blood is not even reaching the left heart, let alone backing up in the pulmonary circuit. Acute right-sided CVP elevation is not dangerous. Were it to continue, edema, ascites, and hepatic engorgement might develop, but with acute tamponade and shock, the patient's life is at stake and a brief elevation of CVP is a small price to pay. Often, volume replacement to

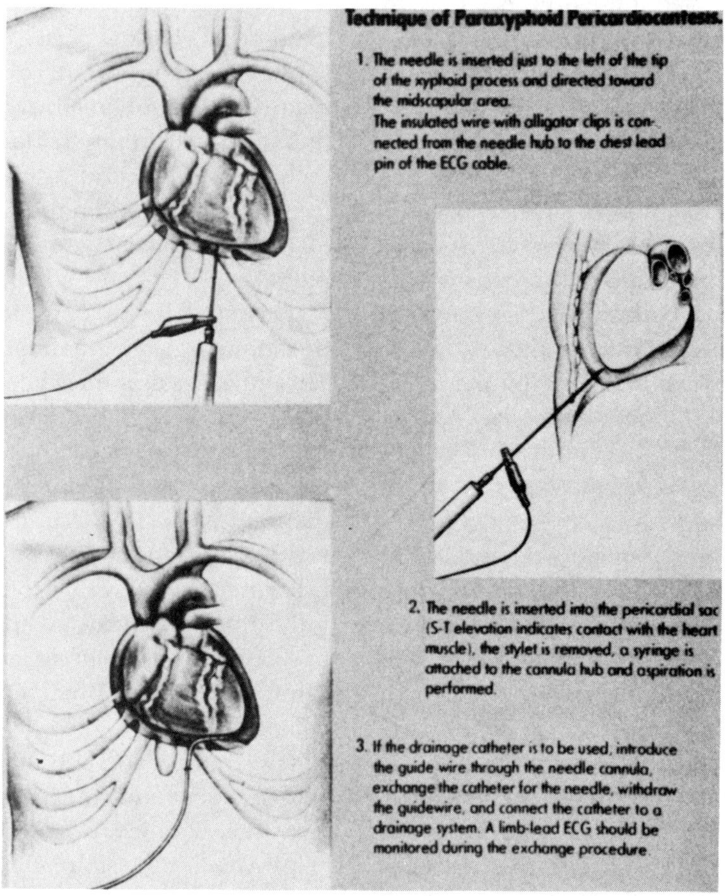

Fig. 9-2. Subxiphoid pericardiocentesis. The needle is shown connected to a V lead of the ECG, for detection of contact with the surface of the heart. (Courtesy of Mansfield Scientific, Inc.)

drive CVP up is successful in restoring some effective circulation in tamponade.

Inotropes are not part of the usual treatment of tamponade because they do not address the underlying physiology, which is failure of the heart to fill. Further, young patients in shock probably will have great release of endogenous catecholamines. Nevertheless, in desperate circumstances, inotropic support can be instituted. While a beta agonist is probably unnecessary, some alpha agonists may raise systemic pressures, albeit at the expense of organ perfusion, and allow better coronary perfusion. This could conceivably improve cardiac performance. Epinephrine or norepinephrine may be used.

The medical interventions discussed are important, but they represent essentially temporizing measures; the defect in tamponade is a mechanical one that requires a mechanical correction.

Pericardiocentesis may be the first step in the surgical management of acute traumatic tamponade. The subxiphoid approach is illustrated in Figure 9-2. As is well appreciated, because of the inelastic nature of the percardium, removal of even a small volume of blood can significantly lower intrapericardial pressures and produce dramatic improvement in vital signs. Pericardiocentesis in this setting is not easy and not always effective. Blood is likely to be thick and partially clotted; it may not draw back through the needle. The heart, coronaries, lungs, and liver may be injured. Most authorities agree that a patient who requires pericardiocentesis for acute traumatic tamponade should be taken for operation to control the injury. The alternative, waiting to see if bleeding recurs, represents unnecessary delay that is unlikely to prevent surgery.

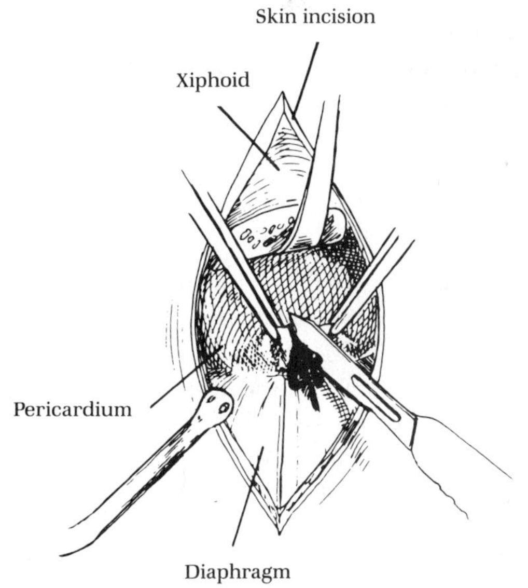

Fig. 9-3. Subxiphoid pericardiotomy. (From D. C. Sabiston, Jr. and F. C. Spencer, *Gibbon's Surgery of the Chest* (7th ed.). Philadelphia: Saunders, 1974.)

There is another technique available for decompressing the pericardium urgently with which the trauma surgeon should be familiar [15]. This is subxiphoid pericardiotomy (Fig. 9-3). This procedure can be done on the emergency ward or in the operating room under local anesthesia (or without anesthesia if vital signs are failing). If vital signs are preserved, this procedure may be performed to prevent the deterioration seen with induction of general anesthesia. The procedure is done by making a midline vertical incision over the lower sternum and the xiphoid process, excising the xiphoid process, and spreading the few diaphragmatic fibers present to visualize the pericardium.

Next, one picks up the pericardium and incises it. This provides immediate, thorough decompression of the pericardial space. A condition of tamponade can be converted in this way to a condition of cardiac injury without tamponade. Once this is performed, the patient will not die of tamponade. However, bleeding may be vigorous. With hemodynamic stability restored by the pericardiotomy, sternotomy or thoracotomy can then be done for definitive control of the injury. The cardiac surgeon usually finds sternotomy convenient, quick, familiar, and exceptionally well suited for access to all parts of the heart.

It is probably the approach of choice except when major associated lung injury is suspected, in which case left or, rarely, right thoracotomy may be chosen. Specific cardiac injuries are then repaired as detailed below.

CHEST WALL

Rib Fracture

Rib fracture is the most common thoracic injury. The resilient ribs of the child are quite immune to fracture, and the atrophic ribs of elderly patients are quite susceptible. Fracture may occur from a direct blow to the rib or from compression of the chest with "snapping" of the rib.

Rib fracture can usually be diagnosed clinically. The patient complains of local pain; this is aggravated by cough or movement. The findings on examination are those of any bony fracture: tenderness, swelling, and ecchymosis. Movement of the bony fragments may be discerned. Chest x-ray may confirm the diagnosis, although it is not uncommon for the x-ray to miss a fracture, especially one in the anterior or lateral ribs. Specialized views are rarely warranted [16].

Rib fractures are most significant because they may point to other important injuries from blunt trauma. Especially pneumothorax or hemothorax may be seen—as a consequence of the blow itself or of the protruding rib fragments. It is well known that fracture of the uppermost ribs—normally protected by the clavicle, scapula, and arm—requires a severe blow and is associated with blunt injury to the descending thoracic aorta, as well as the heart and the major bronchi. Low rib fractures should raise suspicion of splenic or hepatic injury.

The rib fracture itself requires no specific treatment. The major concerns are to rule out significant associated injury and to prevent the atelectasis or pneumonia that can occur from splinting due to pain. Adhesive strapping or belting of the chest is no longer recommended. The elderly or infirm are especially susceptible to complications of hypoventilation from pain, and these patients may on occasion require admission to the hospital for respiratory therapy and intercostal nerve block. Epidural anesthesia by indwelling catheter may also play a role in such patients, similar to its use in the post-thoracotomy surgical patients.

Flail chest has been discussed under General Management.

Subcutaneous Emphysema (and Mediastinal Emphysema)

Subcutaneous emphysema, with its characteristic "crackly" sensation, may occur when a pneumothorax decompresses itself through a defect in the parietal pleura (usually at the site of a rib fracture) into the soft tissues of the chest wall. This can be seen especially when the pleural space is obliterated by prior surgery or inflammatory disease, so that the lung parenchyma at the site of injury leaks air but cannot fall freely away from the chest wall. Subcutaneous emphysema can progress rapidly, especially with positive pressure ventilation, but, though unsightly, is not dangerous.

Often an intrapleural air space (pneumothorax) coexists with subcutaneous emphysema; placement of a tube into this space will prevent future accumulation of air in the tissues. Resolution of air already accumulated will take days to weeks. If subcutaneous emphysema has or threatens to become massive, small skin incisions can be made under the clavicle and the soft tissues spread down to the pectoral fascia. Regular "milking" of subcutaneous air through the incisions will permit early resolution.

When subcutaneous emphysema involves the neck and is associated with the cervical and mediastinal planes by x-ray, bronchial or esophageal injury must be suspected. Bronchoscopy and esophagoscopy may be necessary. In rare cases, when great pressure develops in the mediastinal tissue planes, a tamponade-like effect on the heart may occur. If deterioration in vital signs is felt to be on this basis, decompression can be obtained by performing an "almost tracheostomy" [17]. Dissection is carried out as by tracheostomy, but the trachea itself is not opened. This vents all cervical continuations of mediastinal tissue planes, decompresses the heart, and restores vital signs.

Open Defects

Major defects of the chest wall can occur, especially with high-velocity gunshot wounds and close-range shotgun wounds. Early management of the open chest wound by occlusive dressing is discussed under General Management. Small wounds can be treated just like chest tube sites and will seal within days. Large wounds may require operative debridement and formal closure. Complex muscle and skin flaps may be required, occasionally with artificial materials to restore rigidity of the chest wall. Until experienced personnel are available to carry out such procedures, patients with such wounds can be treated with positive pressure ventilation and open dressings, even directly on the heart and lungs. Transition to spontaneous ventilation will not be possible until an airtight seal of the pleural cavity is accomplished by formal closure.

Sternal Fracture

Sternal fracture occurs much less commonly than rib fracture; considerable force is required. Because of this, there is a considerable mortality in patients with sternal fractures from associated major organ (cardiac, bronchial, great vessel) injury [18].

Physical examination and lateral chest x-ray are usually diagnostic.

Aside from diligent search for associated injuries, no specific treatment is usually required. In the occasional case of complete transverse fracture with overriding of the fragments, operative treatment by open reduction and wiring may hasten recovery and restore the contour of the thoracic wall.

Blunt Injuries

Laceration of the pulmonary parenchyma is commonly seen with blunt injury. This produces pneumothorax or hemothorax, which is usually well controlled by chest tube placement.

Occasionally, blood collects within the pulmonary parenchyma, resulting in a localized hematoma. These are apparent as smooth, rounded fluid collections on x-ray. They usually clear in several weeks without specific therapy. Often a scar remains on the chest x-ray. The patient should be notified so that confusion with a lung cancer does not arise in the future.

Penetrating Injuries

Stab wounds and gunshot wounds of the lung are frequently seen injuries in any busy emergency department. Up to 90 percent of these injuries are adequately managed by simple chest tube insertion. The chest tube corrects the pneumothorax and drains the hemothorax. As the visceral pleura comes up against the parietal pleura with lung reexpansion, the lung "sticks" to the chest wall, and the air leak is sealed and bleeding tamponaded. The pulmonary artery branches in the parenchyma, it should be remembered, are low-pressure vessels; normal pulmonary artery peak pressures are on the order of 25 mm Hg. Bleeding rarely persists after chest tube placement unless a central pulmonary vessel or an arterial chest wall vessel has been injured.

If hemorrhage persists, thoracotomy may be required. At surgery, resection need rarely be performed. Most bleeding parenchymal injuries may be controlled by wide, deep sutures of the entry and exit sites in the parenchyma. The lung may look terrible because of hemorrhage into the alveoli, but it will improve quickly as the blood is cleared postoperatively.

If lobar or hilar vessels or bronchi are injured, resection is required (lobectomy or pneumonectomy). Resection may also be required for high-velocity peripheral lung injuries from military-type weapons, which produce extensive "shock-wave" injury. A recent report emphasizes the high mortality in patients who require emergency pneumonectomy; fully 75 percent of patients died, usually from hemorrhage or right heart failure and pulmonary edema in the remaining lung [19].

Tracheobronchial Tree

Although penetrating injuries of the tracheobronchial tree do occur, most such injuries originate from blunt trauma. These injuries are not terribly common [9], and even major trauma centers see only several cases yearly. The unusual nature of the injuries, especially those of the intrathoracic trachea, is seen in the fact that case reports of repair still appear in the literature [10,20].

Injuries fall into several patterns. In terms of location in the tracheobronchial tree, more than 80 percent occur with 2.5 cm of the carina [21]. In terms of orientation, some occur as vertical tears of the membranous portion of the trachea or main stem bronchi, and others as transversely oriented tears between cartilaginous rings (Fig. 9-4). The circumferentially oriented tears vary from small injuries involving less than one-fourth of the circumference of the trachea to complete transections, often with major distraction of the transected ends.

No clear-cut data exist on the pathologic mechanisms of blunt tracheobronchial rupture. Some propose that if a crush injury occurs while the glottis is closed, intratracheal pressure may rise to tremendous levels, causing essentially a "blow-out" injury of the tissues. Others speculate that sudden deceleration causes a disruption by shearing the tissues.

The presentation can vary greatly among different cases. The worst-case scenario is

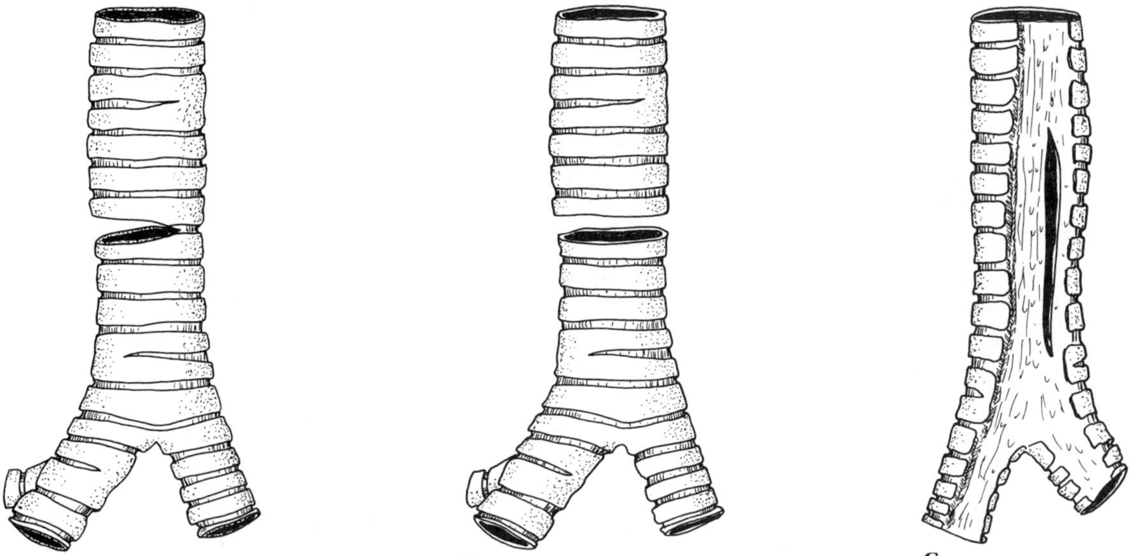

Fig. 9-4. Tracheobronchial injuries. *A.* Circumferential tear, partial. *B.* Circumferential tear, complete. *C.* Longitudinal tear.

that of the patient with complete transection of the intrathoracic trachea. This patient may present with complete airway obstruction and go on to die within minutes. In other patients, even with complete transection and distraction of the ends, the soft tissues around the trachea may maintain the airway perfectly well—without any respiratory symptoms apparent.

Hemoptysis is common, but not absolutely necessary. Subcutaneous emphysema is commonly seen, especially in the neck. This represents air that breaks out from the trachea or bronchi and spreads along mediastinal tissue planes. This is apparent on chest x-ray as mediastinal emphysema. Hemothorax is possible (from bleeding of the bronchial tear), but uncommon. Pneumothorax is common, but not absolutely necessary; pneumothorax occurs when the parietal pleura is torn as well as the bronchus, allowing air to enter the free pleural space. Tension pneumothorax can ensue very quickly. With major tracheobronchial injuries, when the chest tube is placed, the air leak may be seen to be large; in some cases, the lung may not even reexpand with the tube or with suction because the disruption is so large that negative pressure cannot be restored in the pleural space.

The key to diagnosis is to suspect bronchial injury in all patients with major blunt chest trauma, especially if accompanied by any of the above signs. Bronchoscopy is essential if the suspicion of injury is raised. This may be done flexibly if hemoptysis is not massive and ventilation is adequate; otherwise, the rigid bronchoscope may be of critical utility. Bronchoscopic findings are usually clear-cut, with extrabronchial tissues visible from inside the lumen and disrupted cartilage seen out of place. The treatment is prompt thoracotomy for repair. If the airway is secure and other injuries are life-threatening, repair need not be immediate, but it must be recognized that intubation and positive pressure ventilation for general anesthesia may further disrupt the airway or aggravate air leak, emphysema, and pneumothorax. (Some very minor tears without complications can be left to seal untreated [22].)

The approach is by right thoracotomy for tracheal injuries and right or left thoracotomy for bronchial injuries (depending on which lung is involved). Debridement and primary anastomosis with durable but absorbable sutures is recommended. Attention to preserve the lateral blood supply of the trachea is important. Many authorities advocate wrapping the anastomosis with muscle, pleura, or omentum. For these few tears that occur in lobar bronchi, lobectomy is an acceptable alternative to repair.

It should be noted that many tracheobronchial injuries are missed and do not present until later. This is possible because supporting tissues may preserve the airway or because symptoms may be minimal with the more peripheral tears. Patients may present later with obstructive symptoms (wheezing, dyspnea, pneumonitis, atelectasis) from stricture formation. Repair is always indicated, as good functional return can be expected, even with chronic collapse of the lobe or lung beyond the injury; successful restoration of function has been seen as late as 15 years postinjury [23].

Management of the airway during reconstruction of the pericarinal tracheobronchial tree can be a challenge. Direct intubation of a main stem bronchus by way of the operative field is often used. Cardiopulmonary bypass can be employed, allowing suspension of ventilation during the reconstruction [24].

Air Embolism

The fascinating phenomenon of systemic air embolism from parenchymal injuries of the lung was not recognized and reported until 1973 [25]. Subsequently, reports have confirmed the existence of the condition and clarified the pathologic physiology [26] as well as delineated principles of treatment [27]. Even autopsy confirmation of the phenomenon has been published [28].

Parenchymal lung injury often disrupts both *bronchi* and *pulmonary veins*. Especially if the patient is receiving positive pressure ventilation, air from the disrupted bronchi can enter the pulmonary veins. From there it is carried to the left atrium and ejected from the left heart into the systemic circulation. Air that reaches the brain can precipitate sudden neurologic collapse, and air that reaches the coronary arteries, sudden cardiovascular collapse. A hypovolemic state, as exists so often in major trauma, can lower the intravascular pressure in the pulmonary veins and encourage the passage of air from bronchus to systemic circuit. Similar systemic air embolism can occur from iatrogenic procedures on the lung, such as needle biopsy, chest tube place-

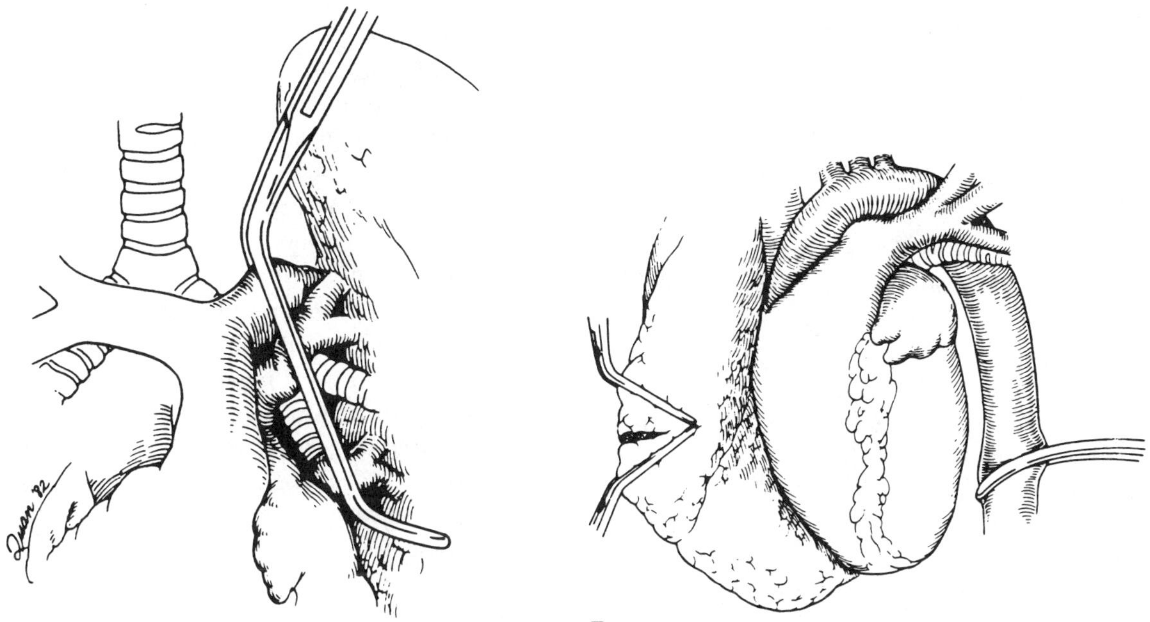

A B

Fig. 9-5. Surgical maneuvers for air embolism. *A.* Mass clamping of hilum. *B.* Control of peripheral parenchymal lung injury by exclusion in clamps. (Note adductive clamping of descending aorta for resuscitation.) (From E. S. Yee, E. D. Verrier, and A. N. Thomas, Management of air embolism in blunt and penetrating thoracic trauma. *J. Thorac. Cardiovasc. Surg.* 85:661, 1983.)

ment, and contrast study of empyema cavities.

The most common clinical picture is one in which the patient with any type of lung injury suffers sudden onset of shock or cardiopulmonary arrest shortly after arrival in the emergency department, especially upon being placed on positive pressure ventilation. Often bleeding into the endotracheal tube is noted before cardiovascular collapse. Also, high inspiratory pressures have frequently been noted.

Chest x-ray excludes common lesions like massive hemothorax and tension pneumothorax. The diagnosis of systemic air embolism is rarely made until resuscitative thoracotomy is performed and air is noted in the coronary arteries and bloody froth seen at the lung injury.

This condition was previously considered uniformly fatal [26]. Recently, some survivors have been reported. Key to attaining survival in this condition is maintaining a high index of suspicion. This injury is probably very overwhelmingly underdiagnosed. When the diagnosis is suspected, urgent thoracotomy is required. This should be on the side of the injury if it is unilateral or on the left initially if bilateral.

Thoracotomy allows confirmation of the diagnosis (by visualization of air in the coronary arteries) and treatment. Aside from open resuscitation, treatment includes

1. Placing the patient in the Trendelenburg position to direct air away from the brain.
2. Interrupting the bronchovenous connection (Fig. 9-5). (This may be done by urgent clamping of the hilum, by isolating the injured parenchyma between clamps, or by advancing the endotracheal tube into the noninjured lung, defunctionalizing the bronchial tree to the injured area.)
3. Venting of air from the heart by making a needle hole in the ascending aorta and aspirating the left ventricular apex.
4. Formal resection of the injured lobe or lung when hemodynamic stability has been restored. Occasionally, a wedge resection of a peripheral laceration may suffice.

Lobar Torsion

A fascinating, rare phenomenon is traumatic lobar torsion of the lung. A number of cases have been reported [29,30]. It is speculated that blunt trauma may tear the inferior pulmonary ligament, tear interlobar bridging tissues, and displace a lobe so severely as to leave it twisted on its pedicle. The radiographic appearance is that of lobar consolidation and displacement. On bronchoscopy, bronchial obstruction is found. The treatment is urgent operation for detorsion or resection.

HEART

Blunt Injury

Myocardial Contusion

Myocardial contusion describes injury to myocardial tissues from blunt trauma. This may include edema, hemorrhage, or necrosis. Recent years have produced a voluminous proliferation of papers addressing the topic of traumatic myocardial contusion [31–37]; much of this literature contains little information of practical importance. There remains confusion even regarding diagnosis of myocardial contusion [38].

Among the diagnostic modalities used are ECG, enzymes, angiography, pyrophosphate scanning, and MUGA (ECG-gated radionuclide angiographic) scanning [31]. Changes on ECG include ST and T wave abnormalities, sinus tachycardia, conduction defects, and premature ventricular contractions. The ECG has been found to be nonspecific and insensitive. Enzyme tests (including lactic dehydrogenase [LDH], aspartate aminotransferase [AST], creatine kinase [CK], and CK-MB band) have been found to be nonspecific, probably because of release of enzyme from noncardiac traumatized tissues. Angiography has been found sensitive and specific but is considered too invasive for widespread use. MUGA scanning has proved specific and sensitive. On MUGA, depressed right ventricular function is seen most commonly; depressed left ventricular function is seen on occasion. The right ventricle is thought most vulnerable because it is located directly behind the sternum and because its thin wall is easily injured transmurally.

Physiologic effects of the contusion can

range from none to ventricular dysfunction severe enough to require the intra-aortic balloon pump [39] or to cause death [31,40]. Severe dysfunction is unusual, however. Full recovery is the rule for patients who survive the associated injuries and the myocardial contusion [41]. One study has shown that regardless of other criteria of contusion, patients are unlikely to suffer significant complications if the CK-MB fraction is not elevated [32].

Management principles may be summarized as follows: All patients with blunt trauma to the chest should be suspected of having myocardial contusion. Serial CK-MB determinations and serial ECGs should be done. Patients with positive tests should be monitored in an intensive care setting, being treated like patients with acute myocardial infarction. Surveillance for complications is carried out, and complications are treated as in the setting of myocardial infarction.

Valvular Injuries

Injury of each of the cardiac valves has been reported from blunt trauma: aortic [42,43], mitral [44–48], pulmonary, and tricuspid [44,49–51]. These injuries should be suspected when congestive heart failure develops unexpectedly or when new murmurs are heard. The aortic valve is the most commonly injured; often, a leaflet is torn or detached from the aortic annulus. With the mitral valve, rupture of the papillary apparatus is the usual injury. It is thought that papillary muscle injury may occur when the traumatic blow occurs during systole, when the left ventricle is firm and the papillary apparatus taut. Left-sided injuries may produce abrupt hemodynamic compromise, as acute aortic insufficiency and mitral regurgitation are poorly tolerated. Right-sided injuries rarely produce early hemodynamic problems. Cardiac catheterization and valve repair or replacement are carried out with whatever urgency is dictated by the clinical setting.

Intracardiac Communications

Blunt trauma can produce ventricular septal defects [52] and cause aortocardiac fistula [43]. Diagnosis by catheterization and appropriate surgical repair are carried out, again with a timing determined by the clinical urgency.

Cardiac Rupture

Rupture of the chambers of the heart from blunt trauma is a well-known phenomenon that is usually immediately lethal in the field. Those few patients who survive commonly present with tamponade (if the pericardium does not decompress) or massive hemothorax (if the pericardium decompresses into the pleural space). All cardiac chambers have been known to rupture, including the right atrium [53–57], left atrium [52], right ventricle [52], left ventricle [54], aortic root, and main pulmonary artery. Most survivors have atrial tears, as ventricular tears are usually rapidly fatal. Most patients have been victims of motor vehicle accidents, but animal kicks to the chest represent another common cause of blunt cardiac rupture. It should be kept in mind that many of the atrial injuries occur at the junction with the feeding veins, SVC and IVC for the right atrium, and pulmonary veins for the left atrium. Diagnosis and treatment parallel those described for penetrating cardiac injuries. Speed in diagnosis and immediate operative intervention are of obvious importance. Cardiopulmonary bypass may be required for repair but usually is not, as most patients with large ventricular injuries die in the field.

Coronary Artery Injury

Coronary arteries can be injured by blunt trauma [58–61]. Bleeding may result in hemopericardium. Acute injury can lead to coronary occlusion and myocardial infarction; later, atherosclerotic narrowing, arteriovenous fistula, or coronary artery aneurysm may follow. Angina may be a late sequel due to atherosclerotic narrowing or "coronary steal" into the venous circulation through an arteriovenous fistula. Diagnosis is by catheterization. Treatment is individualized but may include coronary artery grafting.

Tension Pneumopericardium

In rare cases, air may find its way not only into the pleural space or mediastinum, but also into the pericardium after blunt traumatic lung injury [62–64]. Especially with positive pressure ventilation, tension may develop in the pericardium. Hemodynamic deterioration, analogous to ordinary cardiac tamponade, can develop. A characteristic "small heart" sign may be seen on chest x-ray. Treatment is urgent surgical decompression; subxiphoid pericardiotomy is a good approach.

Pericardial Rupture and Cardiac Herniation

Rupture of the pericardium from blunt trauma is a rare but well-documented condition [64–67]. Acute sequelae include hemorrhage into the thorax (from pericardial vessels or from the vessels in the phrenic neurovascular bundle) and cardiac herniation. Cardiac herniation can be acutely life-threatening. This is similar to the herniation through a pericardial defect that can occur after intrapericardial pneumonectomy. The heart slips into the chest (usually to the left side) through the opening in the pericardium (Fig. 9-6). The marked sudden displacement, with resultant strangulation of the heart, can cause a severe low-output state or sudden cardiac arrest. Late sequelae of pericardial rupture include herniation of intestines into the pericardium and a Dressler's-type pericarditis.

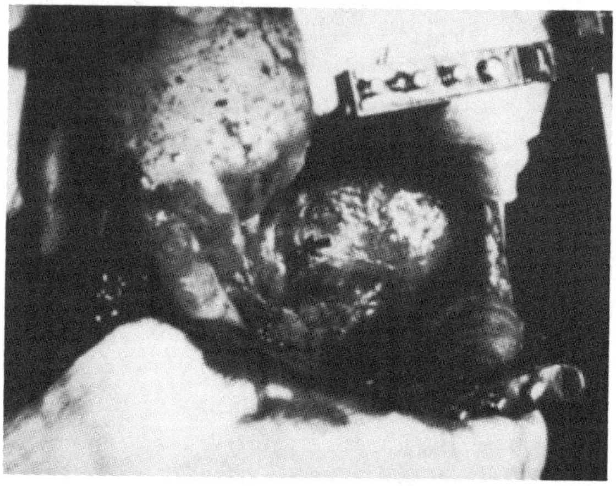

Fig. 9-6. Herniation of the heart through a pericardial rupture (*arrow*).

With rupture of the pericardium and sudden herniation, death may occur before the diagnosis is made. If vital signs are maintained, several clinical and radiologic clues may suggest the diagnosis. Heart sounds may be distant. The cardiac apex may be dislo-

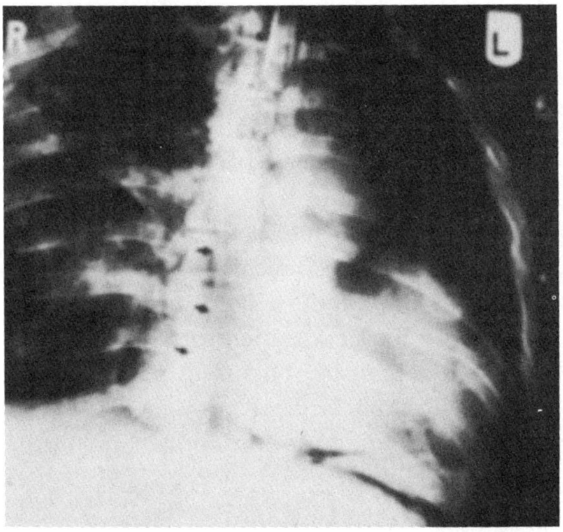

Fig. 9-7. Dislocation of the heart secondary to pericardial rupture shown on chest film.

cated. The ECG may show unusual axis and poor R-wave progression. On chest x-ray, the heart is seen to be dislocated (Fig. 9-7), the right vertebral shadows are seen more clearly than normal, and the left heart border is outlined especially distinctly. Fluoroscopy and echocardiography may provide additional clues. Angiography can confirm the diagnosis but is only indicated if the patient's condition is clinically stable.

The treatment for pericardial rupture with cardiac herniation is immediate thoracotomy for reduction of the heart. Either the pericardial defect is closed or the pericardium is excised widely to prevent further herniation.

Penetrating Injury

Penetrating injuries of the heart have increased in frequency in emergency departments because of increasing incidence of violent crime and improved and more rapid emergency medical systems. Still, up to 80 percent of patients with penetrating cardiac injuries, especially gunshot wounds, die before reaching the hospital. Some of the history of surgical treatment of penetrating cardiac trauma has recently been summarized [68]. Penetrating cardiac wounds are described in Homer's *Iliad.* Pericardiocentesis was first performed in 1829. In 1883, Billroth condemned pericardiocentesis as a "prostitution of the surgical art" and stated that a surgeon who attempted suture of the human heart should "lose the respect of his colleagues." Nonetheless, a German surgeon did successfully repair a human right ventricular stab wound in 1896. It was not until 1903 that the first cardiorraphy for cardiac stab wound was performed in this country.

Knife wounds and bullet wounds are the most common penetrating cardiac injuries. Ice pick wounds are not uncommon. Nails ejected by lawn mowers and [69] frank cardiac impalement [70] have been reported. Knife wounds cause lacerations much like surgical incisions; gunshot wounds create large defects.

The frequency with which each cardiac chamber is affected by penetrating trauma corresponds to the frontal area presented by each chamber to the anterior chest wall (Fig. 9-8); thus, the injured chamber, in decreasing order of frequency, is the right ventricle, left ventricle, right atrium, left atrium, and great vessels. Stab wounds of the right ventricle tend to continue to bleed because of the thin chamber wall; conversely, stab wounds of the left ventricle often seal spontaneously if they

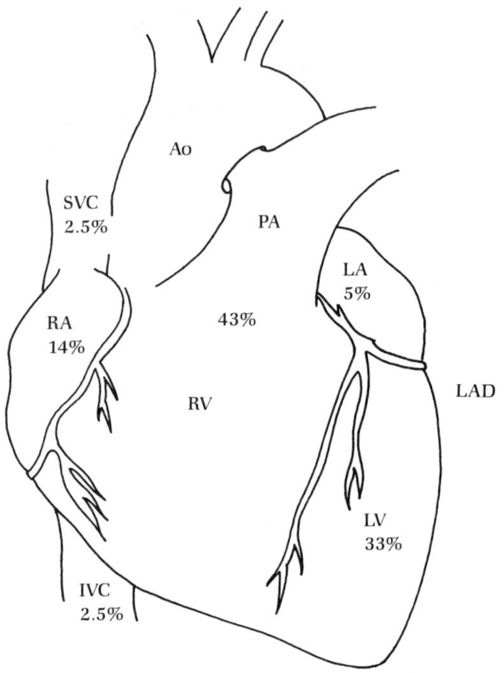

Fig. 9-8. Frequency distribution of penetrating cardiac trauma. Ao = aorta; SVC = superior vena cava; PA = pulmonary artery; LA = left atrium; RA = right atrium; RV = right ventricle; LAD = left anterior descending artery; LV = left ventricle; IVC = inferior vena cava. (Adapted from R. Karrel, M. A. Shaffer, and J. B. Franaszek, Emergency diagnosis, resuscitation, and treatment of acute penetrating cardiac trauma. *Ann. Emerg. Med.* 11:504, 1982.)

are not large, because the thicker wall seals the wound [71]. Atrial stab wounds may seal because of low pressure or may bleed by virtue of the thin wall.

Patients alive on arrival with penetrating cardiac wounds tend to present with one of three scenarios:

1. *Total stability:* This may be the case with a stab wound that seals promptly.
2. *Massive hemothorax:* This is seen when cardiac bleeding continues and empties through an accompanying pericardial defect into the pleural space. This is especially common with gunshot wounds, which tend to decompress into the pleural space because the corresponding pericardial defect is large.
3. *Cardiac tamponade:* This occurs when the cardiac injury continues to bleed but the pericardium seals. This is especially common with knife wounds, in which the pericardial slit may rapidly approximate and be closed by clot.

Management is chosen according to the manner of presentation. Stable patients may safely be observed, usually in an intensive care unit, if cardiac injury is suspected, as sudden bleeding can occur in patients previously stable. Because of the possibility of sudden bleeding, some [72] would advocate prompt pericardial window in all patients with suspected cardiac injury; this allows confirmation of hemopericardium, which in turn mandates surgery for assessment and repair.

A number of principles and techniques should be kept in mind for the repair of penetrating cardiac injuries (these supplement the general approaches discussed in the section on cardiac tamponade):

Stab wounds anywhere within the central thoracic mantle (Fig. 9-9) should be suspected to have incurred cardiac injury. A gunshot wound may produce cardiac in-

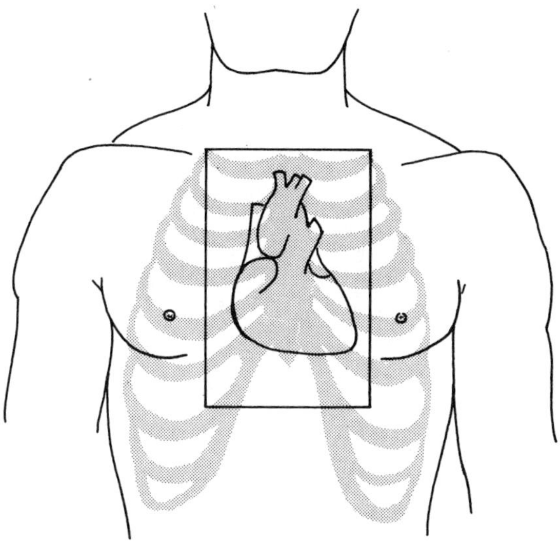

Fig. 9-9. Central thoracic mantle. Stab wounds anywhere in this mantle must be suspected to have produced cardiac injury. (Adapted from R. Karrel, M. A. Shaffer, and J. B. Franaszek, Emergency diagnosis, resuscitation, and treatment of acute penetrating cardiac trauma. *Ann. Emerg. Med.* 11:504, 1982.)

jury despite a distant entry wound, of course.

Most penetrating injuries of the heart can be repaired without cardiopulmonary bypass.

Finger control can stop bleeding from most atrial, ventricular, or aortic wounds (Fig. 9-10A).

Myocardial wounds can be repaired directly by pledgeted sutures (Fig. 9-10A). It is important to take deep bites with heavy suture and to tie just tightly enough to approximate the edges to avoid tearing through tissue and extending the defect.

Larger defects can be approximated by crossed parallel sutures (Fig. 9-10B) to effect hemostasis while multiple pledgeted sutures are placed.

Atrial injuries can often be excluded in a side-biting clamp (e.g., Satinsky, Cooley, Potts) and oversewn (Fig. 9-10C).

A Foley catheter is recommended by some to act as an obturator while repair is effected [73] (Fig. 9-10D).

Sutures can be passed below coronary arteries to close adjacent wounds without coronary occlusion (Fig. 9-10E).

Small, distal coronary branches should be ligated, if injured, rather than repaired.

Injury of major coronary arteries must be treated by ligation with coronary grafting beyond the lesion done on cardiopulmonary bypass.

Inflow occlusion (Fig. 9-10F) may be used to obtain a dry field for large right atrial, right ventricular, or pulmonary artery wounds. (This is similar to the technique used for urgent pulmonary embolectomy when cardiopulmonary bypass is not available.) A vascular clamp is placed on the SVC and one on the IVC, allowing the heart to beat empty. A dry field is thus obtained. Of course, circulation ceases during inflow occlusion, so repair of the injury must be effected within minutes and the clamps removed.

Internal massage is required for patients without adequate circulation. This must be done effectively but atraumatically, otherwise iatrogenic insult will be added to the traumatic injury. This is best performed between the palms of two hands.

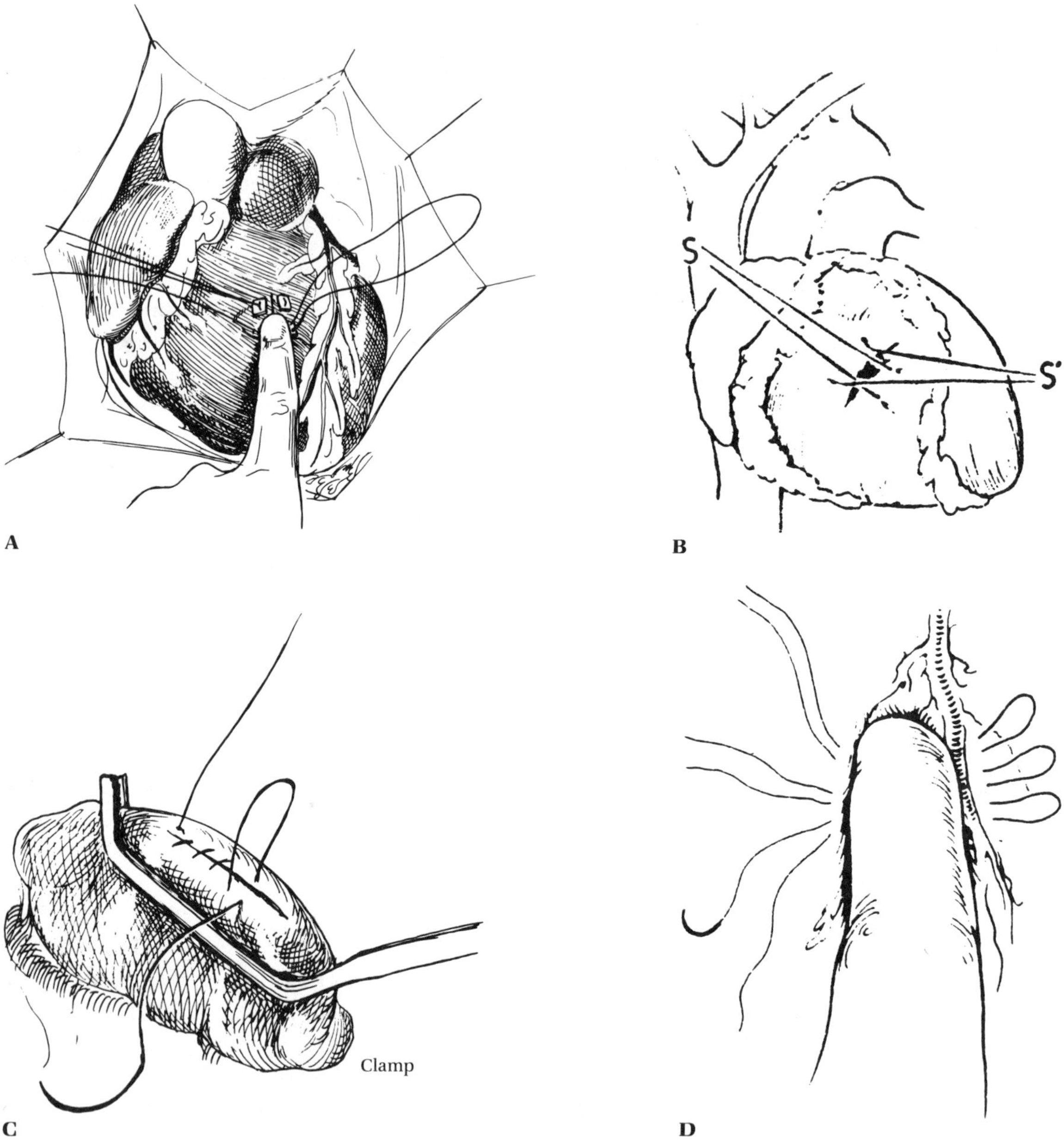

Fig. 9-10. Techniques for control and repair of penetrating cardiac injuries. *A.* Finger control, followed by pledgeted suture repair of myocardial stab wound. *B.* Crossed, parallel sutures for early control of large defects. *C.* Side-biting control and suturing of ascending aorta injury. *D.* Control of myocardial injury using Foley catheter as temporary obturator.

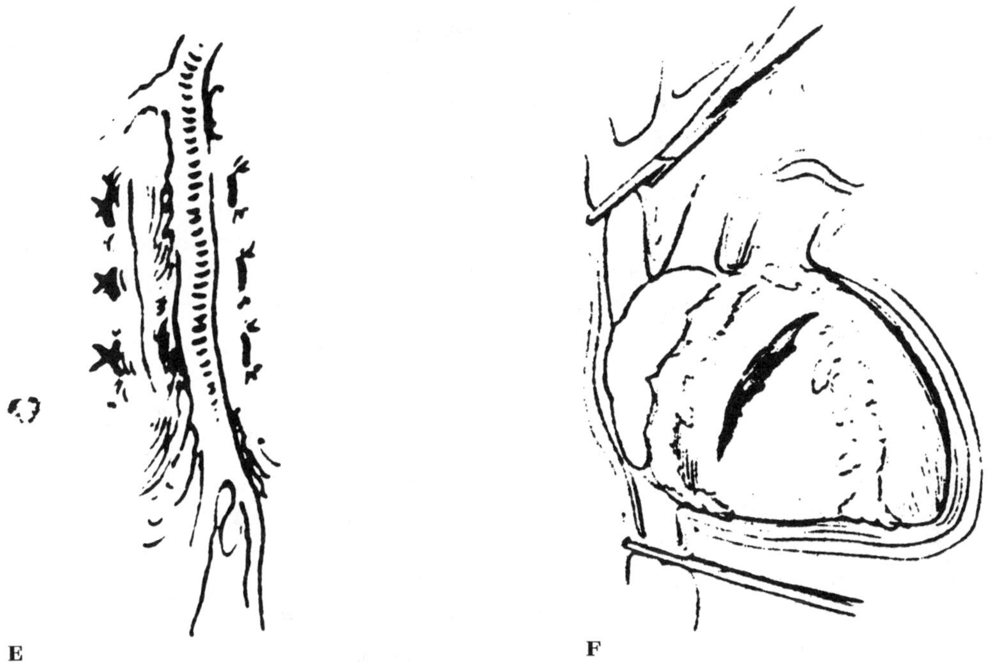

Fig. 9-10 (continued). *E.* Subcoronary suture ligation to spare coronary circulation. Sutures being placed (*left*) and tied (*right*). *F.* Inflow occlusion for large myocardial wound. Note clamps on SVC and IVC. (From D. C. Sabiston, Jr. and F. C. Spencer, *Gibbon's Surgery of the Chest* (4th ed.). Philadelphia: Saunders, 1983; J. K. Trinkle, J. Marcus, F. L. Groner, and L. M. Coello, Management of the wounded heart. *Ann. Thorac. Surg.* 17:230, 1974; J. Asfaw and A. Arbulu, Penetrating wounds of the pericardium and heart. *Surg. Clin. North Am.* 57:37, 1977.)

In certain cases, it may be best to allow ineffective circulation without massage for a minute or two while the injury is repaired, then restore volume, massage, and resuscitate the heart.

Internal defibrillation (10–20 joules only) and internal pacing are essential for open resuscitation. These techniques are described elsewhere [3].

It must be remembered that abdominal injuries may accompany stab wounds anywhere below the nipples, as the diaphragm comes quite high during expiration. Thoracic gunshot wounds always should be suspected to have produced abdominal injury as well, as the missile may travel extensively within the body.

Penetrating trauma can cause intracardiac injuries (septal or valvular) in addition to those injuries detected on the surface of the heart. This is commonly seen with gunshot wounds [74,75]. In most cases, unless hemodynamics are unstable or severe congestive heart failure is manifested, these injuries are best assessed by catheterization after the patient is recovered and treated electively if severe enough to warrant surgery [76].

ESOPHAGUS

Unlike cardiac, pulmonary, or great vessel injuries, esophageal injuries do not produce the serious immediate consequences of hemorrhage or respiratory and circulatory embarrassment. Prompt recognition is required, however, because sepsis can result within hours or days of unrecognized injuries and because problems of reconstruction become even more complex when recognition is delayed and tissues become inflamed.

The esophagus can suffer penetrating injury from knives or bullets. These injuries can occur anywhere along the length of the esophagus. The esophagus may rupture from blunt trauma. This rupture usually occurs in the low esophagus above the cardioesophageal junction, the same location where spontaneous rupture (Boerhaave's syndrome) is known to occur. Blunt rupture of the esophagus is not a commonly seen injury.

Signs and symptoms are usually delayed and are essentially those of mediastinitis, as are seen with iatrogenic instrumental perforations of the esophagus. There may be fever or even frank sepsis. Subcutaneous emphysema in the neck may be seen. A mediastinal "crunch" may be heard on auscultation. Patients who eat may report dysphagia.

On x-ray, air may be seen in the soft tissues of the neck or mediastinum. Pneumothorax or pleural effusion may be seen if the esophageal perforation communicates with the pleural space. Contrast esophagography makes the diagnosis of esophageal injury and indicates the location.

A high index of suspicion is critical in diagnosing esophageal injuries. Esophagography is mandatory whenever a penetrating injury occurs close to the esophagus. Likewise, if clinical or radiographic findings even remotely suggest blunt esophageal injury, contrast study is essential. Diagnosis, unfortunately, is often not made at all premortem or not made until late postinjury in blunt esophageal rupture.

Treatment includes administration of antibiotics and fluids and definitive surgical intervention. Early intervention (within hours) is important, both because sepsis is avoided and because primary repair of smaller injuries can be effected. With severe or neglected injuries, primary repair is not feasible; a variety of procedures to exclude the injured area and provide alternate enteral routes for alimentation have been described [77].

THORACIC DUCT

The thoracic duct can be injured by blunt trauma [78]. There are usually no early consequences. A persistent pleural effusion appears days or weeks later.

Thoracentesis yields a characteristic milky

fluid, which is sterile and shows chylomicrons on laboratory examination.

Treatment may be nonoperative (NPO, tube drainage) or operative (right thoracotomy, with ligation of the thoracic duct at the diaphragm).

SPECIAL TOPICS

Emergency Room Thoracotomy

The literature has seen a considerable debate over the advisability of emergency room thoracotomy for patients with chest injuries [72,79–87]. Several general principles can be extracted:

If the patient has preserved vital signs, transfer to the operating room is preferred. Light, equipment, and personnel are usually better in the operating room than in the emergency ward. Even if vital signs are suboptimal (with tachycardia and moderate hypotension) but stable, transfer to the operating room is preferred.

Emergency room thoracotomy is not only acceptable but *mandatory* for patients in extremis from *penetrating* chest wounds; emergency thoracotomy is *not indicated* for patients with *blunt* chest trauma. Of course, control of the airway, positive pressure ventilation, and volume administration need to be carried out immediately, before or during thoracotomy.

Salvage will be nil in patients without discernible signs of life in the field, in transit, or at any time after arrival in the emergency department. When this is clearly the case, unnecessary thoracotomy can be avoided. If there is any question of there having been signs of life, the patient should be given the benefit of the doubt and emergency thoracotomy performed. One interesting recent paper [88] has found that those patients who present in sinus rhythm, even with shock, do well, while those in agonal rhythms (asystole, ventricular fibrillation, slow ventricular escape rhythm) do poorly.

The technique is quite straightforward (Fig. 9-11). A left anterolateral thoracotomy is performed in the fourth or fifth intercostal space—below the breast in females or the prominence of the pectoral muscle in males—and taken from the sternum anteriorly to the edge of the latissimus muscle posteriorly. The pectoral and serratus muscles are incised parallel to the incision. The intercostal muscles are incised and a finger popped through the pleura; with the lung protected by the finger, the intercostal muscles are opened widely along the length of the incision. The chest retractor is placed. The lung is pushed posteriorly to expose the pericardium. It should be remembered that massive abdominal bleeding may push up the diaphragm, making it appear like the pericardium. The phrenic nerve and its accompanying vessels are visualized and preserved. The pericardium is grasped with toothed forceps and opened sharply—anterior to and parallel to the phrenic nerve. The incision is extended cephalad and caudad. The heart is lifted into position for inspection.

Defibrillation, pacing, internal massage, and repair of cardiac injuries are carried out as appropriate.

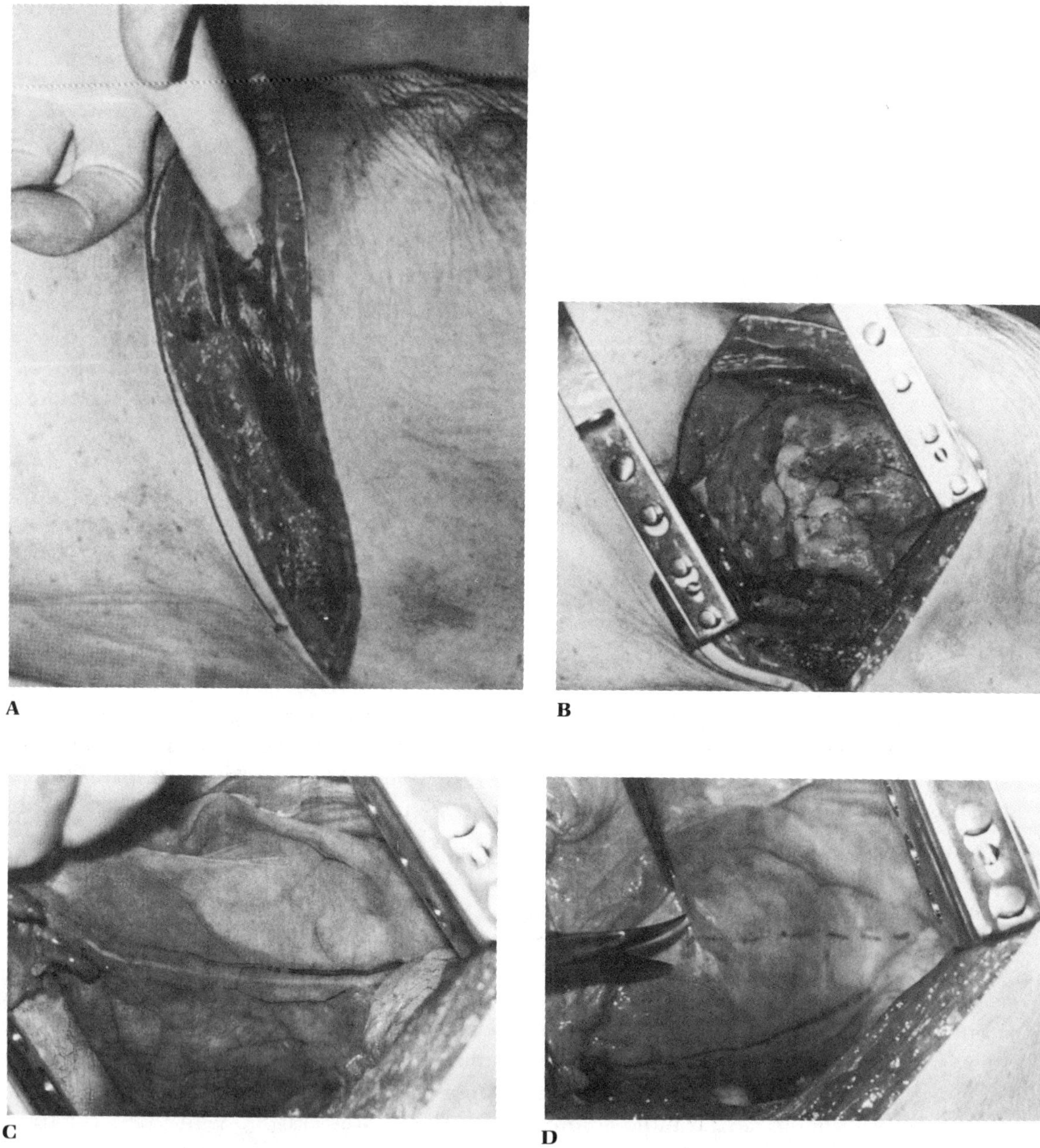

Fig. 9-11. Technique of emergency thoracotomy. *A.* Submammary anterolateral incision, breaking into the pleural space with index finger. *B.* Placement of chest retractor. *C.* Phrenic pedicle visualized. *D.* Incision of pericardium (*dotted line*) anterior and parallel to phrenic pedicle.

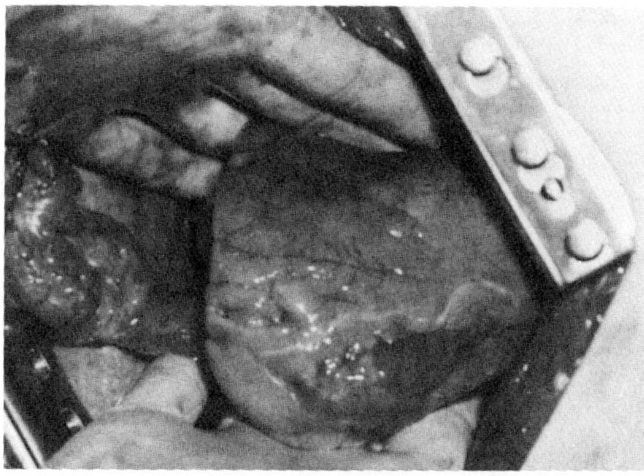

E

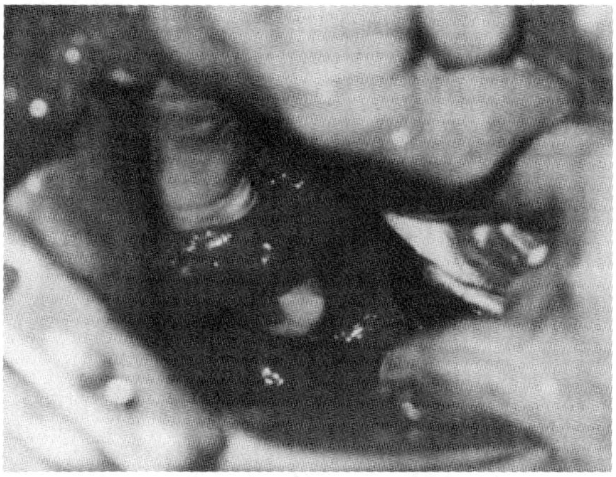

F

Fig. 9-11 (continued). *E.* Mobilization of heart for massage, inspection, and repair. Left anterior descending coronary artery seen. *F.* Mobilization of descending thoracic aorta for adjunctive clamping to facilitate resuscitation. (Adapted from H. E. Wahlstrom, B. J. Carroll, and E. H. Phillips, Emergency thoracotomy: Indications and technique. *Surg. Rounds* 86:23, 1986.)

The descending aorta can be controlled by retracting the lung anteriorly, incising the pleural reflection of the aorta, and mobilizing the aorta by finger dissection. A vascular clamp can be applied. This maneuver may occasionally be useful to raise blood pressure in the upper body.

The esophagus may easily be injured severely by the inexperienced operator, as it lies immediately anterior and medial to the aorta. Placing a nasogastric tube may aid in identifying and preserving the esophagus.

Infectious complications are minimal, even though sterility is often violated by emergency or "crash" thoracotomy.

Care should be taken not to injure the heart or coronary arteries when the pericardium is opened.

Thorough hemostasis (especially of the internal mammary and intercostal arteries) must be attained at the completion of the procedure.

Transmediastinal Gunshot Wounds

Patients with transmediastinal gunshot wounds with unstable vital signs require immediate exploration, as discussed in previous sections. Sternotomy or thoracotomy may be chosen.

Patients who are stable are best served by a specialized, systematic evaluation [89] rather than immediate surgery. Some of these patients may not require surgery at all; it is not uncommon for no vital structures to be injured by a transmediastinal missile. In those patients who do require exploration, the surgical approach may then be tailored to the specific injury uncovered.

The systematic diagnostic evaluation includes

1. *Angiography* to rule out great vessel arterial injury (great vessel venous injury need not be diagnosed if no significant bleeding is occurring).
2. *Esophagography* to rule out penetrating esophageal injury.
3. *Bronchoscopy* to rule out great airway injury.
4. *Subxiphoid pericardial window* to rule out intrapericardial bleeding. (Observation in an intensive care unit may at times substitute for subxiphoid exploration.)

Detection of injury can lead to precise planning of the approach. If all studies are negative, patients do well with general observation without surgery.

Autotransfusion

An elegant report by Symbas [89] has established through animal and subsequent clinical studies the safety and efficacy of autotransfusion of traumatic hemothorax. Blood draining from the chest is routed to a collection device and then reinfused at intervals through a filter. (Many commercial autotransfusion drainage devices are available.) No infection was seen in the study. No other adverse consequences of autotransfusion were noted. Risk of disease transmission from donor blood was avoided. Autotransfused red cells showed normal survival times, in contradistinction to the known shortened survival of donor blood cells.

Autotransfusion probably merits wider use in thoracic trauma, especially as convenient commercial equipment is now available at many centers for use postoperatively after open heart surgery.

Foreign Bodies in and Around the Heart

A colorful literature has developed surrounding foreign bodies in and about the heart [90–94]. The account by Harken [90] of 78 cases operated on in World War II is of great historical interest; specifically, the approaches to foreign body removal in this pre–cardiopulmonary bypass era are fascinating. Harken operated on these patients with *no mortality*.

When objects cause penetrating trauma to the heart with acute sequelae (bleeding or tamponade), urgent intervention is required. On occasion, a bullet (or other airborne particle) lodges in or around the heart without causing any acute problem. It is in such cases that the management of cardiac or pericardiac foreign bodies, per se, arises. It should be noted that there exist other avenues for foreign bodies to get to a position in or around the heart besides direct penetrating wounds: erosion from surrounding structures (esophagus, trachea, diaphragm) or migration through great veins (following a venous or hepatic injury).

The first important distinction is to recognize the precise locations that foreign bodies may occupy: in the parietal pericardium, inside the pericardial cavity but outside the myocardium, inside the myocardium, partially within the myocardium and partially inside a cardiac cavity, and fully within a cardiac cavity. The initial diagnosis of paracardiac foreign body is usually based on routine chest x-ray. It can be difficult to localize the foreign body precisely, to categorize its location among the possibilities mentioned above. Echocardiography, computed tomography (CT), and angiography may help with localization. Fluoroscopy may demonstrate whether the foreign body moves with the contracting heart wall. If the foreign body is freely movable with changes in the patient's position, this is strong evidence for intracavitary position.

Management essentials include the following:

At the time of an initial operation for acute consequences of penetrating cardiac trauma, only easily accessible foreign bodies should be removed. Further efforts may be required at a later date once the patient is stabilized.

At the time of the initial exploration, the pericardium should be searched for foreign bodies lying freely in the pericardium.

When they come to light late after surgery, foreign bodies outside the heart but inside the pericardial space do not necessarily require removal; they usually become encapsulated and remain dormant. On occasion, pericarditis, infection, or migration toward the cardiac chambers may occur, necessitating surgical intervention.

Foreign bodies embedded circumferentially within heart muscle usually become encapsulated and remain dormant; surgical therapy is not essential.

Foreign bodies lying partly within myocardium and partly within a cardiac chamber and those foreign bodies lying entirely within a cardiac chamber are more prone to complications and should be removed. Specifically, these foreign bodies may become involved with endocarditis or may embolize (to the lungs from the right heart and to the systemic circuit from the left heart). On occasion, they do become encapsulated and lie dormant, but this benign course cannot be predicted.

Foreign bodies in the right heart can be observed for a few days, in the hope that they will embolize to the lungs. Such emboli do not usually cause an acute problem; on the contrary, embolization to a pulmonary artery makes possible easier removal by thoracotomy without cardiopulmonary bypass. If they do not embolize, removal on cardiopulmonary bypass is recommended.

Foreign bodies in the left heart should be removed promptly, because of the danger of systemic embolization, especially to the brain.

Before surgery to remove a foreign body from the heart, thorough assessment for intracardiac injury (septal defect or valvular injury) should be carried out. This includes physical examination and possibly saturation runs or cardiac catheterization.

At surgery, for removal of foreign bodies, cardiopulmonary bypass is usually employed in the current day and age. It is important to clamp both the aorta and the pulmonary artery to prevent distal migration of the foreign body during cardiotomy. It is wise to have fluoroscopy available, in case the object is not readily found.

Occasionally, the radiologist may be able to snare and remove small foreign bodies by catheterization, thus avoiding open heart surgery.

REFERENCES

1. Mattox, K. L., and Allen, M. K. Emergency department treatment of chest injuries. *Emerg. Med. Clin. North Am.* 2:783, 1984.
2. Rutherford, R. B. Thoracic Injuries. In W. F. Ballinger, R. B. Rutherford, and G. D. Zuidema, *The Management of Trauma*. Philadelphia: Saunders, 1973.
3. Elefteriades, J. A., and Geha, A. S. *House Officer Guide to ICU Care*. Rockville, Md.: Aspen, 1985.
4. Westaby, S. Injury to the major airways. *Br. J. Hosp. Med.* 34:210, 1985.
5. Maloney, J. V., and MacDonald, L. Paradoxical respiration and "pendelluft." *J. Thorac. Cardiovasc. Surg.* 41:291, 1961.
6. Trinkle, J, Richardson, J., Franz, J., et al. Management of flail chest without mechanical ventilation. *Ann. Thorac. Surg.* 19:355, 1975.
7. Shackford, S., Virgilio, R., and Peters, R. Selective use of ventilator therapy in flail chest injury. *J. Thorac. Cardiovasc. Surg.* 81:194, 1981.
8. Worthley, L. I. Thoracic epidural anesthesia in the management of chest trauma. *Intens. Care Med.* 11:312, 1985.
9. Kelly, J. P., Webb, W. R., Moulder, P. V., and Everson, C., et al. Management of airway trauma I: Tracheobronchial injuries. *Ann. Thorac. Surg.* 40:551, 1985.
10. Lazar, H. L., Thomashow, B., and King, T. C. Complete transection of the intrathoracic trachea due to blunt trauma. *Ann. Thorac. Surg.* 37:505, 1984.
11. Rutherford, R. B., Hurt, H. H., Brichman, R. D., and Tubb, J. M. The pathophysiology and treatment of progressive tension pneumothorax. *J. Trauma* 8:212, 1968.
12. Isaacs, J. P., Berglind, E., and Sornoff, S. J. Ventricular function: III. Pathologic physiology of acute cardiac tamponade studied by means of ventricular function curves. *Am. Heart J.* 38:66, 1954.
13. Shabetai, R., Fowler, N., and Guntheroth, W. G. The hemodynamics of cardiac tamponade and constrictive pericarditis. *Am. J. Cardiol.* 26:480, 1920.
14. Shoemaker, W. Pericardial Tamponade. In W. Shoemaker, W. Thompson, and P. Holbrook (eds.), *Textbook of Critical Care*. Philadelphia: Saunders, 1984.
15. Arom, D. V., Richardson, J. D., Webb, G., et al. Subxiphoid pericardial window in patients with suspected traumatic pericardial tamponade. *Ann. Thorac. Surg.* 23:545, 1977.
16. Thompson, B. M., Finger, W., Tonsfeldt, D., et al. Rib radiograms for trauma: Useful or wasteful? *Ann. Emerg. Med.* 15:261, 1986.
17. von Hippel, A. *Chest Tubes and Chest Bottles*. Springfield, Ill.: Thomas, 1975.
18. Buckman, R., Trooskin, S. Z., Flankbaum, L., and Chandler, J. The significance of stable patients with sternal fracture. *Surg. Gynecol. Obstet.* 164:261, 1987.
19. Bowling, R., Mavroudis, C., Richardson, J. D., et al. Emergency pneumonectomy for penetrating and blunt trauma. *Ann. Surg.* 51:136, 1985.
20. Martinez, M. J., Hotzman, R. S., Salcedo, and Garcia-Rinaldi, R. Successful repair of a transected intrathoracic trachea after chest trauma. *J. Thorac. Cardiovasc. Surg.* 91:307, 1986.
21. Ecker, R. R., Libertini, R. V., Rea, W. J., et al. Injuries of the trachea and bronchi. *Ann. Thorac. Surg.* 11:289, 1971.
22. de la Rocha, A. G., and Kayler, D. Traumatic rupture of the tracheobronchial tree. *Can. J. Surg.* 28:68, 1985.
23. Neugebauer, M. K., Fine, J. B., and Hurt, T. W. Traumatic rupture of the trachea and mainstem bronchus. *J. Trauma* 14:265, 1974.
24. Bricher, D. L., Parker, T. M., and Dalton, M. L., Jr. Cardiopulmonary bypass in anesthetic management of resection: Its use for severe tracheal stenosis. *Arch. Surg.* 114:847, 1979.
25. Thomas, A. N., and Roe, B. B. Air embolism fol-

lowing penetrating lung injuries. *J. Thorac. Cardiovasc. Surg.* 66:533, 1973.
26. Graham, J. M., Beall, A. C., Mattox, K. L., and Vaughan, G. D. Systemic air embolism following penetrating trauma to the lung. *Chest* 72:449, 1977.
27. Yee, E. S., Verrier, E. D., and Thomas, A. N. Management of air embolism in blunt and penetrating thoracic trauma. *J. Thorac. Cardiovasc. Surg.* 85:661, 1983.
28. King, M. W., Aitchison, J. M., and Nel, J. D. Fatal air embolism following penetrating lung trauma: On autopsy study. *J. Trauma* 24:753, 1984.
29. Felson, B. Lung torsion: Radiographic findings in nine cases. *Radiology* 162:631, 1987.
30. Moser, E. S., Jr., and Proto, A. V. Lung torsion: Case report and literature review. *Radiology* 162:639, 1987.
31. Sutherland, G. R., Calvin, J. E., Driedger, A. A., et al. Anatomic and cardiopulmonary responses to trauma with associated blunt chest injury. *J. Trauma* 21:1, 1981.
32. Michelson, W. B. CPK-MB isoenzyme determinations: Diagnostic and prognostic valve in evaluation of blunt chest trauma. *Ann. Emerg. Med.* 9:562, 1980.
33. Sutherland, G. R., Driedger, A. A., Holliday, R. L., et al. Frequency of myocardial injury after blunt chest trauma as evaluated by radionuclide angiography. *Am J. Cardiol.* 52:1099, 1983.
34. Kron, J. L., and Cox, P. M., Jr. Cardiac injury after chest trauma. *Crit. Care Med.* 11:524, 1983.
35. Soliman, M. H., and Waxman, K. Value of a conventional approach to the diagnosis of traumatic cardiac contusion after chest injury. *Crit. Care Med.* 15:218, 1987.
36. Waxman, K., Soliman, M. H., Braunstein, P., et al. Diagnosis of traumatic cardiac contusion. *Arch. Surg.* 121:689, 1986.
37. Torres, M., Gruenberg, J. C., Brown, R. S., and Obeid, F. N. Spectrum of myocardial contusion. *Am Surg.* 48:383, 1982.
38. Tenzer, M. L. The spectrum of myocardial contusion: A review. *J. Trauma* 25:620, 1985.
39. Snow, N., Lucas, A. B., and Richardson, J. D. Intra-aortic balloon counterpulsation for cardiogenic shock from cardiac contusion. *J. Trauma* 22:426, 1982.
40. MacDonald, R. C., O'Neil, D., Hanning, C. D., and Ledingham, I. M. Myocardial contusion in blunt chest trauma: A ten-year review. *Inten. Care Med.* 7:365, 1981.
41. Sturaitis, M., McCallum, D., Sutherland, G., Cheung, H. W., et al. Lack of significant long-term sequelae following traumatic myocardial contusion. *Arch. Intern. Med.* 146:1765, 1986.
42. Devineni, R., and McKenzie, F. N. Avulsion of a normal aortic valve cusp due to blunt chest trauma. *J. Trauma* 24:910, 1984.
43. Rehr, R. B., Mack, M., and Firth, B. G. Aortic regurgitation and sinus of Valsalva–right atrial fistula after blunt thoracic trauma. *Br. Heart J.* 48:410, 1982.
44. Pellegrini, R. V., Copeland, C. E., DiMarco, R. F., et al. Blunt rupture of both atrioventricular valves. *Ann. Thorac. Surg.* 42:471, 1986.
45. Cuadros, C. L., Hutchinson, J. E., and Mogtader, A. H. Laceration of a mitral papillary muscle and the aortic root as a result of blunt trauma to the chest: Case report and review of the literature. *J. Thorac. Cardiovasc. Surg.* 88:134, 1984.
46. Mazzucco, A., Rizzoli, G., Faggion, G., et al. Acute mitral regurgitation after blunt chest trauma. *Arch. Intern. Med.* 143:2326, 1983.
47. Pillai, R., Fountain, S. W. Qureshi, S. A., et al. Avulsion of the anterior papillary muscle of the mitral valve due to non-penetrating trauma to the chest. *Thorax* 37:943, 1982.
48. Devineni, R., and McKenzie, F. N. Acute mitral insufficiency resulting from blunt chest trauma. *J. Thorac. Cardiovasc. Surg.* 85:797, 1983.
49. Katz, N. M., and Pallas, R. S. Traumatic rupture of the tricuspid valves: Repair by chordal replacements and annuloplasty. *J. Thorac. Cardiovasc. Surg.* 91:310, 1986.
50. Fracasso, A., Pothen, P., and Gallucci, V. Tricuspid regurgitation caused by blunt chest trauma in association with pericardial agenesis: Surgical correction after eight years. *Thorax* 37:75, 1982.
51. Sheikhzadeh, A., Langbehn, A. F., Ghabusi, P., et al. Chronic traumatic tricuspid insufficiency. *Clin. Cardiol.* 7:299, 1984.
52. Merzel, D. I., Sterling, M. C., and Custer, J. R. Massive fatal ventricular septal defect due to non-penetrating chest trauma in a six-year old boy: The role of early invasive monitoring in

an evolving lesion. *Pediatr. Emerg. Care* 1:138, 1985.
53. Tobin, H. M., Hirazka, L. F., and Vangish, T. Ruptured right atrium from non-penetrating trauma of the chest. *South. Med. J.* 79:499, 1986.
54. Martin, T. D., Flynn, T. C., Rawlands, B. J., et al. Blunt cardiac rupture. *J. Trauma* 24:287, 1984.
55. Parmlee, L. F., Manson, W. C., and Mattingly, T. W. Nonpenetrating traumatic injury to the heart. *Circulation* 18:371, 1958.
56. DiMarco, R. F., Layton, T. R., Manzetti, G. W., and Dellagrini, R. V. Blunt traumatic rupture of the right atrium and the right superior pulmonary vein. *J. Trauma* 23:353, 1983.
57. Getz, B. S., Davies, E., Steinberg, S. M., et al. Blunt cardiac trauma resulting in right atrial rupture. *J.A.M.A.* 255:761, 1986.
58. Loss, D. M., MacMillan, R. M., and Maranhao, V. Coronary artery obstruction due to blunt chest trauma with residual angina pectoris. *Cathet. Cardiovasc. Diagn.* 9:297, 1983.
59. Lascault, G., Komajda, M., Drobinski, G., and Grosgogeat, Y. Left coronary artery aneurysm and anteroseptal acute myocardial infarction following blunt chest trauma. *Eur. Heart J.* 7:538, 1986.
60. Stone, D. L., and Fleming, H. A. Aneurysm of left ventricle and left coronary artery after non penetrating chest trauma. *Br. Heart J.* 50:495, 1983.
61. Lowe, J. E., Adams, D. H., Dummings, R. G., et al. The natural history and recommended management of patients with traumatic coronary artery fistulas. *Ann. Thorac. Surg.* 36:295, 1983.
62. Mirvis, S. E., Indek, M., Schorr, R. M., and Diaconis, J. N. Post-traumatic tension pneumopericardium: The "small heart" sign. *Radiology* 158:663, 1986.
63. McDougal, C. B., Muldur, G. A., and Hoffman, J. R. Tension pneumopericardium following blunt chest trauma. *Ann. Emerg. Med.* 14:167, 1985.
64. Cummings, R. G., Wesby, R. L., Adams, D. H., and Lowe, J. E. Pneumopericardium resulting in cardiac tamponade. *Ann. Thorac. Surg.* 37:511, 1984.
65. Clifford, R. P., and Gill, K. S. Traumatic rupture of the pericardium with dislocation of the heart. *Injury* 16:123, 1984.
66. Kyriakidis, M., Vassiliadis, J., Kyriakidis, C. R., and Toutouzas, P. Rupture of the pericardium presenting as postpericardial trauma syndrome late after blunt chest injury. *Clin. Cardiol.* 9:467, 1986.
67. Tulasne, P. A., Gaudias, J., Laporte, B., et al. Cardiac arrest caused by pericardial heart dislocation. *Ann. Fr. Anesth. Reanim.* 5:78, 1986.
68. Shaffer, K. R., and Franaszek, J. B. Emergency diagnosis, resuscitation and treatment of acute penetrating cardiac trauma. *Ann. Emerg. Med.* 11:504, 1982.
69. David, C., Schecter, D. C., and Gilbert, L. Injuries to the heart and great vessels due to pins and needles. *Thorax* 24:246, 1969.
70. McGill, J. W., Moore, E. B., and Marx, J. A. Successful management of cardiac impalement: The result of an integrated EMS-trauma system. *J. Trauma* 26:702, 1986.
71. Asfaw, J., and Agustin, A. Penetrating wound of the pericardium and heart. *Surg. Clin. North Am.* 57:37, 1977.
72. Karrel, R., Shaffer, M. A., and Franaszek, J. B. Emergency diagnosis, resuscitation and treatment of acute penetrating cardiac trauma. *Ann. Emerg. Med.* 11:504, 1982.
73. Wilson, S. M., and Au, F. C. In extremis use of a Foley catheter in a cardiac stab wound. *J. Trauma* 26:400, 1986.
74. Hardy, J. D., and Timmis, H. Repair of intracardiac gunshot injuries: Report of three cases. *Ann. Surg.* 169:906, 1969.
75. Borkon, A. M., Schneider, R., Serr, M., and Reutz, B. Immediate mitral valve replacement following gunshot wound to the heart. *J. Trauma* 27:96, 1987.
76. Wilson, R. F. Trauma. In W. C. Shoemaker, W. L. Thompson, and P. R. Holbrook, *Textbook of Critical Care*. Philadelphia: Saunders, 1984.
77. Urschel, H. C., Razzuk, M. A., Wood, R. E., et al. Improved management of esophageal perforation: Exclusion and diversion in continuity. *Ann. Surg.* 179:587, 1974.
78. Pai, G. P., Bhatt, N. A., Ellison, R. G., et al. Thoracic injury from blunt trauma. *South. Med. J.* 77:667, 1984.
79. Krome, R. L., and Dalbec, D. L. Emergency thoracotomy. *Emerg. Med. Clin. North Am.* 4:459, 1986.
80. Wahlstrom, H. E., Carroll, B. J., and Phillips, E. H. Emergency thoracotomy: Indications and technique. *Surg. Rounds* 9:23, 1986.

81. Tavares, S., Henkins, J. R., Moulton, A. L., et al. Management of penetrating cardiac injuries: The role of emergency room thoracotomy. *Ann. Thorac. Surg.* 38:183, 1984.
82. Washington, B., Wilson, R. F., Steiger, Z., and Gassett, J. S. Emergency thoracotomy: A four-year review. *Ann. Thorac. Surg.* 40:188, 1985.
83. Cogbill, T., Moore, E. E., Millikan, J. S., and Cleveland, H. C. Rationale for selective application of emergency department thoracotomy in trauma. *J. Trauma* 23:453, 1983.
84. Beaver, B. L., Colombani, P. M., Buck, J. R., et al. Efficacy of emergency room thoracotomy in pediatric trauma. *J. Pediatr. Surg.* 22:19, 1987.
85. Feliciano, D. V., Bitando, C. G., Cruse, P. A., et al. Liberal use of emergency center thoracotomy. *Am. J. Surg.* 152:654, 1986.
86. Schwab, C. W., Adcock, O. T., and Max, M. H. Emergency department thoracotomy: A 26 month experience using an "agonal" protocol. *Am. Surg.* 52:20, 1986.
87. Baker, C. C., Thomas, A. N., and Trunkey, D. D. The role of emergency room thoracotomy in trauma. *J. Trauma* 20:848, 1980.
88. Brautigan, M. W., and Tictz, G. Emergency thoracotomy in an urban community hospital: Initial cardiac rhythm as a new predictor of survival. *Am. J. Emerg. Med.* 3:311, 1985.
89. Symbas, P. N. Extraoperative autotransfusion from hemothorax. *Surgery* 84:722, 1978.
90. Harken, D. E. Foreign bodies in, and in relation to, the thoracic blood vessels and heart. *Surg. Gynecol. Obstet.* 83:117, 1946.
91. Bland, E. F., and Beebe, G. W. Missiles in the heart: A twenty year followup report of World War II cases. *U.S. Navy Med. News Lett.* 48:3, 1966.
92. Symbas, P. N. Blunt and Penetrating Trauma to the Heart. In W. W. L. Glenn (ed.), *Thoracic and Cardiovascular Surgery.* Norwalk, Conn.,: Appleton-Century-Crofts, 1983.
93. Symbas, P. N., and Harlaftis, N. Bullet emboli in the pulmonary and systemic arteries. *Ann. Surg.* 185:318, 1977.
94. Schechter, D. C., and Gilbert, L. Injuries of the heart and great vessels due to pins and needles. *Thorax* 24:246, 1969.

10
Abdominal Trauma

Liver Injuries

Evan R. Geller and Alexander J. Walt

Injury to the liver remains a major challenge to the surgeon caring for the injured patient. Despite extensive military and civilian experience, morbidity from these injuries continues to exceed 25 percent, with mortality rates ranging between 6 and 15 percent depending on the severity of the injuries treated. These statistics have prompted reevaluation of the techniques utilized to manage liver trauma and stimulated new approaches to the management of more complex injuries. In practice, surgical decisions are straightforward and management uncomplicated in about 80 percent of patients. In the remaining 20 percent, however, the surgeon's actions will very clearly determine the incidence of morbidity and mortality. Regarding these patients, the surgeon is required to possess a broad knowledge of the various techniques available as well as the wisdom with which to apply them.

ETIOLOGY

The liver is the most frequently injured solid organ in patients suffering abdominal trauma. The spectrum of injury is broad, with the majority of parenchymal injuries requiring little or no treatment. Life-threatening hepatic injury may be sustained following either penetrating or blunt trauma. In the United States, penetrating injuries to the liver are the type most frequently encountered in the setting of the major urban trauma center. In the accumulated series from Detroit Receiving Hospital, penetrating injuries accounted for approximately 85 percent of the patients undergoing operation (Table 10-1). Stab wounds and low-velocity gunshot wounds usually

Table 10-1. Mechanism and Mortality of Liver Injuries, Wayne State University 1980–1985

Agent	No. of patients	Deaths
Gunshot wound	137	11 (8%)
Stab wound	110	4 (4%)
Blunt trauma	26	9 (35%)
Shotgun wound	7	1 (14%)
Iatrogenic	2	0
	282	25 (8.9%)

seen in civilian practice most commonly result in relatively minor parenchymal injury requiring modest treatment; the outcome is almost uniformly excellent. Occasionally, associated major vascular injury to the hilar or juxtahepatic vessels, colon, or intrathoracic organs may render the patient unsalvageable. The hepatic parenchymal injury, however, is the injury of fatal consequence in about one-third of deaths. Despite this fact, it should be noted that the poorly managed liver injury, leading to intra-abdominal hematoma or biliary collection, may combine with associated injuries to result in significant morbidity or even the demise of an otherwise salvageable patient.

In contrast, blunt abdominal trauma not infrequently results in severe, even fatal, liver injury. Next to the spleen, the liver is the most commonly injured solid organ in blunt trauma. Extensive destruction of hepatic parenchyma, often in the form of stellate lacerations or major fractures extending across anatomic planes of resection, may be so severe as to be fatal in their own right. Such injuries require a thorough knowledge of hepatic anatomy and challenge the surgeon's ability to combine techniques of resection and debridement with those of repair, hemostasis, and appropriate management of biliary disruption. Concomitant injuries, the need for massive transfusion, and shock raise exponentially the rate of morbidity and mortality in this challenging group of injured patients.

As invasive radiologic procedures become increasingly common and aggressive, the surgeon is being called on to treat a new and increasing population of patients with iatrogenic liver injury. These patients, having undergone percutaneous liver biopsy, computed tomography (CT)–guided placement of drainage catheters, or the insertion of biliary stents, may suffer complications of parenchymal injury such as hemorrhage or biliary disruption. These complications are more frequently encountered when invasive procedures are applied to patients with preexisting liver disease, such as cirrhosis. Other disease states, such as sickle cell disease, peliosis, coagulopathy, or pregnancy [1] may lead to apparently spontaneous hemorrhage from the liver, requiring operation.

DIAGNOSIS

The variability in presentation of patients suffering liver trauma reflects the broad range of underlying injury. Relatively minor injuries or injuries resulting in minimal bleeding may be asymptomatic. Most such injuries are detected incidentally at laparotomy performed specifically for nonhepatic injury. Those individuals suffering more extensive hepatic injury may present with the clinical picture of intra-abdominal hemorrhage, deepening hypotension, abdominal tenderness, and perhaps expanding hemoperitoneum. Such a presentation leads to early diagnosis and prompt surgical intervention. There exists between these extremes, however, a population of patients harboring injuries to the liver that may be subtle in presentation but nonetheless significant and requiring operation. It is this group that challenges the diagnostic abilities of the examining physician and demands a high degree of suspicion.

CASE STUDY

A 40-year-old driver involved in a high-speed motor vehicle accident presented to the emergency department alert with stable vital signs. Abdominal examination was unremarkable. Twenty minutes after admission, the patient developed deepening hypotension and rapidly expanding abdominal distention. Emergency laparotomy initially revealed only splenic rupture. The liver was free of obvious injury, and there was no evidence of retroperitoneal hematoma. Prior to closure, however, a persistent trickle of venous blood from the area below the xyphoid was noted. Further exploration was greeted with sudden, massive bleeding. Median sternotomy and division of the diaphragm revealed a 6-cm tear of the retrohepatic vena cava.

Any recent history of trauma to the right upper abdominal quadrant or lower thorax should immediately signal the presence of possible hepatic injury. Right-sided rib fractures, right pleural effusion, and penetrating injury at or below the fourth intercostal space are frequent indirect indications of liver trauma. Similarly, injury to the diaphragm and underlying liver may be reflected in bilious drainage from a tube thoracostomy or by pain referred to the right shoulder. As in all aspects of medicine, a careful history and thorough physical examination are of paramount importance in diagnosing hepatic injury.

Laboratory examinations, with the exception of serial hematocrit determinations, are rarely helpful. These studies are not sensitive indicators of acute injury and should not be relied on to rule out significant liver injury.

Currently, gunshot wounds to the abdomen are routinely explored at most institutions and therefore do not present a diagnostic dilemma as regards liver injury. However, blunt abdominal trauma may be a testing diagnostic challenge in the most experienced hands, particularly in association with obtundation secondary to head injury or inebriation. Stab wounds may present a similar problem in regard to diagnosis of significant associated intra-abdominal injury. In these settings, several diagnostic modalities have proved invaluable. Diagnostic peritoneal lavage has been shown repeatedly to be 95-percent sensitive and at least 90-percent specific in the diagnosis of significant intra-abdominal injury [2]. Peritoneal lavage is a simple and effective method of quickly diagnosing significant intra-abdominal hemorrhage. It may be employed early in the selective evaluation of patients suspected of liver injury but is losing popularity with the availability of the CT scan. A positive lavage with a red blood cell count greater than 100,000 cells/μl, the aspiration of 10 ml of gross blood on initial tap, or the inability to read newsprint through the IV tubing should prompt serious consideration of surgical exploration.

While diagnostic peritoneal lavage may indicate the presence of significant intra-abdominal hemorrhage, it cannot indicate the anatomic source of hemorrhage. If necessary, the injury may be determined preoperatively by means of CT scan. While plain radiologic examinations of the abdomen have little diagnostic value in the setting of liver trauma, CT scan has proved to be uniquely suited to the evaluation of solid organ injury. Preoperative CT scan is gaining increasing popularity in the diagnosis of intra-abdominal injury, as it has proved to be an accurate, noninvasive method of determining liver injury [3]. CT scan enjoys the added advantage of demonstrating associated injuries to the spleen, pancreas, kidney, and retroperitoneum with excellent sensitivity. The CT scan provides information concerning the anatomy of the liver, as well as allowing estimation of the quantity of intraperitoneal blood, provided peritoneal lavage has not been performed prior to CT scan (Fig. 10-1). The sensitivity of CT scanning in detecting intraparenchymal hematomas has permitted the selective nonoperative management of this lesion with serial CT scan monitoring. This diagnostic technique, however, should only be employed in the setting of a cooperative and hemodynamically stable patient. Patients requiring continued fluid resuscitation or demonstrating clinical deterioration require urgent operation, and CT scan is contraindicated.

Fig. 10-1. CT scan of 19-year-old motorcycle rider involved in a high-speed collision. Scan reveals major disruption of the right hepatic lobe and spleen as well as the hemoperitoneum.

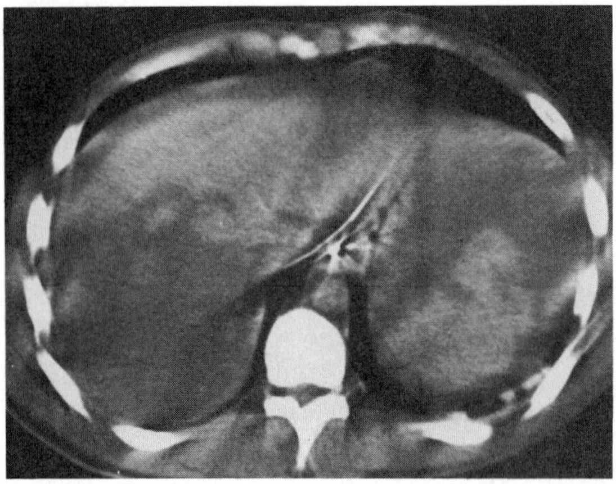

TREATMENT

The single greatest danger attending liver injury is hemorrhage. Therefore, initial evaluation of the injured patient is directed toward the prompt diagnosis and aggressive treatment of ongoing blood loss from the liver injury. Patients presenting with hypotension require the rapid placement of several large-bore intravenous cannulas and resuscitation with isotonic crystalloid solution. Rapid access to the central venous circulation may be gained through the percutaneous placement of subclavian or internal jugular venous catheters, but the potential hazard of an iatrogenic pneumothorax in the shocked patient must be recognized. Alternatively, large volumes of resuscitative solutions may be administered rapidly through sterile intravenous extension tubing introduced directly into the saphenous vein by means of a cutdown at the ankle. Those patients responding promptly to replacement volumes of less than 3 liters of the crystalloid infusion may be carefully monitored while the infusion rate is decreased and evaluation continued; patients remaining hypotensive after 3 liters of rapid crystalloid infusion, or those patients who again become hypotensive after initial normalization of blood pressure, require initiation of blood transfusion and emergent operative intervention. In these latter patients, it has been our policy at Detroit Receiving Hospital to begin transfusion with type-specific blood through multiple IV lines as the patient is rapidly transported to the operating suite. Nasogastric and Foley catheters are inserted. Tetanus and antibiotic prophylaxis is initiated. A regimen of either a second-generation cephalosporin or a combination of penicillin, gentamicin, and clindamycin is begun in anticipation of possible concomitant gastrointestinal injury.

On the operating room table, the patient is prepped from chin to knees and draped widely in anticipation of possible drainage sites or ostomies. An upper midline incision provides rapid and adequate exposure of most injuries and is easily extended into either side of the chest or, more likely, as a median sternotomy if this should prove necessary. Once the abdomen is entered, any hemoperitoneum is rapidly evacuated. Packs are placed about the injured liver and may be required in each of the abdominal quadrants as well. As each quadrant is subsequently explored, injuries are evaluated and hemorrhage controlled. With the possible exception of injuries to the inferior vena cava or juxtahepatic veins, this initial perihepatic packing, perhaps supported by a firmly applied deep retractor, is almost always effective in obtaining adequate hemostasis while the urgent injuries lying in other quadrants are attended to.

After adequate hemostasis in the other quadrants has been obtained and points of intestinal disruption controlled, the pack is removed from the right upper quadrant. Commonly, significant bleeding has ceased. If the wound is easily visualized, attention may be directed to definitive repair of associated injuries and the hepatic wound observed. When the liver wound is not directly visible, adequate mobilization is mandatory to expose it clearly. Mobilization is usually begun by division of the round ligament of the falciform ligament over the superior aspect of the liver. This maneuver allows traction on the liver in a posterior and inferior direction and should be performed early and routinely for all significant liver injuries. Further mobilization of the individual hepatic lobes may be afforded by division of the right or left triangular ligaments, leading to exposure of the anterior and superior surfaces of the respective lobes. The left triangular ligament is usually easily divided under direct vision. The right triangular ligament, however, often must be divided blindly, at times in the face of obscuring hemorrhage. Care must be taken to palpate the tips of the scissors with the opposite and retracting hand to protect the inferior vena cava and right hepatic vein from injury as the dissection is continued posteriorly. One must also be cautious to avoid injury to the inferior phrenic vessels coursing along the underside of the diaphragm as the triangular ligament is divided on either side.

Division of the ligamentous attachments between the liver and diaphragm allows mobilization of the liver toward the midline where hemostasis and debridement of the parenchymal injury may be more easily performed. Extensive debridement of ischemic liver up to 400 gm of tissue or more with preservation of venous drainage to the extent possible may be the optimal technique. In parallel with this, direct ligation of large intraparenchymal vessels under direct vision may be accomplished and obviate the use of an atriocaval shunt.

Mobilization alone will not usually provide adequate exposure of injuries to the retrohepatic vena cava. In the face of such an injury, extension of the abdominal incision into the chest is necessary. Extension into a median sternotomy is the preferred approach, as this may be accomplished rapidly and provides excellent exposure. Following division of the sternum, the diaphragm is divided in the sagittal plane from the xyphoid to the inferior vena cava. This approach also affords the exposure needed for the placement of an atriocaval shunt should this be required. An alternative approach is the extension of the midline abdominal incision obliquely across the costal cartilages into the right thorax. This thoracoabdominal approach with division with the right hemidiaphragm provides excellent access to the posterior aspect of the right lobe of the liver and juxtahepatic veins but is tolerated less well than median sternotomy in the postoperative period, resulting in a higher incidence of pulmonary complications. Left thoracotomy may occasionally be necessary in the massively bleeding patient to allow cross clamping of the descending aorta. In the patient exhibiting unrelenting shock and a tense hemoperitoneum, initial thoracotomy and aortic clamping prior to laparotomy has been utilized in an effort to avert the sudden and fatal shock often accompanying the release of the abdominal tamponade [4].

The majority of hepatic parenchymal injuries encountered will either have stopped bleeding totally at the time of operation or be easily controlled with pack compression for the period necessary to complete the abdominal survey and deal with associated major injuries. Failure of a properly placed perihepatic pack to control bleeding from the right upper quadrant should strongly suggest injury to the retrohepatic vena cava or juxtahepatic veins. In this event, efforts to obtain adequate exposure as described above are rapidly undertaken. In the absence of injury to these major vascular structures, a perihepatic pack will afford excellent hemostasis. Upon subsequent removal of the pack and mobilization of the liver to afford exposure of the injuries, the majority of hepatic wounds will be found to be bleeding modestly or not at all. In those instances where removal of the pack is greeted by significant hemorrhage, a Pringle maneuver should be performed. This maneuver involves occlusion of the portal triad by application of a vascular clamp to the margin of the hepatoduodenal ligament [5]. Failure of such inflow occlusion to control hemorrhage adequately again suggests the possibility of retrohepatic caval or juxtahepatic venous injury; occasionally, an anomalous hepatic artery may be responsible. When the Pringle maneuver affords adequate hemostasis, the vascular clamp is left in place until adequate exposure and local hemostasis at the wound site are accomplished. Traditionally, the clamp was released every 15 to 20 minutes during operation to allow periods of hepatic perfusion. More recently, periods of inflow occlusion have been extended to more than an hour without evidence of complication. Currently, it is common practice to continue inflow occlusion until local hemostasis is obtained [6].

A multitude of techniques have evolved to achieve hepatic hemostasis (Table 10-2). Difficult lesions will often require a combination of several such techniques. The placement of hepatic parenchymal sutures is the most frequently employed hemostatic method. While the subject of some condemnation of late, the careful placement of sutures, usually 2-0 chromic on a blunt-tipped liver needle in a mattress fashion about or across the site of injury, will frequently provide hemostasis. Care must be taken to avoid undue tension, which risks necrosis of hepatic tissue. While this technique is effective for controlling hemorrhage from relatively superficial lesions, it is ineffective and hazardous when employed inappropriately in efforts to control significant bleeding from within the depths of a hepatic lobe, leading to necrosis of large areas of parenchyma and possible intrahepatic hematoma formation.

Table 10-2. Method of Treatment of Liver Injuries, Wayne State University 1980–1985 (282 Patients)

Treatment	No. of patients
Laparotomy alone	71 (25%)
Local pressure	136 (48%)
Suture	68 (24%)
Hepatotomy/ligation	12 (4%)
Hepatic artery ligation	5 (2%)
Nonanatomic debridement	11 (4%)
Lobectomy	8 (3%)
Atrial-caval shunt	7 (2%)
Packing	9 (3%)

When the depth of the wound precludes safe employment of simple hepatic suture, the actively bleeding hepatic wound must be exposed through a hepatotomy to permit direct ligation of injured intrahepatic vessels and biliary radicles [7]. Exposure may be accomplished through hepatotomy by finger-fracture or other blunt dissection techniques. Once the full extent of the wound is exposed and adequate hemostasis is obtained, the margins of the injury may then be reapproximated through the use of liver sutures. While ideally all actively bleeding hepatic wounds would be treated by means of hepatotomy and ligation of bleeding points, there are times when this is not practical. Such a case is encountered when an actively bleeding penetrating injury tract traverses the depths of a hepatic lobe. While superficial tracts should be opened and direct vascular control obtained, the large volume of normal hepatic tissue that must be divided to expose adequately the deeply placed injury tract precludes the early application of this technique. The temptation to close the bleeding ends of the penetrating tract with deeply placed hepatic sutures should be eschewed due to the substantial risk of subsequent hematoma formation [8]. Alternative techniques must therefore be employed.

More recently, the technique of packing bleeding hepatic wounds with pedicled omentum has been advocated in facilitating hemostasis and has been enjoying increased utilization. Such a pack may be used to fill a parenchymal crack or otherwise obliterate parenchymal dead space, affording control of venous bleeding [9,10], but is not applicable to unopened missile tracks.

When the bleeding wound is not amenable to the aforementioned techniques, or when active arterial bleeding recurs from the depths of a laceration upon release of the Pringle maneuver, the technique of selective hepatic artery ligation may effect hemostasis [11,12]. The technique is not without risk and is employed in less than 3 percent of all cases. Hepatic artery ligation is reserved for those instances where bleeding is stemmed with compression of the appropriate hepatic artery and where hemostasis cannot otherwise be obtained. The ligation should be performed as close as possible to the liver to preserve collateral flow. While usually safe, this technique does entail a risk of hepatic necrosis, particularly when employed in combination with extensive mobilization of the bleeding lobe and placement of perihepatic packs.

When these relatively simple techniques have failed to achieve adequate hemostasis, the surgeon must ultimately consider resorting to the placement of a perihepatic pack and abdominal closure or lobectomy to avert death from exsanguination. If the former is selected, dry laparotomy packs are placed above and below the liver to achieve compression of the bleeding parenchyma, but excessive pack compression must be avoided following extensive mobilization and hepatic artery ligation, as this combination may lead to hepatic ischemia and necrosis. Posterior compression of the inferior vena cava by the pack is also carefully avoided. Postoperatively, the patient is maintained on mechanically assisted ventilation, as diaphragmatic movement is impaired. Antibiotic coverage is maintained during the period that the packs are in place. Approximately 36 to 96 hours later, when the patient has recovered from the perioperative hemodynamic and metabolic insult, the packs are removed at formal laparotomy. There is usually little or no bleeding at this time. If necessary, other techniques of hemostasis may be applied now that the patient has recovered from the metabolic derangements of shock, such as a direct transhepatic approach to the bleeding site.

While the technique of perihepatic packing is often reserved as a last-ditch effort to get the patient off the operating table, recent experiences support earlier employment of the technique prior to massive blood loss and its attendant morbidity [13–15]. Certainly the development of the diffuse bleeding seen secondary to coagulopathy should be an indication to proceed quickly to perihepatic packing and closure [16,17]. The technique of perihepatic packing has also been employed in the treatment of large, nonexpanding intraparenchymal hematoma. This technique allows compression to prevent expansion of hematoma and avoids deep hepatotomy for selective vessel ligation or the need for a large hepatic resection.

No current discussion of the management of liver injuries would be complete without mention of a nonoperative approach. With the development of high-resolution CT scanning, it has become possible to diagnose liver injury short of exploratory laparotomy. In patients with blunt abdominal trauma who have evidence of liver injury by CT scan but who do not demonstrate clinical signs of significant continuing hemorrhage, nonoperative management with close observation and serial CT or ultrasonographic scanning has been demonstrated to be safe in selected cases [18–20]. While such an approach to penetrating injury of the liver has been recently advocated by some, most centers still employ routine exploration due to the high frequency of associated injuries. In patients in whom a nonoperative approach is pursued, close in-hospital observation with the patient at bed rest for 1 to 2 weeks is essential. If serial CT scan and hematocrit determinations show no evidence of expansion of the hematoma, the patient is discharged on limited activity to be followed closely with serial scanning. As resolution of the hematoma is demonstrated, activity is slowly increased over 6 to 8 weeks. The development of peritoneal signs or evidence of hematoma expansion at any time mandates prompt surgical exploration. The technique appears most applicable to the pediatric population.

Injury to the Retrohepatic Vena Cava and Juxtahepatic Vasculature

Injury to the retrohepatic vena cava remains a formidable challenge. The injury may be suspected preoperatively by the trajectory of a penetrating missile and cannot be excluded by a preoperative clinical picture that suggests negligible bleeding. Massive hemorrhage may be delayed for many hours. In such cases, massive bleeding may be encountered from the right upper quadrant as soon as the abdomen is opened. Not uncommonly, however, initial bleeding may be only moderate until further mobilization of the liver for better exposure is greeted by massive dark hemorrhage. Major venous injury is also suggested by posterior bleeding that is not abated by the placement of compressive packs. Indeed, the usual practice of placing a pack above the diaphragmatic surface of the liver to achieve compression may cause distraction of the cava at the point of injury and initiate or exacerbate the bleeding. When such a circumstance is encountered, the diagnosis of retrohepatic caval injury must be assumed and efforts undertaken immediately to achieve adequate exposure. As noted earlier, the preferred method is the immediate extension of the midline abdominal incision into a median sternotomy with division of the diaphragm in the sagittal plane from xyphoid to cava. While exposure is being obtained, hemostasis may often be effected by maintaining posteriorly directed pressure on the liver against the cava rather than by attempting to control the bleeding primarily with packs. Efforts at encircling the inferior vena cava from an infradiaphragmatic approach often require retraction of the liver, leading to increased hemorrhage. Once adequate exposure is obtained, local control of the bleeding point may allow direct repair of the cava or hepatic vein. Alternatively, an atriocaval shunt may be placed to afford control of the bleeding point while venous return to the heart is maintained [21,22]. The experience with this technique is not encouraging, and the placement of such a shunt will not salvage the patient already in deep shock following substantial transfusion and incipient or established disseminated intravascular coagulation.

Injuries to the porta hepatis are best treated by repair or vascular reconstruction. This may be facilitated by a Pringle maneuver during initial dissection and isolation of the injury. With a patient in dire straits and the surgeon faced with a technically difficult repair of the common hepatic artery, this artery may be ligated provided that portal blood flow is intact and the liver is not otherwise compromised from prolonged hypotension or cirrhosis. Ligation of the proper hepatic artery, however, may not be tolerated. Injury to the portal vein leads to massive hemorrhage and is often fatal. Simple ligation is associated with an unacceptably high mortality rate and is reserved as a desperate last resort. Lateral repair or reconstruction with a patch or panel vein graft should be aggressively pursued.

Debridement and Drainage

Adequate debridement of devitalized tissue is required in the treatment of the traumatized liver to avoid subsequent fluid collections and septic complications. Such debridement should be limited to removal of obviously ischemic tissue and may be accomplished with electrocautery or blunt fracture techniques. Precise anatomic lobar or segmental resection is seldom indicated except in those few instances where hepatic artery ligation leads to obvious lobar ischemia. Rarely, an injury that cannot be treated by the usual methods of hemostasis may be dealt with by resection [23–25]. Resection in the face of hemorrhage is a considerable challenge, however, and one may be better advised to proceed to perihepatic packing where feasible [26].

Drainage of the injured liver has been an area of much debate. Dogmatic adherence to a policy of draining all parenchymal injuries is no longer appropriate [27,28]. Small lesions treated with simple techniques of hemostasis and showing no evidence of bleeding or biliary leakage at the end of the operation may be safely left undrained. More extensive injuries, or injuries requiring complex hemostatic maneuvers, should be adequately drained because of the high risk of postoperative hematoma formation. Such a hematoma may combine with biliary leakage to lead to septic complications. Adequacy of hemostasis may only be evaluated in the normotensive state, and closure in the presence of hypotension mandates drainage. Such drains will not prevent formation of hematoma but serve only to signal the presence of ongoing or recurrent hemorrhage. The issue of Penrose drainage versus closed sump drainage continues to be much debated. A lesser incidence of septic complications has been claimed for closed sump drains, but these devices are more prone to failure from obstructing hematoma. The use of multiple large Penrose drains left in the perihepatic region in the area of injury and dressed on the operating table with a sterile wound drainage bag has proved quite satisfactory. This technique allows continual monitoring of the volume and character of the drainage fluid, including the presence of bile or blood clots. When properly managed, the risk of sepsis is equivalent to that of closed drainage. Drains are left in place until output is negligible and there is no gross evidence of bile in the drainage fluid. Drains are usually removed on the third or fourth postoperative day after an initial shortening of the drain. Any leakage of bile from the injured liver should be readily apparent by the third postoperative day if the drain is properly placed. The use of T-tube drainage in the absence of biliary tract injury has been associated with an increased rate of septic complications and is to be condemned [29].

Biliary Tract Injuries

Injuries to the extrahepatic biliary tree accompany liver trauma in approximately 15 percent of cases. The most common association is injury to the gallbladder. Cholecystectomy is generally preferable to cholecystorrhaphy, for the injured gallbladder has been demonstrated to be nonfunctional in most cases and prone to complication. Cholecystectomy may also be indicated to obtain adequate exposure of wounds on the inferior hepatic surface and is a requirement whenever the right hepatic artery is ligated. Injuries to the common bile duct may be either partial or complete. Partial injuries are repaired over a T-tube stent. An end-to-end anastomosis of the completely transected common bile duct is prone to late stenosis, and this injury is preferably managed by a choledochoenteric anastomosis.

COMPLICATIONS OF LIVER INJURY

The most common complication of liver injury is bleeding and consequent hematoma formation. At operation, intraperitoneal blood and clots are evacuated and adequate drains placed in proximity to the wound. This allows postoperative assessment of the quantity and character of the drainage fluid as an indication of recurrent hemorrhage. Serial hematocrit determinations on the drainage fluid may aid in the assessment of any voluminous drainage. Blood clot seen within the drainage bag is evidence of rapid and continuing hemorrhage, suggesting insufficient time for intra-abdominal fibrinolysis.

Postoperative bleeding may not be of such magnitude as to prompt reoperation and yet result in hematoma formation. Any hematoma, in association with bile leakage or concomitant injury to the gastrointestinal tract, predisposes to the development of intra-abdominal sepsis. The development of a perihepatic abscess is usually manifested in 7 to 14 days following operation, although it may occur earlier in the patient suffering prolonged shock or massive transfusion. The diagnosis is confirmed with the finding of a subdiaphragmatic or subhepatic fluid collection on ultrasonography or CT scan. Management may consist of exploration and open drainage, twelfth rib resection and posterior drainage, or percutaneous drainage utilizing CT scan–guided placement of drainage catheters. The choice of technique will depend on the patient's condition, the location of the abscess, and the consistency of the purulent material. Appropriate antibiotic coverage is provided based on cultures obtained from the drainage.

Hemobilia, though a rare condition, is most often caused by liver trauma [30]. Classically, the triad of right upper quadrant abdominal pain, jaundice, and gastrointestinal tract bleeding in the form of hematemesis or melena marks the development of a fistula between the hepatic vasculature and biliary tree. Small communications may present less dramatically. Arteriography will usually confirm the diagnosis and delineate the anatomy for intervention [31]. Angiographic embolization is usually effective in occluding the bleeding point. Failing this, hepatotomy with direct ligation of the offending vessel, resection, packing, or selective hepatic artery ligation may be employed but is rarely necessary today.

Spleen Injuries

Peter Mucha, Jr., and William L. Buntain

Historically, the management of splenic trauma has always been characterized by controversy [1]. Although conflicting opinions continue to exist, there is, in fact, considerable unanimity as to the modern management of such injuries. Nowhere is this more exemplified than in the experience of the authors, both of whom have expressed viewpoints on certain aspects of splenic trauma that were not only in opposition to the mainstream of their respective specialties, but also to each other [2–9]. As our discussions in this collaborative effort progressed, the more we were impressed with how little we actually differed. The objective of this section is hopefully to clarify some of the present confusion and promote a more uniform approach toward splenic trauma management.

INCIDENCE

The exact incidence of splenic trauma is unknown. Its common occurrence has been suggested by reports from several centers in this country managing 20 to 100 cases per year [3,8,10–23]. In the only controlled general population study addressing the issue of sepsis following splenectomy for any reason, an incidence rate based on the United States population of 1980 was projected at more than 40,000 splenectomies per year [9]. The age-adjusted incidence of splenectomy per 100,000 person-years in this upper Midwest study population was 20.5 for men, 15.3 for women, and 17.7 overall. Only 25 percent of these splenectomies, however, were performed for trauma. Excluding primary splenic disease or hematologic malignancies, 46 percent were incidental at the time of abdominal surgery. Exactly how many of these incidental splenectomies represent iatrogenic injury is unknown.

Demographically, a peak incidence of splenic injury is noted in the second and third decades of life with males predominating, while a secondary small peak is observed in women over the age of 70 (Fig. 10-2). Mortality appears to parallel age. Patients with splenomegaly secondary to any number of conditions (e.g., infectious mononucleosis, hemolytic anemia, leukemia, agnogenic myeloid metaplasia) are felt to be more susceptible, with splenic rupture having been reported following trivial mechanisms of injury or occurring even spontaneously.

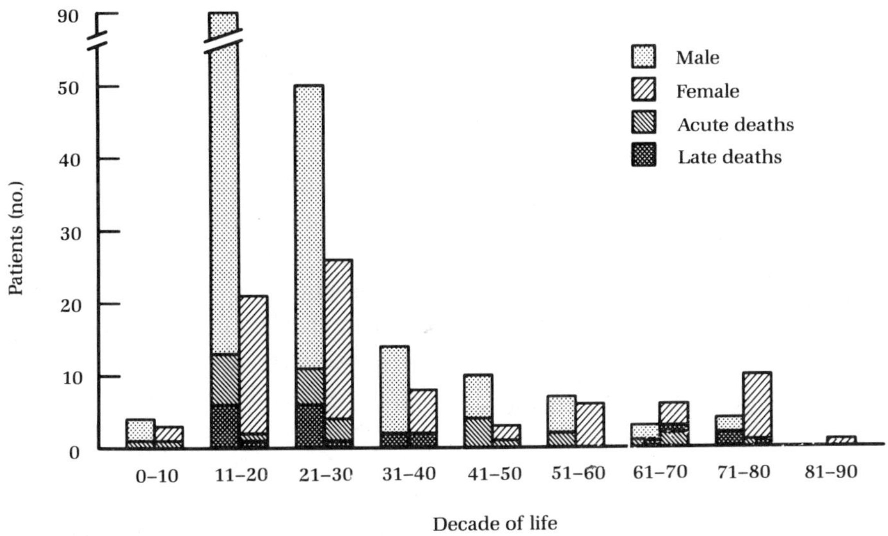

Fig. 10-2. Demographic data (sex, age, and mortality) of 273 consecutive blunt splenic trauma victims.

MECHANISMS OF INJURY

Blunt

Following blunt mechanisms of abdominal trauma, the spleen is consistently the most commonly injured organ requiring operative intervention [24]. If all trauma victims with nonpenetrating injuries to the spleen are included (dead on arrival and expired in the emergency room), mortality ranges from 18 to 25 percent [1,12,13,22–24]. This alarmingly high death rate reflects the magnitude of multisystem injury and, in particular, associated injuries to the head and chest. Until the advent of diagnostic peritoneal lavage (DPL) and more recently computed tomography (CT), part of this high mortality was also attributed to difficulties in diagnosis and delays in operative intervention.

The mechanism of injury most often responsible for blunt trauma continues to be motorized vehicles. Such high-speed and energy-dissipating events account for the high incidence of extra-abdominal injuries (80–85 percent) associated with splenic injuries [8,12,13,22,23]. Associated intra-abdominal injuries have been reported in 30 to 61 percent of blunt splenic trauma cases and remain the strongest argument for those supporting abdominal exploration in all cases of blunt splenic injury [8,14,15,22,25]. As an advocate of nonoperative management in selected cases, one of the authors (P.M.) acknowledges this high incidence of associated intra-abdominal injuries but argues that only 20 percent of these injuries or 10 percent of all blunt splenic trauma victims in his reported experience actually sustained other intra-abdominal injuries that by themselves required operative intervention [8]. However, in a recent study by this section's other author (W.L.B.), 33 percent of patients had associated injuries requiring surgical correction [2]. Both authors would agree that with the current emphasis of aggressively identifying any and all potential organ injuries through the application of newer diagnostic modalities, especially CT, the vast majority of these associated abdominal injuries requiring operation should be readily apparent.

Isolated blunt splenic injury occurs in less than one-fourth of cases and usually involves less destructive forces of energy such as direct blows to the left upper abdomen following minor falls and contact sports. With access to effective emergency care systems, the mortality of isolated blunt splenic trauma, regardless of the definitive method of management, should ideally be less than 1 percent.

Penetrating

The incidence of splenic injury in reported series of operative penetrating abdominal trauma approximates less than 10 percent [24]. The frequency of penetrating splenic injury reflects the volume of intraperitoneal space occupied by the spleen as compared to that of other intra-abdominal organs. Mortality of penetrating splenic trauma varies with the mechanism of injury, ranging from 0 to 1 percent with stab wounds to 10 percent with gunshot wounds [12,14,24]. High-velocity weapons and shotgun wounds would be expected to cause higher mortality rates. Noteworthy with penetrating splenic trauma is the reported 90-percent incidence of associated intra-abdominal injury [12,14,22]. The majority of these associated injuries require surgical correction, thereby justifying the universal consensus that every case of penetrating splenic trauma demands operative intervention.

Iatrogenic

Any number of maneuvers or procedures anatomically related to the left upper quadrant have resulted in splenic injury, including external cardiac massage, the Heimlich maneuver, pericardiocentesis, and chest tube thoracostomy. Undoubtedly, the most common cause of iatrogenic injury is that occurring at the time of abdominal surgery. The spleen is especially vulnerable when operating on the proximal stomach (fundoplication and vagotomy), left kidney, and adrenal gland and when mobilizing the splenic flexure of the colon. Awareness of the consequences of the asplenic state has prompted an attitude change among most practicing surgeons to now, whenever possible, repairing the incidentally injured spleen, rather than resorting to splenectomy [26].

ANATOMY

The spleen becomes morphologically mature during the first year of life, reaching its maximal weight at puberty and thereafter decreasing in weight by 25 to 30 percent in a normal adult. Accessory spleens have been reported in 14 to 30 percent of patients, being more commonly encountered in patients operated on for hematologic disorders [27]. The close anatomic relationship of the spleen to the diaphragm, stomach, splenic flexure of the colon, and left kidney and adrenal gland, along with its several suspensory ligaments, should be familiar to all practicing surgeons.

Of importance with the renewed interest in splenorrhaphy is awareness of the vascular segmentation of the spleen. Gupta and coworkers [28] demonstrated that 84 percent of adult human spleens had two segments (superior and inferior), while the remaining had three (superior, intermediate, and inferior). Anastomotic communication between segments is absent. The arterial pedicle at the splenic hilum generally adopts a Y shape in 70 percent or more [29], with the splenic artery dividing into two major vessels some distance away from the hilum, and each branch subsequently dividing into smaller segmental branches at the edge of the spleen itself. The second most common pattern is described as the T type, occurring in about 20 percent of patients, where the splenic artery leads straight up to the hilus of the spleen and then superiorly and inferiorly into two major branches, each giving off branches. A comparable segmentation of splenic veins has also been demonstrated.

The internal architecture or splenic stroma is described as a rich blood vessel network consisting of *white pulp* containing lymphocytes and macrophages; *red pulp*, a storage area for red blood cells, granulocytes, and platelets; additional macrophages and plasma cells in what is referred to as the *marginal zone* where cellular interaction takes place; and lastly, ellipsoids containing dense periarteriolar concentrations of phagocytes [27]. Awareness of this highly organized morphologic arrangement has led some authorities to question the practicality of autotransplanting fragments of splenic tissue. Unlike documented successful piecemeal autotransplantation of endocrine tissue (parathyroid, islet cells), autotransplanting fragments of spleen with the goal of preserving splenic function would be analogous to autotransplanting pieces of kidney or liver. Although immunologic benefits in humans have yet to be absolutely confirmed, experimentally precisely reimplanted slices of splenic tissue do demonstrate revascularization and viability for long periods and can restore many of the functional abnormalities seen postsplenectomy, including higher levels of pneumococcal antibody production following immunization [4,30,31].

PHYSIOLOGY

Total circulation of the spleen is estimated at between 150 and 250 ml per minute, representing 5 percent of the total cardiac output. Intimately related to the architectural anatomy is the ability of the spleen to remove blood-borne particulate matter and abnormal red blood cells. However, the historical concept of the spleen functioning only as a filter is somewhat obsolete. Although total understanding of the physiologic importance of the spleen is far from complete, data thus far unequivocally demonstrate that the regulatory functions exerted by the spleen and, in particular, its immunologic role are extensive [1,32,33]. The spleen contains 25 percent of the total lymphoid body mass and has been shown to have a direct impact on distinct populations of lymphocytes, that is, T and B cells [34–37]. Impaired capacity for clearance of blood-borne particles [35], decreased phagocytic activity directed against encapsulated bacteria [38,39], decreased antibody response to specific antigens [31,40,41] and decreased opsonization of bacteria [42,43], together with an absence of circulating tuftsin [44–46], other decreased antibody responses [41,47], and decreased properdin [48], have all been demonstrated in the asplenic state.

Of particular importance clinically has been the recognition of the phenomenon of "overwhelming postsplenectomy sepsis" [1,49–56]. Regardless of the reason for removing the spleen, the mortality rate for overwhelming postsplenectomy sepsis is in excess of 50 percent with infection occurring 50 to 200 times more than the incidence in the normal population at large [2,9,55,56]. Healthy individuals splenectomized for trauma appear to be at slightly lesser risk than those splenectomized for hematologic disease, and young children seem to fare worse than older children and adults [57]; however, the severity of sepsis appears to be worse in older patients [5]. The majority of serious infections following splenectomy are said to occur within 24 months, with almost 50 percent within 12 months [2,57], but there is no time limit beyond which an asplenic person can be considered safe, with overwhelming sepsis having been reported as late as 15 years postsplenectomy.

In addition to overwhelming sepsis, an increased susceptibility to almost any type of infection appears to be evident following splenectomy [25,33,57,58]. Of potential concern is the unexpectedly high incidence of viral illness in asplenic individuals [2,25,33], providing evidence that the phenomenon of postsplenectomy sepsis is not confined to encapsulated bacteria. Early postoperative septic morbidity and mortality in splenectomized trauma patients are also believed to be greater than in a comparable group of nonsplenectomized trauma patients [25]. Long-term follow-up of 740 American servicemen splenectomized for trauma during World War II (1939–1945) revealed a statistically significant excess mortality from pneumonia and ischemic heart disease [59]. The mortality from cirrhosis in this same study was also interestingly increased, but not significantly so. Postsplenectomy thrombocytosis and hypercoagulability have been postulated as reasons for the increased risk of fatal myocardial ischemia, while an increased susceptibility to viral illness might account for the observed increase in cirrhosis.

At present, there is considerable evidence supporting a much more conservative surgical attitude toward the spleen. The main controversy remains as how best to accomplish splenic preservation following injury. The enthusiasm of those espousing either splenic repair at all cost, nonoperative management, or autotransplantation must be balanced against the immediate threat of exsanguination and the sequelae following a missed associated injury or delayed diagnosis of a severe splenic injury. Paramount is the need to confirm that these different management techniques accomplish what is intended, that is, preservation of normal or near normal splenic function without jeopardizing the trauma victim's chances for a full and complete recovery.

DIAGNOSIS

Prior to the advent of radionuclide imaging and, more recently, DPL and CT, the diagnosis of splenic injury was based largely on clinical findings. Signs and symptoms suggestive of a ruptured spleen are those associated with intra-abdominal bleeding from any cause and vary according to the severity and degree of hemorrhage, associated injuries, and the temporal relationship to the traumatic event. Generalized abdominal pain and nausea are common. Pain localized to the left upper quadrant is reported in about 30 percent of patients. The reported incidence of pain at the tip of the left shoulder (Kehr's sign) has varied from 15 to 75 percent and can be enhanced by placing the patient in the Trendelenburg position. Tachycardia, hypotension, or both may be evident. Palpation of the abdomen usually reveals tenderness and muscle spasm, while signs of peritoneal irritation secondary to hemoperitoneum are not uncommon. On occasion, a tender mass may be palpated at the left costal margin in association with an area of fixed dullness that can be outlined by percussion (Ballance's sign). Leukocytosis (> 12,000) is common. Initial reliance on hematocrit levels may not be helpful; however, a decrease may be suggestive of ongoing blood loss.

The astute clinician should be extremely cautious in avoiding the temptation to dismiss any patient with trauma to the left upper abdomen as a trivial injury. A minimum 3- to 4-hour period of observation is recommended, rather than having the patient dismissed only to return later in profound shock. However, it should be remembered that less severe injuries are diagnosed by physical examination alone in only 42 to 87 percent of cases [3].

If any concern exists, clinicians have any number of fairly accurate diagnostic modalities now at their disposal. In keeping with the modern philosophy of aggressively identifying any and all organ injuries as soon as possible to optimize a trauma victim's care, delayed diagnosis of splenic injury should be the exception rather than the rule. This approach primarily explains the rather marked reduction in the reported frequency of "delayed rupture" (period de latance) of the spleen, previously reported to occur in up to 30 to 40 percent of splenic injuries to less than 2 percent in more recent series [8,11,60].

Radionuclide Imaging

Splenic scintigrams are highly sensitive and specific indicators of splenic injury and were quite popular in the late 1960s and early to mid 1970s [61–64]. They have proved particularly valuable in the follow-up of nonoperatively managed patients and those undergoing partial splenectomy or splenorrhaphy [65–67]. Major disadvantages in the evaluation of acute abdominal trauma, however, include the time required for nuclear scanning and its qualitative limitation in assessing other intra-abdominal structures, with the possible exception of the liver.

Diagnostic Peritoneal Lavage

DPL is considered by many as the gold standard in the assessment of blunt abdominal trauma (98-percent sensitive) and, with modification of the diagnostic criteria, has proved to be of increasing value with penetrating wounds to the abdomen, flank, and lower thorax whenever there is a question of violation of the peritoneal cavity. One of the major limitations of DPL in the assessment of splenic trauma has been its qualitative lack of specificity as to exactly what organs might be injured. Additional criticisms include its invasive nature and the inability of DPL consistently to identify injury to retroperitoneal structures (duodenum, pancreas, kidneys) and the diaphragm. There is little argument that DPL represents a most efficient and economical diagnostic tool in identifying abdominal trauma requiring operative intervention, particularly when there is any degree of urgency such as encountered with hemodynamically unstable trauma victims. With stable patients, many institutions today place comparable emphasis on CT.

Angiography

Invasive arteriography has demonstrated a high degree of accuracy in the diagnosis and delineation of splenic injury, with excellent correlation with operative and autopsy specimens. Fisher and associates [68] formulated a classification scheme based on arteriographic findings that allowed a better understanding of the different patterns of splenic trauma. Most centers, however, do not advocate routine angiography for the purposes of diagnosing splenic trauma unless the patient already requires angiography for other suspected conditions such as traumatic transection of the aorta, diagnostic and therapeutic embolization of pelvic fracture bleeding, or peripheral vascular trauma. In patients requiring arteriography, advantage should be taken to assess the spleen, thereby avoiding unnecessary duplication of diagnostic effort.

Computed Tomography

At most major centers, the ready availability of CT has proved especially useful in the objective evaluation of splenic injury, both quantitatively as well as qualitatively. Criticisms include the financial cost of CT and its impractical application in patients requiring aggressive resuscitative efforts. However, with stable patients, CT does represent a most accurate and noninvasive diagnostic modality, and there is little question that many splenic injuries are now being identified that previously would have gone unnoticed.

A major advantage of CT is its ability to evaluate other abdominal structures. Diagnostic accuracy is greatly improved with contrast enhancement (intravenous, orogastric, and in selected cases, retrograde colon). Many believe [69–73] that CT reduces the number of ancillary tests required for evaluation of traumatized patients, provides accurate information regarding the extent and severity of injury, and results in more appropriate decisions regarding the need for exploration versus nonoperative management. CT provides clear, understandable evaluation of findings in the third dimension, including assessment of the retroperitoneum, in a short period of time. As experience has been gained with CT, imaging classification has now been correlated with operative findings, enabling an even more accurate assessment as to the degree and extent of splenic injury [3].

Ultrasonography

Ultrasonography should be mentioned as an additional noninvasive diagnostic modality useful in the assessment of splenic trauma. Popular in European centers, a positive feature is its bedside (cart) application. Free intraperitoneal blood and splenic capsular disruption can be readily identified, but limitations again include a lack of specificity as well as decreased sensitivity when compared to other diagnostic measures, especially CT. In a controlled study comparing ultrasonography to CT for abdominal trauma in children [74], ultrasound had an unacceptable false-negative rate of 50 percent.

CLASSIFICATION

A number of different classification schemes have been suggested for splenic injury. Arteriography [68] has allowed classification into major areas of injury according to the anatomic location: superior, polar, hilar, or peripheral, while dividing hematomas into subcapsular and intraparenchymal, and if the spleen is in several pieces, termed fragmentation. These injuries are then classed as massive, major, or minor and further subdivided into 11 subclasses within each of these three. Although a high degree of correlation with the severity of injury can be achieved both clinically and prognostically, angiography has unfortunately proved cumbersome and is not presently recommended for routine evaluation of abdominal trauma victims except when already indicated for some other reason.

Several intraoperative classifications have been devised. The simplest, that of Oakes and Charters [18], defines the injuries as either *minor* (damage limited to a small area of capsular disruption) or *major* (damage consisting of deep fractures extending to the splenic parenchyma, large subcapsular hematomas, total avulsion, and/or fragmentation). Traub and Perry [22] classified the extent and nature of injury into splenic injury only, splenic injury with concomitant intra-abdominal injury, and splenic injury with concomitant extra-abdominal injury. Although helpful as general prognosticators, both of these classifications are based on operative findings, and neither therefore contributes to the decision-making process as to how specifically to manage an injured spleen.

Shackford and colleagues [109], with slight modification [12], have developed a much more detailed classification of splenic injury, again based on the operative findings:

Grade 1 Capsular tear or minor parenchymal laceration often requiring no treatment

Grade 2 Minor capsular avulsion requiring only a topical hemostatic agent

Grade 3 Major parenchymal fracture or laceration or a through-and-through gunshot or stab wound necessitating suture repair alone or in combination with a topical hemostatic agent

Grade 4 Severe parenchymal stellate fracture, crush, bisection, or hilar injury usually requiring partial splenic debridement or, often, splenectomy

Grade 5 Shattered or avulsed spleen nearly always requiring splenectomy

It has been suggested that splenic salvage should be achievable in over 90 percent of grade 1 and 2 injuries, 60 to 65 percent of grade 3, and 5 to 10 percent of grade 4 injuries, with ultimate success dependent on the surgeon's experience, ingenuity, and persistence [12].

Barrett and associates [10], Buntain and Gould [2], and Buntain and Lynn [5], independent of one another, have outlined workable and remarkably similar classifications based on CT (Table 10-3). Type I injuries consist of localized capsular disruption or subcapsular hematomas, without significant parenchymal injury. Type II injuries consist of single or multiple capsular disruptions with parenchymal injury that does not extend into the hilum or involve major vessels, with or without intraparenchymal hematoma. Type III injuries consist of deep fractures, single or multiple, that extend into the hilum and involve major vessels. Type IV injuries are those in which the spleen is completely shattered, fragmented, or separated from its normal blood supply. To this classification has been added the subclassification A—splenic injury without other associated injuries within the abdomen; B—splenic injury with associated intra-abdominal injuries (B_1 for those that involve a solid viscus, B_2 for those involving a hollow viscus); and E—splenic injury with associated extra-abdominal injuries. Hence, for a parenchymal injury not involving the hilum or major splenic vessels but with an associated renal injury and pulmonary contusions, the injury would be classified as a Type IIB_1E injury. Usefulness of this classification for preoperative evaluation has been recently confirmed, with correlation both qualitatively and quantitatively, with CT and operation [3]. Universal adoption of this standardized classification is recommended to help clarify our future understanding of splenic trauma.

Table 10-3. Classification of Spleen Injuries

Type I	Localized capsular disruption or subcapsular hematoma, without significant parenchymal injury
Type II	Single or multiple capsular and parenchymal disruptions, transverse or longitudinal, that do not extend into the hilum or involve major vessels; intraparenchymal hematoma may or may not coexist
Type III	Deep fractures, single or multiple, transverse or longitudinal, extending into hilum and involving major segmental blood vessels
Type IV	Completely shattered or fragmented spleen, or separated from its normal blood supply at the pedicle
A	Without other associated intra-abdominal injury
B	With other associated intra-abdominal injury
B_1	Solid viscus
B_2	Hollow viscus
E	With associated extra-abdominal injury

DEFINITIVE CARE

The ultimate manner in which any splenic injury will be managed must be dictated by the patient's needs. With increased awareness of the consequences of the asplenic state, every surgeon should make a concerted effort to conserve splenic tissue and resist splenectomy. At times, there is no other recourse, especially if the spleen has been shattered or avulsed from its blood supply. Many variables may affect the final decision, including the mechanism of injury, associated intra-abdominal injuries, other life-threatening associated injuries, the patient's hemodynamic status, and of course the status of the spleen itself.

Splenectomy

The technical aspects of splenectomy are well-known. As far back as 1908, John Gibbon [75], speaking before the Philadelphia Academy of Surgery, stated, "... If the spleen were not so easily removed, fewer splenectomies for rupture would be reported. ..." The dispatch with which splenectomy can be safely performed in experienced hands has been well documented; however, attention to technical detail is essential.

In most trauma situations, a midline incision is employed to ensure adequate exposure of the entire peritoneal cavity. Although free intraperitoneal blood is often encountered with splenic injury, especially in the pelvis and paracolic gutters, initial inspection will usually reveal partially clotted blood in the left upper quadrant. Adequate mobilization and exposure are the keys to any operation on the spleen. Following careful manual extraction of blood and clot from the left upper quadrant, visual assessment should be made as to the extent of ongoing splenic hemorrhage. The finding of either a totally shattered spleen or one avulsed from the splenic pedicle may leave the surgeon no alternative but to gain immediate control of the splenic vasculature by manually compressing the distal pancreas. Most often, however, lesser degrees of hemorrhage will be evident. In fact, minimal ongoing bleeding is usually present.

Care must be taken at all times to avoid compounding an already existing splenic injury. For mobilization and assessment, the lienocolic attachments are usually divided first, permitting a downward displacement of the splenic flexure of the colon. The left lobe of the liver is retracted to the right by the assistant, while the surgeon applies medial traction on the greater curve of the stomach and gastrocolic ligament. A moist sponge or laparotomy pad on the anterior surface of the spleen facilitates anteromedial rotation of the spleen by the surgeon's left hand to enable visualization of the posterior peritoneum, which in turn is incised or cauterized 2 cm from the posterior edge of the spleen. The surgeon's right hand manually helps to elevate the lower half of the spleen and its vascular pedicle, including the tail of the pancreas, with care taken to avoid injury to the more deeply positioned left kidney and adrenal gland. Frequently, the superior half of the spleen cannot be adequately mobilized without transection and ligation of the short gastric vessels. Extreme care is required to avoid incorporation of the serosa and wall of the stomach in clamps, which might result in necrosis and subsequent gastric perforation [76]. The spleen may now be delivered up through the wound.

Once mobilized, it is helpful to place two large packs in the splenic bed to help support the elevated structures and avoid the annoying problem of having the spleen slip back into the left upper quadrant, as well as to tamponade small-vessel oozing from raw surfaces in the splenic fossa. If splenectomy is deemed necessary, the splenic artery and vein should be isolated. A concerted effort must be made to identify clearly the tail of the pancreas and its relationship to the splenic hilum. Theoretically, if conditions permit, the splenic artery should be clamped first and the spleen squeezed in an attempt to autotransfuse any splenic blood back into the circulation. In severely traumatized spleens, however, this is usually not possible. Separate ligation of the splenic artery and vein is also advisable to prevent development of a possible arteriovenous fistula. Most surgeons either suture ligate or at least doubly ligate the splenic artery as well as the short gastric vessels. Care should be taken to avoid deep suture ligation of the pancreatic parenchyma. Two or three clean large packs are then placed in the left upper quadrant while the surgeon evaluates the remainder of the peritoneal cavity and performs any additional surgery as indicated. As the operation nears completion, attention is again focused on the left upper quadrant. After the packs are removed, the finding of clotted blood is suggestive of ongoing bleeding and demands careful reexamination of all raw surfaces in the splenic fossa as well as reinspection of all ligatures.

The question of routine drainage of the splenic bed has been challenged by Cohn [77], who demonstrated an 11-fold increase in complications when drainage was employed. Obviously, if the splenic bed is dry and there is no concern about the pancreas or other associated injuries in the left upper quadrant, one should not drain. However, if there is concern, Pachter and coworkers [19] demonstrated that there are no apparent increased complications among patients drained with closed systems (Jackson-Pratt or Hemovac) as compared to patients who are not drained. Pachter also noted that the type of drains (Penrose) and the length of time that drains were left in place probably accounted for the higher complication rate noted in earlier studies. If drains are employed, they can and usually should be removed within 72 to 96 hours, unless deemed necessary for longer.

Following splenectomy for trauma, several issues warrant discussion. The first is that of nasogastric tube decompression of the stomach. Popular at many centers a decade or two ago was the rationale to maintain gastric decompression for a minimum of 5 days to avoid distention and the potential consequence of short-gastric-vessel ligatures slipping off with resultant hemorrhage. At present, most would agree that there is little need for such prolonged decompression unless dictated by the patient's clinical status (e.g., associated gastrointestinal injuries, ileus). The complications of prolonged nasogastric decompression far outweigh the risk of a tie coming off a short gastric vessel, especially if one has taken the time to ensure secure ligation at the time of splenectomy. Hence, we recommend nasogastric decompression for only 36 to 48 hours, unless dictated otherwise.

A second issue is that of the expected thrombocytosis following splenectomy. The practice of checking routine platelet counts at specific intervals during the postoperative period to recognize significant thrombocytosis (in excess of 1 million) as a guide for institution of prophylactic anticoagulation has fallen in disrepute. Although the immediate consequences of hypercoagulability appear real based on the observed thrombocytosis, patients in fact have not demonstrated any immediate increased risk. However, such hypercoagulability may explain the higher incidence of ischemic heart disease and perhaps carotid occlusive disease reported several years after splenectomy [7,59]. Most surgeons still periodically check platelet counts out of interest, but rarely is there any reason to alter one's postoperative management.

Of importance with any splenectomized patient, and in particular the otherwise healthy trauma patient with an expected normal longevity, are the consequences of the asplenic state.

Asplenic Registry

It is recommended that every institution (if not every individual surgeon) caring for trauma victims maintain an "asplenic registry." There is a responsibility to address splenectomized patients as to their awareness of the potential long-term consequences of splenectomy (i.e., ischemic heart disease, carotid occlusive disease, cirrhosis, and of course increased susceptibility to infection, including overwhelming postsplenectomy sepsis). Such reevaluation and reassessment would then allow splenectomized patients to be updated of recent developments and reminded of the importance of seeking early medical attention for what may seem like even a minor viral illness. Several institutions routinely provide Medic Alert bracelets for splenectomized patients.

Pneumovax

Even though only 50 percent of all cases of overwhelming postsplenectomy sepsis are attributed to pneumococcal organisms, there is general agreement that pneumococcal vaccine (Pneumovax) should be employed in all splenectomized patients [78]. Ideally, it would be preferable to administer the initial vaccination presplenectomy, but this is usually not possible in trauma patients. The vaccine is administered in a dosage of 0.5 ml SQ or IM, and at present, there seems to be no advantage or disadvantage whether it is given during the acute phase or once the patient has begun to convalesce. Patients should be warned against a false sense of security in that the vaccine does not protect against all strains of pneumococcal or other commonly incriminated encapsulated organisms (*Escherichia coli, Haemophilus influenzae, Neisseria meningitidis*) in the pathogenesis of overwhelming sepsis [79–82]. Revaccination is not presently recommended for adults; however, after 5 years or more, pending long-term data, some authors recommend revaccination for children [4]. Contraindications include children less than 2 years, pregnant females, and anyone with a febrile illness, especially respiratory.

In children, *N. meningitidis* and *H. influenzae* vaccines are additionally recommended by most pediatric surgeons [4,83]. Dosage, administration, and contraindications are similar to Pneumovax.

Prophylactic Penicillin

Low-dose suppressive prophylactic penicillin therapy has been advocated for splenectomized children [4,65,84,85]. Zarrabi and Rosner [58,86] have demonstrated similar protection with adults. Although several authorities recommend routine penicillin prophylaxis in all patients, the practicality of this approach is questioned by the documented low rate of sustained patient compliance. It is recommended that all patients (adults and children) should ideally receive penicillin or erythromycin prophylaxis for 2 to 4 weeks after pneumococcal vaccinations. Young asplenic patients who suffer acute febrile illnesses should be considered for penicillin or erythromycin prophylaxis even if previously vaccinated.

Autotransplantation

An important consideration in any trauma patient requiring splenectomy is autotransplantation. Experimental studies have confirmed the viability of reimplanted revascularized splenic tissue capable of phagocytizing pneumococcal organisms and contributing to a higher level of antibody formation following pneumococcal vaccination [30,31,87,88]. Several sites of autotransplantation [30,88–91] have been described, the most popular technique being where splenic fragments (20 × 20 × 5 mm) are strategically implanted into a greater omental pouch [15]. The amount of protection afforded by autotransplantation has been questioned because of cases of overwhelming sepsis reported in patients who have undergone autotransplantation [92] and following the natural phenomenon of splenosis [93,94]. Preservation of total splenic function appears to require both an inherent blood supply [95] and retention of at least one-third of the splenic mass [96]. Experimentally in rats, some degree of immunologic protection is afforded, with an inverse linear relationship between the amount of tissue successfully transplanted and subsequent susceptibility to infection [88,90,97].

It is the lack of complete preservation of function that has led many not to consider autotransplantation as a practical clinical alternative at this time. A justifiable concern is the false sense of security. In fact, evidence would suggest that patients who have undergone autotransplantation of splenic fragments should still receive Pneumovax and possibly penicillin prophylaxis and probably should be registered into a subcategory within each institution's asplenic registry. Several centers, however, routinely employ autotransplantation, especially if the splenic injury is isolated or associated injuries are minor. In addition, some would argue that perhaps the more severely injured and those at most risk are the ones who should be offered the most protection and hence should undergo autotransplantation. To date, there appears to be no significant adverse sequelae from autotransplantation as originally theorized, such as a propensity for bowel obstruction or spontaneous rupture of regenerated fragments. Nevertheless, at present the clinical application of splenic autotransplantation in humans must be considered experimental.

Splenorrhaphy

There is little disagreement today that if and when operative intervention is indicated for splenic trauma, splenorrhaphy, rather than splenectomy, is preferred [2,5,7,12–14,16,18,19, 65,84,98–100]. Several technical options are available. Most often, exposure will be gained through a standard midline incision, in keeping with the urgency of operation in most trauma situations and the need to explore the intra-abdominal contents thoroughly. Initial inspection and evaluation are the same as described for splenectomy. Morgenstern and Shapiro [101] have advocated gaining routine vessel loop control of the splenic artery through the lesser sac, except when the rate of bleeding from the injured spleen precludes any delay in delivering the traumatized organ. Although theoretically appealing, this is almost never necessary and can be very dangerous and not without complication. Others have advocated selective control of the splenic artery at the hilum, again a sometimes difficult and time-consuming task. We would suggest temporary sponge-stick compression of the splenic artery where it crosses the vertebral body, followed by prompt mobilization and finger control at the hilum for extensive ongoing hemorrhage. As previously emphasized, aside from extremely simple avulsions on the anterior capsule of the spleen, effective splenic repair demands meticulous atraumatic mobilization. Thorough assessment of the extent and severity of the splenic injury can only be achieved by direct visualization and inspection of the entire organ [2,5,101].

Topical Hemostasis

When a superficial avulsion (type I injury) has stopped bleeding spontaneously, no further treatment is required. If bleeding persists, several materials are available for topical control and include microcrystalline collagen (Avitene), Surgicel, Gelfoam, and topical thrombin. Avitene is most popular, either by itself or in combination with Surgicel. A thin (2 mm) layer of Avitene should be applied with pressure for approximately 3 minutes. If continued surface bleeding results, the procedure may be repeated with a secondary application to remaining areas of breakthrough bleeding. Electrocautery may be effective when applying an arc current to avoid deep penetration of the splenic parenchyma with the cautery tip; however, electrocautery is often of little or no help. Others have advocated ultrasonic scalpels [102,103] and fibrin glue [104,105].

Suture Techniques

Following adequate mobilization, superficial clots are gently removed, actively bleeding vessels ligated or controlled with mattress sutures, and loose and devitalized tissue gently debrided. Five basic suture techniques, alone or in combination, seem sufficient to manage most cases of splenic injury [4]: (1) direct suture of the splenic parenchyma and capsule with simple or mattress sutures, with or without buttressing pledgets or omentum (Fig. 10-3); (2) suture ligation of individual splenic vessels; (3) ligation of segmental vessels in the hilum; (4) application of an absorbable suture hemostatic "ladder" or "net"; and (5) large entire organ through-and-through absorbable mattress sutures (Figure 10-4). Splenorrhaphy meticulously accomplished by knowledgeable and competent surgeons should take little more time to accomplish than splenectomy, the management of associated intra-abdominal injuries being the major determinant of operative time. Although some reluctance has been voiced about suture repair of the spleen because of the potential complications of delayed rupture, the development of traumatic splenic cysts, and the phenomenon of abdominal splenosis, these problems have

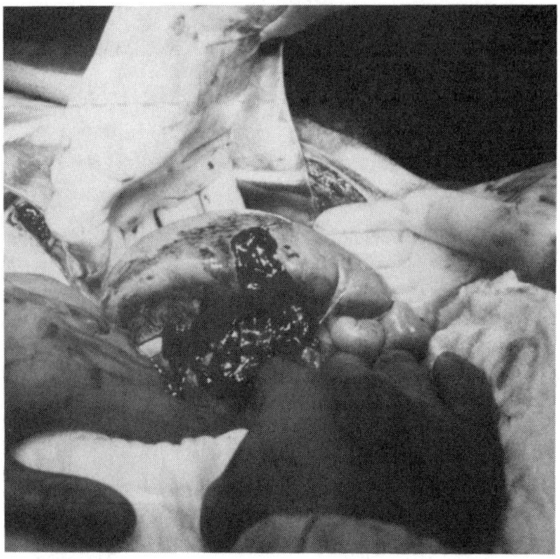

A

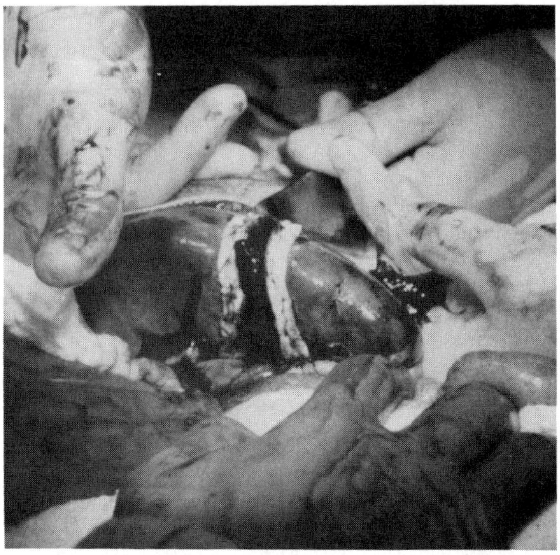

B

Fig. 10-3. ***A and B.*** **Type III injury repaired with buttressing mattress sutures and Teflon pledget. (From W. L. Buntain and H. R. Gould, Splenic trauma in children and techniques of splenic salvage.** ***World J. Surg.*** **9:398, 1985. With permission.)**

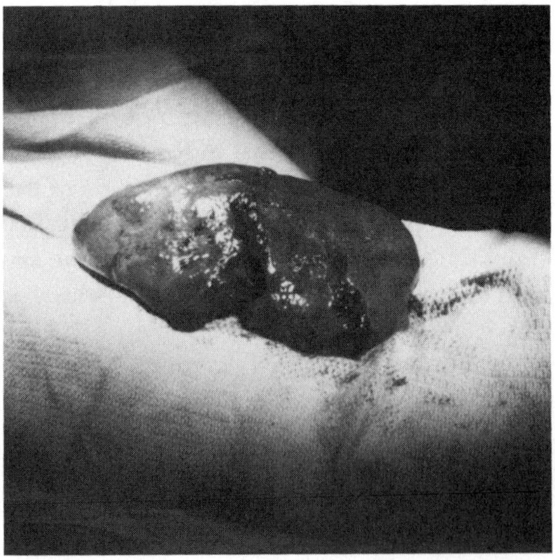

A

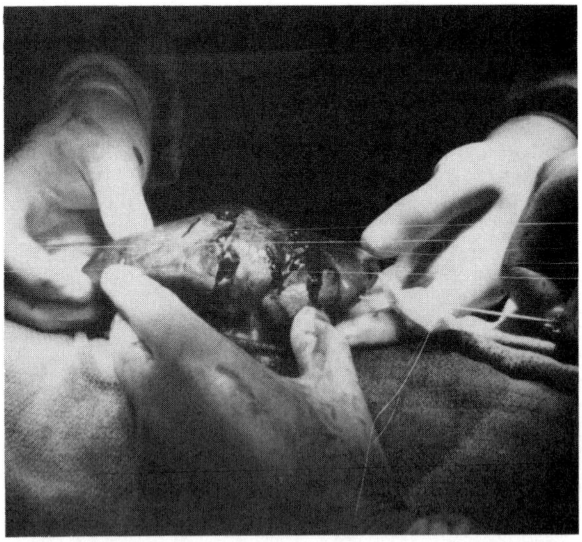

B

Fig. 10-4. ***A. to F.*** **Type III injury repaired with through-and-through parenchymal sutures. (From W. L. Buntain and H. R. Gould, Splenic trauma in children and techniques of splenic salvage.** ***World J. Surg.*** **9:398, 1985. With permission.)**

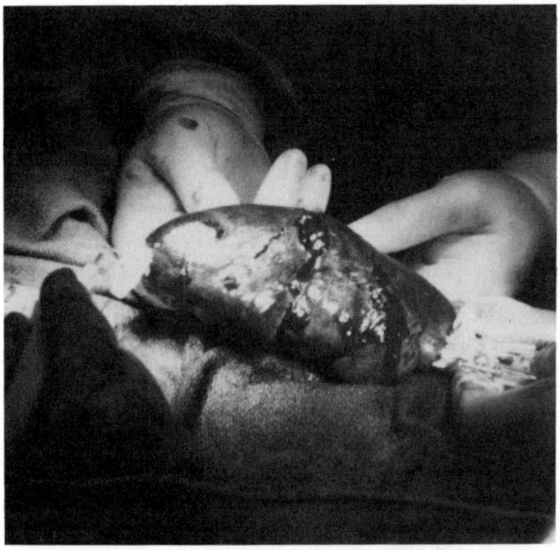

C

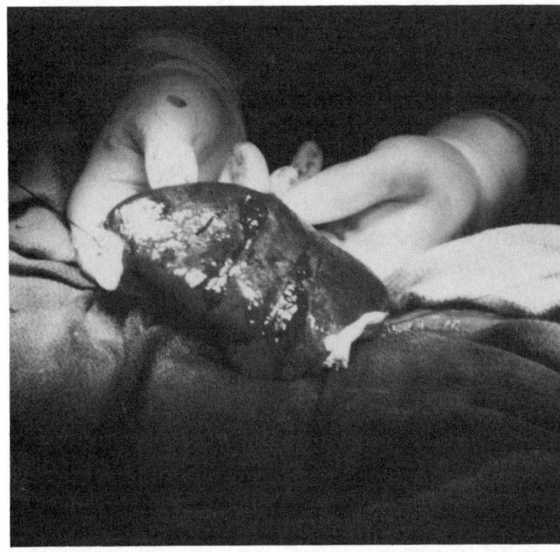

D

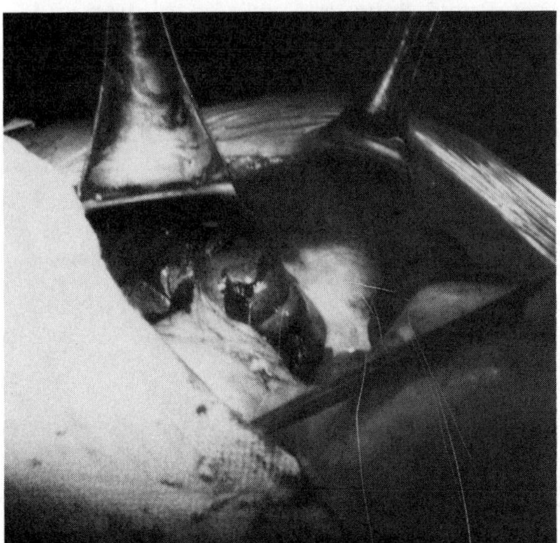

E

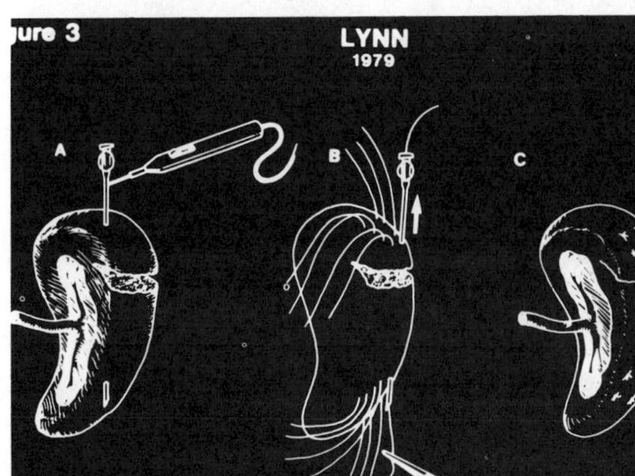

F

Fig. 10-4. (continued).

been virtually nonexistent following splenorrhaphy. Dulchavsky and associates [106] have actually demonstrated a higher wound breaking strength involving suture-repaired wounds of the spleen in dogs and pigs as compared to uninjured sites when measured 3 weeks postinjury. Interestingly, at 6 weeks postinjury, the wound breaking strength is the same for normal spleen, repaired spleen, and unrepaired but healed splenic injuries.

Partial Splenectomy

With an obvious devitalized segment of spleen damaged beyond repair, partial or hemisplenectomy can be expeditiously and safely performed because of the segmental vascular arrangement of the spleen [3,4,107,108]. Control of either the splenic artery proper or its major branches facilitates resection. Vessels identified in the retained cut surface of the spleen are individually ligated with fine suture. Horizontal mattress sutures help compress the raw edges, while the raw surface itself can be controlled with a topical hemostatic agent if necessary (Figure 10-5). Ideally, when contemplating partial resection, one would want to retain at least one-third but preferably more of the splenic mass along with its inherent vascular supply.

Fig. 10-5. Type III injuries managed by partial splenectomy (*A*) and hemisplenectomy (*B*). Note topical hemostatic agent control of raw splenic surface in *B*. (From W. L. Buntain and H. R. Gould, Splenic trauma in children and techniques of splenic salvage. *World J. Surg.* 9:398, 1985. With permission.)

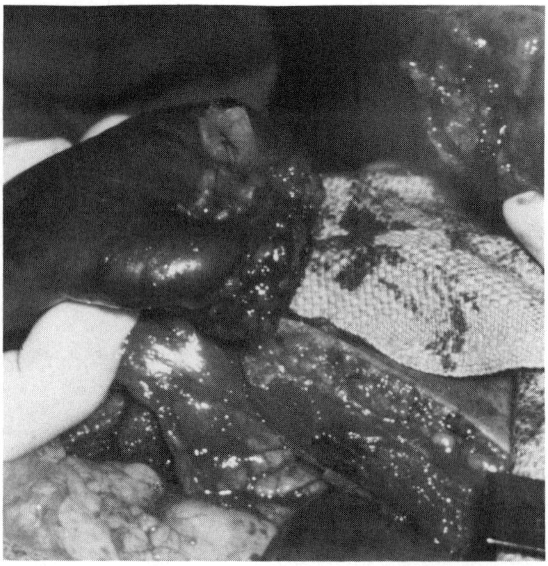

A

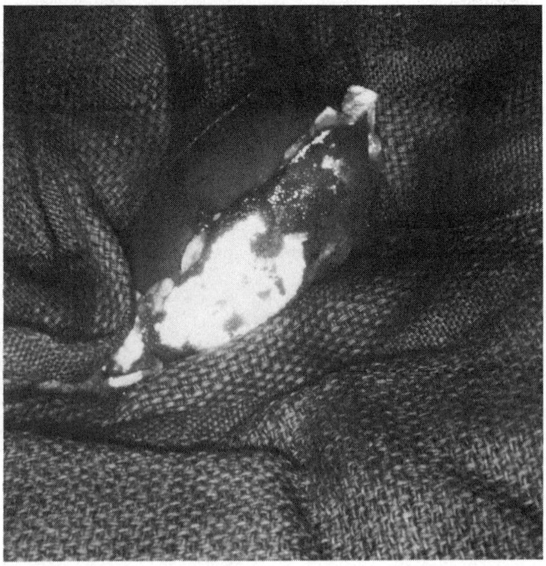

B

Splenic Artery Ligation
Splenic artery ligation, either alone or in combination with topical hemostatic agents and/or suture techniques, has been proposed in much the same manner as hepatic artery ligation (HAL) for liver trauma [109,110]. A major concern is devascularization of the spleen, especially if the short gastric vessels have been compromised at the time of splenic mobilization. Pabst and colleagues [111] experimentally demonstrated in piglets that arterial ligation produced no evidence of infarction, and at 6 months the spleen maintained its normal size with enlarged vessels in the gastrolineal ligament. When the splenic remnant was left attached only to the ligated splenic artery, no obvious growth could be demonstrated, while splenic tissue left in contact with smaller vessels (short gastrics and peritoneal) increased in size. Sherman and Asch [112] have reported similar findings in children.

Capping Techniques
Self-made buttressing Vicryl ladders have been described for holding the injured spleen together [5]. Others have employed omentum or the falciform ligament of the liver [101]. More recently, Delany and coworkers [113] and Lange and associates [114] have employed commercially available polyglycolic acid (Dexon) mesh, in essence a hair-netting effect holding together pulverized pieces of spleen (Fig. 10-6). The actual number of times that such a capping technique might be indicated are quite infrequent but in selected patients may represent the only alternative to splenectomy.

Postoperative Care
Following splenic repair, by whatever technique, the remainder of the operation and immediate postoperative care are essentially the same as following splenectomy. Although successful repair has been performed in the face of fecal or enteric contamination, some degree of reluctance is only natural, especially if it entails leaving behind foreign material (e.g., Dexon or Vicryl mesh, felt or Teflon pledgets). Initial monitoring in an intensive care unit for 24 to 48 hours permits early recognition of splenic hemorrhage. Thereafter, an additional 5 to 6 days of routine postoperative care usually suffices, with the patient dismissed and followed on an outpatient basis unless longer hospitalization is required for associated injuries. After 6 weeks, gradual and complete return to full activity is encouraged. Depending on the severity of injury, a postoperative CT or radionuclide scan (6 weeks) may be obtained to assess splenic healing [4].

With all the current enthusiasm over splenorrhaphy, the practicing surgeon may feel compelled to pursue repair at all costs, since failure, in the view of some armchair theorists, seems to imply technical shortcomings. Nothing is further from the truth. A realistic approach in achieving what is best for any given patient recognizes that not all spleens can be repaired, nor should they, especially if one is going to leave behind nothing more than a mass of devitalized splenic tissue.

Although a major criticism directed toward splenorrhaphy has been the additional time required for repair, several comparative studies have revealed very little difference in the actual duration of surgery for splenorrhaphy

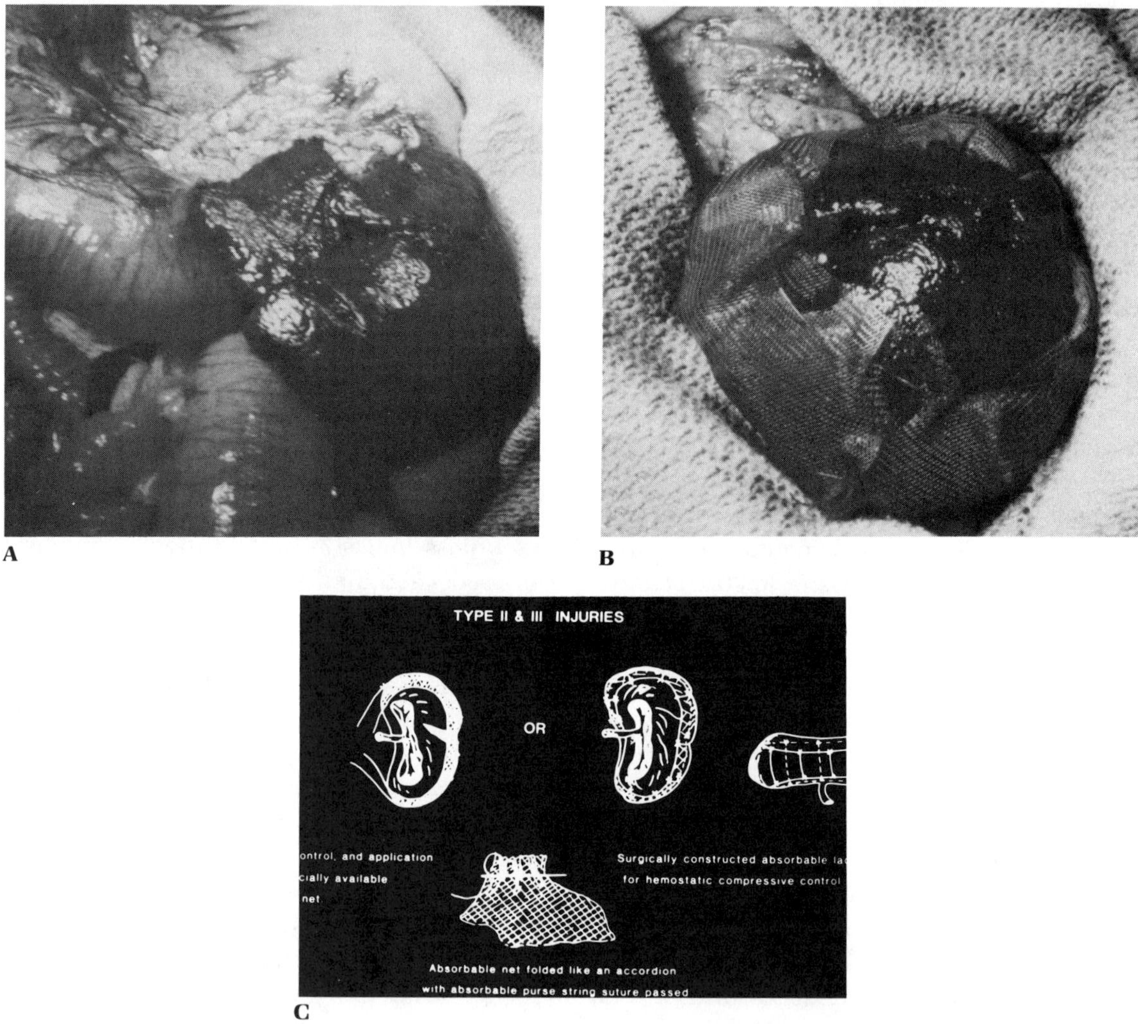

Fig. 10-6. ***A to C.*** **Type III injury held together with absorbable mesh. (From W. L. Buntain and H. R. Gould, Splenic trauma in children and techniques of splenic salvage.** ***World J. Surg.*** **9:398, 1985. With permission.)**

as compared to splenectomy [2,8,12,13,16,18]. Similarly, there appears to be no greater risk in regard to mortality and morbidity, and in fact, patients who undergo repair appear to have fewer complications than those subjected to splenectomy. Still, on occasion, a patient's other associated injuries (intra- and extra-abdominal) are of such a life-threatening nature that persistent attempts at splenic repair would be hazardous. It is also agreed that one should not hesitate to abandon repair if, in the surgeon's judgment, splenic hemostasis is inadequate. Finally, if one cannot salvage at least one-third of the functioning splenic mass along with its inherent vascular supply, splenorrhaphy should be abandoned.

Nonoperative

For many reasons, including the technical ease of splenectomy and reports of nonoperative management of blunt splenic trauma dating back to the turn of the century resulting in greater than 90-percent mortality [115], the prevailing attitude toward splenic trauma has remained one of operative intervention. Pediatric surgeons, however, primarily concerned about the risks of the asplenic state in children, reintroduced the concept of nonoperative management in the late 1970s. Since that time, well over a thousand nonoperatively managed pediatric splenic trauma patients have been collectively reported during the past two decades [5,85,98,112,116–122]. Although stringent criteria are not well defined, there appears to be general agreement in the objective requirement of less than 40 ml of blood/kg (or half of the total blood volume) over 24 hours to maintain hemodynamic stability as an acceptable guide for continued but close observation of splenic injuries [2,4]. A review of published series now reveals that up to 68 percent of children are being successfully managed nonoperatively without apparent significant risk or the need for later surgery [2,5,98,104,117,120].

Several investigators [8,17,21,23] have independently published a cumulative experience with over 100 adult splenic trauma patients managed nonoperatively, representing from 24 to 38 percent of all adult blunt splenic trauma cases seen at their respective institutions. To date, standardized selection criteria have not yet been adopted for adults, but one report admitted a failure rate of nonoperative management of 29 percent early in its experience before specific selection criteria were defined [8]. Malangoni and coworkers [123] have stated that nonoperative management of adult splenic trauma has uniformly failed in their hands, and others have expressed similar caution [2,99].

In the few series of nonoperative management of adult splenic trauma available for review, similar conclusions have been reached. As in children, nonoperative management of adult splenic trauma appears to be most applicable to patients who are hemodynamically stable. Even with transient post-traumatic hypotension rapidly responsive to fluid resuscitation, it is felt that operative intervention is preferable to nonoperative management. Among a subset of seven adult patients who had exhibited hypotension postinjury and who were intentionally treated nonoperatively, five (71 percent) subsequently required splenic surgery, while none of the successful nonoperatively managed adults in the same series ever exhibited any hemodynamic instability [8]. Although some have accepted transfusion requirements of upward to half the estimated blood volume for nonoperative management of adult splenic injury, Mucha and colleagues [8] and Morgenstern and Uyeda [17] have independently established a maximum transfusion requirement of two and three units respectively for ensuring successful nonoperative management. Patients with isolated blunt splenic injury most often fulfill these criteria. Nevertheless, there can be no substitute for experienced surgical judgment in assessing the magnitude of total body injury, establishing priorities, and noting subtle signs and symptoms of other intra-abdominal injuries that, by themselves, might demand operation.

One of the most consistently voiced arguments against nonoperative management, in both adults and children, has been the reported high incidence of associated abdominal injuries [2,4,14,22,100]. The reported incidence of associated abdominal injuries with blunt splenic trauma varies from 35 to 50 percent. However, if one looks at those associated abdominal injuries that by themselves would have actually necessitated surgery, the incidence varies from 10 percent in adults [8] to 33 percent in children [2]. With increasing reliance on CT in evaluating hemodynamically stable splenic trauma, experienced interpretation greatly reduces the risk of missing significant associated abdominal injuries. Unquestionably, part of the current success of nonoperative management of blunt splenic trauma is as much a manifestation of diagnostic technology as the boldness of its proponents. The sensitivities and ease of application of noninvasive imaging techniques are such that many splenic injuries are now being diagnosed that heretofore would have gone unrecognized. Surely, the diagnosis of a splenic injury, in and of itself, is no longer an indication for mandatory operation unless dictated by the patient's needs.

Another argument voiced against nonoperative management in adults has been the theorized decreased contraction and retraction of injured splenic vessels with age [100]. Supporting the presumed difference in vascular integrity is the fact that nonoperative management is more often successful in the pediatric age group. Nevertheless, nonoperative management in selected adults has been well documented [8,17,21,23].

A third argument against nonoperative management has been the need for prolonged hospitalization and restriction of the patient's physical activity. Although admittedly somewhat misleading because those patients subjected to splenic trauma surgery more often have multisystem trauma and associated injuries that account for longer hospitalization and convalescence, nonoperatively managed patients generally require hospitalization for a shorter period of time than those undergoing surgery, simply because their overall injuries are less severe [8]. However, patients hospitalized and convalescing from long-bone fractures, for example, or other associated injuries with minor nonoperatively managed spleen injuries diagnosed by CT also do well and could be home were it not for their other problems.

Nonoperative management of splenic trauma is being increasingly embraced as a viable option, but many feel that more precise criteria are needed to ensure the safety of such an approach to be elucidated. Nonoperative management should not simply be a matter of "luck" but rather a planned course of action applicable to selected situations with an expected high degree of success and minimal risk to the patient.

We concur with the opinion that nonoperative management should be reserved for patients who remain absolutely hemodynamically stable. Beyond this, application of a standardized classification scheme as presented in Table 10-3, when correlated with abdominal CT and blood transfusion requirements, should facilitate decision making as to the need for operative intervention. The same classification when correlated with operative findings at the time of surgery should also assist in determining the feasibility and optimum method of repair.

A spectrum of splenic injuries is well recognized, ranging from simple type I, superficial capsular avulsions or subcapsular hematomas, to type IV, shattered or avulsed spleens. There is also a spectrum in the magnitude of the traumatic insult to the body as a whole, ranging from low-energy, isolated splenic injuries to tremendous kinetic energy forces resulting in severe multisystem trauma. There is little question that the actual manner in which any splenic injury is definitively managed has to take into account the total patient. All too often recent innovations or new approaches in management may fall victim to any one individual's most recent anecdotal experience. Failure to take into account the full spectrum of possible injury that might be encountered can sometimes result in a somewhat overzealous enthusiasm to the exclusion of all other options. Variations in the mix of patients with blunt splenic trauma have been clearly demonstrated and should be expected (Fig. 10-7). The surgeon best suited for caring for any splenic trauma victim must be knowledgeable and well versed in all therapeutic options.

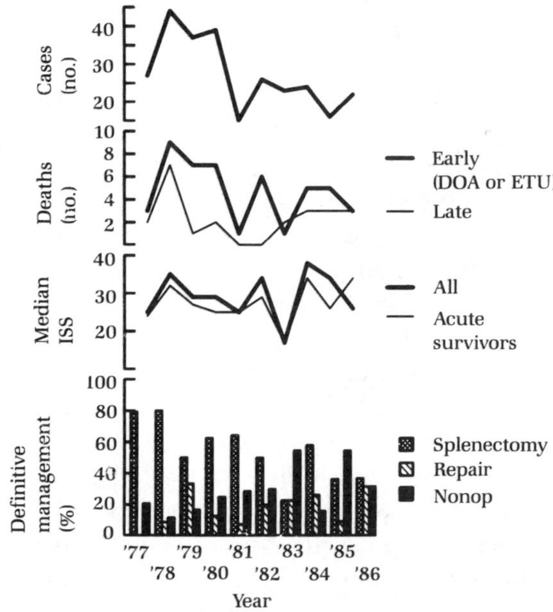

Fig. 10-7. Annual variations in the mix of 273 blunt splenic trauma patients as based on number of cases, mortality, injury severity scores, and definitive method of management. ISS = injury severity score.

Injuries of the Stomach, Duodenum, Pancreas, and Small Intestine

Timothy C. Fabian and
C. Richard Patterson

ANATOMY

Injuries of the duodenum are of particular consequence because of the unique anatomic and functional features of the duodenum. The first part of the duodenum lies at the level of the first lumbar vertebra, the second or descending part parallels the second and third lumbar vertebrae, and the third part crosses the midline at this level to end at the fourth or ascending part slightly to the left of the aorta. This location brings the respective parts of the duodenum into intimate relationship with the liver, bile duct, portal vein, pancreas, right kidney, vena cava, aorta, superior mesenteric artery and vein, the transverse colon, and the left kidney. Any of these nearby structures may be injured concomitantly with the duodenum, and those injuries may significantly alter the method of therapy employed for the duodenal injury. The duodenum is also partially retroperitoneal beginning at the second portion, with the result that it lacks total circumferential serosa for the majority of its length. Repair in the absence of a serosa is less certain, and injuries have a relatively greater propensity for dehiscence.

Dehiscence of any gastrointestinal suture line can have serious consequences, but duodenal leakage can be particularly devastating because the duodenum is the immediate common conduit for gastric, biliary, and pancreatic secretions. The components of these individual organ secretions include powerful digestive compounds that are activated by their admixture. The result of the combination is an autodigestive capacity that greatly exceeds that of the individual components and makes the management of duodenal dehiscence more difficult and urgent than isolated injuries of the stomach, pancreas, or biliary system. Preventing leakage of the duodenal contents is therefore the major principle underlying successful treatment of duodenal injuries, and the nature and location of the injury may dictate diversion of those contents rather than simple repair alone (see Operative Management of Duodenal Injuries).

The duodenum is best exposed by the Cattel maneuver, a reflection of the right colon and its mesentery beginning with incision of the line of peritoneal fusion at the right border of the colon. This reflection is limited only by the origin of the mesenteric vessels and allows full exposure of the duodenum except in its most distal extent. The exposure is completed by a similar reflection of the duodenum, which can be extended to the point where the left renal vein crosses the aorta (Kocher maneuver). This manner of exposure is recommended for the complete inspection of the duodenum and the head of the pancreas and as a preliminary to tension-free repair of the duodenum. The fourth portion of the duodenum can be completely evaluated by mobilizing the ligament of Treitz.

The surgeon should bear in mind that the duodenum and head of the pancreas share a common blood supply, the superior and inferior pancreaticoduodenal arteries, derived from the gastroduodenal and the superior mesenteric arteries, respectively. This vascular arcade is located in the pancreaticoduodenal groove, which parallels the medial wall of the second portion of the duodenum. Injury or manipulation of one organ can therefore adversely affect the other, and resection or ligation should only be carried out after consideration of the consequences for the contiguous organ. The gastroduodenal artery can be isolated in the hepatoduodenal ligament by blunt and sharp dissection at the superior border of the duodenum. The origin of the gastroduodenal artery from the common hepatic artery should be positively identified by exposing the common hepatic, the gastroduodenal, and the proper hepatic arteries. Confusion among the three and subsequent inappropriate ligation can result from a less than complete revelation of the anatomy, particularly for the surgeon relatively inexperienced in the dissection of the porta hepatis. The superior mesenteric artery and vein exit from behind the neck of the pancreas and cross the third portion of the duodenum. The artery is to the left and slightly posterior to the vein. Full exposure of the artery is rarely necessary in injuries of the pancreas and duodenum, but when necessitated by proximal arterial injury, it should not be attempted by this anterior approach. The appropriate approach to the superior mesenteric artery is retroperitoneal, by reflection of the left colon, spleen, pancreas, and left kidney. Exposure of the superior mesenteric vein is more commonly required, usually as a prelude to distal pancreatic resection or transection of the pancreas for the control of portal vein injuries. After complete transection of the gastrocolic ligament to the right, the vein is revealed by rotation of the pancreas superiorly and incision of the inferior, primarily avascular peritoneal attachment of the pancreas in the region of its neck. Once the anterior perivenous plane is achieved, it can be extended superiorly by blunt dissection to separate the vein from the pancreas. Although the anterior surface of the vein is free of tributaries, careful dissection is required in obtaining circumferential control to avoid the thin-walled and high-flow lateral tributaries. Circumferential control of the superior mesenteric vein is usually not necessary in operations for trauma.

We explore the pancreas and duodenum in every laparotomy for blunt trauma. Bile, hematoma, or crepitance in the region of the duodenum multiplies the necessity for complete exploration, and injuries to the bile duct should also be suspected. After rotation of the duodenum, the common bile duct is exposed by incision of the peritoneum and areolar tissue, which compose the inferolateral border of the hepatoduodenal ligament. Too extensive a dissection may devascularize the duct, and circumferential dissection should be avoided. Operative cholangiography augments inspection and is superior to dissection in the evaluation of the intrapancreatic duct. Cholangiography can be accomplished by direct needle stick into the common duct, compression of a dye-filled gallbladder, or cannulation of the transected cystic duct. The last method should be used only if the gallbladder will not be required for reconstruction. Localization of the ampulla of Vater is often possible by palpation through the wall of the intact duodenum. It is located on the medial wall of the middle third of the second portion of the duodenum, and intraoperative estimates of its position most often err on the superior side. The ampulla can be definitely identified without duodenotomy by introduction of a Fogarty catheter through either the cystic duct or the supraduodenal common bile duct. The orifice of the pancreatic duct is usually located distal and anteromedial to that of the bile duct at the ampulla, and care should be exercised to avoid its injury. The pancreatic duct angles upward and to the left from its origin at the ampulla, then courses more obliquely to the left near the junction of the upper and middle thirds of the pancreatic body and tail. The duct is relatively superficial in the normal pancreas.

DIAGNOSIS OF PANCREATIC AND DUODENAL TRAUMA

Mechanism of Injury

The mechanism of injury has important implications in the diagnosis of pancreaticoduodenal trauma. At our institution, we routinely explore all patients with suspected penetrating abdominal trauma, and the issue in such patients is one of intraoperative rather than preoperative diagnosis. The result of injuries missed at laparotomy can be devastating, and the exploration must be careful and thorough. The apparent path of a bullet or blade can be misleading, and there must be close attention to indicators of injury.

Hematoma is the most common indicator and requires mobilization and inspection of the organ. All intra-abdominal hematomas due to penetrating injury should be explored, and in large, central hematomas, major vascular injury should be suspected and the technique of exploration altered accordingly (see Anatomy). The hematomas associated with injury of the duodenum and particularly the pancreas may be misleadingly subtle. Any hematoma overlying the duodenum or pancreas must be completely explored to rule out visceral injury [1]. In the cases of equivocal duodenal exploration, Brotman and his associates [2] have recommended the instillation of methylene blue through the nasogastric tube. The staining of periduodenal tissues with the blue-green dye is irrefutable evidence of duodenal rupture, and the lack of staining, in their hands, has proved reliable in ruling out full-thickness duodenal injury. We have little experience with this technique and are ordinarily able to satisfy ourselves by dissection and irrigation of the duodenal hematoma. Dissection of pancreatic hematomas is more frequently equivocal than in duodenal hematomas, and in these cases, the surgeon should reflect on the major issue: whether there is major ductal injury or not. This issue is usually more easily resolved by dissection than whether there is merely pancreatic parenchymal injury. In ductal injury, resection is often required, whereas in patients with *possible* parenchymal injury, simple drainage will suffice (see Operative Management). We do not recommend routine intraoperative pancreatography, either retrograde or prograde. The former requires distal pancreatectomy, the latter requires duodenotomy, and either may inflict more injury and morbidity than the original wounding agent.

The diagnosis of blunt pancreaticoduodenal trauma is more complex than that of penetrating trauma. Victims of blunt trauma are not so frequently explored as victims of penetrating wounds, and preoperative diagnosis assumes great importance. Delay in diagnosis and treatment is uniformly recognized as the leading cause of morbidity and mortality in patients with blunt injuries of the pancreas and duodenum [3–5]. This circumstance is compounded by the lack of specific signs of pancreaticoduodenal trauma and by the fact that these injuries are sometimes not accompanied by other significant organ injuries that might prompt early exploration and their incidental discovery [4,6]. Attention to the specific mechanism of injury may heighten suspicion, for these injuries most often occur in unrestrained drivers in motor vehicle accidents [4,7], presumably by contact with the steering wheel. Other forms of trauma, no matter how trivial, can produce pancreaticoduodenal injury. Handlebar injuries are common among children and motorcycle riders, and we have treated patients with surprisingly extensive injuries from being struck by a foot or fist. The pancreas is injured by direct impact or compression. The duodenum is probably injured in one of three ways: by deceleration and resulting sheer forces produced by the points of fixation of the duodenum, by direct compression against the vertebral column, or by the production of high intraluminal pressures in the closed loop formed between the contracted pylorus and the angulation at the ligament of Treitz. Direct impact is more likely to result in injury in patients whose abdominal musculature is relaxed secondary to either altered sensorium or the suddenness and surprise of the blow [8].

Physical Examination

Initial physical examination is notoriously inexact in determining the presence of pancreaticoduodenal trauma. In patients with combined intra-abdominal injuries, the associated injuries almost always dominate the clinical picture and serve as the indication for exploration. Physical findings in isolated retroperitoneal injuries range from frank peritonitis to mild tenderness, with the latter decidedly more common than the former. Upper abdominal tenderness of any degree associated with an appropriate mechanism of injury should raise the suspicion of pancreaticoduodenal injury. Lucas [9] has described a transient diminution in abdominal tenderness in patients with such injuries. He has found that the tenderness at 2 hours following admission is less than that found on admission and is replaced by an increased tenderness at 6 hours following admission. Proper utilization of this characteristic profile requires, of course, serial examinations conducted by the same physician throughout the early hours of the patient's hospitalization. Distinction between deep tenderness and the tenderness of isolated abdominal wall trauma may be aided by asking the patient to raise his head from the mattress. The flexion of the abdominal musculature may ameliorate deep tenderness, while abdominal wall tenderness should remain essentially unchanged. Physical examination, no matter how benign, cannot rule out significant injury.

Laboratory and Radiographic Examination

Laboratory and radiographic examination share the inexactness of initial physical examination. Serum amylase is probably the most widely discussed laboratory test. While the value was elevated in 70 percent of our patients with duodenal injuries [4], and Lucas [9] recommends rising amylase levels as an indicator of pancreatic injury, many investigators have found amylase to be an unreliable test [7,10,11]. Furthermore, the source of hyperamylasemia in patients with facial trauma or recent ethanol ingestion may be obscure. One thing is certain: Pancreatic and/or duodenal injury occurs frequently without a concomitant rise in serum amylase levels. Monitoring serum amylase levels during the early postinjury phase seems prudent, but the clinician should regard normal levels as inconclusive.

Plain films of the abdomen may be more helpful, but only if interpreted carefully. Missed roentgenographic signs are frequently reported in retrospective series. Lucas [9] describes scoliosis or obliteration of the right psoas shadow in 18 of 20 patients with duodenal rupture and air bubbles around the psoas or kidney in 10 of those 18. The presence of retroperitoneal air is sufficient evidence to compel exploration, and Lucas recommends water-soluble contrast examination in patients with the less specific signs of scoliosis and psoas obscuration. Flint and coworkers [7] emphasize the tendency of surgeons and particularly radiologists to overlook the evidence present on plain films, but their experience with contrast studies has been disappointing, with two false-negative studies in three patients with full-thickness duodenal injury. A false-negative contrast study is doubly dangerous because of the sense of security it inspires. Plain films and contrast studies, like serum amylase determinations, should be used to prompt early exploration, not to dismiss the possibility of pancreaticoduodenal injury.

Lavage, Tomography, and Endoscopy

Diagnostic peritoneal lavage (DPL) has been widely employed in the evaluation of blunt and, to a lesser extent, penetrating abdominal trauma [12]. Its sensitivity in retroperitoneal injuries is rightfully suspect, however. While Flint and his associates [7] are enthusiastic about DPL, the associated injuries in their series rather than the duodenal injuries are probably responsible for its apparent sensitivity. We are convinced that DPL is currently the best ancillary means of evaluating the victim of blunt abdominal trauma [13], but we share the reservations of others concerning its efficacy in detecting retroperitoneal injuries [6,9].

Our reservations extend to computed tomography of the abdomen (CTA), despite the enthusiasm of others. We are aware of no convincing evidence that CTA is very accurate in the early diagnosis of pancreatic and duodenal injuries. CTA may be capable of diagnosing pancreatic trauma reliably at 24 hours after injury, but that after all is the time when clinical deterioration should be evident and prompting exploration rather than further diagnostic tests. Contrast CTA examinations may be more sensitive for duodenal injury than conventional studies, but our experience with this technique is sufficient only to indicate that false-negative and false-positive results are possible. We currently employ CTA in patients with predisposing mechanisms of injury who are without other indications of retroperitoneal injury, in an effort to shorten the preoperative delay.

Duodenoscopy and endoscopic pancreatography have been suggested as means of improving the diagnostic rate for pancreaticoduodenal injuries. Most of these suggestions are casual and not derived from broad clinical experience. We have not employed duodenoscopy in this manner, and our experience with endoscopic pancreatography has been restricted to patients with persistent hyperamylasemia or pseudocysts following known pancreatic trauma.

Summary

The diagnosis of pancreaticoduodenal trauma is more often made by the astute clinician than by any laboratory test or x-ray. The major principle in diagnosis is awareness of the initial subtlety of these injuries, and the major requirement for success is that the diagnostic possibility be borne in mind. All ancillary measures may be collectively characterized as reliable only when they suggest or identify an injury of the pancreas or duodenum. The "normal" study is perfidious. The solution to the diagnostic quandary is the conscientious examination and reexamination of the patient at risk for pancreatic and duodenal injury combined with a readiness to explore carefully when there is a change for the worse. One should not be cavalier about negative laparotomies, but they are preferable to neglected injury.

OPERATIVE MANAGEMENT OF DUODENAL INJURIES

There are two major considerations to be taken into account when deciding on operative management of duodenal injuries. The first is degree of tissue injury, and the second is whether the injury is intraperitoneal or extraperitoneal. Those wounds to the intraperitoneal duodenum occur through a serosal surface and are well managed by simple primary closure with one or two layers of suture. The retroperitoneal duodenum has no serosal covering and is therefore at greater risk of leak from primary repair. Stab wounds and small-caliber, low-velocity weapons often produce intraperitoneal, nondestructive wounds. Wounds to the duodenum produced by most blunt trauma and larger-caliber or high-velocity weapons generally have more tissue injury and involve the retroperitoneal area of the duodenum. Simple repair of these injuries has been demonstrated to yield a high incidence of complications [14]. Dehiscence of these suture lines is caused in part and made more ominous by the nature of the duodenal contents (see Anatomy). The stomach produces 2 to 3 liters of fluid rich in hydrochloric acid and pepsin, the liver produces 800 to 1200 ml of bile, while the pancreas adds 600 to 1000 ml of fluid rich in the enzymes required for carbohydrate, fat, and protein digestion.

Various methods of managing complex duodenal injuries have been developed, and decompression of some or all of the digestive fluids is a significant component of these approaches. Decompression lowers intraduodenal pressure and should decrease suture line failure. One of the earliest described approaches to the management of these injuries was duodenal diverticulization [6] (Fig. 10-8). Diverticulization involves repair of the duodenal wound combined with gastric resection and Billroth II reconstruction. This procedure diverts the gastric contents from the area of the repair. Three shortcomings of the procedure are the requirement for gastric resection, the creation of a gastrointestinal suture line, and the lack of diversion of pancreatic and biliary secretions. The last shortcoming can be at least partially overcome with the addition of a duodenostomy tube.

A similar approach, but one not requiring gastric resection, is that of pyloric exclusion [15] (Fig. 10-9). After duodenal repair, the pylorus is sutured closed through a distal

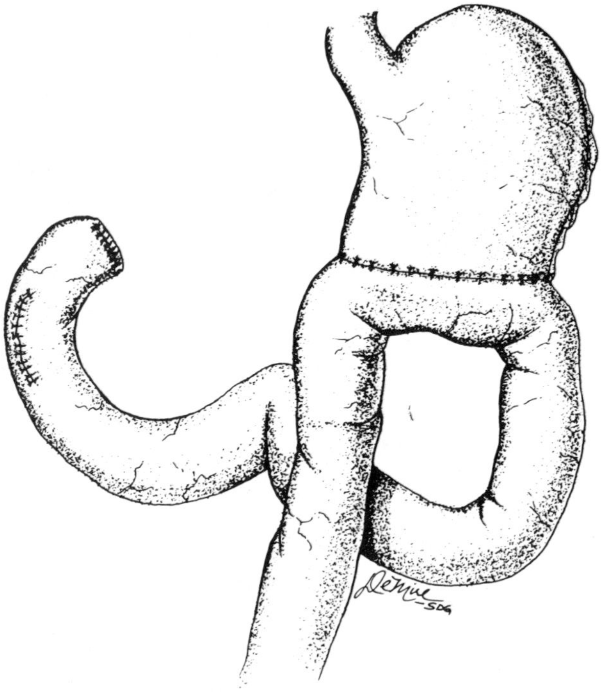

Fig. 10-8. Treatment of duodenal injury by the application of duodenal diverticulization.

greater curvature gastrotomy. The gastrotomy is then utilized to create a side-to-side gastrojejunostomy. As with diverticulization, this procedure only diverts gastric secretions and, although not requiring resection, does entail a gastrointestinal anastomosis. In a report by Martin and colleagues [16] in which absorbable polyglycolic acid or catgut suture was used for pyloric closure, 39 of 44 patients had a patent pylorus after 3 weeks. Even among the patients sutured with nonabsorbable polypropylene, nearly all patients studied had a patent pylorus. Vagotomy has not been necessary because of the temporary nature of the occlusion and a low incidence of marginal ulceration [15].

A third approach, extensively applied at our institution for complex or retroperitoneal duodenal wounds, employs retrograde jejunostomy, feeding jejunostomy, and gastrostomy [17] (Fig. 10-10). After duodenal repair, a proximal loop of jejunum is selected, and Witzel jejunostomies are created utilizing 16 Fr rubber catheters. One catheter is passed retrograde into the second portion of the duodenum and placed on gravity drainage to decompress the pancreatic and biliary secretions. The second jejunostomy is threaded distally and provides for feeding and reinstil-

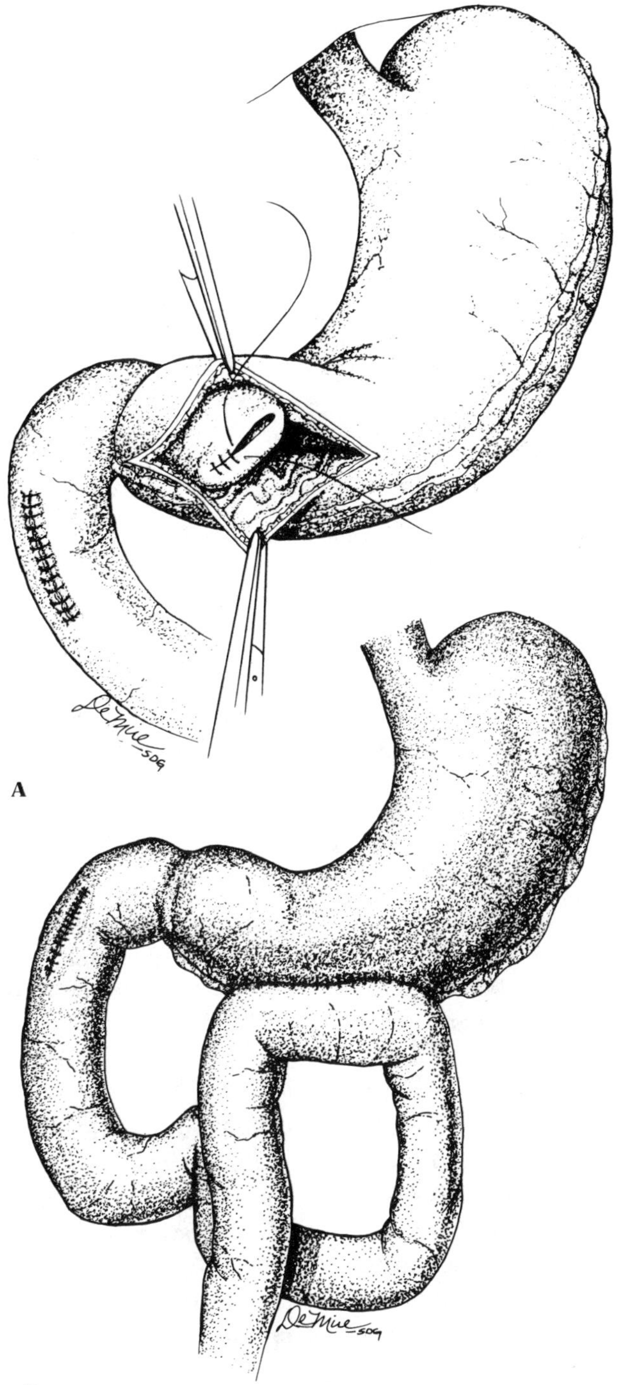

A

B

Fig. 10-9. Treatment of duodenal injury by the application of duodenal exclusion.

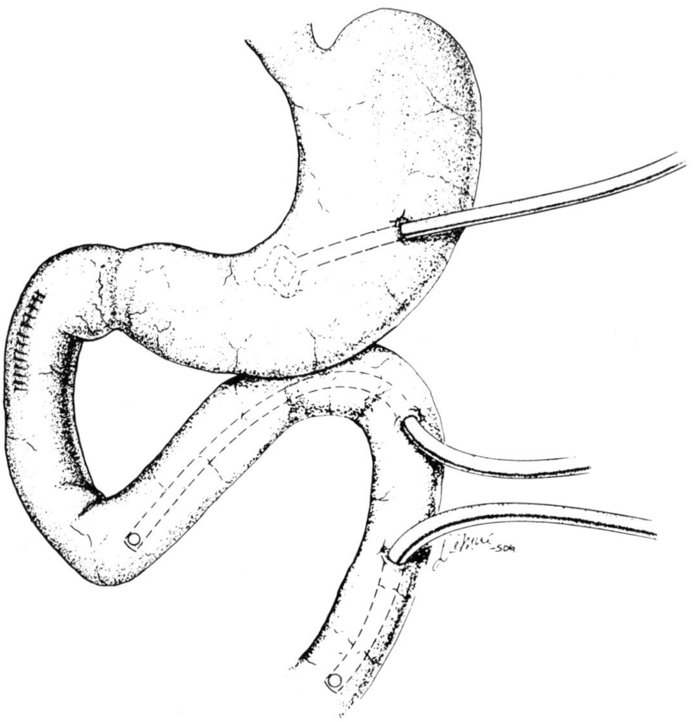

Fig. 10-10. Treatment of duodenal injury by duodenal decompression by retrograde jejunostomy, use of a feeding jejunostomy, and gastrostomy.

lation of the pancreatic and biliary secretions, avoiding electrolyte disturbances and enhancing digestion. A gastrostomy is frequently employed to avert the problems of reflux and poor pulmonary toilet associated with prolonged nasogastric intubation. This approach to management of duodenal wounds has produced excellent results, yielding only one duodenal leak in 237 patients so treated [17].

Occasionally a patient will be encountered with more extensive loss of duodenal substance. Such injuries to the third and fourth portions of the duodenum can be managed by distal duodenectomy and end-to-end duodenojejunostomy, Roux-Y. These injuries are relatively uncommonly managed because of the lethality of associated vascular injuries. A serosal patch has also been reported to be efficacious in treating patients in whom a large area of duodenal wall is destroyed in a noncircumferential fashion. An onlay of a jejunal loop is applied, utilizing the serosal surface of the onlay patch to provide the lost area of duodenal wall.

The Whipple procedure is reserved for patients in whom there is extensive devitalization of the C-loop of the duodenum and head of the pancreas, most often due to a close-range shotgun blast. It is a truism that bears repeating that the Whipple procedure is performed for trauma only when the injury has accomplished the resection. The surgical procedure becomes one of hemostasis and reestablishing gastrointestinal and biliary-enteric continuity. Nondevitalizing wounds of both the second or third portion of the duodenum and the head of the pancreas are managed as though they occurred separately. The pancreatic wound is generally drained and the duodenal wound handled according to the extent of injury, by either simple repair or duodenal decompression.

Biliary decompression by means of a T-tube has no place in the management of pancreatic or biliary injury. A prospective study [18] has demonstrated their lack of utility and suggests they create a risk because of placement in a normal common bile duct. Placing external drains in the vicinity of the duodenal repair is not encouraged, although little data are available either to support or condemn their application. A study by Stone and Fabian [17] did report a 23 percent duodenal leak rate when drains were used, compared to 8 percent when they were not. It would seem that placing a foreign body around a suture line might predispose toward dehiscence.

OPERATIVE MANAGEMENT OF PANCREATIC INJURIES

The options for management of pancreatic wounds include external drainage, internal drainage, resection, or a combination of these. More than 88 percent of penetrating pancreatic wounds do not involve the main pancreatic duct [19], and they are successfully managed by external drainage alone. The same is true of any pancreatic injury in which there is no major ductal involvement, but blunt pancreatic injuries are more commonly complete transections.

Acceptable external drainage systems include sump and closed suction drains. Passive drains of the Penrose variety are not advocated, since dependent drainage cannot usually be obtained and inadequate drainage of pancreatic juices occurs. A 37-percent complication rate has been reported with Penrose drains, as compared to 2 percent with sump drains [19]. The disadvantage of sump drainage is that no matter which system is applied, bacterial contamination from the environment occurs. This contamination can occasionally produce a peripancreatic abscess and commonly produces bothersome drain tract infections that prolong hospitalization. Placing filters on the sumps does not appear to impact this problem. Closed suction systems should significantly reduce the incidence of bacterial colonization, but closed suction systems have been observed to become plugged rapidly in other clinical applications. Controlled experience is lacking with their use in pancreatic drainage, and we are currently involved in a prospective randomized trial of sump versus closed suction pancreatic drainage at our trauma center. Pancreatic drains should be left in place for at least 10 days because pancreatic leakage often does not develop until that time [19,20].

Internal drainage of pancreatic injuries through a Roux-Y loop of jejunum has been reported [20,21]. This offers the potential advantages of preservation of pancreatic tissue [20] as well as improved drainage of secretions [22]. This technique has been applied in pancreatic wounds, resulting in division of the main pancreatic duct. Those authors most concerned with preservation of pancreatic substance have anastomosed the proximal pancreatic remnant to one side of the jejunal loop and the distal remnant to the opposite side. Pancreaticojejunostomy has also been combined with resection of the distal pancreatic remnant. We do not practice this technique of internal drainage. Five of seven patients reported with this approach had major complications, including three deaths from pancreatic infection [19]. There are two problems that may contribute to the difficulties experienced with this procedure. The first problem is that of sewing the bowel to the normal pancreas, which is not fibrotic as is the case with internal drainage for chronic pancreatic disease. Secondly, the jejunum supposedly functions as a "living vacuum," but these patients generally are severely injured and have an ileus that may last several days. This allows for colonization by gastrointestinal flora and may produce pancreatic sepsis. It has also been reported that resections of up to 80 percent result in no exocrine or endocrine insufficiency in the otherwise healthy gland [20,23].

The remaining option for management of the pancreatic wound is resection. Distal resection is our preferred approach for lesions of the body and tail. Splenic salvage is attempted when the patient is stable, although associated injuries from both penetrating and blunt trauma frequently demand expeditious management, prohibiting the meticulous dissection required to separate the tail of the pancreas from the splenic vessels and hilum. The technique is outlined in Figure 10-11. After the pancreas is mobilized from the retroperitoneum, the splenic vein and artery are individually doubly ligated. A vascular clamp is placed across the proximal pancreas, and the gland is divided. The vascular clamp is applied because of the extensive bleeding resulting from division of the normal pancreas. After division of the pancreas, a series of U-sutures of polypropylene are placed at close intervals to provide hemostasis. These should be placed right against the clamp to avoid a large cuff of devitalized pancreas. After the sutures have been placed, the clamp is removed and an attempt is made to ligate the pancreatic duct individually. The duct can be readily ligated if it is identified prior to tying the U-sutures. After resection, individual vessels are ligated as necessary. An apron of omentum is placed beneath the resected pancreas to prevent the ligated vessels from being digested by pancreatic enzymes, and a suction drain is placed at the resected edge. The technique of pancreatic resection has also been accomplished with the GI anastomosis type of stapling device.

Wounds to the head of the pancreas are usually a result of penetrating trauma. Major vascular injuries often occur due to the proximity of the superior mesenteric vessels, portal vein, aorta, and vena cava. The greater part of the operative effort is directed at controlling these vascular injuries, which are the major reason for the high mortality associated with penetrating wounds of the head of the pancreas. Occasionally a relatively isolated wound will occur from a low-caliber missile

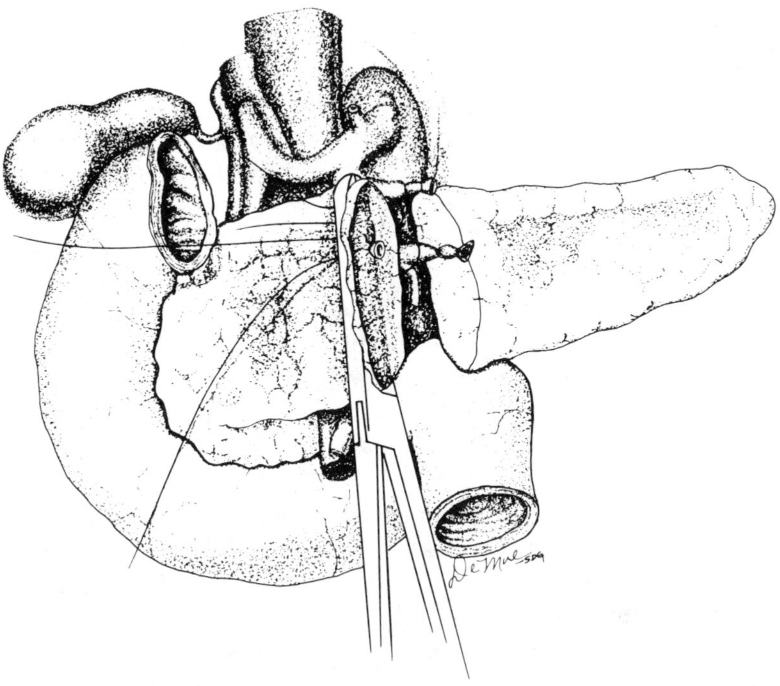

Fig. 10-11. Technique for distal pancreatectomy for trauma.

or stab wound. We manage these injuries by drainage, even if the main duct is suspected to be involved. If a pancreatic fistula develops, it can be managed as a chronic fistula and treated at a second, elective exploration if necessary.

A blunt pancreatic injury occasionally occurs in which the base of the small bowel mesentery including the mesenteric vessels is thrust forward from deceleration and the uncinate process is torn at the point where the mesenteric vessels enter the peritoneal cavity from behind the pancreas. We have treated two such patients in the last 2 years. Both developed pseudocysts postoperatively and did well following internal drainage procedures.

COMPLICATIONS OF PANCREATIC AND DUODENAL TRAUMA

Complication rates among patients with pancreatic injuries range from 36 to 50 percent [21,22]. The complications are attributable to both the function and location of the gland. Enzyme and fluid production provide a setting for autolytic tissue destruction, and the location of the gland in the upper abdomen surrounded by a number of major vessels predisposes to the life-threatening complications associated with hemorrhagic shock: bleeding diathesis, sepsis, and multiple organ failure. Although never completely avoidable, pancreatic complications can be minimized by appropriate and expeditious operative management of both the pancreatic and vascular wounds.

The commonest pancreatic complications are pancreatitis, peripancreatic abscess, drain tract infections, postoperative hemorrhage, fistula, and pseudocyst. Traumatic pancreatitis is generally a self-limited process that is treated symptomatically, resolving within a week or so. Occasionally the symptoms will completely resolve while the serum amylase remains mildly elevated. These patients can often be fed without exacerbation of their pain. If pain develops, or the amylase rises, symptomatic therapy can be reinstituted. In some patients, the post-traumatic pancreatitis will last up to a few weeks and require nutritional support before resolution. Persistent pancreatitis is more frequently the harbinger of other complications including pseudocyst and infection, however.

The colonization required for pancreatic infection generally comes from associated gastrointestinal injuries, especially following penetrating trauma. Aerobic gram-negative rods and gram-positive cocci are the usual infecting organisms, and antibiotics covering these should be started, pending sensitivity testing of any recovered infectious specimen. The stage for infection is further set in these patients because inadequately drained pancreatic secretions will locally digest tissue, providing an excellent culture medium for the colonizing organisms. The infections may develop as lesser sac abscesses, infected pseudocysts, or phlegmons, necrotizing collections in the retroperitoneum. Drain tract infections, which are nosocomial, are seldom life-threatening but result in morbidity, prolonged antibiotic therapy, and hospitalization. Many of the organisms are gram-negative rods typical of intensive care unit–acquired infections: *Enterobacter, Escherichia coli, Acinetobacter, Pseudomonas,* and *Klebsiella.* Proper management of drains can reduce these infections. All sump drains have some colonization at their base. When they are removed, a second drainage tube such as a sterile rubber or large Foley catheter should be reinserted in the tract. The secondary drain is advanced over a few days as the tract heals, averting closed space infections. Using closed suction drains might avoid some of these infections, but first they must be proved to be effective in adequately draining the pancreatic secretions.

Pancreatic fistulas occur in nearly one-third of patients with pancreatic wounds [21,24]. Nearly all of these will close spontaneously within 2 to 4 weeks and occasionally will close after longer periods of time. The enzymes are usually not activated and produce little problem with skin excoriation. In the occasional patient whose fistula does not close, there is usually an injury to the duct of Wirsung. Fistulography will generally demonstrate the injury. Resection or internal Roux-Y drainage will provide definitive management.

Pseudocysts are reported in 1.5 to 2.2 percent of pancreatic injuries [21,25]. They are the consequence of either inadequate drainage or injury to the duct of Wirsung. Infected pseudocysts should be drained externally. Uninfected traumatic pseudocysts can be managed by either internal drainage or resection. Endoscopic retrograde pancreatography should be performed to aid in the selection of procedure.

Another complication associated with pancreatic duct disruption is that of "pancreatic sequestrum," a chronic condition that has been described in patients long after a missed pancreatic injury [26]. These patients are among the apparent few who do not develop the fulminant sequelae of untreated pancreatic injury but develop rather a chronic pancreatitis or pseudocyst. The condition can be prevented by the identification of pancreatic injuries primarily and should be suspected in patients presenting with abdominal pain following remote trauma. Treatment may require internal drainage, resection, or pancreaticojejunostomy and can be guided by endoscopic pancreatography.

Postoperative hemorrhage can be a serious, early complication following pancreatic injury. It most commonly occurs following pancreatic resection and results from the autodigestive capacity of the liberated pancreatic secretions. Salvage requires early reoperation to obtain hemostasis and wide pancreatic drainage. The omentum should be used as already described to isolate the pancreatic remnant. This is a complication to which the surgeon must remain alert from the earliest postoperative moment and throughout the patient's hospitalization.

Duodenal complications include fistula and dehiscence. The occurrence of dehiscence may be signalled by the patient's general deterioration or by bile staining the dressings. In the case of deterioration, reoperation is necessary, and the injury should be treated as a complex, retroperitoneal duodenal injury, as previously described. Some duodenal fistulae are well tolerated, however, and in those selected patients, observation and parenteral nutrition can be expected to result in spontaneous closure. Tolerance is defined as no sign of sepsis, no digestion of the abdominal wall, and the maintenance of adequate nutrition and fluid and electrolyte balance.

STOMACH AND SMALL INTESTINE

Blunt gastric disruption occurs very uncommonly; the incidence of isolated small bowel disruption is 1 to 2 percent among victims of blunt abdominal trauma. Physical examination is the mainstay of diagnosis in the patient with an unaltered sensorium. The chemical peritonitis produced by gastric injuries is more fulminant than that of bowel perforation, and serial examination is often necessary to detect the patient with isolated small-bowel injury. Both organs harbor relatively low bacterial contents, but if the chemical peritonitis is allowed to persist before repair, it will be superseded by a bacterial peritonitis that significantly complicates the patient's course.

Physical examination cannot be relied on in the patient with an altered sensorium due to injury or intoxication. Plain films are of little utility, although gastric injuries result in detectable pneumoperitoneum more frequently than injuries of the intestine. Peritoneal lavage remains the most reliable diagnostic aid, although timing may be a critical determinant of accuracy. Lavage performed within 2 to 4 hours of injury may precede the establishment of the peritoneal inflammatory response that is necessary for a positive study [27,28].

In patients at risk and in whom the initial lavage is equivocal, the catheter may be left in place for a delayed repeat lavage. The lavage effluent is usually tested for white blood cell count and the presence of bile and vegetable matter. Bile and vegetable fibers are so uncommonly found among patients with intestinal perforation that a good argument can be made for omitting these assays. A white blood cell count equal to or greater than 500 cells/μl is considered positive [28]. In a recent series of 13 patients at our institution with blunt small-bowel injury, 9 underwent preoperative peritoneal lavage. Six lavages were positive on the basis of red blood cell counts due to bleeding from concomitant injuries; three lavages were positive by white cell criterion alone [29]. The white cell count should never be omitted from effluent evaluation.

Some authors have reported utilizing alkaline phosphatase levels in the lavage effluent as a means of diagnosing small-bowel injuries [27,30]. This assay is more costly than white cell count, and because of the relative infrequency of isolated intestinal perforation in blunt trauma, it is difficult to prove that enzyme analysis significantly improves diagnostic yield. This technique requires more controlled experience before routine application. The same can be said for computed tomography; although the technique has been reported useful [31], our experience suggests a lack of sensitivity in isolated intestinal injuries [13].

The repair of gastric and intestinal injuries is usually straightforward. Both are amenable to primary repair, and resection and diversion are usually not required. The sine qua non of successful repair is recognition of the injury. The injuries are usually obvious at exploration, but several areas require particularly careful attention: the fat-infiltrated greater and lesser gastric curvatures, the proximal posterior gastric wall, the gastric fundus and cardia, and the mesenteric border of the small bowel. Injuries in these areas may be overlooked if the surgeon is not conscientious with exposure and dissection. In penetrating trauma, the discovery of an odd number of perforations should prompt the surgeon to a redoubled effort to find further injury.

Isolated mesenteric injuries are usually of little consequence, but early hemorrhage and late intestinal infarction are two potential problems. The former is detected routinely, but the latter may be subtle, and patients may not become symptomatic for 4 or 5 days following injury. The apparent viability of the bowel at exploration can be misleading, and the diagnosis of intestinal ischemia should be suspected in all victims of blunt trauma who develop delayed abdominal findings and sepsis. The proper course in this setting is exploration or reexploration. The intraoperative Doppler device is useful in determining the extent of devitalized bowel.

Injuries of the Colon and Rectum

Roger Sherman and Christina Rehm

Wounds of the colon and rectum can be highly lethal when they are not recognized and treated expediently. The history of management of colon and rectal injuries in the wars of this century is an example par excellence of how improved management of a specific injury evolves over time as experience is gained with large numbers of cases.

Death from these once highly lethal injuries can virtually always be avoided today because of modern advances in medicine as well as improvement in surgical techniques. Major factors contributing to improved survival are shorter intervals from injury to the operating room, use of preoperative antibiotics for both aerobic and anaerobic coverage, and development of safe techniques for treatment of these injuries in all circumstances.

EARLY DIAGNOSIS

Successful management begins preoperatively with early diagnosis. There is no reliable method for identification of colon injuries other than exploratory laparotomy. Unstable patients automatically undergo prompt exploratory laparotomy, which easily uncovers colon injuries, if present. Since colon injuries, per se, produce little in the way of initial symptoms, patients without obvious need for prompt laparotomy are at much greater risk for the dreaded late complications of an undiagnosed colonic wound. In these patients, indications for exploratory laparotomy include a high index of suspicion in blunt trauma, all patients with penetrating wounds with entrance or exit wounds below the fifth intercostal space, and patients with x-ray evidence of bullets below the diaphragm.

Patients with abdominal stab wounds require selective laparotomy for criteria similar to those for patients with blunt trauma or with evidence of penetration of the peritoneal cavity on exploration of the wound. Patients with gunshot wounds of the abdomen require routine laparotomy.

Rectal injuries can easily be missed at laparotomy and should be diagnosed preoperatively. All patients with injuries to or in the proximity of the pelvis and perineum need a careful proctosigmoidoscopy examination, a cystourethrogram, and speculum inspection of the vagina.

Preoperative Antibiotics

Patients with suspected colon or rectal injury should receive preoperative parenteral antibiotics for aerobe and anaerobe coverage so that adequate blood levels can be achieved before the laparotomy incision is made.

Technique of Exploration

In most instances, a standard midline incision is the operative approach of choice in laparotomy. To limit fecal contamination, all obvious injuries of the bowel should be controlled initially by noncrushing clamps or running sutures that will also achieve hemostasis if necessary.

If there are no associated injuries demanding immediate attention, all gross fecal material should be removed at this time, followed by careful inspection of the entire colon. Hematomas, fecal staining, and air in the retroperitoneum are important indications of possible colonic injury. It is mandatory to include exploration of the retroperitoneal portions of the ascending and descending colon by complete division of the lateral peritoneal attachments of both the left and right colon.

Opening the peritoneum of the pelvic floor to explore the extraperitoneal rectum from above is not recommended.

MANAGEMENT OF COLON INJURIES

Once wounds of the colon have been identified, there are a number of options available for management, depending on the circumstances in each individual patient (Table 10-4).

Table 10-4. Options for Treatment of Colon Injuries

Primary repair
Colostomy with injured colon as the stoma
Resection with end colostomy and mucous fistula
Resection with end colostomy and Hartmann's pouch
Repair with proximal diversion
Primary repair with exteriorization

Penetrating Injuries

On review of the extensive literature concerning colon wounds, a long list of factors has been suggested as influencing the success or failure of primary colon repair in patients with these injuries [1–6]. The presence of shock, age of the patient, site and extent of injury, number, degree and kind of associated injuries, time interval from injury to surgery, and degree of fecal contamination are included among others. More important than assessing multiple "risk factors" is to realize which of these factors affect the management of the injury per se and which should be attributed to the traumatic insult on the patient as a whole. The anatomic, physiologic, and bacteriologic differences between the various segments of the large intestine have been overemphasized as determinants of success of colon repair, and in fact, many injuries of all segments of the colon can be managed primarily [1,7,8]. The type of injury is of much more importance than location in selecting the appropriate method of management.

The extent of the colon injury has consistently been found to be the most important factor in deciding the most appropriate form of repair. Attention to the colon injury alone allows successful primary repair in 50 to 60 percent of patients. The majority of civilian colon injuries are caused by knives or small-caliber, low-velocity missiles that cause limited tissue destruction. Accordingly, primary repair should be the method of choice for the majority of these injuries.

A "protective" colostomy proximal to a primary repair is not indicated. The fate of a primary repair of a colon anastomosis is not influenced by a proximal colostomy. All this diversion of the fecal stream does is protect from the consequences of a fecal leak [1].

When all of the factors that influence the method of management of colon injuries are taken into consideration, the circumstances under which primary repair is indicated are clear (Table 10-5).

Although no one specific type of associated injury is a contraindication to primary repair, if a short operating time in a severely traumatized patient is lifesaving, primary repair should not be carried out. Other contraindi-

Table 10-5. Indications for Primary Repair

Wound less than ⅓ of circumference
Mesenteric aspect uninvolved
Good blood supply
No peritonitis
Injury < 8 hours old
No rectal injury
Will not prolong management of severe or multiple associated injuries

cations to primary repair include multiple wounds to one area of the colon, significant hematomas of the wall of the colon, and mesenteric injury with vascular compromise.

As a rule, when primary repair is not indicated, the affected colon can be resected. Primary ileocolostomy following resection of injuries of the right colon is a most satisfactory procedure. After resection of left colon lesions, we prefer not to perform a colocolostomy with unprepared bowel, but rather to exteriorize the proximal bowel as an end colostomy and either bring out the distal bowel as a mucous fistula or close it with a Hartmann's procedure.

The Hartmann's procedure is safe, and a mucous fistula is only necessary in the rare trauma patient in whom a distal colonic or rectal obstruction is present. Location of the distal colon at the time of colostomy closure is facilitated by tagging the closed distal colon by a long proline suture and by insertion of a large rectal tube through the anus prior to laparotomy.

When lifesaving measures are more important than specific management of colon wounds, the injured segment of the colon can simply be exteriorized for definitive management at a later time.

An alternative method to primary repair advocated by some is primary repair with exteriorization of the sutured segment of the colon [9,10]. The colon can be exteriorized over a glass rod or by creating a window in the mesocolon with suture of the fascia behind the colon. The advantage of this method is that a repair that breaks down is easily converted into a loop colostomy without the risk of peritonitis. If a leak does not develop, the repaired bowel can be easily returned to the peritoneal cavity in a few days.

Our experience with this method of management is limited, as our results have included a large number of disruptions of the repair as well as obstruction of the colon at the site of fascial closure [11,12]. It is our contention that a colonic suture line for primary repair is surrounded and protected by omentum and loops of bowel when it remains in the peritoneal cavity and is far less likely to leak than when it is placed under dressings on the abdominal wall.

Colostomy

The purpose of a colostomy is the controlled diversion of the fecal stream. The only colostomy that can reliably achieve this goal is an end colostomy. In an emergency situation, it should be brought out through a separate incision and not "matured." Maturing is not wise in the emergency situation, as the bowel is likely to become edematous, and postoperative abdominal distention secondary to ileus can cause disastrous retraction of the stoma. A loop colostomy, although easier to construct and easier to close, will not achieve reliable complete fecal diversion. Under emergency conditions, however, by stapling across the efferent limb, a loop colostomy can be turned into an end colostomy.

Finally, it is important to emphasize that a colostomy is not an innocuous procedure [13]. The mere presence of a colostomy or an exteriorized bowel segment is a source of morbidity in itself. It is a source of contamination of incision and of the abdominal cavity. It is associated with a longer hospital stay compared with primary repair and requires reoperation for closure, which is associated with a morbidity of 10 to 30 percent.

Drains

Drainage of a colon repair or colon anastomosis is not recommended. Drains placed close to an intestinal suture line lead to increased colonic leaks and abscess formation. Drains placed elsewhere in the abdominal cavity in the face of generalized fecal contamination serve no purpose and are also not indicated.

Peritoneal Irrigation

In treating colon wounds, it is important to remove all possible particulate matter from the peritoneal cavity. Bacterial contamination, per se, is handled well by the peritoneal cavity, whereas gross fecal matter is not. It is a potentiating factor to simple bacterial contamination that leads to peritonitis and abscess formation. Mechanical cleansing of the abdomen is best achieved by irrigation with copious amounts of warm saline solution. Irrigation with various antibiotic solutions has been suggested, but their efficacy is doubtful when compared to the protective effect of adequate blood levels of appropriate antibiotics achieved prior to laparotomy.

Wound Closure

When there has been gross contamination of the skin and subcutaneous tissue as is common in colon injuries, the fascia should be closed and the wound packed open. Primary skin closure will be successful only if there is minimal contamination and adequate hemostasis has been achieved. In these instances, irrigation of the incision before closure should be routine. A colostomy or exteriorized repair is not a contraindication for primary wound closure, but they should be separated from the incision by an occlusive dressing or a well-fitting appliance.

Blunt Colon Injuries

Injuries to the colon from blunt abdominal trauma are particularly dangerous [14,15]. As mentioned earlier, there is no reliable method to establish early diagnosis of these injuries other than exploratory laparotomy. This is the inherent danger in the present trend to treat stable patients with hemoperitoneum nonoperatively. A high index of suspicion of colon injury is essential.

Certain types of blunt abdominal trauma, such as seat belt injuries, carry a high risk of injury to the intestine as well as to the mesentery. The lap-type seat belt slips over the anterior superior iliac spines, and the full force of impact is transmitted to the viscera trapped between the belt and the spinal column. These blunt visceral injuries frequently lead to delayed perforation as a result of ischemia secondary to either contusion or extensive hematoma formation of the bowel wall or the mesenteric vessels. Careful observation of the patient for the early diagnosis of these occult but potentially lethal types of injuries is essential.

Early and persistent ileus or the onset of adult respiratory distress syndrome are both good indicators of possible occult intra-abdominal sepsis.

Treatment of blunt colon injuries depends on the type of injury produced. Blunt trauma may cause damage by laceration, contusion, hematoma of the bowel wall, stripping off the seromuscular layer, necrosis of the bowel from compression by hematoma, or avulsion of the mesentery.

Injuries from blunt trauma usually are not appropriate for primary repair. Since contused and devitalized colon may extend beyond the obvious injury, primary repair is risky. Superficial seromuscular tears can be repaired by simple suture, but most full-thickness wounds should be resected and an end colostomy performed. Hematomas should be evacuated and clear demonstration of adequate blood supply to the colon obtained prior to closure of the abdomen. Early reexploration should be entertained if further necrosis of the bowel is suggested by pain, fever, leukocytosis, persistent ileus, or the onset of adult respiratory distress syndrome.

RECTAL INJURIES

Injuries of the rectum are the most serious of all intestinal injuries because of its extraperitoneal location [9–12,16]. The rectum is surrounded by poorly vascularized fatty tissue without fixed anatomic boundaries so that wounds of the rectum permit rapid spread of infection in the virtually unlimited retroperitoneal space.

Diagnosis

Since the rectum is entirely extraperitoneal, laparotomy often fails to demonstrate rectal injury. All penetrating wounds of the perineum, buttocks, and lower abdomen are suspect for rectal injury. Careful digital examination of the rectum that shows blood on the examining finger is highly suggestive of rectal injury. Demonstration of blood by proctoscopy or sigmoidoscopy virtually confirms the diagnosis. Visualization of the injury itself is not always possible and is not necessary. In addition to proctosigmoidoscopy, a retrograde cystourethrogram should be obtained and a careful vaginal examination done in females to rule out concomitant injury to the urogenital system. Indications for proctosigmoidoscopy to rule out rectal injuries are listed in Table 10-6 [17]. If a rectal injury is suspected from proximity of penetrating wounds or in conjunction with severe pelvic fractures, it is wise to manage as if rectal injury is present. A completely diverting colostomy should be performed.

Treatment

There is little controversy over the management of rectal injuries. The distal colon and rectum should be defunctionalized by complete diversion by end colostomy and performance of a Hartmann's pouch (Fig. 10-12) [18]. A semicircular incision is made through the median raphe posterior to the anus, through

Table 10-6. Indications for Proctosigmoidoscopy

Penetrating	Blunt
Rectal blood	Rectal blood
Perianal, perineal wounds; trajectory of missile below pelvic brim, above upper thigh, or crossing of pelvis at any point	Pelvic fractures with displaced symphysis pubis
Hematuria	Perianal or perineal lacerations
Vaginal blood	Bladder or urethral tear
Extraperitoneal pelvic hematoma adjacent to rectum at laparotomy	Extraperitoneal pelvic hematoma adjacent to rectum at laparotomy

which bilateral, presacral, Penrose drains are placed (Fig. 10-13) [18]. Sacral fractures or other pelvic bony defects should be avoided because of the risk of osteomyelitis. Saline irrigation of the defunctionalized distal rectal stump to wash out retained feces, although not absolutely necessary, completes the management of these injuries.

Repair of the rectal injury itself is not mandatory and should be done only if it can be visualized and performed easily transanally. Occasionally, an easily visualized, distal, par-

Fig. 10-12. The essential steps of rectal trauma management: Completely diverting colostomy, presacral drainage, closure of easily accessible rectal injury (for proximal lesion), or healing by secondary intention (for distal lesion). (From D. Trunkey et al., Management of rectal trauma. *J. Trauma* 13:411, © by Williams & Wilkins, 1973.)

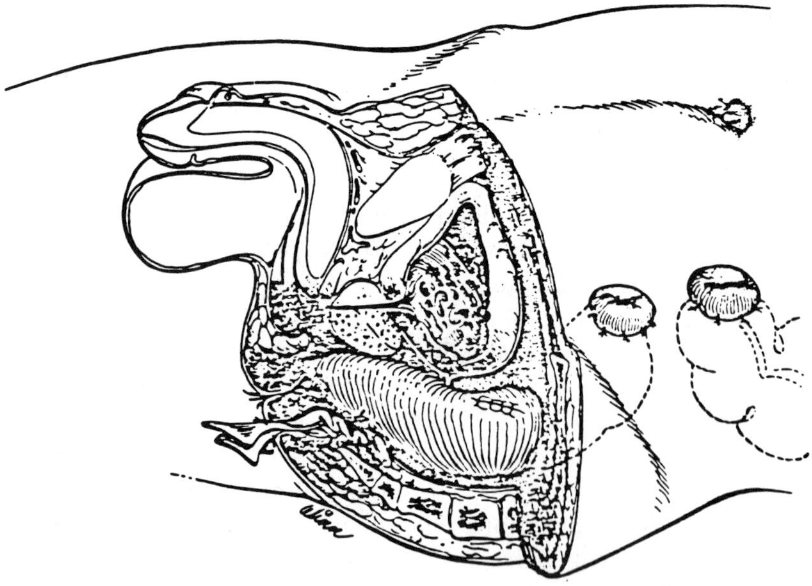

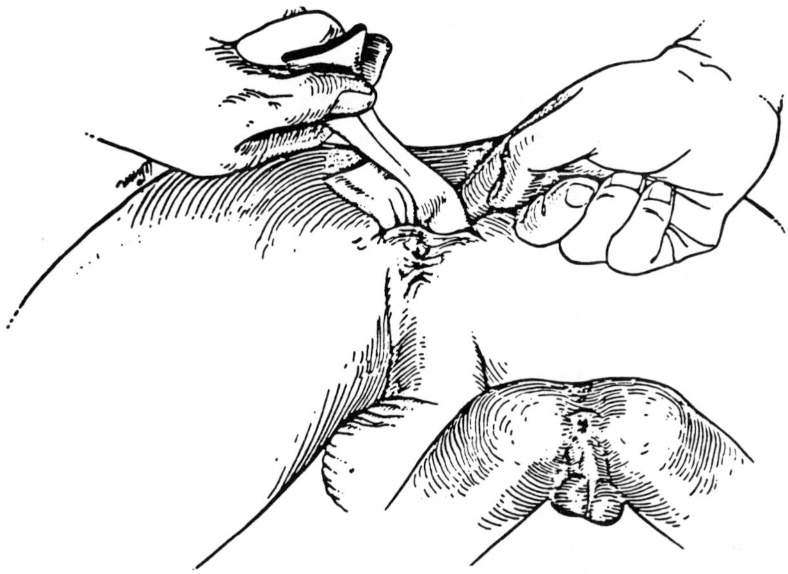

Fig. 10-13. Technique of presacral drainage in rectal injuries: A semicircular incision is made through the median raphe posterior to the anus. By blunt dissection, the presacral space is entered, and Penrose drains are placed bilaterally. (From D. Trunkey et al., Management of rectal trauma. *J. Trauma* 13:411, © by Williams & Wilkins, 1973.)

tial-thickness injury of the rectum can be repaired without proximal diversion.

Rectal Foreign Bodies

Patients who present with retained foreign bodies of the rectum are nearly always males and are the subject of a form of sexual practice [19,20]. Rarely, retained rectal foreign bodies are the result of violence. The former patients usually seek medical attention late, after multiple attempts at removal of the object. This usually produces swelling and edema of the rectum and perianal region.

The presence of a rectal foreign body can be documented by digital examination, proctoscopy, or x-ray examination. Digital examination of the rectum should be done with care, as the foreign object is sometimes glass, which may injure the examiner. The majority of the objects will be lodged in the sacral hollow and can be removed transanally once the anal sphincter has been relaxed. General anesthesia is often required to facilitate removal.

Prior to removal of the foreign body, appropriate antibiotics should be administered in addition to adequate antitetanus prophylaxis. In some patients, a trial of removal in the emergency room under sedation and local anesthesia can be carried out. If this is unsuccessful, removal in the operating room under general anesthesia will be required. Careful proctosigmoidoscopy postextraction to rule out a perforation is mandatory for all patients. As most of these patients routinely give themselves enemas, should a tear have occurred, fecal spillage is usually not extensive. Rectal perforations should be managed as a rectal injury from any other cause.

Rectal injuries as the result of violent insertion of a foreign body into the rectum are true impalement wounds. They occur from falls on a sharp object or by forceful insertion of a foreign body into the rectum as an act of violence. Because of the anatomic relationship of the rectum and bladder, true impalement injuries of the rectum penetrate the anterior rectal wall and frequently enter the urinary bladder. Accordingly, associated injury to the urinary bladder must always be ruled out in these patients.

Patients who present with perforation of the bowel secondary to sexual practices may give a history of an impalement injury to hide the true etiology; however, perforations in these patients are nearly always above the peritoneal reflection and are without urinary bladder injury. These perforations are suspected in the presence of peritoneal signs and reliably documented by free air on abdominal x-rays, sigmoidoscopy, or a water-soluble contrast enema.

These patients all require laparotomy. The general principles of management of full-thickness colon injuries apply. If the tear is small and without gross fecal spillage, primary repair is indicated.

Patients with perforations below the peritoneal reflection require total fecal diversion and presacral drainage. Mucosal tears may bleed significantly but usually stop spontaneously. Perianal and anal disruptions can usually be handled like obstetric injuries and may be primarily repaired without fecal diversion. If seen late and significant inflammation is present, they are best left open and repaired secondarily if incontinence results.

Injuries of the Diaphragm

O. LaWayne Miller and Frederick L. Grover

The first reported injury to the diaphragm was accredited to Sennertus in 1541 [1,2]. In 1578, Ambroise Paré [2] described two patients who were found to have diaphragmatic injuries at autopsy. The first antemortem diagnosis of traumatic diaphragmatic hernia was made by Bowditch in 1853 [1]. The first successful surgical repair was by Riolfi in 1886 [2,3]. The majority of these early reports were related to traumatic diaphragmatic hernia, which is relatively rare compared to injury without hernia [4]. Traumatic injury of the diaphragm, however, is not uncommon and should be suspected in all patients with severe blunt torso or penetrating injuries of the lower chest, upper abdomen, flank, or back.

ETIOLOGY

Traumatic injuries of the diaphragm can be divided into blunt and penetrating injuries. The most common cause of blunt injury to the diaphragm is motor vehicle accidents.

Other forms of blunt trauma responsible for diaphragm injuries include falls or crush injuries. As many as 5 percent of patients who undergo laparotomy for blunt abdominal trauma will have a rupture of the diaphragm [5–8].

Penetrating injuries of the diaphragm are usually either the result of stab wounds or gunshot wounds. Rarely, iatrogenic penetration of the diaphragm can occur during subdiaphragmatic surgical procedures and occasionally from the introduction of a chest tube. The incidence of diaphragmatic involvement from penetrating combat wounds varies from 10 to 20 percent [9]. The incidence of diaphragmatic injury in civilian penetrating injuries is usually much lower, in the range of 5 percent; however, it can be as high as 23 percent in some series [9].

DIAGNOSIS

Symptoms

The most common symptoms include shortness of breath, chest pain, and abdominal pain [5]. The symptoms are often due to the space-occupying effects of the abdominal viscera when large diaphragmatic defects are present. This can cause diaphragmatic dysfunction, and it can also compress the lung and mediastinum. Some patients may have few symptoms at all, and others will not be able to give a history because of either severe shock or mental obtundation [10].

Physical Signs

Physical findings may be minimal in an early phase if abdominal herniation has not occurred or in penetrating trauma where the diaphragmatic defect is small [11]. Often physical findings are nonspecific and are usually related to associated injuries [12]. Positive physical findings usually include decreased breath sounds on the side of injury and are due to herniation of abdominal contents, pneumothorax, or hemothorax. A shift of the mediastinum can sometimes be seen when the amount of herniation is large and can cause cardiac insufficiency from obstruction of venous return [6]. Other signs include dullness or tympany to percussion, the presence of bowel sounds in the thorax, and chest and abdominal wall contusions. Hypotension or shock is seen in a large number of patients with blunt traumatic injuries of the diaphragm, indicating a very severe injury. This was present in our series in 44 percent of patients [10]. In penetrating trauma, there is evidence for external entrance and/or exit wounds usually in the lower chest or upper abdomen, back, or flank (Table 10-7). This should cause suspicion of a possible diaphragmatic injury.

Diagnostic Studies

Chest radiographs are usually obtained if the trauma victim is stable enough. The chest x-ray is almost always abnormal with blunt diaphragmatic injury [10]. The findings may be nonspecific, such as rib fractures, pneumothorax, hemothorax, pulmonary contusion or infiltrate, or an elevated diaphragm. The x-ray can be diagnostic of any acute diaphragmatic injury in blunt trauma if the herniated abdominal contents are seen in the chest or if a nasogastric tube is present in the left chest. This can be seen in up to approximately 30 percent of patients with blunt injury to the

Table 10-7. Location of External Injuries in Penetrating Injuries to Diaphragm in San Antonio Series

	Chest		Abdomen		Flank		Back			
	R	L	R	L	R	L	R	L	Multiple	Total
Stab	12	12	6	10	2	4	1	3	12	62
Gunshot wounds	8	5	3	3	2	2	2	4	2	31
Total	20	17	9	13	4	6	3	7	14	93

R = right; L = left.

Table 10-8. Radiographic Findings on Chest X-ray Patients (102)—San Antonio Series

	Blunt	Penetrating	Totals
Hemo- and/or pneumothorax	6	51	57
Normal chest x-ray	0	40	40
Herniated abdominal contents	3	1	4
Pneumoperitoneum	0	1	1
Total	9	93	102

diaphragm (Table 10-8, Fig. 10-14). In contrast, patients with penetrating injuries more commonly have a chest x-ray that is interpreted as normal [10,13] (Fig. 10-15). The most common finding in penetrating trauma is a hemo- or pneumothorax, which is seen in approximately 50 percent of patients [10]. These are very nonspecific findings, however, and are not diagnostic of diaphragmatic injury (Fig. 10-16). Herniated abdominal contents are rarely seen on x-rays of patients with penetrating injuries because of the small size of the injury, and when noted they are usually in delayed cases.

Diagnostic peritoneal lavage [14] is often used to determine if intra-abdominal injury is present and if laparotomy is necessary in blunt or penetrating trauma, particularly in blunt trauma. Some centers [10] consider penetrating trauma to the abdomen or thorax below the fifth intercostal space an indication for exploratory laparotomy, while others observe these patients [15,16]. Diagnostic peritoneal lavage is often positive in patients with penetrating trauma to the abdomen, usually due to associated intra-abdominal injuries rather than the diaphragmatic injury. When positive, it is an indication for operation. Several reports have shown that the most common injury associated with a false-negative peritoneal lavage is isolated diaphragmatic injury [17,18]. Therefore, a negative lavage in pa-

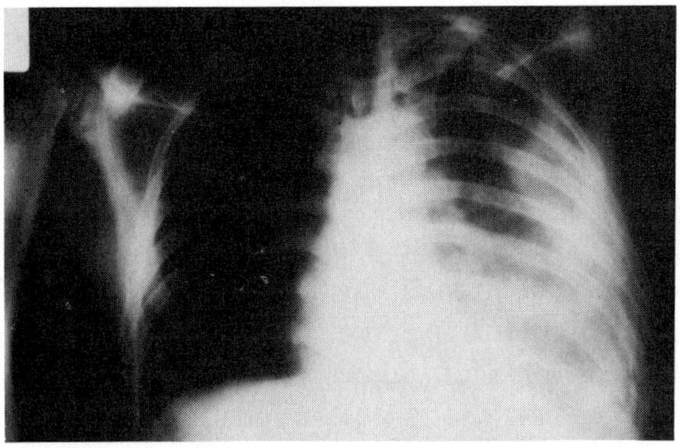

Fig. 10-14. This chest roentgenogram is of a 26-year-old man admitted following a motorcycle accident who complained of left chest pain and shortness of breath. On examination, he was noted to be in moderate respiratory distress and had a large hematoma over the left lateral chest wall with palpable rib fractures. Note the gastric bubble in the left hemithorax. At laparotomy, a posterior lateral rupture of the left hemidiaphragm was closed in two layers with nonabsorbable suture.

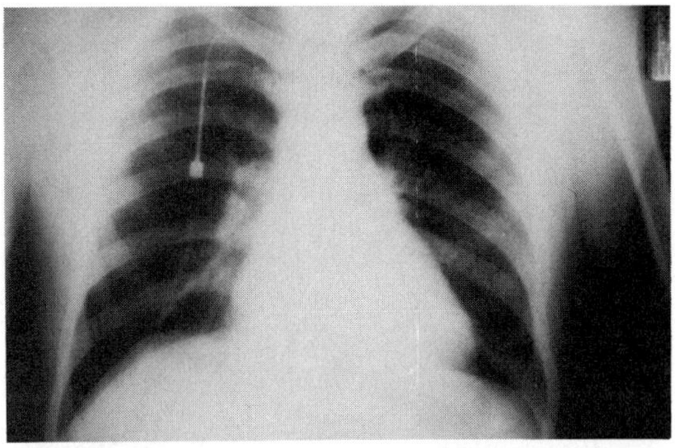

Fig. 10-15. This chest roentgenogram of a 22-year-old man admitted with multiple stab wounds to the abdomen and chest was interpreted as normal. At operation, he was found to have a left diaphragmatic injury. Forty of the 93 San Antonio patients with penetrating injury had normal chest x-rays in spite of their injury.

tients with penetrating injuries should not rule out the possibility of diaphragmatic injury [11,18].

A diagnostic pneumoperitoneum [5,17] has been suggested as a method to diagnose diaphragmatic injuries, especially those on the left side in which a pneumothorax is not present. However, it is not routinely recommended.

When a delay in diagnosis has occurred and there is suspicion of a diaphragmatic hernia, an upper gastrointestinal contrast radiograph or barium enema may be helpful in the diagnosis. Ultrasonography [19], CT scanning, and fluoroscopy have also been used to diagnose diaphragmatic injuries. More recently, radionuclide liver/spleen scanning using technetium 99–sulfur colloid has been utilized to diagnose right-sided diaphragmatic injuries [2,20].

Some authors have noted that an elevated central venous pressure should suggest the possibility of an acute diaphragmatic rupture [21], especially in blunt trauma, although other diagnostic considerations such as tamponade or tension pneumothorax should also be suspected.

TREATMENT

Immediate operative repair is indicated for all injuries of the diaphragm. As noted, the preoperative diagnosis of diaphragmatic injury

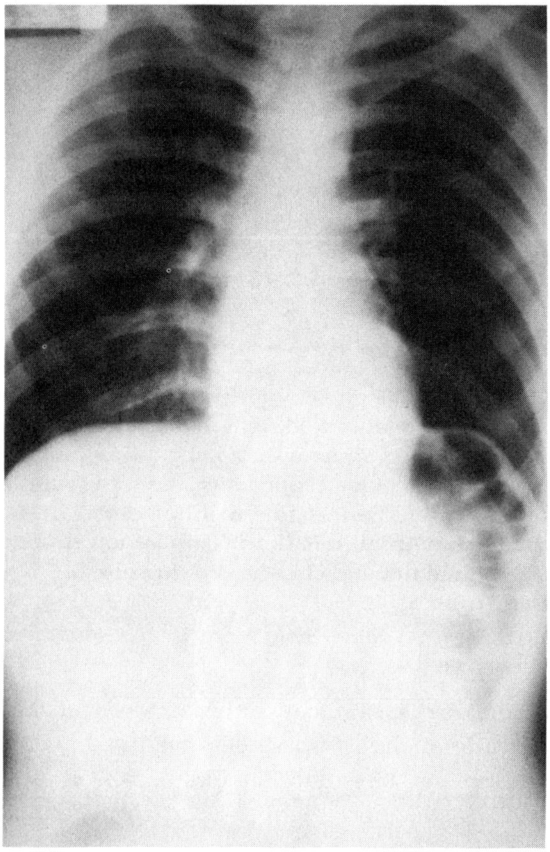

Fig. 10-16. This chest roentgenogram of a 21-year-old man who was stabbed in the left upper quadrant shows an elevated left hemidiaphragm over a gas-filled colon. The patient had a laceration of the left diaphragm and of the splenic flexure of the colon. Although the x-ray was abnormal, it is not diagnostic.

can be elusive, and many of these injuries are discovered at laparotomy performed because of suspected abdominal injury or by thoracotomy for intrathoracic injury or bleeding. At our institution, as previously mentioned, all patients with penetrating injuries below the nipple line in the chest and back and all abdominal and flank wounds receive laparotomy (Table 10-9). The initial operative approach for acute injuries should be laparotomy [8,11–13,18,21–24]. Even if the diagnosis has not been made before exploratory laparotomy, most injuries of the diaphragm can be repaired through the abdominal approach. Approximately 90 percent of patients with diaphragmatic injuries will have significant intra-abdominal injury that will also need to be repaired, which is most easily accomplished by laparotomy. Either the abdominal or thoracic approach may be used for chronic injuries when there is no evidence of strangulation, depending on the preference of the surgeon. Right-sided diaphragmatic injuries may be approached by a right thoracotomy incision and a laparotomy if acute or by thoracotomy alone if chronic (Table 10-10).

At the time of laparotomy, a careful examination of both leaves of the diaphragm should be performed [22]. Two patients in both Ebert and coworkers' [4] and our series [10] had diaphragmatic injuries missed at laparotomy. Occasionally, a bilateral injury will be seen. All defects, no matter how small, should be repaired, since spontaneous closure is rare and herniation, incarceration, and strangulation may occur. Usually the defects can be closed primarily with nonabsorbable sutures. Rarely, it may be necessary to use autogenous tissue

Table 10-9. Indications for Operations*—San Antonio Series

	Blunt	Penetrating	Total
Penetrating wounds to lower chest or upper abdomen	0	91	91
Positive diagnostic peritoneal lavage	6	3	9
Herniated abdominal viscera	3	1	4
Pericardial tamponade	1	1	2
Intrathoracic hemorrhage	0	10	10

*Several patients had more than one indication for operation.

Table 10-10. Operative Approach—San Antonio Series

	Blunt	Penetrating	Total
Laparotomy	8	81	89
Thoracotomy	0	4	4
Sternotomy	0	1	1
Laparotomy and thoracotomy	0	6	6
Laparotomy and sternotomy	1	1	2
Total	9	93	102

grafts such as pericardial flaps or synthetic material to repair the diaphragmatic defects.

The left diaphragm is the most commonly injured diaphragm in blunt trauma, occurring in approximately 90 percent of such injuries. Some recent reports, however, reveal a 30-percent incidence of right-sided diaphragmatic ruptures [21,25]. It has been suggested that the incidence of right-sided disruption is rising because of an increased severity of accidents with a greater number of patients reaching the emergency center alive due to more rapid transportation and resuscitation [25]. There may be a somewhat higher incidence of left-sided injuries in penetrating injuries of the diaphragm, but in some series there is an almost equal incidence of left- versus right-sided penetrating diaphragmatic injuries [10,24] (Table 10-11).

Associated injuries are seen in almost 90 percent of patients with diaphragmatic injuries [1,7,8,10,22,23]. Frequently, the associated injuries have precipitated the exploratory laparotomy, and the diaphragmatic injury is found and diagnosed during the operation. Care must be taken not only to repair the associated injuries but also to examine the diaphragm very compulsively so as not to overlook an injury. The most common associated injuries are to the liver, spleen, and stomach (Table 10-12). An increased incidence of blunt diaphragmatic disruption has been reported in association with pelvic fracture. In one report, more than 50 percent of patients with diaphragmatic injury had pelvic fractures [21]. It is likely that the force required to disrupt the pelvis is also severe enough to raise the intra-abdominal pressure to a level to rupture the diaphragm.

PROGNOSIS

The morbidity and mortality of patients with diaphragmatic injury is usually related to associated injuries [1,7,8,10,18,21,23–25]. Postoperative complications are frequently high and most commonly are pulmonary in nature, followed by septic complications. These patients may require prolonged postoperative ventilator support owing to the diaphragmatic injury as well as to the high incidence of trauma to the lung and chest wall. Other major complications are related to failure to diagnose, leading to delayed treatment, or to missing the lesion at operation (Table 10-13).

The mortality for blunt diaphragmatic rupture is approximately 25 percent [21,23,24], although it varies from 0 to 50 percent. The deaths are almost entirely due to associated injuries [1,7,10,18,21,23–25]. The mortality for penetrating diaphragmatic injuries is much lower than for blunt trauma [1,10,12,24] and usually is dependent on whether the injury is from a gunshot wound or a stab wound. Stab wound injuries have a much lower mortality and morbidity than gunshot wounds because of less frequency and magnitude of associated injuries.

It must be emphasized that early exploratory laparotomy for suspected diaphragmatic injury is important to prevent the complications and sequelae of a missed diaphragmatic

Table 10-11. Hemidiaphragm Injured—102 Patients/122 Injuries

	Right	Left	Total
Penetrating	54	59	113
Blunt	1	8	9
Total	55	67	122

Table 10-12. Associated Injuries (89 Patients)—San Antonio Series

Abdominal		Thoracic	
Liver	50	Hemo/pneumothorax	57
Spleen	22	Lung	5
Stomach	18	Heart	3
Kidney	8	Intercostal artery	3
Colon	6	Internal mammary artery	2
Small bowel	6		
Pancreas	2		
Mesentery	2	Orthopedic	8
Esophagus	1		
Bladder	1	Neurologic	2
No associated injury	9		

Table 10-13. Complications—San Antonio Series (102 Patients)

Death	1
Missed injury at exploration	2
Delay in diagnosis of injury	3
Other complications unrelated to diaphragm injury	9

injury and hernia with possible strangulation [10]. It has been shown that if strangulation of the viscera occurs in the chest secondary to a diaphragmatic hernia, the mortality ranges from 25 to 66 percent [11].

Retroperitoneal Hematoma

A. Enrique Whittwell and David J. Kreis, Jr.

Retroperitoneal hematoma is a common finding in the trauma victim, and the general surgeon in the care of the patient must be familiar with its management. It should be emphasized that retroperitoneal hematoma is a manifestation of an injury to a retroperitoneal structure, the magnitude of which will depend on the vascularity of the organs involved. The objective of this section is to describe the general approach to a retroperitoneal hematoma and not to discuss the specific treatment of the injured retroperitoneal organ, which is discussed in detail elsewhere.

Blunt trauma is responsible for 70 to 80 percent of cases of retroperitoneal hematoma and penetrating trauma for the remainder [1–3]. Although the incidence of retroperitoneal hematoma in trauma is difficult to establish, its presence has been reported in 13 to 44 percent of patients with blunt abdominal trauma [4–6] and 11 percent of patients with penetrating abdominal trauma [7].

Retroperitoneal hematoma due to automobile accidents or pedestrian injuries carry mortalities from 30 to 83 percent [1–3]. Patients who require more than 10 units of blood during the first 24 hours have mortalities above 50 percent [2,3]. Development of respiratory failure carries a mortality of 35 percent [1].

During the last decade, controversies regarding the operative management of retroperitoneal hematomas seem mostly limited to the perinephric or flank area. The decision to open or leave undisturbed the hematoma in this area will be discussed later in this section.

A few years ago, Kudsk and Sheldon [4] proposed a classification for retroperitoneal hematomas by zones that has important clinical implications. The retroperitoneum can be classified by zones: zone I—central, medial; zone II—perirenal, flank; and zone III—pelvis (Fig. 10-17).

The boundaries of zone I include superior (from the diaphragmatic hiatus of the aorta and esophagus), inferior (to the sacral promontory), and lateral (to the medial aspect of both kidneys). The important organs present in this area include the esophagus, duodenum, pancreas, inferior vena cava and branches, aorta and visceral branches, and portal vein and tributaries.

The boundaries of zone II extend from the diaphragm to the iliac wings, medial to the

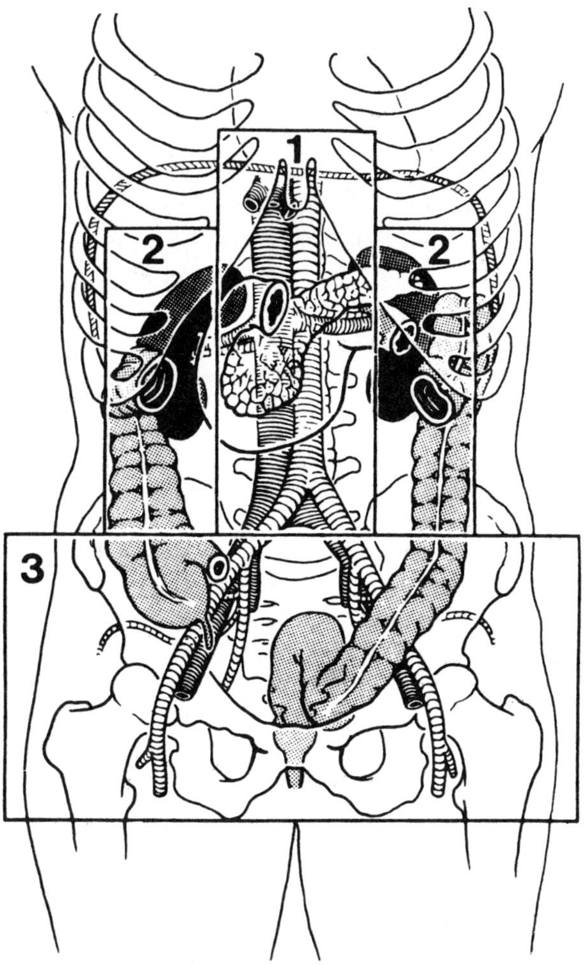

Fig. 10-17. Retroperitoneal hematomas are best classified into three zones: zone 1 (central), zone 2 (flank), and zone 3 (pelvic). (Reprinted by permission from *Abdominal Trauma*, F. W. Blaisdell, D. D. Trunkey, "Trauma Management" series, Volume I. New York: Thieme Medical Publishers, Inc., 1982.)

hilum of both kidneys, and lateral to the abdominal wall. This area contains the adrenals, kidneys, ureters, and right and left hemicolon.

Zone III is limited by the pelvic bones. The retroperitoneal organs in this area include distal ureters, iliac vessels, bladder, and rectum.

ASSESSMENT

The initial assessment starts with the general assessment of the trauma victim. Adequate information regarding mechanism of injury should be obtained. In penetrating injuries, entrance and exit wounds may help to predict organs injured, especially for those affecting the back and flank. Any blunt injury to the epigastric area, including from the steering wheel and seat belt, can lead to duodenal or pancreatic injury. Since the retroperitoneal space may act as a reservoir and conceal large quantities of internal hemorrhage, initially the symptoms are often nonspecific, and the diagnosis is frequently delayed. Depending on the number of associated injuries and the magnitude and rate of bleeding, patients will be assessed in one of two ways.

Unstable Patients

The majority of patients have associated intraperitoneal injuries that require immediate exploration. Retroperitoneal hematoma is discovered during laparotomy. The presence of shock at admission in this group has been reported to be as high as 50 to 60 percent [4].

This group of patients requires a rapid assessment and minimal workup before exploration is undertaken. If the patient's condition permits, x-rays of the chest, abdomen, and pelvis should be obtained in blunt trauma. If the patient has hematuria and shock, an intravenous pyelogram or cystogram can be taken intraoperatively if required.

Stable Patients

If the patient does not have an associated intra-abdominal injury, there still may be abdominal or back pain. Physical findings may be unremarkable, although this is unusual. Occasionally, a Grey Turner's sign is seen. Laboratory data may show low hematocrit, increased amylase, or hematuria, which occurs in 50 percent of patients [2].

If the patient's condition permits, further workup can proceed. Plain x-ray of the abdomen may show retroperitoneal air, secondary to duodenal or colonic injury, or a mass effect due to the hematoma displacing or deforming the retroperitoneal viscera may be seen. An obliterated psoas shadow can be seen if the hematoma overlies this muscle. Pelvic x-ray may discover fractures. If hematuria is present, a cystogram should be obtained. In males, a urethrogram should be done also, particularly if blood is coming from the urethral meatus. Intravenous pyelography should follow to visualize the kidneys and ureters.

If an abnormal result or insufficient information is provided by these contrast studies, then the next recommended test is computed tomography (CT) in the stable patient. Additional contrast material will be required. CT scan is an accurate, noninvasive method for directly imaging abnormalities of the retroperitoneal space [8]. Hemorrhage is detectable on the CT scan as an abnormal soft-tissue density, with resultant obstruction, displacement, or compression of normal retroperitoneal structures. CT scan can detect, quantitate, and localize retroperitoneal hemorrhage. It also may provide an etiologic explanation, thus directing appropriate clinical management (Figs. 10-18 and 10-19). CT scanning is an excellent modality to evaluate the retroperitoneum in a stable patient. Retroperitoneal organ injuries are not well evaluated by peritoneal lavage [9].

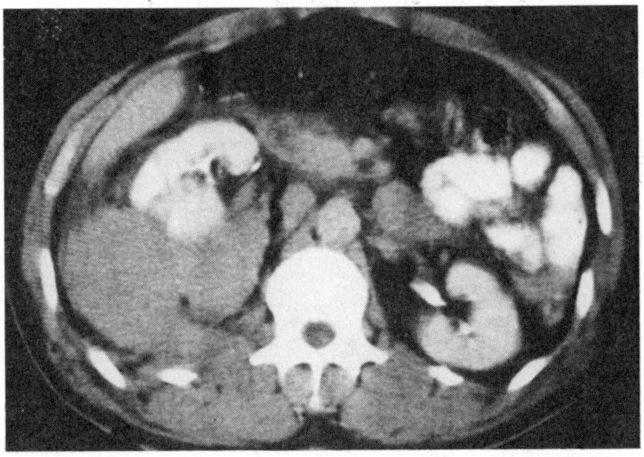

Fig. 10-18. Large zone II or flank retroperitoneal hematoma in a patient with stab wound to the back.

Angiography also has a role in the assessment of occasional patients with retroperitoneal hematoma. In one study [10], angiography was used when CT scan showed a retroperitoneal hematoma that obscured or was in proximity to significant retroperitoneal vessels. Of particular interest is the central hematoma that extends through the aortic diaphragmatic hiatus. An aortogram may detect tears of the thoracic aorta with subsequent hematoma extending down to the retroperitoneum. Other indications include suspicion of arteriovenous fistula, nonvisualization of a

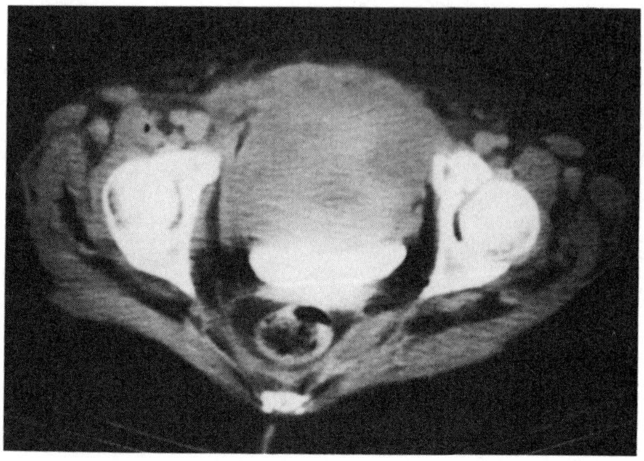

Fig. 10-19. Large zone III or pelvic hematoma in a patient with blunt trauma and pelvic fracture.

kidney on intravenous pyelogram, and unilateral concentration of IV contrast, seen on the CT scan.

Angiogram for pelvic hematomas or zone III injuries has an important role in the management of these patients [11], as will be emphasized later in this chapter.

MANAGEMENT

The management of the patient with a retroperitoneal hematoma will depend on the mechanism of the injury, condition of the patient, associated injuries, behavior of the hematoma (expanding or not), and anatomic localization of the hematoma. Controversies on the decision for exploration or not persist, particularly for those localized to zone II. Retroperitoneal hematoma is usually discovered during exploratory laparotomy for other intra-abdominal injuries.

Zone I Hematomas

Central hematomas (zone I) are associated with high mortality rates [2,3], basically due to associated major-vessel injury. There may be difficulty in achieving adequate exposure and control of the hemorrhage. Different studies [1–3] have reported mortality rates greater than 30 percent when major-vessel injuries were present.

Most trauma surgeons would agree that all central retroperitoneal hematomas found either by CT scan or during exploratory laparotomy must be explored irrespective of etiology, since there is a high incidence of visceral and major vascular trauma associated with them [4,12,13]. Central hematomas are easily identified through the gastrohepatic ligament or by opening the lesser sac, or they can dissect to the root of mesentery, displacing the small bowel (Fig. 10-20). Rarely one will find a central hematoma extending to the periesophageal area. One should remember that disruption of the descending thoracic aorta may dissect down to the retroperitoneum. Grieco and Perry [3] reported two patients with this presentation. The recommended approach in a stable patient with a nonexpanding hematoma in this situation is to close the abdomen and, while maintaining anesthesia, obtain an aortogram. The patient is then returned to the operating room for thoracotomy if the aortogram is positive, followed by completion of the laparotomy.

When a hematoma in zone I is found, proximal control of the major vessels must be obtained prior to the exploration. The aorta may be controlled either by an anterolateral left thoracotomy or subdiaphragmatically as described by Veith and Gupta [14].

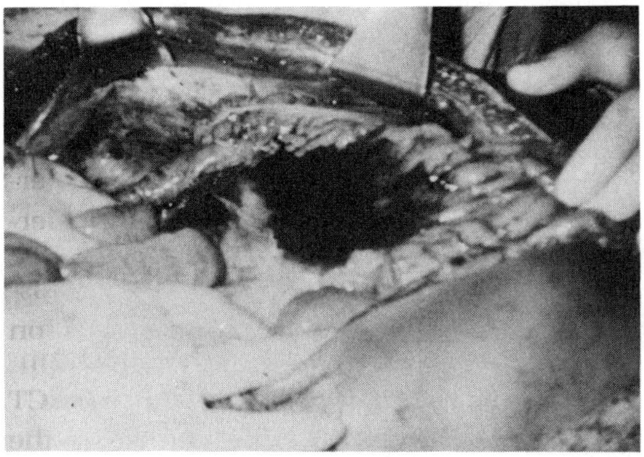

Fig. 10-20. Large zone I or central hematoma in a patient with blunt trauma.

The aortic compressor can also be used [15] without preliminary dissection, by placing the device into the lesser sac above the stomach until the area of trauma is dissected free and an appropriate atraumatic clamp is applied. The inferior vena cava can be difficult to control, especially above the renal veins. The inferior vena cava shunt can be inserted from the saphenous-femoral venous junction as described by Pilcher and associates [16]. In our experience, it is best to inflate the balloon and tamponade the area of possible injury. Other approaches have been described, but most of them are obtained through sternotomy or thoracotomy or by opening the retroperitoneum for placement of clamps or tapes.

After proximal control of the aorta and/or vena cava is obtained, exploration of the hematoma is started. Medial mobilization of the right hemicolon or left hemicolon and spleen will depend on the anatomic localization of the hematoma and the index of suspicion for the vessel or organ affected. If major-vessel injury is excluded as a source of retroperitoneal hematoma, careful exploration of the duodenum and pancreas should be performed. If the hematoma is over the second portion of the duodenum, medial mobilization by severing its lateral attachments is indicated (Kocher maneuver). The third and fourth portion of the duodenum can be inspected by mobilization of the right hemicolon and small-bowel mesentery in a medial and upward direction, as described by Cattell and Braasch [17]. The lesser sac should be opened through the gastrocolic omentum to assess the pancreas for injury. Medial mobilization of the left hemicolon, spleen, and pancreas (Mattox maneuver [18]) should be performed if one suspects an aortic or major visceral vascular injury. Injuries to the retrohepatic inferior vena cava may present with a central hematoma. If the peritoneum is intact, these may dissect to the flank. Prior to opening the hematoma, we recommend placement of an inferior vena cava shunt from the saphenous femoral junction, as described by Pilcher and associates [16].

Zone II Hematomas

Major controversy still surrounds the management of zone II or flank hematomas.

Surgical exploration of zone II retroperitoneal hematoma must be carefully decided after analyzing a number of factors, which include mechanism of injury (blunt or penetrating), clinical status, associated injuries, magnitude of renal injury as seen on intravenous pyelogram, CT scan or arteriogram, and intraoperative increase in hematoma size (Fig. 10-21).

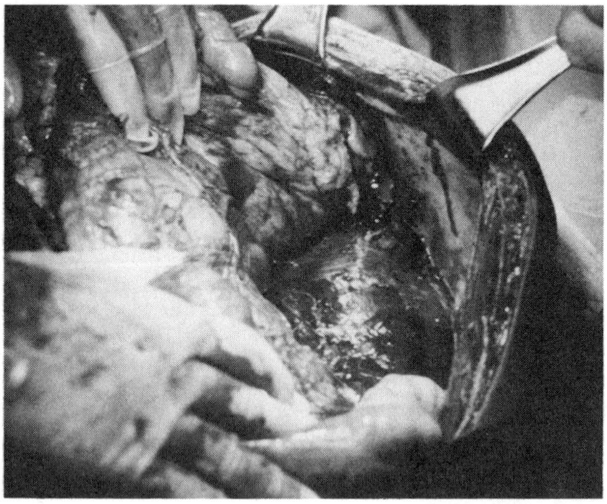

Fig. 10-21. Large zone II or flank hematoma in a patient with gunshot wound to the flank.

The controversy concerns those retroperitoneal hematomas found at laparotomy that are associated with the injured kidney but not with any of the other retroperitoneal organs [19,20]. Advocates of routine exploration state that this permits direct control of bleeding, and renal injuries can be specifically identified and treated. Theoretically, this should minimize the chances of developing postinjury complications like prolonged or delayed hemorrhage, loss of functioning renal tissue, infection, and hypertension. Opponents of such a policy feel that interference with the hematoma may result in disruption of effective tamponade. A nonviolated Gerota's fascia may allow healing of the kidney to proceed with relatively little loss of parenchyma, and the intact fascia confers a degree of protection by containing both bleeding and urine extravasation.

Most of the authors [13,19,21–23] are in the opinion that surgical exploration must be performed for all penetrating injuries when Gerota's fascia has been violated and the benefits of effective tamponade are lost. Others disagree and recommend selective exploration based on clinical status, presence of hematuria, preoperative intravenous pyelogram, CT scan, and renal angiography behavior of the retroperitoneal hematoma in the operating room [24–26]. Hematomas that are pulsatile, uncontained (violated Gerota's fascia), or expanding should be explored [19,23,26] regardless of mechanism of injury.

In blunt trauma when these criteria are absent and a nephrogram denotes adequate renal function, exploration may be avoided with successful results [19,26].

In general, if the decision is made to explore zone II hematomas, prevention and control of renal hemorrhage before exploration should be obtained by achieving proximal renal vascular control as described by Scott and Selzman [27]. An incision is made over the aorta, and loops are placed around the renal vessels of the involved kidney to maintain instant control of bleeding but allow constant renal perfusion. McAninch and Carrol [28] demonstrated that nephrectomy rates in trauma were reduced from 56 to 18 percent when this approach was used.

Zone III Hematomas

Pelvic, or zone III, hematomas are usually not explored unless they are the result of penetrating injury or found to be pulsatile, expanding, or uncontained, as frequently happens with penetrating injuries. About 95 percent of pelvic hematomas are the result of blunt trauma [2], and most of them are the result of pelvic fractures. Certain types of fractures have been associated with specific vascular injuries. Massive crushing pelvic injuries with disruption of the ilium or separation of the sacroiliac joint are associated with lacerations or avulsions of the common or external iliac vessels [29,30]. Disruption of the posterior pelvis has been associated with avulsion of the superior gluteal artery [31,32]. Disruption of the anterior pelvis has been associated with avulsion of the obturator artery [33]. It is accepted that hematomas in the majority of patients are related to disruption of multiple venous tributaries in the vicinity of the fracture site. Since this is a low-pressure system, the intact peritoneum will effectively tamponade the bleeding in most patients. Occasionally, arterial bleeding is present, and hemorrhage will persist. The site of hemorrhage is usually a branch of the internal iliac artery, most frequently the superior gluteal, internal pudendal, or obturator artery [4,34]. Pelvic fractures due to blunt trauma require a multisystem assessment. The number of associated injuries is usually high, and simultaneous steps are taken to rule out associated injuries.

Peritoneal lavage or abdominal CT scanning can be used; the decision for one or the other will depend on the stability of the patient. If peritoneal lavage is performed, an open supraumbilical technique should be used. Since hematomas can dissect anteriorly to the level of the umbilicus, puncture of the hematoma will lead to a false-positive result or a decompression of the hematoma. If the patient's condition permits, an abdominal CT scan can be performed. Pelvic CT scan can be obtained simultaneously to assess pelvic fracture. This may help in determining whether early fixation of the pelvis, using either external [35] or internal [36] methods, is indicated.

In general, all patients with pelvic fractures due to blunt injury should be considered to have a pelvic hematoma. The magnitude of the hematoma is usually directly related to the magnitude of the pelvic fracture. As a rule, posterior pelvic ring fractures have the most bleeding problems. It is important to mention that bladder injuries are seen with disruption of the anterior pelvis. The management of pelvic fractures is discussed elsewhere. Most zone III hematomas are contained by the peritoneum and resolve spontaneously. Attempting to unroof these hematomas may result in catastrophic bleeding.

When zone III hematomas are detected by CT scan and associated with unstable pelvic fractures, pelvic fixation should be strongly considered. This will result in controlling the bleeding and will improve the patient's mobility. Early mobilization of the patient reduces morbidity and mortality. When an orthopedic team is not available, temporizing maneuvers can be utilized, namely, monitoring the patient in the intensive care unit and using the Military Anti-Shock Trousers (MAST) suit. Life-threatening bleeding from closed pelvic fractures is often controlled with this external compression-immobilization device [11].

Peritoneal lavage or CT scanning is recommended early in the workup of the patient with severe pelvic fracture to rule out an intraperitoneal injury. It is very common to observe a decrease in the hematocrit of the patient with pelvic fracture. It is therefore important to rule out intraperitoneal injury early. Numerous authors [11,37] have emphasized that the potential disadvantage of the MAST suit is the development of temporary hemodynamic improvement leading to a false sense of security. A major intraperitoneal injury may be missed if an early workup with either peritoneal lavage or CT scanning is not accomplished. The MAST suit will stop bleeding in 90 percent of patients [11].

Patients who have associated arterial bleeding usually do not stabilize during the first few hours. If bleeding fails to stop within 3 to 6 hours after MAST placement or if blood requirements are larger than 6 units, the patient should be taken to the angiographic suite for diagnostic and therapeutic pelvic angiography.

Control of hemorrhage by selective catheterization of a branch of the hypogastric artery is attractive because it may avoid exploration of the hematoma. With its attendant risks, successful embolization has been accomplished by using autologous clot, muscle, absorbable gelatin sponge, "biologic glue," or metal coils. The angiogram should be repeated after embolization has been completed to prove success.

If arteriographic embolization is unsuccessful in controlling hemorrhage, but the bleeding artery is shown, the patient should be taken to the operating room, and pelvic packing should be performed with closure of the abdomen. If bleeding persists, an attempt to pass a Fogarty balloon catheter into the distal branch of the affected side may be tried in conjunction with proximal ligation of the hypogastric artery [31,38].

If the arteriogram fails to show arterial bleeding but the patient persists with hemorrhage, in general the patient should be taken to the operating room and pelvic packing performed. Usually the peritoneum covering the pelvis is lacerated and has lost its tamponade effect over the pelvic hematoma, resulting in continuous bleeding.

If the patient is found during laparotomy to have an expanding zone III hematoma as a result of blunt trauma, we also recommend pelvic packing and closure of the abdomen, followed by placement of the MAST suit and pelvic angiography to rule out any major arterial injury. Opening of the hematoma in this setting usually results in uncontrollable bleeding. We use as many surgical laps as possible to compress the pelvis and control the bleeding.

The timing for removal of the packing has not been established, but we have found pack removal between 2 and 4 days a successful approach.

Isolated reports of the usefulness of internal iliac artery ligation for control of hemorrhage in fractures of the pelvis have appeared in the past [32,39]. Extensive collateral blood supply of the pelvis precludes consistently obtaining successful results with this technique, and for this reason, we have discontinued its routine use.

Figures 10-22 and 10-23 summarize our management for zone III hematomas associated with pelvic fractures.

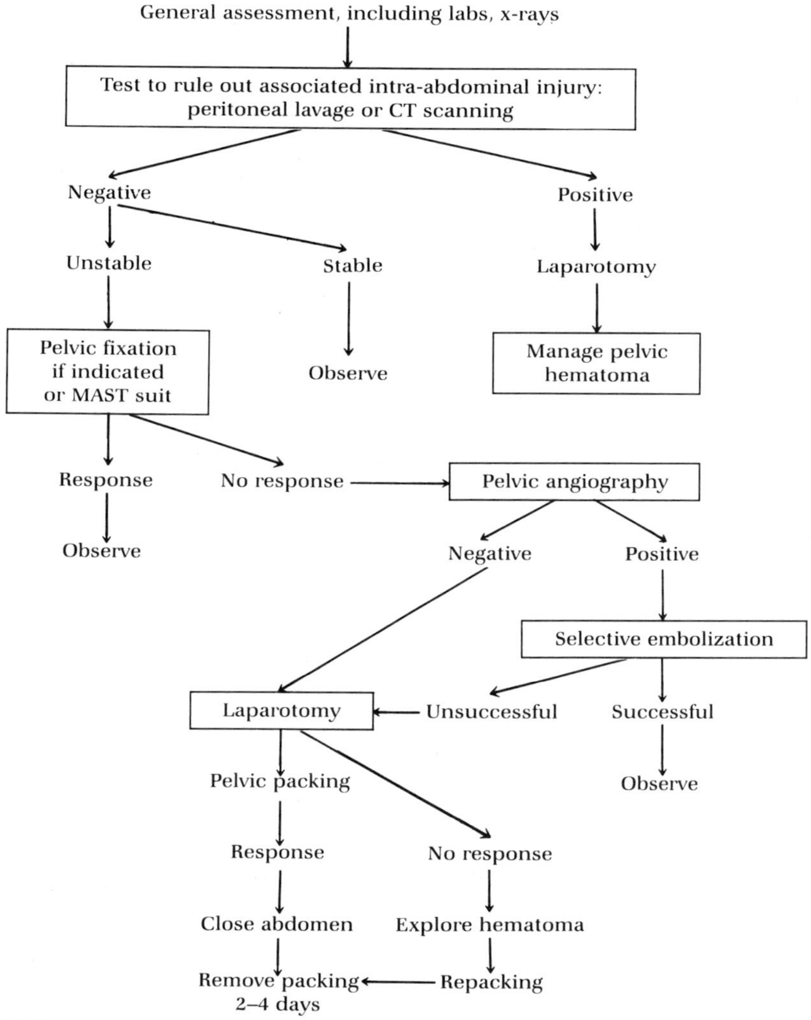

Fig. 10-22. Management of pelvic fracture due to blunt trauma.

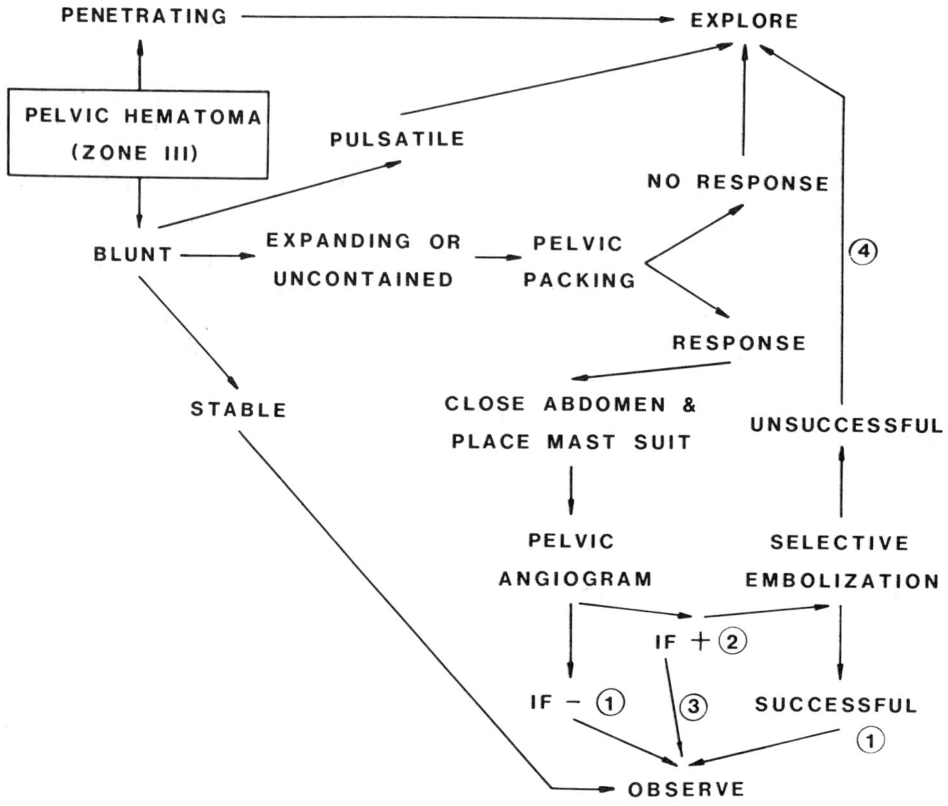

(1) CONSIDER PELVIC FIXATION IF INDICATED, PRIOR TO REMOVING PACKING.

(2) IF A BRANCH OF INTERNAL ILIAC ARTERY SHOWS INJURY.

(3) IF ILIAC ARTERIES ARE INJURED, BUT ADEQUATE DISTAL RECONSTITUTION, DEFERRED REEXPLORATION UNTIL STABILITY IS ACHIEVED.

(4) CONSIDER PLACEMENT OF INTRA-ARTERIAL BALLOON IN THE INJURED BRANCH.

Fig. 10-23. Management of pelvic hematoma.

REFERENCES

Liver Injuries

1. Golan, A., and White, R. G. Spontaneous rupture of the liver associated with pregnancy: A report of five cases. *S. Afr. Med. J.* 56:133, 1978.
2. Olsen, W. R., Redman, H. C., and Hildreth, D. H. Quantitative peritoneal lavage in blunt abdominal trauma. *Arch. Surg.* 104:536, 1972.
3. Moon, K. L., and Federle, M. P. Computed tomography in hepatic trauma. *A.J.R.* 141:309, 1983.
4. Ledgerwood, A. M., Kazmers, M., Lucas, C. E. The role of thoracic aortic occlusion for massive hemoperitoneum. *J. Trauma* 16:610, 1976.
5. Pringle, J. H. Notes on the arrest of hepatic hemorrhage due to trauma. *Ann. Surg.* 48:541, 1908.
6. Feliciano, D. V., Jordan, G. L., Mattox, K. L., et al. Management of 1000 consecutive cases of hepatic trauma (1979–1984). *Ann. Surg.* 204:437, 1986.
7. Pachter, H. L., Spencer, F. C., Hofstetter, S. R., et al. Experience with the finger fracture technique to achieve intra-hepatic hemostasis in 75 patients with severe injuries of the liver. *Ann. Surg.* 197:771, 1983.
8. Mays, E. T. The hazards of suturing certain wounds of the liver. *Surg. Gynecol. Obstet.* 143:201, 1976.
9. Fabian, T. C., and Stone, H. H. Arrest of severe liver hemorrhage by an omental pack. *South. Med. J.* 73:1487, 1980.
10. Stone, H. H., and Lamb, J. M. Use of pedicled omentum as an autogenous pack for control of hemorrhage in major injuries in the liver. *Surg. Gynecol. Obstet.* 141:92, 1975.
11. Flint, L. M., and Polk, H. C. Selective hepatic artery ligation: Limitations and failures. *J. Trauma* 19:319, 1979.
12. Mays, E. T., Conti, S., Fallahzadeh, H., and Rosenblatt, M. Hepatic artery ligation. *Surgery* 86:536, 1979.
13. Calne, R. Y., McMaster, P., Pentlow, B. D. The treatment of major liver trauma by primary packing with transfer of the patient for definitive treatment. *Br. J. Surg.* 66:338, 1979.
14. Carmona, R. H., Peck, D. Z., and Lim, R. C., Jr. The role of packing and planned reoperation in severe hepatic trauma. *J. Trauma* 24:779, 1984.
15. Feliciano, D. V., Mattox, K. L., Jordan, G. L., Jr. Intra-abdominal packing for control of hepatic hemorrhage: A reappraisal. *J. Trauma* 21:285, 1981.
16. Clagett, G. P., and Olsen, W. R. Non-mechanical hemorrhage in severe liver injury. *Ann. Surg.* 187:369, 1978.
17. Svobada, J. A., Peter, E. T., Dang, C. V., et al. Severe liver trauma in the face of coagulopathy: A case for temporary packing and early re-exploration. *Am. J. Surg.* 144:717, 1982.
18. Cheatham, J. E., Smith, E. I., Tunell, W. P., et al. Nonoperative management of subcapsular hematomas of the liver. *Am. J. Surg.* 140:852, 1980.
19. Geis, W. P., Schulz, K. A., Giacchino, J. L., et al. The fate of unruptured intrahepatic hematomas. *Surgery* 90:689, 1981.
20. Lambeth, W., and Rubin, B. E. Nonoperative management of intrahepatic hemorrhage and hematoma following blunt trauma. *Surg. Gynecol. Obstet.* 148:507, 1979.
21. Kudsk, K. A., Sheldon, G. F., Lim, R. C., Jr. Atrial-caval shunting (ACS) after trauma. *J. Trauma* 22:81, 1982.
22. Schrock, T., Blaisdell, W., Mathewson, C., Jr. Management of blunt trauma to the liver and hepatic veins. *Arch. Surg.* 96:698, 1968.
23. Balasegaram, D. M. Hepatic resection in trauma. *Adv. Surg.* 17:129, 1984.
24. Donovan, A. J., Michaelian, M. J., and Yellin, A. E. Anatomical hepatic lobectomy in trauma to the liver. *Surgery* 73:833, 1973.
25. McClelland, R., Shires, T., and Poulos, E. Hepatic resection for massive trauma. *J. Trauma* 4:282, 1964.
26. Moore, F. A., Moore, E. E., and Seagraves, A. Nonresectional management of hepatic trauma: An evolving concept. *Am. J. Surg.* 50:725, 1985.
27. Fischer, R. P., O'Farrell, K. A., Perry, J. F., Jr. The value of peritoneal drains in the treatment of liver injuries. *J. Trauma* 18:393, 1978.
28. Mullins, R. J., Stone, H. H., Dunlop, E. W., and Strom, P. R. Hepatic trauma: Evaluation of routine drainage. *South. Med. J.* 78:259, 1985.
29. Lucas, C. E., and Walt, A. J. Analysis of randomized biliary drainage for liver trauma in 189 patients. *J. Trauma* 12:925, 1972.
30. Goodnight, J. E., and Blaisdell, F. W. Hemobilia. *Surg. Clin. North Am.* 61:973, 1981.

31. Sandblom, P. Hemorrhage into biliary tract following trauma: Traumatic hemobilia. *Surgery* 24:571, 1948.

Spleen Injuries

1. Sherman, R. Perspectives in management of trauma to the spleen: 1979 Presidential Address, American Association for the Surgery of Trauma. *J. Trauma* 20:1, 1980.
2. Buntain, W. L., and Gould, H. R. Splenic trauma in children and technique of splenic salvage. *World J. Surg.* 9:398, 1985.
3. Buntain, W. L., Gould, H. R., and Maull, K. I. Predictability of splenic salvage by computed tomography. *J. Trauma* 28:24, 1988.
4. Buntain, W. L., Lynch, F. P., and Ramenosfsky, M. L. Management of the Acutely Injured Child. In K. I. Maull (ed.), *Advances in Trauma* (vol II). Chicago: Year Book, 1987. Pp. 43–86.
5. Buntain, W. L., and Lynn, H. B. Splenorrhaphy: Changing concepts for the traumatized spleen. *Surgery* 86:748, 1979.
6. Lee, J., and Mucha, P., Jr. Appropriate management of splenic trauma (letter to the editor). *Mayo Clin. Proc.* 61:836, 1986.
7. Mucha, P., Jr. Changing attitude toward the management of blunt splenic trauma in adults. *Mayo Clin. Proc.* 61:472, 1986.
8. Mucha, P., Jr., Daly, R. C., and Farnell, M. B. Selective management of blunt splenic trauma. *J. Trauma* 26:970, 1986.
9. Schwartz, P. E., Sterioff, S., Mucha, P., Jr., et al. Postsplenectomy sepsis and mortality in adults. *J.A.M.A.* 248:2279, 1982.
10. Barrett, J., Scheaff, C., Abuabara, S., et al. Splenic preservation in adults after blunt and penetrating trauma. *Am. J. Surg.* 145:313, 1983.
11. Benjamin, C. I., Engrav, L. H., and Perry, J. F. Delayed rupture or delayed diagnosis of rupture of the spleen. *Surg. Gynecol. Obstet.* 142:171, 1976.
12. Feliciano, D. V., Bitondo, C. G., Mattox, K. L., et al. A four-year experience with splenectomy versus splenorrhaphy. *Ann. Surg.* 201:568, 1985.
13. Hebeler, R. F., Ward, R. E., Miller, P. W., et al. The management of splenic injury. *J. Trauma* 22:492, 1982.
14. Livingston, C. D., Sirinek, K. R., Levine, B. A., et al. Traumatic splenic injury: Its management in a patient population with a high incidence of associated injury. *Arch. Surg.* 117:670, 1982.
15. Millikan, J. S., Moore, E. E., Moore, G. E., et al. Alternatives to splenectomy in adults after trauma: Repair, partial resection, and reimplantation of splenic tissue. *Am. J. Surg.* 144:711, 1982.
16. Moore, F. A., Moore, E. E., Moore, G. E., et al. Risk of splenic salvage after trauma: Analysis of 200 adults. *Am. J. Surg.* 148:800, 1984.
17. Morgenstern, L., and Uyeda, R. Y. Nonoperative management of injuries of the spleen in adults. *Surg. Gynecol. Obstet.* 157:513, 1983.
18. Oakes, D. D., and Charters, A. C. Changing concepts in the management of splenic trauma. *Surg. Gynecol. Obstet.* 153:181, 1984.
19. Pachter, H. L., Hofstetter, S. R., and Spencer, F. C. Evolving concepts in splenic surgery: Splenorrhaphy versus splenectomy and postsplenectomy drainage; experience in 105 patients. *Ann. Surg.* 194:262, 1981.
20. Shackford, S. R., Sise, M. J., Virgilio, R. W., et al. Evaluation of splenorrhaphy: A grading system for splenic trauma. *J. Trauma* 21:538, 1981.
21. Tibi, P., Ouriel, K., and Schwartz, S. I. Splenic injury in the adult: Splenectomy, splenorrhaphy, or nonoperative management. *Contemp. Surg.* 26:73, 1985.
22. Traub, A. C., and Perry, J. F., Jr. Injuries associated with splenic trauma. *J. Trauma* 21:840, 1981.
23. Zucker, K., Browns, K., Rossman, D., et al. Nonoperative management of splenic trauma: Conservative or radical treatment? *Arch. Surg.* 119:400, 1984.
24. Schwartz, S. I. Spleen. In S. I. Schwartz et al. (eds.), *Principles of Surgery.* New York: McGraw-Hill, 1974. P. 1281.
25. Sekikawa, T., and Shatney, C. H. Septic sequelae after splenectomy for trauma in adults. *Am. J. Surg.* 145:667, 1983.
26. Boda, G. R., and Verzosa, E. S. Incidental splenic injury: Is splenectomy always necessary? *Am. J. Surg.* 113:303, 1967.
27. William, P. L., and Warwick, R. *Gray's Anatomy* (36th ed.). Philadelphia: Saunders, 1980. Pp. 773–779.
28. Gupta, C. D., Gupta, S. C., Arora, A. K., et al. Vascular segments in the human spleen. *J. Anat.* 121:613, 1976.

29. Huu, N., Person, H., Hong, R., et al. Anatomical approach to the vascular segmentation of the spleen (lien) based on controlled experimental partial splenectomies. *Anat. Clin.* 4:265, 1982.
30. Cooney, D. R., Swanson, S. E., Dearth, J. C., et al. Heterotopic splenic autotransplantation in prevention of overwhelming postsplenectomy infection. *J. Pediatr. Surg.* 14:336, 1979.
31. Fasching, M. D., and Cooner, D. R. Reimmunization and splenic autotransplantation: A long-term study of immunologic response and survival following pneumococcal challenge. *J. Surg. Res.* 28:449, 1980.
32. King, H., and Shumaker, H. B. Splenic studies: I. Susceptibility to infection after splenectomy performed in infancy. *Ann. Surg.* 136:239, 1952.
33. Llende, M., Santiago-Delpin, E. A., and Lavergne, J. Immunobiological consequences of splenectomy: A review. *J. Surg. Res.* 40:85, 1986.
34. Amsbaugh, D. F., Prescott, B., and Baker, P. J. Effect of splenectomy on the expression of regulatory T cell activity. *J. Immunol.* 121:1483, 1978.
35. Ford, W. L., and Smith, M. E. Lymphocyte Recirculation Between the Spleen and the Blood. In *Role of the Spleen in the Immunology of Parasitic Diseases.* Basel: Schwabe, 1979. Pp. 29–41.
36. Sy, M. A. Splenic requirement for the generation of suppressor T-cells. *J. Immunol.* 119:2095, 1977.
37. Wells, W. L., and Battisto, J. R. Splenic Regulation of Humoral and Cellular Immunological Responses in Other Domains. In *Role of the Spleen in the Immunology of Parasitic Diseases.* Basel: Schwabe, 1979. Pp. 59–84.
38. Bogart, D., Biggar, W. D., and Good, R. A. Impaired intravascular clearance of pneumococcus type-3 following splenectomy. *J. Reticuloendothel. Soc.* 11:77, 1972.
39. Whitaker, A. N. Effect of previous splenectomy on the course of pneumococcal bacteremia in mice. *J. Pathol. Bacteriol.* 95:357, 1968.
40. Chaimoff, C., Douer, D., Pick, I. A., et al. Serum immunoglobulin changes after accidental splenectomy in adults. *Am. J. Surg.* 136:332, 1978.
41. Church, J. A., Mahour, G. H., and Lipsey, A. I. Antibody responses after splenectomy and splenic autotransplantation in rats. *J. Surg. Res.* 31:343, 1981.
42. Hosea, S. W., Brown, E. J., Hamburger, M. I., et al. Opsonic requirements for intracellular clearance after splenectomy. *N. Engl. J. Med.* 304:245, 1981.
43. Likhite, V. V. Opsonin and leukophilic γ-globulin in chronically splenectomized rats with and without heterotropic autotransplanted splenic tissue. *Nature* 253:742, 1975.
44. Chu, D. Z. J., Nichioka, K. El-Hagin, T., et al. Effects of tuftsin on postsplenectomy sepsis. *Surgery* 97:701, 1985.
45. Constantopoulos, A., Najjar, V. A., Wish, J. B., et al. Defective phagocytosis due to tuftsin deficiency in splenectomized subjects. *Am. J. Dis. Child.* 125:663, 1973.
46. Najjar, V. A., and Nishioka, K. "Tuftsin": A physiological phagocytosis stimulating peptide. *Nature* 228:672, 1970.
47. Downey, E. C., Catanzaro, A., Ninnemann, J. C., et al. Long term depressed immunocompetence of patients splenectomized for trauma. *Surg. Forum* 29:41, 1980.
48. Carlisle, H. N., and Soslaw, S. Properdin levels in splenectomized persons. *Proc. Soc. Exp. Biol. Med.* 102:150, 1959.
49. Bisno, A. L., and Freeman, J. C. The syndrome of asplenia, pneumococcal sepsis and disseminated intravascular coagulation. *Ann. Intern. Med.* 72:389, 1970.
50. Diamond, L. K. Splenectomy in childhood and the hazard of overwhelming infection. *Pediatrics* 43:886, 1969.
51. Dickerman, J. D. Traumatic asplenia in adults: A defined hazard? *Arch. Surg.* 116:361, 1981.
52. Ein, S. H., Shandling, B., Simpson, J. S., et al. The morbidity and mortality of splenectomy in childhood. *Ann. Surg.* 185:307, 1977.
53. Eraklis, A. J., Kevy, S. V., and Diamond, L. K. Hazard of overwhelming infections after splenectomy in childhood. *N. Engl. J. Med.* 276:1225, 1967.
54. Erikson, W. D., Burgert, E. O., and Lynn, H. B. The hazard of infection following splenectomy in children. *Am. J. Dis. Child.* 116:1, 1968.
55. Francke, E. L., and Neu, H. C. Postsplenectomy infection. *Surg. Clin. North Am.* 61:135, 1981.
56. Singer, D. B., Postsplenectomy Sepsis. In A. D. Rosenburg and R. P. Bolande (eds.), *Perspectives in Pediatric Pathology.* Chicago: Year Book, 1973. Vol. 1, pp. 285–311.

57. Holschneider, A. M., Kreiz-Klimeck, H., Strasser, B., et al. Complications of splenectomy in childhood. *Z. Kinerchir.* 35:130, 1982.
58. Zarrabi, M. H., and Rosner, F. Serious infections in adults following splenectomy for trauma. *Arch. Intern. Med.* 144:1421, 1984.
59. Robinette, C. D. Splenectomy and subsequent mortality in veterans of the 1935–45 war. *Lancet* 2:127, 1977.
60. Berlatzky, Y., Shiloni, E., Anner, H., et al. "Delayed rupture of the spleen" or delayed diagnosis of the splenic injury? *Isr. J. Med. Sci.* 16:659, 1980.
61. Gold, R. E., and Redman, H. C. Splenic trauma: Assessment of problems in diagnosis. *Am. J. Radiol.* 116:413, 1972.
62. Mishalany, H. G., Miller, J. H., and Woolley, M. M. Radioisotope spleen scan in patients with splenic injury. *Arch. Surg.* 117:1147, 1982.
63. Wener, L., and Boyle, C. D. Splenic scintiscanning in the preoperative diagnosis of subcapsular hematoma. *N. Engl. J. Med.* 277:35, 1967.
64. Witek, J. T., Spencer, R. P., Pearson, H. A., et al. Diagnostic spleen scans in occult splenic injury. *J. Trauma* 14:197, 1974.
65. Haller, J. A. A new philosophy of pediatric splenic surgery: Save our spleens. *Surg. Rounds* 3:23, 1980.
66. Howman-Giles, R., Gilday, D. L., Venugopal, S., et al. Splenic trauma: Nonoperative management and long-term follow-up by scintiscan. *J. Pediatr. Surg.* 13:121, 1978.
67. Lutzker, L. G., and Chun, K. J. Radionuclide imaging in the nonsurgical treatment of liver and spleen trauma. *J. Trauma* 21:382, 1981.
68. Fisher, R. G., Foucar, K., Estrada, R., et al. Splenic rupture in blunt trauma: Correlation of angiographic and pathologic records. *Radiol. Clin. North Am.* 19:141, 1981.
69. Fuchs, W. A., and Robotti, G. The diagnostic impact of computed tomography in blunt abdominal trauma. *Clin. Radiol.* 34:261, 1983.
70. Jeffrey, R. B., Laing, F. C., Federle, M. P., et al. Computed tomography of splenic trauma. *Radiology* 141:729, 1981.
71. Karp, M. P., Cooney, D. R., Berger, P. E., et al. The role of computer tomography in the evaluation of blunt abdominal trauma in children. *J. Pediatr. Surg.* 16:316, 1981.
72. Sherck, J. P., and Oakes, D. D. Computed tomography in the management of thoracic, abdominal, and pelvic trauma. *Infect. Surg.* 505, July 1985.
73. Toombs, B. D., Lester, R. G., Ben-Menachem, Y., et al. Computed tomography in blunt trauma. *Radiol. Clin. North Am.* 19:17, 1981.
74. Kaufmann, R. A., Towbin, R., Babcock, D. S., et al. Upper abdominal trauma in children: Imaging evaluation. *A.J.R.* 142:449, 1984.
75. Gibbon, J. H. Rupture of the spleen (a reported discussion). *Ann. Surg.* 48:152, 1908.
76. Bryk, D., and Petigrow, N. Postsplenectomy gastric perforation. *Surgery* 61:239, 1967.
77. Cohn, L. H. Local infections after splenectomy: Relationship of drainage. *Arch. Surg.* 90:230, 1965.
78. Lennard, E. S. Pneumococcal vaccine: A surgeon's overview (editorial). *Am. J. Surg.* 137:283, 1979.
79. Brivet, F. Herer, G., Fremaux, A., et al. Fatal post-splenectomy pneumococcal sepsis despite pneumococcal vaccine and penicillin prophylaxis. *Lancet* 2:356, 1984.
80. Evans, D. I. K. Fatal post-splenectomy sepsis despite prophylaxis with penicillin and pneumococcal vaccine. *Lancet* 1:1124, 1984.
81. Hostetter, M. K., Schwartz, A. L., Siber, G. R., et al. Pneumococcal vaccine failure. *Am. J. Dis. Child.* 135:1149, 1981.
82. Zarrabi, M. H., and Rosner, F. Pneumococcal sepsis and meningitis in vacinated subjects: A review of 55 reported cases. *J. Natl. Med. Assoc.* 79:372, 1987.
83. Hedges, J. R. Commentary "infocus" splenectomy and sequelae. *E. D. News* 14, Aug., 1980.
84. Cooney, D. R., Michalak, W. A., Michalak, D. M., et al. Comparative methods of splenic preservation. *J. Pediatr. Surg.* 16:237, 1981.
85. Orland, J. C., and Moore, T. C. Splenectomy for trauma in childhood. *Surg. Gynecol. Obstet.* 134:94, 1972.
86. Zarrabi, M. H., and Rosner, F. Rarity of failure of penicillin prophylaxis to prevent postsplenectomy sepsis. *Arch. Intern. Med.* 146:1207, 1986.
87. Cooney, D. R., Dearth, J. C., Swanson, S. E., et al. Relative merits of partial splenectomy, splenic reimplantation, and immunization in preventing postsplenectomy infection. *Surgery* 86:561, 1979.

88. Steely, W. M., Satava, R. M., Brigham, R. A., et al. Splenic autotransplantation: Determination of the optimal amount required for maximal survival. *J. Surg. Res.* 45:327, 1988.
89. Annexton, M. Autotransplantation of the spleen tissue after trauma: Encouraging evidence. *J.A.M.A.* 241:437, 1979.
90. Livingston, C. D., Levine, B. A., and Sirinek, K. R. Site of splenic autotransplantation affects protection from sepsis. *Am. J. Surg.* 146:734, 1983.
91. Patel, J., Williams, J. S., Shmigel, B., et al. Preservation of splenic function by autotransplantation of traumatized spleen in man. *Surgery* 90:683, 1981.
92. Moore, G. E., Stevens, R. E., Moore, E. E., et al. Failure of splenic implants to protect against fatal postsplenectomy infection. *Am. J. Surg.* 146:413, 1983.
93. Rice, H. M., and James, P. D. Ectopic splenic tissue failed to prevent fatal pneumococcal septicaemia after splenectomy for trauma. *Lancet* 1:565, 1980.
94. Sass, W., Bergholz, M., Kehl, A., et al. Overwhelming infection after splenectomy in spite of some spleen remaining and splenosis: A case report. *Klin. Wochenschr.* 61:1075, 1983.
95. Horton, J., Ogden, M. E., Williams, S., et al. The importance of splenic blood flow in clearing pneumococcal organisms. *Ann. Surg.* 195:172, 1982.
96. Van Wyck, D. B., Witte, M. H., Witte, C. L., et al. Critical splenic mass for survival from experimental pneumococcemia. *J. Surg. Res.* 28:14, 1980.
97. Steely, W. M., Satava, R. M., Harris, R. W., et al. Comparison of omental splenic transplants to partial splenectomy: Protective effect against septic death. *Am. Surg.* 53:702, 1987.
98. Kakkasseril, J. S., Stewart, D., Cox, J. A., et al. Changing treatment of pediatric splenic trauma. *Arch. Surg.* 117:758, 1982.
99. Medina, M., Staht, W. M., and Reynolds, B. M. Is splenorrhaphy safe in the multiple trauma patient? *J. Trauma* 23:651, 1983.
100. Morgenstern, L. Conservation of the injured spleen. *Surg. Rounds,* July 1980. Pp. 13–20.
101. Morgenstern, L., and Shapiro, S. J. Techniques of splenic conservation. *Arch. Surg.* 114:449, 1979.
102. Derderian, G. P., Walshaw, R., and McGehee, J. Ultrasonic surgical dissection in the dog spleen. *Am. J. Surg.* 143:269, 1982.
103. Hodgson, W. J. B., and McElhinney, A. J. Ultrasonic partial splenectomy. *Surgery* 91:346, 1982.
104. Brands, W., Mennicken, C., and Beck, M. Preservation of the ruptured spleen by gluing with highly concentrated human fibrinogen: Experimental and clinical results. *World J. Surg.* 6:366, 1982.
105. Scheele, J. Gentsch, H. H., and Matteson, E. Splenic repair by fibrin tissue adhesive and collagen fleece. *Surgery* 95:6, 1984.
106. Dulchavsky, S. A., Ledgerwood, A. M., Lucas, C. E., et al. Wound healing of the injured spleen with and without splenorrhaphy. *J. Trauma* 27:1155, 1987.
107. Campos, C. M. Segmental resection of the spleen. *Hosp. Rio.* 62:575, 1962.
108. Morgenstern, L. The avoidable complications of splenectomy. *Surg. Gynecol. Obstet.* 145:525, 1977.
109. Høivik, B., and Solheim, K. Splenic artery ligation in splenic injuries. *Injury* 15:1, 1983.
110. Keramidas, D. C. The ligation of the splenic artery in the treatment of traumatic rupture of the spleen. *Surgery* 85:530, 1979.
111. Pabst, R., Kamran, D., and Creutzig, H. Splenic regeneration and blood flow after ligation of the splenic artery or partial splenectomy. *Am. J. Surg.* 147:382, 1984.
112. Sherman, N. H., and Asch, M. J. Conservative surgery for splenic injuries. *Pediatrics* 61:267, 1978.
113. Delany, H. M., Porreca, F., Mitsudo, S., et al. Splenic capping: An experimental study of a new technique for splenorrhaphy using woven polyglycolic acid mesh. *Ann. Surg.* 196:187, 1982.
114. Lange, D., Zaert, P. H., Merlotti, G. J., et al. The use of absorbable mesh in splenic trauma. *J. Trauma* 28:269, 1988.
115. Berger, E. Die Verletzungen der Milz und ihre Chirurgische Behandlung. *Arch. Klin. Chir.* 68:56, 1902.
116. Aronson, D. Z., Scherz, A. W., Einhorn, A. H., et al. Non-operative management of the splenic trauma in children: A report of six consecutive cases. *Pediatrics* 60:482, 1977.

117. Cohen, R. C. Blunt splenic trauma in children: A retrospective study of nonoperative management. *Aust. Paediatr. J.* 18:221, 1982.
118. Douglas, G. J., and Simpson, J. S. The conservative management of splenic trauma. *J. Pediatr. Surg.* 6:565, 1971.
119. Ein, S. H., Shandling, B., Simpson, J. S., et al. Nonoperative management of traumatized spleen in children: How and why. *J. Pediatr. Surg.* 13:117, 1978.
120. King, D. R., Lobe, T. E., Haase, G. M., et al. Selective management of injured spleen. *Surgery* 90:677, 1981.
121. Weinstein, M. E., Govin, G. G., Rice, C. L., et al. Splenorrhaphy for splenic trauma. *J. Trauma* 19:692, 1979.
122. Wesson, D. E., Filler, R. M., Ein, S. H., et al. Ruptured spleen: When to operate? *J. Pediatr. Surg.* 16:324, 1981.
123. Malangoni, M. A., Levine, A. W., Droege, E. A., et al. Management of injury to the spleen in adults: Results of early operation and observation. *Ann. Surg.* 200:702, 1984.

Injuries of the Stomach, Duodenum, Pancreas, and Small Intestine

1. Campbell, R., and Kennedy, T. The management of pancreatic and pancreaticoduodenal injuries. *Br. J. Surg.* 67:845, 1980.
2. Brotman, S., Cisternino, S., Myers, R. A., and Cowley, R. A. A test to help diagnosis of rupture in the injured duodenum. *Injury* 12:464, 1981.
3. Corley, R. D., Norcross, W. J., and Shoemaker, W. C. Traumatic injuries to the duodenum. *Ann. Surg.* 181:92, 1974.
4. Fabian, T. C., Mangiante, E. C., and Millis, M. Duodenal rupture due to blunt trauma. *South. Med. J.* 77:1078, 1984.
5. Lucas, C. E., and Ledgerwood, A. M. Factors influencing outcome after blunt duodenal injury. *J. Trauma* 15:839, 1975.
6. Berne, C. J., Donovan, A. J., White, E. J., et al. Duodenal "diverticulation" for duodenal and pancreatic injuries. *Am. J. Surg.* 127:503, 1974.
7. Flint, L. M., McCoy, M., Richardson, J. D., and Polk, H. G. Duodenal injury: Analysis of common misconceptions in diagnosis and treatment. *Ann. Surg.* 191:697, 1980.
8. King, W. L., and Provan, J. L. Diagnosis and management of duodenal injuries. *Can. J. Surg.* 15:269, 1972.
9. Lucas, C. E. Diagnosis and treatment of pancreatic and duodenal injury. *Surg. Clin. North Am.* 57:49, 1977.
10. Davis, J. J., Cohn, I., and Nance, F. C. Diagnosis and management of blunt abdominal trauma. *Ann. Surg.* 183:677, 1976.
11. Talbot, W. A., and Shuck, J. M. Retroperitoneal duodenal injury due to blunt abdominal trauma. *Am. J. Surg.* 130:659, 1975.
12. Fischer, R. P., Beverlin, B. C., Engrav, L. H., et al. Diagnostic peritoneal lavage—fourteen years and 2,586 patients later. *Am. J. Surg.* 136:701, 1978.
13. Fabian, T. C., Mangiante, E. C., White, T. J., et al. A prospective study of 91 patients undergoing both computed tomography and peritoneal lavage following blunt abdominal trauma. *J. Trauma* 26:602, 1986.
14. Morton, J. R., and Jordan, G. L. Traumatic duodenal injuries. *J. Trauma* 8:127, 1968.
15. Vaughn, G. D., Frazier, O. H., Graham, D. Y., et al. The use of pyloric exclusion in the management of severe duodenal injuries. *Am. J. Surg.* 134:785, 1977.
16. Martin, T. D., Feliciano, D. V., Mattox, K. L., and Jordan, G. L. Severe duodenal injuries. *Arch. Surg.* 118:631, 1983.
17. Stone, H. H., and Fabian, T. C. Management of duodenal wounds. *J. Trauma* 19:334, 1979.
18. Lucas, C. E., and Walt, A. J. Analysis of randomized biliary drainage for liver trauma in 189 patients. *J. Trauma* 12:925, 1972.
19. Stone, H. H., Fabian, T. C., Satiani, B., and Turkleson, M. L. Experiences in the management of pancreatic trauma. *J. Trauma* 21:257, 1981.
20. Jones, R. C., Management of pancreatic trauma. *Am. J. Surg.* 150:698, 1985.
21. Graham, J. M., Mattox, K. L., and Jordan, G. L. Traumatic injuries to the pancreas. *Am. J. Surg.* 136:744, 1978.
22. Northrup, W. F., and Simmons, R. L. Pancreatic trauma: A review. *Surgery* 71:27, 1972.
23. Frey, C. Trauma to the Pancreas and Duodenum. In F. W. Blaisdell and D. D. Trunkey (eds)., *Trauma Management: Abdominal Trauma.* New York: Thieme-Stratton, 1982.
24. Werschky, L. R., and Jordan, G. L. Surgical man-

agement of traumatic injuries to the pancreas. *Am. J. Surg.* 116:768, 1968.
25. Tayiem, A. K. Pancreatic/duodenal trauma. *J. Kan. Med. Soc.*, May 1979. P. 247.
26. Kudsk, K. A., Temizer, D., Ellison, E. C., et al. Post-traumatic pancreatic sequestrum: Recognition and treatment. *J. Trauma* 26:320, 1986.
27. Marx, J. A., Moore, E. E., and Bar-Or, D. Peritoneal lavage in penetrating injuries of the small bowel and colon: Value of enzyme determination. *Ann. Emerg. Med.* 12:68, 1983.
28. Mueller, G. L., Burney, R. E., and Mackenzie, J. R. Leucocytosis in peritoneal lavage effluent after selected abdominal organ injury in an experimental model. *Ann. Emerg. Med.* 11:343, 1982.
29. Troop, B. R., Fabian, T. C., Distretti, J., et al. Unpublished data, 1987.
30. Marx, J. A., Bar-Or, D., Moore, E. E., et al. Utility of lavage alkaline phosphatase in detection of isolated small intestinal injury. *Ann. Emerg. Med.* 14:10, 1985.
31. Donohue, J. H., Federle, M. P., Griffiths, B. G., et al. Computed tomography in the diagnosis of blunt intestinal and mesenteric injuries. *J. Trauma* 27:11, 1987.

Injuries of the Colon and Rectum

1. Abcarian, H., and Lowe, R. Colon and rectal trauma. *Surg. Clin. North Am.* 58:519, 1978.
2. Beall, A. C., Bricker, D. L., and Alessi, F. J. Surgical considerations in the management of civilian colon injuries. *Am. J. Surg.* 173:971, 1971.
3. Burch, J. M., Brock, J. C., Gevirtzman, L., et al. The injured colon. *Am. J. Surg.* 203:701, 1986.
4. Freeark, R. J. The injured colon. *J. Trauma* 17:563, 1977.
5. Haygood, D., and Polk, H. C. Gunshot wounds of the colon. *Am. J. Surg.* 131:213, 1976.
6. Lo Cicero III, J., Tajima, T., and Drapanas, T. A half century of experiences in the management of colon injuries: Changing concepts. *J. Trauma* 15:575, 1975.
7. Schrock, T. R., Deveney, C. W., and Dunphy, J. E. Factors contributing to leakage of colonic anastomoses. *Am. J. Surg.* 177:513, 1977.
8. Thompson, J. S., Moore, E. E., and Moore, J. B. Comparison of penetrating injuries of the right and left colon. *Am. J. Surg.* 193:414, 1981.
9. Dang, C. V., Peter, E. T., and Parks, S. N. Trauma of the colon. *Arch. Surg.* 177:652, 1982.
10. Kirkpatrick, J. R. Injuries of the colon. *Surg. Clin. North Am.* 57:67, 1977.
11. Schrock, T. R., and Christensen, N. Management of perforating injuries of the colon. *Surg. Gynecol. Obstet.* 135:65, 1972.
12. Thompson, J. S., and Moore, E. E. Factors affecting the outcome of exteriorized colon repairs. *J. Trauma* 22:403, 1982.
13. Thal, E. R., and Yeary, E. C. Morbidity of colostomy closure following colon trauma. *J. Trauma* 20:287, 1980.
14. Bubenik, O., Meakins, J. L., and McLean, A. P. Delayed perforation of the colon in blunt abdominal trauma. *Can. J. Surg.* 23:473, 1980.
15. Winton, T. L., Girotti, M. J., and Manley, P. N. Delayed intestinal perforation after nonpenetrating abdominal trauma. *Can. J. Surg.* 28:437, 1985.
16. Vitale, G. C., Richardson, J. D., and Flint, L. M. Successful management of injuries to the extraperitoneal rectum. *Am. J. Surg.* 49:159, 1983.
17. Trunkey, D., Hays, R. J., and Shires, J. T. Management of rectal trauma. *J. Trauma* 13:411, 1973.
18. Barone, J. E., Yee, J., and Nealon, T. F. Management of foreign bodies and trauma of the rectum. *Surg. Gynecol. Obstet.* 156:453, 1983.
19. Crass, R. A., Tranbaugh, R. F., and Kudsk, K. A. Colorectal foreign bodies and perforation. *Am. J. Surg.* 142:85, 1981.

Injuries of the Diaphragm

1. Estera, A. S., Platt, M. R., and Mills, L. J. Traumatic injuries of the diaphragm. *Chest* 75:306, 1979.
2. Harman, P. K., Mentzer, R. M., Weinberg, A. C., et al. Early diagnosis by liver scan of right-sided traumatic diaphragmatic hernia. *J. Trauma* 21:489, 1981.
3. Pomerantz, M., Rodgers, B. M., and Sabiston, D. C. Traumatic diaphragmatic hernia. *Surgery* 64:529, 1968.
4. Ebert, P. A., Baertner, R. A., and Zuidema, J. D. Traumatic diaphragmatic hernia. *Surg. Gynecol. Obstet.* 125:59, 1967.
5. Brooks, J. W. Blunt traumatic rupture of the diaphragm. *Ann. Thorac. Surg.* 26:199, 1978.
6. Jones, K. W. Thoracic trauma. *Surg. Clin. North Am.* 60:957, 1980.

7. Ward, R. E., Flynn, T. C., and Clark, W. P. Diaphragmatic disruption secondary to blunt abdominal trauma. *J. Trauma* 21:35, 1981.
8. Wise, L., Connors, J., and Hwang, Y. H. Traumatic injuries to the diaphragm. *J. Trauma* 13:946, 1987.
9. Sandrassagra, F. A. Penetrating thoracoabdominal injuries. *Br. J. Surg.* 64:638, 1977.
10. Miller, O. L., Bennet, E. D., Root, H. D., et al. Management of penetrating and blunt diaphragmatic injury. *J. Trauma* 24:403, 1984.
11. Grimes, O. F. Traumatic injuries of the diaphragm. *Am. J. Surg.* 128:175, 1974.
12. Adamthwaite, D. N. Penetrating injuries of the diaphragm. *Injury* 14:151, 1982.
13. Dajee, A., Schepps, D., and Hurley, E. J. Diaphragmatic injuries. *Surg. Gynecol. Obstet* 153:31, 1981.
14. Perry, J. F., Demeules, J. E., and Root, H. D. Diagnostic peritoneal lavage in blunt abdominal trauma. *Surg. Gynecol. Obstet.* 131:742, 1970.
15. Jackson, G. L., and Thal, E. R. Management of stab wounds of the back and flank. *J. Trauma* 19:660, 1979.
16. Thal, E. R. Evaluation of peritoneal lavage and local exploration of lower chest and abdominal stab wounds. *J. Trauma* 17:642, 1977.
17. Aronoff, R. J., Reynolds, J., and Thal, E. R. Evaluation of diaphragmatic injuries. Presented at the 34th Annual Meeting of the Southwestern Surgical Congress. April 26–29, 1982, Coronado, California.
18. Flancbaum, L., Morgan, A. S., and Esposito, T. Non left sided diaphragmatic rupture due to blunt trauma. *Surg. Gynecol. Obstet.* 161:266, 1985.
19. Ammann, A. M., Brewer, W. H., and Maull, K. I. Traumatic rupture of the diaphragm: Real time sonographic diagnosis. *A.J.R.* 140:915, 1983.
20. Kim, A. E., McConnel, B. J., McConnel, R. W., et al. Radionuclide diagnosis of diaphragmatic rupture with hepatic herniation. *Surgery* 94:35, 1983.
21. Rodriquez-Morales, G., Rodriquez, A., and Shatney, C. H. Acute rupture of the diaphragm in blunt trauma. *J. Trauma* 26:438, 1986.
22. Drews, J. A., Mercer, E. C., and Benfield, J. R. Acute diaphragmatic injuries. *Ann. Thorac. Surg.* 16:67, 1973.
23. Morgan, A. S., Flancbaum, L., Esposito, T., et al. Blunt injury to the diaphragm. *J. Trauma* 28:565, 1986.
24. Symbas, P. N., Blasis, S. E., and Hatcher, C. Blunt and penetrating diaphragmatic injuries with or without herniation of organs into the chest. *Ann. Thorac. Surg.* 42:158, 1986.
25. Estera, A. S., Landay, M. J., and McClelland, R. N. Blunt traumatic rupture of the right hemidiaphragm. *Ann. Thorac. Surg.* 39:525, 1985.

Retroperitoneal Hematoma

1. Selivanou, V., Hoon Sang, C. H. I., Alverdy, J., et al. Mortality in retroperitoneal hematoma. *J. Trauma* 24:1022, 1984.
2. Henao, F., and Aldrete, J. Retroperitoneal hematomas of traumatic origin. *Surg. Gynecol. Obstet.* 161:106, 1985.
3. Grieco, J., and Perry, J. Retroperitoneal hematoma following trauma: Its clinical importance. *J. Trauma* 20:733, 1980.
4. Kudsk, K. A., and Sheldon, G. F., Retroperitoneal hematoma. In F. W. Blaisdell, and D. D. Trunkey (eds.), *Abdominal Trauma.* Trauma Management, Vol. I. New York: Thieme-Stratton, 1982. P. 281.
5. Allen, R., Eastmen, B., Halter, B., and Conolly, W. Retroperitoneal hemorrhage secondary to blunt trauma. *Am. J. Surg.* 118:558, October 1969.
6. Nick, W. V., Zollinger, R. W., and Pace, W. G. Retroperitoneal hemorrhage after blunt abdominal trauma. *J. Trauma* 7:652, 1967.
7. Zuidema, G. D., Rutherford, R. B., and Ballinger, W. *The Management of Trauma* (4th ed.). Philadelphia: Saunders, 1985.
8. Sagel, S. S., Siegel, M. J., Stanley, R. J., and Jost, R. G. Detection of retroperitoneal hemorrhage by computed tomography. *Am. J. Roentgenol.* 129:403, 1977.
9. Jackson, G. L., and Thal, E. R. Management of stab wounds of the back & flank. *J. Trauma* 19:660, 1979.
10. Phillips, T., Sclafani, S. J. A., Goldstein, A., et al. Use of the contrast-enhanced CT enema in the management of penetrating trauma to the flank and back. *J. Trauma* 26:593, 1986.
11. Flint, L., Brown, A., Richardson, S. D., et al. Definitive control of bleeding from severe pelvic fractures. *Ann. Surg.* 189:709, 1979.

12. Steichen, F. M., Dragon, E. L., Pearlman, D. M., and Weil, P. H. The management of retroperitoneal hematoma secondary to penetrating injuries. *Surg. Gynecol. Obstet.* 123:581, 1966.
13. Scott, R., Jr., Carlton, C. E., Jr., and Goldman, M. Penetrating injuries of the kidney: An analysis of 181 patients. *J. Urol.* 101:247, 1969.
14. Veith, F. J., and Gupta, S. Technique for occluding the supraceliac aorta through the abdomen. *Surg. Gynecol. Obstet.* 151:427, 1980.
15. Conn, J. discussion of: L. C. Buscaghia et al., Penetrating abdominal vascular injuries *Arch. Surg.* 99:768, 1969.
16. Pilcher, D. B., Harman, P. R., and Moore, E. E., Jr. Retrohepatic vena cava balloon shunt introduced via the sapheno-femoral junction. *J. Trauma* 17:837, 1977.
17. Cattell, R. B., and Braasch, J. W. A technique for the exposure of the third and fourth portions of the duodenum. *Surg. Gynecol. Obstet.* 111:378, 1960.
18. Mattox, K. L., McCollum, W. B., Beall, A. C., et al. Management of penetrating injuries of the suprarenal aorta. *J. Trauma* 15:808, 1975.
19. Holcroft, J. W., Trunkey, D. D., Minagi, H., et al. Renal trauma and retroperitoneal hematomas: Indications for exploration. *J. Trauma* 15:1045, 1975.
20. McClelland, R. N., Jones, R. C., Shires, G. T., et al. *Trauma to the Abdomen: Care of the Trauma Patient.* New York: Blakiston Div., McGraw-Hill, 1966. Pp. 400–403.
21. Osios, M. G., Hole, S. D., and Lytton, B. The management of renal injuries. *J. Trauma* 16:954, 1976.
22. Shaftan, G. W. Retroperitoneal trauma. *Contemp. Surg.* 16:25, 1980.
23. Weil, P. H. Management of retroperitoneal trauma. *Curr. Probl. Surg.* 20:541, 1983.
24. Costa, M., and Robbs, T. V. Management of retroperitoneal hematoma following penetrating trauma. *Br. J. Surg.* 72:662, 1985.
25. Sagalowsky, A. I., McConnell, J. D., and Peters, P. C. Renal trauma requiring surgery: An analysis of 185 cases. *J. Trauma* 23:128, 1983.
26. Blaisdell, F. W., and Trunkey, D. D. (ed.), McAninch J. W. (Guest ed.) *Urogenital Trauma.* Trauma Management, Vol. II. Thieme-Stratton, 1985.
27. Scott, R. F., Jr., and Selzman, H. M. Complications of nefrectomy: Review of 450 patients and a description of a modification of the transperitoneal approach. *J. Urol.* 95:307, 1966.
28. McAninch, J. W., and Carrol, P. R. Renal trauma: Kidney preservation through improved vascular control—a refined approach. *J. Trauma* 22:285, 1982.
29. Stone, H. H., Rutledge, B. A., and Martin, J. D., Jr. Massive crushing pelvic injuries. *Am. Surg.* 34:869, 1968.
30. Motsay, G. J., Manlove, C., and Perry, J. F. Major venous injury with pelvic fracture. *J. Trauma* 9:343, 1969.
31. Sheldon, G. F., and Winestock, D. P. Hemorrhage from open pelvic fracture controlled intraoperatively with balloon catheter. *J. Trauma* 18:68, 1978.
32. Miller, W. E. Massive hemorrhage in fractures of the pelvis. *South. Med. J.* 56:933, 1968.
33. Margolies, M. N., Ring, E. J., Waltman, A. C., et al. Arteriography in the management of hemorrhage from pelvic fractures. *N. Engl. J. Med.* 287:217, 1972.
34. Brotman, S., Soderstrom, C. A., Oster-Granite, M., et al. Management of severe bleeding in fractures of the pelvis. *Surg. Gynecol. Obstet.* 153:823, 1981.
35. Mears, D. External fixation of pelvic fractures. *Orthop. Clin. North Am.* 11:465, 1980.
36. Goldstein, A., Phillips, T., Sclafani, S. J. A., et al. Early open reduction and internal fixation of the disrupted pelvic ring. *J. Trauma* 26:325, 1986.
37. Ravitch, M. M. Clinical experience with the G-suit (letter to the editor). *Arch. Surg.* 101:544, 1970.
38. Davidson, A. T. Direct intralumen balloon tamponade: A technique for the control of massive retroperitoneal hemorrhage. *Am. J. Surg.* 136:396, 1978.
39. Honton, R. E., and Hamilton, S. G. I. Ligature of the internal iliac artery for massive hemorrhage complicating fracture of the pelvis. *J. Bone Joint Surg.* [Br.] 50B:376, 1968.

11

Genitourinary Trauma

Alexander S. Cass

Urologic injuries occur in approximately 3.4 percent of trauma cases [1]. Most of them (91 percent of all urinary injuries and 94 percent of renal injuries) are caused by blunt trauma. The organ most frequently injured is the kidney (84 percent of all injuries). Overall, the bladder and urethra are injured with equal frequency (approximately 8 percent), but as would be expected, there is a sharp difference by sex in the frequency of urethral injuries. For example, in one series of 200 patients with fractured pelves, there were urethral injuries in 17 of the 121 men but in none of the 79 women [2]. Ureteral trauma is almost entirely iatrogenic, although it occurs occasionally as the result of a knife or gunshot wound.

Although the most long-term consequences of trauma are often of genitourinary origin, few of these injuries are immediately life-threatening. Therefore, in the earliest stages of management, the role of the urologist is often to stay out of the way. In particular, the urologist must firmly resist the temptation to perform a retrograde urethrogram in the male patient with a fractured pelvis until the angiographers approve. Patients do not die immediately of a ruptured urethra, but they can die quickly of a ruptured internal iliac artery, and angiography and embolization, generally the preferred immediate treatment for an arterial tear, will be difficult or impossible if the pelvis is filled with contrast medium from urologic studies [3–5]. The generally lower priority for the treatment of urologic injuries should be borne in mind throughout the following discussion.

EMERGENCY MANAGEMENT

History of the Accident

A thorough description of the accident should be obtained, in part to help the physician understand the mechanism of the injury. For example, because the tip of the knife blade is triangular, a 2-cm laceration of the renal capsule at the bottom of a stab wound marks a parenchymal laceration at least 2 cm deep. Ben-Menachem and coworkers [5] describe two patients in whom this fact was not appreciated and the renal capsule was simply reunited. Both patients had stormy postoperative courses, as a result of a strangulating subcapsular hematoma in one patient and continued hemorrhage in the other that could be controlled only by nonselective embolization that caused infarction of most of the kidney.

Physical Examination

The presence and location of ecchymosis, local tenderness, masses, and pain should be ascertained. A rectal or vaginal examination must be made. The presence of blood at the urethral meatus must be noted, as must the presence of hematuria.

Radiologic Evaluation

Indications

A retrograde cystogram is indicated in patients with hematuria (gross or microscopic) or a pelvic fracture. Although most patients with significant urethral or bladder injuries generally have gross hematuria [2], this must not be assumed. A retrograde urethrogram is indicated in the patient with blood at the urethral meatus.

Excretory urography is indicated if there is hematuria (gross or microscopic), flank or lateral abdominal pain, tenderness, or a mass; if there are fractures of transverse processes of the lumbar vertebrae; if a deceleration injury has occurred; or if a perirenal hematoma is found at laparotomy. It may also be indicated in patients with fractured ribs or unexplained gross hematuria [2].

A computed tomography (CT) scan is indicated if excretory urography shows extravasation, distortion of the calices, incomplete collecting-system filling, or delayed opacification. If no renal function is apparent on urography, arteriography is indicated. In the patient who has sustained a stab wound in the flank and is clinically unstable, it may be possible to embolize a bleeding vessel during the same procedure, obviating operation. Cystoscopy and retrograde urography may be needed to delineate a rupture of the collecting system.

Techniques

For a retrograde cystogram in an adult, the bladder should be filled with 400 ml of radiopaque medium. Use of smaller amounts, so that the bladder is not fully distended, will lead to failure to diagnose some bladder tears. After the films have been made, the bladder is drained and rinsed with saline, after which postdrainage films are obtained and examined for extravasated contrast medium.

Excretory urography should be performed as an infusion intravenous urogram (IVU) or with a large bolus of contrast medium. This study is not a substitute for cystography [6,7]; in one series, the IVU revealed only 5 of 23 proven bladder ruptures [6].

In patients with known or suspected urethral rupture, a retrograde urethrogram is performed, and conventional catheter passage is ill-advised. In some of these patients, it may be appropriate to perform cystography through a suprapubic puncture.

INJURIES OF THE KIDNEY

The kidney may be injured by blunt trauma (which accounted for 94 percent of the injuries in one series [1]) or by knives or guns. In most cases of blunt trauma (83 percent in one series [1]), there are other injuries, and in 20 to 30 percent, these other injuries are serious [8]. The presence of fractures of the vertebral processes or the eleventh or twelfth rib is common. Abnormal kidneys, such as those with congenital anomalies, tumors, or hydronephrosis, are more susceptible to injury. Indeed, in an unfortunate number of children, rupture of a Wilms' tumor after a seemingly minor injury is the first sign of the tumor's presence.

Types of Injury

Four types of renal injury are recognized. In increasing order of severity they are

1. *Contusion:* bruises or minor tears of the renal parenchyma without capsular tears
2. *Lacerations:* parenchymal disruption with capsular or caliceal damage or both
3. *Fragmentation:* rupture or shattering of the parenchyma with multiple deep lacerations
4. *Pedicle injuries:* tears or occlusion of the renal arteries or vein

Assessment

The pain caused by renal injuries is usually a dull ache in the flank, which may be obscured by the pain of other injuries. Hematuria, usually gross, is present in 90 percent of patients with renal injuries other than those of the pedicle. However, the amount of blood does not correlate with the severity of the injury. In one series, 40 percent of patients with gross hematuria had contusion or simple lacerations, whereas 3 of the 11 patients with severe injuries had only microhematuria [1]. Local tenderness, muscle rigidity, ecchymosis, and a flank mass may be present. Retroperitoneal bleeding may cause nausea, vomiting, and paralytic ileus.

A plain film of the abdomen may show loss of the renal and psoas shadows; scoliosis; fracture of the transverse processes, ribs, and spine; or altered bowel-gas patterns. An IVU will show incomplete filling, distortion of the calices, and extravasation in the presence of a laceration or rupture and nonfunction if there is a pedicle injury. Tomography is a helpful adjunct. Both plain films and the IVU are often normal when a simple contusion is the only injury.

CT scan will accurately demonstrate the site and extent of renal lacerations and ruptures. Some believe renal arterial occlusion can be diagnosed on CT by the lack of enhancement or opacification. Arteriography is indicated whenever vascular injury is suspected.

Treatment

Contusions and superficial lacerations can be managed expectantly with monitoring of the hemoglobin and hematocrit levels. All penetrating injuries and deep lacerations require exploration. Immediate surgical management involves an anterior approach with incision of the peritoneum in the lateral colonic gutter. The colon and its mesentery are reflected medially to expose the area of the renal artery and renal vein. Dissection is carried out through the retroperitoneal tissues to isolate

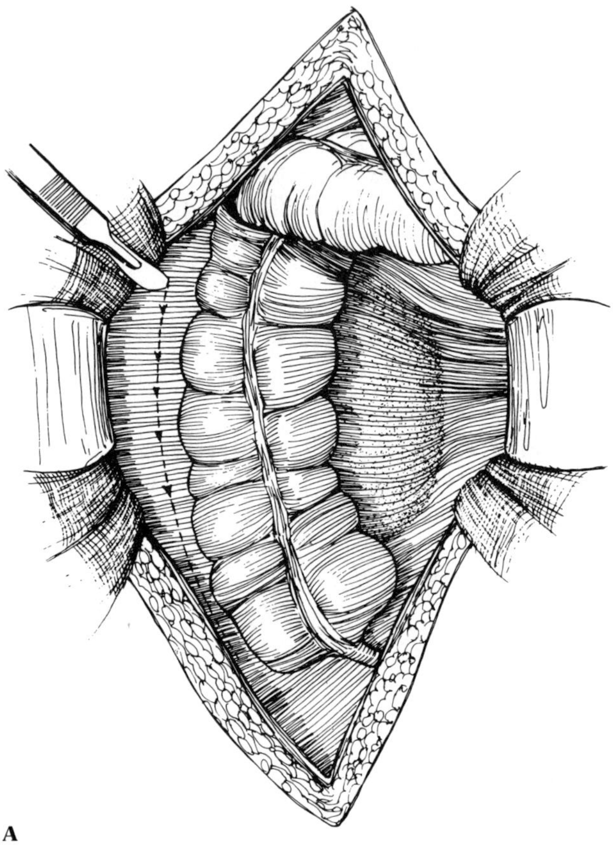

A

Fig. 11-1. Operative approach to the kidney. *A.* Incision in the peritoneum to reflect colon from perirenal hematoma. *B.* Preliminary pedicle control with vascular clamps on renal artery and renal vein before incision of Gerota's fascia, which releases renal tamponade. (From L. M. Nyhus and R. J. Baker, *Mastery of Surgery*. Boston: Little, Brown, 1984.)

the renal vein and then the renal artery lying behind it. Vascular clamps are applied to give preliminary vascular control, then Gerota's fascia is opened with evacuation of the perirenal clot (Fig. 11-1). With preliminary vascular control, deliberate surgical repair of the laceration is performed with either renorrhaphy or nephrectomy, depending on the extent of renal laceration found. When all ischemic or macerated tissue is debrided, the collecting system, if open, is closed with con-

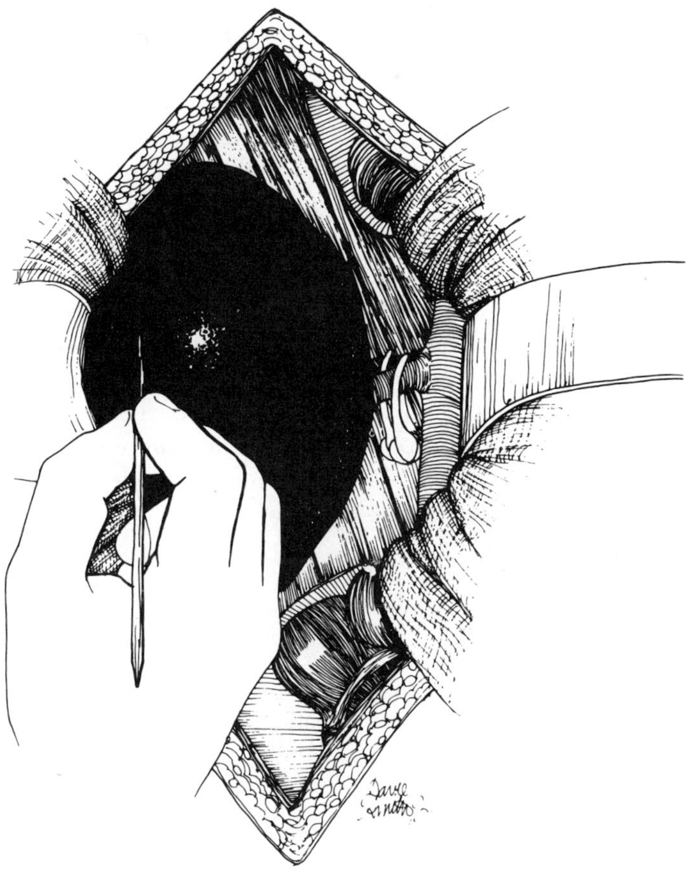

B

Fig. 11-1. (continued).

tinuous suture. If a partial nephrectomy is performed, the renal surface is left open and the kidney replaced in Gerota's fascia. Retroperitoneal drains are placed in position. As an alternative or adjunct, segmental embolization of the bleeding area may be helpful. Renal pedicle injuries should be repaired promptly if appropriate, but frequently necessitate nephrectomy. A fragmented kidney must be removed.

Long-Term Problems

Occasionally, a hematoma is not properly absorbed and becomes infected or forms a perirenal cyst. Atrophy follows impairment of the blood supply and may cause renovascular hypertension. Fibrosis in response to extravasation of blood or urine may obstruct the kidney or ureter, leading to hydronephrosis.

Perinephric abscesses require surgical drainage, although it may be appropriate to drain noninfected cysts percutaneously. Atrophy or hydronephrosis may necessitate nephrectomy or repair.

INJURIES OF THE URETER

Ureteral injuries differ from those elsewhere in the urinary tract in that most of them are iatrogenic; the depth and mobility of the ureter protect it from most other types of injury. Ureteral injuries are said to occur in 2.5 to 3.0 percent of abdominal hysterectomies [9] and were reported in 0.94 percent of 1900 patients from whom renal or ureteral stones were removed endourologically [10–12].

Pathology

Iatrogenic Injuries

During any intra-abdominal operation, a ureter may be severed, lacerated, ligated, kinked, crushed, or devitalized. Such injuries are especially likely in patients with pelvic tumors, infection, or prior radiation [9,13]. If the injury is not identified and repaired immediately, it may present as hydronephrosis, peritonitis, cellulitis, a retroperitoneal mass, urinary fistula, or extravastion on an IVU.

Ureteral catheterization or endourologic procedures such as ureterorenoscopy and stone basketing may cause ureteral perforation, avulsion, or rarely, separation [11,14].

External Trauma

External trauma to the ureter can be classified as penetrating or blunt. Penetrating injuries are usually caused by knives or gunshot wounds and may produce lacerations, contusions, or complete severance. Contusions are often the result of gunshot wounds, the blast effect from which damages the intima of the small blood vessels in the ureteral wall. In severe cases, thrombosis, ischemia, necrosis, and leakage follow in turn [15].

Blunt injuries of the ureter usually take the form of rupture or avulsion of the ureteropelvic junction or of a renal pelvic tear. They may be caused by hyperextension injury in a child or by traffic accidents. Injuries of the ureteropelvic junction are often associated with fractures of the lower ribs and diaphragmatic rupture [8].

Assessment

Iatrogenic Injuries

If the injury is not recognized intraoperatively, the postoperative period may be complicated by flank and abdominal pain, unexplained fever, vomiting, and paralytic ileus. Pyelonephritis or peritonitis may complicate the picture. Urine may leak from the incision. If the injury is bilateral, anuria is possible.

Slight extravasation of contrast medium is common after endourologic stone removal and probably indicates small tears. However, if the kidney is adequately drained, as is routine, these leaks appear to be of no importance.

If it is not clear intraoperatively whether the ureter has been injured, indigo carmine can be given intravenously. Appearance of the blue dye in the operating field indicates leakage from the urinary tract. Postoperatively, an IVU will show extravasation, and cystoscopy with retrograde pyelography will identify the site. Injuries during endourologic procedures are usually identified by nephroscopy or ureteroscopy during the procedure or by a post-procedure nephrostogram.

External Injuries

A ureter lacerated or severed by a gunshot produces the same signs and symptoms as one similarly injured by a scalpel, that is, a mass, abdominal distention, extravasation, vomiting, paralytic ileus, and cellulitis. In contrast, contusion often produces no immediate signs, although hematuria will be present. When the ureter is ruptured, hematuria is usually absent, as the blood and urine are draining into the retroperitoneum.

Treatment

Injuries Recognized Intraoperatively

The type of repair that is appropriate depends on the amount and site of damage and the patient's condition. For example, for laceration or severance of the ureter within 4 cm of the ureterovesical junction in a patient without regional infection who has not had pelvic radiation, Fry and associates [9] recommend ureteroneocystostomy, with a psoas hitch if appropriate. More distant injuries can be repaired by ureteroureterostomy. However, if a long segment of the ureter has been removed, or if the area is infected or has been irradiated, nephrectomy, ileal substitution, or autotransplantation may be required. A ureter that has been crushed should not be ignored; insertion of a stent is advised [9].

Delayed Recognition

Prompt recognition of the significance of the signs and symptoms of ureteral injury is both important and difficult, as the symptoms are often mild. An IVU is the primary means of evaluation. Ureterectasis, pyelectasis, a dense nephrogram, or delayed or absent opacification of the collecting system indicates obstruction; extravasation or a mass effect suggests leakage. Ultrasonography can be a useful screen for hydronephrosis or a urinoma. CT can precisely locate a urine collection and may suggest the cause, although CT probably is unnecessary in most cases. Retrograde pyelography can reveal the site of injury. After the diagnosis has been made, a percutaneous nephrostomy tube should be inserted to drain the kidney while the treatment approach is being selected [16].

Most endourologic ureteral injuries heal nicely if the ureter is stented and the urine is thoroughly diverted.

Contusion of the ureter secondary to gunshot wounds might be an excellent indication for simple stenting.

Ureteral or ureteropelvic junction avulsions and ruptures generally occur only in conjunction with other severe injuries that take priority. As a result, optimal management of the ureter is often impossible [17]. Percutaneous nephrostomy may be advisable as a temporizing measure and should reduce the number of cases in which nephrectomy becomes the only option.

INJURIES OF THE BLADDER

Bladder injuries are often associated with fractures of the pelvis and long bones [1,6,7]. Predisposing factors include bladder distention, fixation (e.g., by tumor or scar), obstruction, and youth—children are more susceptible [7].

Bladder injuries are classified as ruptures, which may be intraperitoneal, or extraperitoneal, or both, and contusions. Intraperitoneal and extraperitoneal ruptures occur with approximately equal frequency, and approximately 10 percent of patients with bladder ruptures have both types. Intraperitoneal ruptures usually occur on the posterior superior wall as a result of blunt trauma to a full bladder. Extraperitoneal ruptures are usually on the anterior or anterolateral bladder wall near the bladder neck and are almost always associated with pelvic fractures [7]. (Conversely, 5 percent of patients with pelvic fractures have extraperitoneal ruptures [7].) Extraperitoneal ruptures are generally caused by spicules of bone from the pelvis or, less often, the femur. A few cases are caused by knives or guns. Bladder ruptures are seldom immediately life-threatening, although MacMahon and colleagues [6] describe a fatal case. However, untended, they can often be lethal.

Pathology

Intraperitoneal rupture of the bladder leads to peritonitis, which is worse if the urine is infected. Extraperitoneal extravasation of infected urine leads to spreading pelvic cellulitis and sepsis.

Assessment

These patients often have multiple injuries, and shock may be profound. Lower abdominal pain and tenderness with rebound tenderness are common. Pain in the shoulder suggests urine in the peritoneal cavity. If the patient can urinate, hematuria is nearly always seen. A suprapubic mass may be palpated.

Bladder injury should be considered probable in any patient with a pelvic-arch fracture or abdominal trauma with local pain and inability to void [7]. In the absence of urethral injury, retrograde cystography with postwashout films is indicated. Enough contrast medium should be used to distend the bladder (400 ml in adults); otherwise, a significant number of penetrating injuries and extraperitoneal ruptures will be overlooked [6,7]. An IVU is not adequate to diagnose bladder ruptures.

Treatment

Bladder contusions and small extraperitoneal tears can be managed by drainage alone [1,6,7,18]. Intraperitoneal ruptures require primary repair with adequate drainage of urine away from the site. Prevesical drainage is also required.

INJURIES OF THE URETHRA

Urethral injuries occur in male patients far more often than in females, as would be expected. The injuries range in severity from simple contusions, which usually can be managed nonoperatively and can be expected to heal without sequelae, to complete ruptures, which are difficult to manage and often lead to stricture or even obliteration of the urethra. Serious urethral injuries are most often associated with pelvic fractures that displace the bones and with anterior arch fractures. Published reports show a range in the frequency of urethral and bladder injury accompanying pelvic fractures of 0.7 to 25 percent [2,7,8,18,19]. In approximately one-half of these patients, only the urethra is injured. In only 5 percent of patients are the urinary tract injuries the only injuries [18].

In female patients, pelvic fractures are seldom associated with urethral injuries. When these do occur, vaginal lacerations are also present. Most instances of trauma to the female urethra are secondary to obstetric complications, vaginal operation, or foreign bodies [20].

Injuries of the male urethra may affect the membranous (posterior) portion or the bulbous and penile (anterior) portion, with the former outnumbering the latter approximately 3 : 1 [6]. The two types require different management.

Injuries of the Membranous Urethra

Injuries of the membranous urethra should be suspected in any male patient with a pelvic fracture. They arise because of the enclosure and immobilization of the membranous urethra by the urogenital diaphragm. Generally, there are injuries to other organs as well. Blood or urine extravasates into the periprostatic and perivesical spaces and, if the urogenital diaphragm is badly damaged, into the perineum. Extravasation may not be apparent if the patient is seen soon after the injury, so the physician should not make too much of its absence if other signs and symptoms and the nature of the accident and other injuries suggest injury of the membranous urethra [2]. Extravasation leads to cellulitis and sepsis, and urethral stricture is a common long-term problem no matter what is done immediately after the injury. Urinary incontinence will follow if the urinary sphincter is injured. Approximately one-third of patients will suffer erectile impotence, probably as the result of nerve injury.

Assessment

The nature of the pelvic fracture is a valuable guide to the nature of the urethral injury. For example, Blandy and King [21] classify such fractures as spring-back, in which the fracture is in the rami of the pubic or ischial bones, and dislocations, in which as much as one-half of the pelvic girdle is displaced—for example, as the result of force of impact being transmitted upward along the femur. In the former type of injury, the injury to the urethra is usually a bruise, kink, or perhaps a partial tear. In contrast, patients with a fracture dislocation generally have a disrupted membranous urethra, with the extent of bony displacement indicating the extent of dislocation of the soft tissues, including the urethra. Devine and Devine [19] have developed a more elaborate classification of pelvic fractures and the accompanying urethral injuries.

The symptoms of urethral injury are pain in the perineum and lower abdomen and inability to void. The signs include urethral bleeding and hematuria, which is seldom microscopic if the injury is serious [2]. A tender suprapubic mass may represent a distended bladder or extravasated blood and urine. Rectal examination may identify a large boggy mass of extravasated fluid and upward dislodgement of the prostate, although a free-floating prostate can be difficult to identify. Plain films of the abdomen will show the nature and extent of pelvic fractures. Lateral views are often important in identifying spring-back fractures of the pubis, which often have a nearly normal appearance on anteroposterior views

[21]. An IVU or cystogram usually reveals a teardrop-shaped bladder. A retrograde urethrogram will show the location and extent of the injury, but one should not pass a catheter through a badly traumatized urethra, particularly if a partial tear is suspected.

Treatment

The proper treatment of posterior urethral injuries is still a contentious issue, probably because the results are so often unsatisfactory no matter what is done. Blandy and King [21] have offered a useful listing of the goals one should seek, a list that is a helpful guide to selecting treatment procedures:

1. Save the patient's life.
2. Prevent stricture.
3. If (2) is not possible, ensure that the stricture can be managed by the simplest and least invasive means.
4. If (3) is not possible, ensure that only a simple urethroplasty will be needed.
5. Prevent other complications: incontinence, impotence, deformity, pelvis instability.

In most patients with multiple trauma and complete urethral rupture, other injuries take priority, and the urologist's efforts will be confined to inserting a suprapubic cystostomy tube. Further approaches to the urethra may often then be delayed until the orthopedic surgeons have reduced the fracture and, as a consequence, brought the severed ends of the urethra closer together [21].

Opinion is divided on whether urethral continuity should then be restored by open end-to-end anastomosis or use of interlocking sounds or catheters through urethra and bladder neck simultaneously (Fig. 11-2) or whether suprapubic drainage with later urethroplasty is optimal [19,22,23]. The last-mentioned method has become more appealing with the recent demonstration that urethral continuity can often be reestablished by a combination of transurethral and endoscopic means without open operation [24]. In my experience, most of these patients require pelvic surgery to exclude bladder rupture and to insert a suprapubic tube, and one should realign the urethra at the same time after cutting the puboprostatic ligaments. I suspect, as do others [21], that the patient's long-term problems such as impotence are determined primarily by the nature of the injury rather than by anything the urologist does, with one exception: It is possible to cause ischemic necrosis of the bladder neck, and consequent incontinence, with overenthusiastic traction on a Foley catheter to align the urethral ends [21].

Partial ruptures of the urethra are managed by a combination of suprapubic cystostomy and perivesical drainage or by urethral catheter drainage. Only the experienced should attempt to pass a urethral catheter in these patients, as there is considerable risk of converting a partial rupture to a complete one.

Injuries of the Bulbous or Penile Urethra

Injuries of the bulbous or penile urethra, which involve the urethra below the urogenital diaphragm, are caused by direct blows, straddle accidents, or urethral instrumentation. Blood and urine extravasate into the perineum initially and may spread to the scrotum, penis, and abdominal wall, where their spread is limited by Colles' fascia. Serious in-

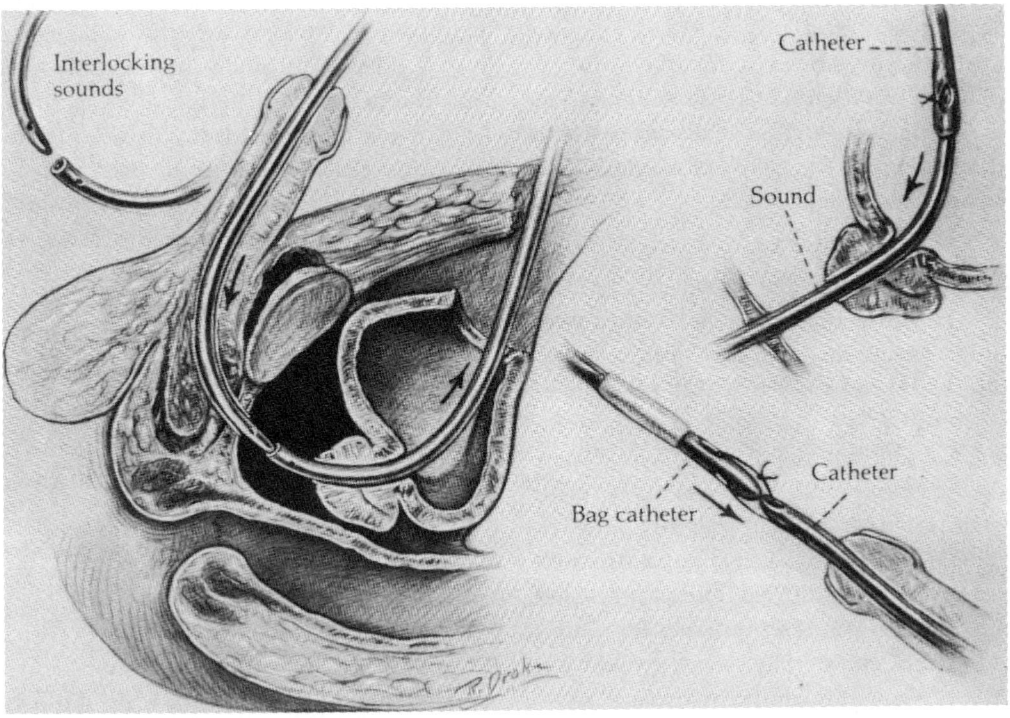

Fig. 11-2. Use of interlocking sounds to effect immediate realignment of the urethra after traumatic disruption. Male sound is used to draw a whistle-tipped latex catheter through the urethra in an antegrade manner. In turn, a balloon catheter of approximate size is drawn in a retrograde direction to serve as a realigning stent. (From J. H. DeWeerd, *J.A.M.A.* 165:1916, 1957.)

fection often ensues, and a stricture may form.

Assessment

There is local pain, and an attempt to micturate is painful and causes perineal or penile swelling. Urethral bleeding and a tender perineal mass are to be expected. Swelling and discoloration of the skin of the scrotum, penis, and lower abdomen are a late sign. A retrograde urethrogram will reveal the site and degree of injury.

Treatment

Complete ruptures are repaired by end-to-end anastomosis with evacuation of the hematoma, suprapubic cystostomy drainage, and adequate antibiotic coverage. Partial ruptures can be managed by a combination of suprapubic cystostomy and prevesical drainage or by urethral catheterization.

For both types of urethral injury, the resulting strictures can often be corrected by cold-knife urethrotomy. The procedure can be repeated if it fails. Provided the stricture is less than 2 cm long, this technique is successful in more than 90 percent of patients, obviating repeated urethral dilatations [25].

Injuries of the Female Urethra

Complete ruptures of the female urethra produce much the same signs and symptoms as do those in the male urethra. Those injuries are frequently accompanied by pelvic fractures, genital lacerations, or both. Distal injuries may be approached transvaginally, with catheterization of the distal segment and suturing of the vaginal incision around the neomeatus. If the urethra has been detached from the bladder, the anatomy can be reconstructed over a catheter by a retropubic approach. Any vaginal lacerations must also be repaired to avert fistula formation. Suprapubic cystostomy drainage generally is used postoperatively. The same precautions against overenthusiastic catheter traction are to avoid damage to the bladder neck that can cause incontinence [20].

INJURIES OF THE TESTIS

The mobility of the testis, cremaster muscle contraction, and the tough capsule of the testis (tunica albuginea) are responsible for its infrequent injury in the patient multiply injured from a traffic accident. A direct blow with impingement of the testis against the symphysis pubis results in a testicular injury. The testicular injury is either contusion or a testicular rupture. In both cases, the tunica vaginalis sac is filled with blood (hematocele) resulting in a large, swollen, tender, blue scrotal mass (Fig. 11-3). Early exploration with evacuation of blood clots in the tunica vaginalis and repair of the testicular rupture, if present, result in a shorter hospital stay, a greatly reduced period of disability, and a faster return to normal activity compared with patients managed conservatively. Conservative management is complicated by secondary infection of the hematocele or the injured testis, and the pressure effect of the tense hematocele can result in subsequent atrophy of the testis after the hematocele resolves.

SCROTAL AVULSION

If at all possible, the scrotum should be reconstructed around the testes even if the closure is under considerable tension. The scrotum usually regains nearly normal size within a few months. If scrotal reconstruction is impossible, the testicles should be placed in thigh pockets superficial to the subcutaneous fat, where the temperature is similar to that inside the scrotum.

INJURIES OF THE PENIS

Injuries of the penis include blunt trauma, which may cause penile fracture (rupture of the corpora cavernosa, frequently with urethral rupture [26]) or rupture of the suspensory ligaments, strangulation (tourniquet syndrome), suction (e.g., by a vacuum cleaner),

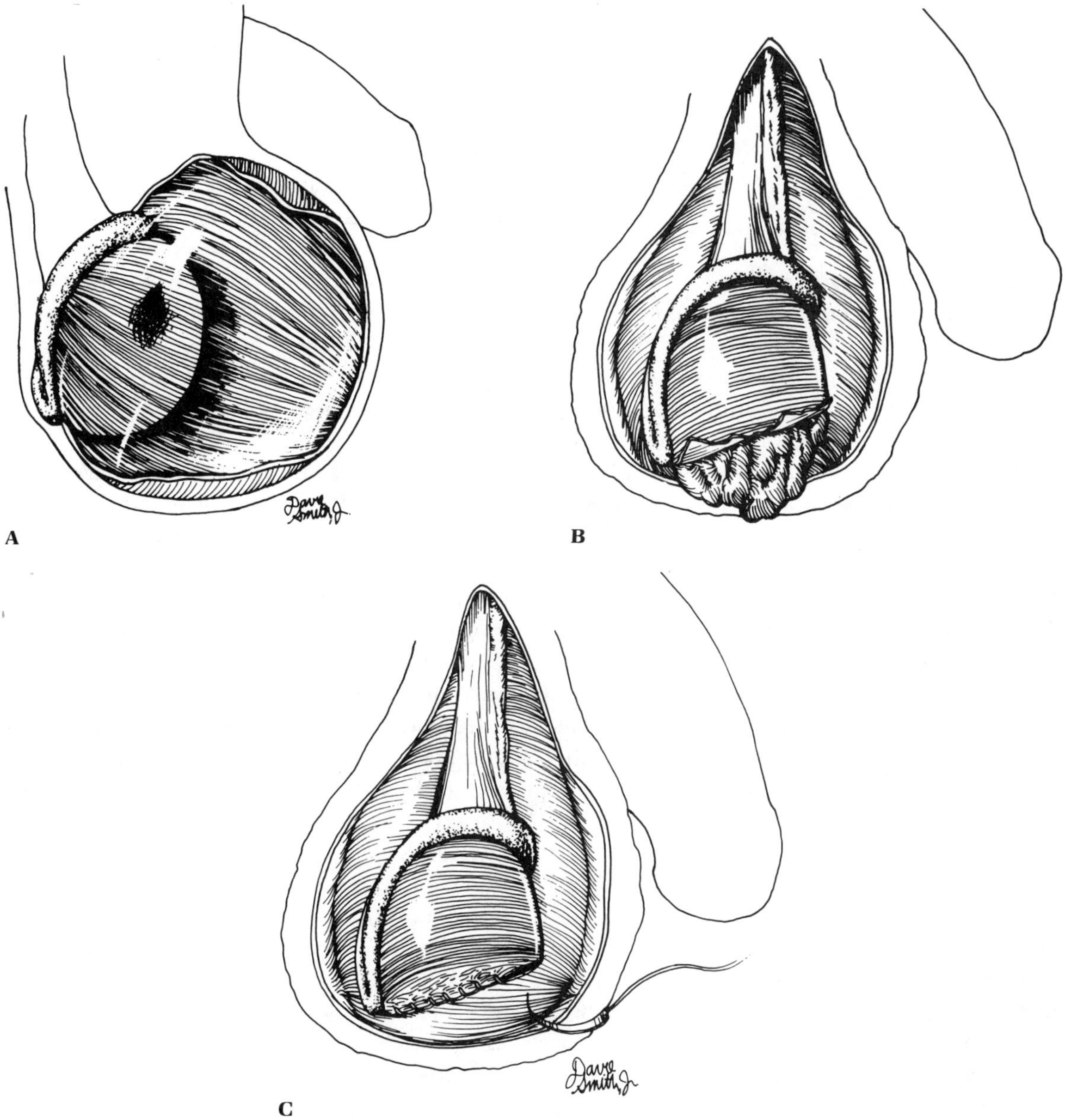

A

B

C

Fig. 11-3. Testicular injuries and their correction. *A.* Sagittal section of testicular contusion with surrounding hematocele. *B.* Ruptured testicle before repair. *C.* Repair of ruptured testicle after debridement with closure of tunica albuginea. (From L. M. Nyhus and R. J. Baker, *Mastery of Surgery*. Boston: Little, Brown, 1984.)

amputation, and skin injuries as a result of burns or zippers. None of these injuries is common.

Management of Blunt Trauma

Penile fractures occur when the erect penis strikes a hard object, receives a direct blow, or is bent abnormally. This causes a cracking sound followed by pain, immediate detumescence, rapid swelling, discoloration, and distortion, with eventual deviation of the penis away from the rupture. The lesion itself is a tear in the tunica albuginea, with hemorrhage and hematoma formation. Urethral bleeding, hematuria, and urinary extravasation will be present in the one-third of the patients in whom the urethra is ruptured.

There are two schools of thought on the appropriate treatment of penile fracture. One advocates conservative measure: urethral catheter or suprapubic cystostomy drainage, ice packs, anti-inflammatory and sedative drugs (e.g., oxyphenbutazone and diazepam [27]), and oral streptokinase [28]. The other school of thought advocates immediate surgical evacuation of the hematoma and primary repair of the corpus [26,29]. This approach appears to produce better long-term results, as conservative management has led to infection of the hematoma, painful penile lumps, permanent deformity, suboptimal erections, and difficulty with coitus [27,30–33].

Traumatic rupture of the suspensory ligament has resulted from ventral deflation of the erect penis and from multiple pubic fractures. Pain and swelling occur at the base. In two of three reported cases, when erectile function returned after many months, the erect position was abnormal because of an extensive defect between the symphysis pubis and the penile base. To avert this, Pryor and Hill [34] recommend open repair with nylon sutures between the symphysis and the tunica albuginea. The penis is then inflated with saline, and if the resulting erection is not normal, another row of sutures is placed more distally on the shaft.

Management of Strangulation Injuries

The patient with penile tourniquet syndrome may present early, with pain and swelling distal to the constricting device, or late, with urethral fistula, partial amputation, or both. Necrosis of the glans does not occur because slow constriction allows deep collateral circulation to develop.

Human hair is a particularly common culprit. Because human hair is stretchable when wet and contracts when dry, it may become buried in the swollen skin to the point of near invisibility. A hair injury should be suspected in any circumcised boy with a swollen gland. If the condition is untreated, the hair may cut dorsally into the shaft, sparing the urethra but damaging the neurovascular bundle, or it may transect the urethra but spare sensation in the glans.

A single-stage repair may be adequate, as it was in a patient of ours. However, for more severe injuries, a staged repair is advisable because the blood supply may be precarious.

Management of Vacuum Cleaner Injuries

Vacuum cleaner injuries to the penis are more common than the number of published cases would lead one to think; there have been seven cases in our hospital alone. Eleven of the first 13 cases reported involved multiple lacerations of the glans, shaft, prepuce, or urethral meatus, and only suturing was needed. In only two patients were the corpora involved. In our series, simple lacerations were the exception: five patients had extensive injury of the glans with the loss of 1 to 2 inches of the urethra. Reconstruction will be necessary in these patients.

Management of Traumatic Amputation

The treatment of choice in traumatic amputation is reattachment if the distal segment is available and in good condition and if the ischemia time is 18 hours [35] (longer if the detached segment is kept in iced saline). Microneurovascular repair is advisable. Local reshaping measures, with closure of open corpora and meatoplasty, will be necessary if the amputated segment is lost or severely damaged. Plastic repair may be considered later.

The proper management of the penile skin after a reattachment is controversial. Some authorities advocate reapproximation, but there is a high incidence of skin necrosis if the amputation was complete. Other authorities suggest removing the skin and burying the penis in the scrotum, although it has been argued that this maneuver causes tension on the corporal and urethral suture lines and reduces corporal blood flow. It may be best to choose the approach individually on the basis of the condition of the phallus and the duration of ischemia.

Patients who have undergone amputation require the cooperative efforts of the urologist, plastic surgeon, and psychiatrist or psychologist.

Management of Skin Injuries

Avulsion or burns require removal of the damaged skin with split-thickness grafts after the denuded area is clean and free of infection. Avulsed skin should not be reattached, as it invariably becomes necrotic and infected.

Penile skin trapped in a zipper can sometimes be freed by manipulation under local anesthesia. Alternatively, the zipper can be destroyed by applying bone-cutting pliers to the median bar or diamond [36].

REFERENCES

1. Krieger, J. N., Algood, C. B., Mason, J. T., et al. Urological trauma in the Pacific Northwest: Etiology, distribution, management and outcome. *J. Urol.* 132:70, 1984.
2. Fallon, B., Wendt, J. C., and Hawtrey, C. E. Urological injury and assessment in patients with fractured pelvis. *J. Urol.* 131:712, 1984.
3. Ben-Menachem, Y. Logic and logistics of radiography, angiography, and angiographic intervention in massive blunt trauma. *Radiol. Clin. North Am.* 19:9, 1981.
4. Kam, J., Jackson, H., and Ben-Menachem, Y. Vascular injuries in blunt pelvic trauma. *Radiol. Clin. North Am.* 19:171, 1981.
5. Ben-Menachem, Y., Handel, S. F., Ray, R. D., et al. Embolization procedures in trauma: A matter of urgency. *Semin. Intervent. Radiol.* 2:107, 1985.
6. MacMahon, R., Hosking, D., and Ramsey, E. W. Management of blunt injury to the lower urinary tract. *Can. J. Surg.* 26:415, 1983.
7. Bonavita, J. A., and Pollak, H. M. Trauma of the adult bladder and urethra. *Semin. Roentgenol.* 18:299, 1983.
8. Campbell, J. E. Urinary tract trauma. *J. Can. Assoc. Radiol.* 34:237, 1983.
9. Fry, D. E., Milholen, L., and Harbrecht, P. J. Iat-

rogenic ureteral injury. *Arch. Surg.* 118:454, 1983.
10. Reddy, P. K., Hulbert, J. C., Lange, P. H., et al. Percutaneous removal of renal and ureteral calculi: Experience with 400 cases. *J. Urol.* 134:662, 1985.
11. Segura, J. W., Patterson, D. E., LeRoy, A. J., et al. Percutaneous removal of kidney stones: Review of 1,000 cases. *J. Urol.* 134:1077, 1985.
12. Lee, W. J., Smith, A. D., Cubelli, V., et al. Percutaneous nephrolithotomy: Analysis of 500 consecutive cases. *Urol. Radiol.* 8:61, 1986.
13. Smith, A. D. Ureteral Obstruction in the Female. In S. Raz (ed.), *Female Urology.* Philadelphia: Saunders, 1983. P. 394.
14. Winfield, H. N., and Clayman, R. V. Complications of percutaneous removal of renal and ureteral calculi: I and II. *World Urol. Update Series* 2(37 and 38), 1985.
15. Cass, A. S. Ureteral contusion with gunshot wounds. *J. Trauma* 24:59, 1984.
16. Demos, T. C., Churchill, R., Flisak, M. E., et al. The radiologic diagnosis of complications following gynecologic surgery: Radiography, computed tomography, sonography, and scintigraphy. *CRC Crit. Rev. Diagn. Imaging* 22:43, 1984.
17. Cass, A. S. Blunt renal pelvic and ureteral injury in multiple-injured patients. *Urology* 22:268, 1983.
18. Palmer, J. K., Benson, G. S., and Corriere, J. N., Jr. Diagnosis and initial management of urological injuries associated with 200 consecutive pelvic fractures. *J. Urol.* 130:712, 1983.
19. Devine, P. C., and Devine, C. J., Jr. Posterior urethral injuries associated with pelvic fractures. *Urology* 20:467, 1982.
20. Rodrigues Netto, N., Jr., Ikari, O., and Zuppo, V. P. Traumatic rupture of the female urethra. *Urology* 22:601, 1983.
21. Blandy, J. P., and King, J. B. Management of the fractured pelvis with urethral injury in the male. *World Urol. Update Series* 1(37):2, 1983.
22. Webster, G. D., Mathes, G. L., and Selli, C. Prostatomembranous urethral injuries: A review of the literature and a rational approach to their management. *J. Urol.* 130:898, 1983.
23. Al-Ali, I. H., and Husain, J. Disrupting injuries of the membranous urethra: The case for early surgery and catheter splinting. *Br. J. Urol.* 55:716, 1983.
24. Gonzalez, R., Chiou, R. K., Hekmat, K., et al. Endoscopic reestablishment of urethral continuity after traumatic disruption of the membranous urethra. *J. Urol.* 130:785, 1983.
25. Clayman, R. V. Diagnostic and Therapeutic Applications of Outpatient Cystourethroscopy. In K. W. Kaye (ed.), *Outpatient Urologic Surgery.* Philadelphia: Lea & Febiger, 1985. P. 111.
26. Nymark, J., and Kristensen, J. K. Fracture of the penis with urethral rupture. *J. Urol.* 129:147, 1983.
27. Julla, A., Wani, N. A., and Rashid, P. A. Fracture of the penis. *J. Urol.* 123:285, 1980.
28. Creecy, A. A., and Beazlie, F., Jr. Fracture of the penis: Traumatic rupture of corpora cavernosa. *J. Urol.* 78:620, 1967.
29. Gross, M., Arnold, T. L., and Peters, P. Fracture of the penis with associated laceration of the urethra. *J. Urol.* 117:725, 1977.
30. Farah, R., and Cerny, J. C. Penis tourniquet syndrome and penile amputation. *Urology* 2:310, 1973.
31. Walton, J. K. Fracture of the penis with laceration of the urethra. *Br. J. Urol.* 51:308, 1979.
32. Pryor, J. P., Hill, J. T., Packham, D. A., et al. Penile injuries with particular reference to injury to the erectile tissue. *Br. J. Urol.* 53:42, 1981.
33. Bergner, D. M., Wilcox, M. E., and Frentz, G. D. Fracture of penis. *Urology* 20:278, 1982.
34. Pryor, J., and Hill, J. T. Abnormalities of the suspensory ligament of the penis as a cause of erectile dysfunction. *Br. J. Urol.* 51:402, 1979.
35. Engelman, E. R., Polito, G., Perley, J., et al. Traumatic amputation of the penis. *Urology* 112:774, 1974.
36. Saraf, P. Zipper injury of the foreskin. *Am. J. Dis. Child.* 136:557, 1982.

12

Vascular Trauma

Cervical Vascular Trauma

Evan R. Geller and James Maurer

The casualties of cervical trauma once associated with military conflict are seen with increasing frequency in civilian urban centers. With the proliferation of efficient prehospital care and transport systems, the patient with serious cervical injury is more often surviving to present to the emergency department. In this population of patients suffering from life-threatening injury, outcome is often dependent on the expeditious and knowledgeable response of the treating physician. It is incumbent upon the physician, therefore, to possess the working knowledge and skill required to accurately diagnose and treat trauma to the vital structures of the neck.

HISTORY

The first successful treatment of a cervical vascular injury is generally attributed to Fleming, who in 1803 ligated an injured carotid artery aboard the H.M.S. Tonnant [1]. With rare exception, simple ligation remained the primary treatment of these injuries for the next 150 years. Such treatment, however, was accompanied by a mortality rate during World War I of 44 percent, with almost a third of survivors suffering significant neurologic deficit [2]. Such dismal results led to the recommendation that penetrating cervical injury be best managed by observation [2]. It was not until the advancement of vascular surgical technique during the Korean conflict that repair of carotid arterial injuries replaced ligation. The observed improvement in outcome following vascular repair subsequently led to the recommendation that all patients suffering from penetrating neck injury undergo surgical exploration and repair [3]. Thus, the experience over 25 years led to a complete swing in the therapeutic pendulum from strict observation to mandatory surgical exploration. Not surprisingly, the subsequent decades have seen the pendulum reverse somewhat, with an increasing literature supporting a policy of selective exploration.

ANATOMY

The significance of trauma to the neck is related to the close anatomic relations of the contained vital structures. Diagnostic and therapeutic maneuvers are dependent on anatomic considerations of the injury.

Classically, the anatomy of the neck is divided into triangles. The sternocleidomastoid muscle serves to divide the neck into posterior and anterior triangles. The carotid arteries rise from the thoracic inlet to enter the anterior neck. Here they ascend in a lateral and posterior course, enveloped in a sheath formed by the deep cervical fascia. Within this sheath, the carotid artery is accompanied by the vagus nerve and internal jugular vein. At the level of the superior margin of the thyroid cartilage, the common carotid artery bifurcates into the internal and external arteries. The aerophagic structures course along the midneck between the carotid sheaths, in anatomic continuity with the mediastinum (Fig. 12-1).

Besides the anatomic division of the neck into anterior and posterior triangles, a clinical classification of injury has been based on the level of injury. This classification defines three zones in the neck: Zone I is defined as the base of the neck below the level of the cricoid cartilage, zone II extends from the cricoid to the angle of the mandible, and zone III rises above the angles of the mandible. While the structures of the neck course in a vertical manner and therefore exist across all three zones, the surgical exposure and technique demanded at each zone make this classification a useful one.

Fig. 12-1. Anatomy of the neck in cross section. (From N. Rich and F. Spencer [eds.], *Vascular Trauma*. Philadelphia: Saunders, 1978. With permission.)

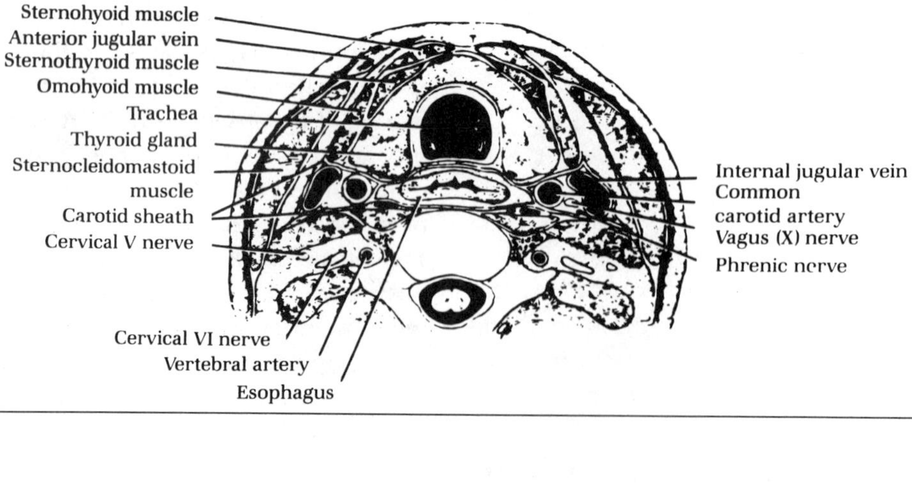

INJURIES AND THEIR TREATMENT

Significant cervical injury generally results from penetrating trauma and involves the major structures discussed above. Blunt trauma may involve critical flexion and extension forces leading to vertebral injury and often spinal cord injury as well. Such trauma demands prompt diagnosis and immobilization until stability can be reestablished; emergent surgical intervention is rarely required, however. Serious vascular injury as a consequence of blunt trauma is rare; when present, outcome is comparatively poor [4]. Blunt injury to the trachea or laryngeal cartilages may rapidly lead to catastrophic loss of airway unless promptly diagnosed and appropriately managed.

In the far more common setting of penetrating trauma to the neck, the integrity of the patient's airway remains of prime importance. Direct injury to the structures of the airway may present with respiratory distress and demand prompt intervention. Injuries to vascular structures in the neck may, as a result of hemorrhage, lead to loss of the airway more or less rapidly. Therefore, in the face of any and all injuries to the neck, it is incumbent upon the treating physician first and foremost to evaluate and secure an adequate airway. This may require early endotracheal intubation; emergent tracheostomy is to be avoided, as violation of cervical fascial planes may lead to inadvertent decompression of hematoma.

Once the airway is assured, attention turns to the basic resuscitation of breathing and circulation. Most importantly, one must be aware of the frequent association of thoracic trauma with injuries of the neck. Such injuries may impair ventilation by way of pneumothorax or hemothorax. Similarly, significant hemorrhage may occur at either the cervical or thoracic sites of injury. Basic principles of trauma resuscitation relate to the management of these associated injuries.

Finally, attention is turned to evaluation of the neurologic status and to clinical and radiologic evaluation of the cervical spine. Evidence of cervical injury, whether blunt or penetrating in nature, demands early immobilization until cervical spine injury can be excluded by clinical and radiologic assessment.

Evaluation

The diagnostic evaluation of the patient with cervical trauma is dependent on both anatomic site of injury and clinical presentation. The patient exhibiting active life-threatening hemorrhage requires emergent surgical exploration as the only diagnostic and therapeutic intervention. In the patient with isolated cervical injury, however, such massive bleeding is unusual even in the face of arterial injury. Patients exhibiting adequate response to resuscitation may be subjected to evaluation dictated by the site of injury.

Injuries at the level of the base of the neck, that is, zone I injuries, in the stable patient require adequate preoperative angiographic assessment to determine presence and site of injury. Failure to perform such assessment may lead to the inability to secure adequate proximal control of the injured vascular structures at the base of the neck.

Similarly, injuries in zone III may present great difficulties of exposure and vascular control and are therefore best assessed preoperatively with angiography. Injuries confined to the posterior triangle of the neck rarely involve major anatomic structures and are therefore also amenable to radiologic evaluation.

Controversy exists as to the proper management of injuries to the anterior triangle of the neck at the level of zone II. The density of vital structures in this region leads to a significant incidence of injury. Intraoperative exposure and evaluation are easily accomplished. Historically, the routine and mandatory exploration of all injuries penetrating the platysma muscle in this region has been standard practice. While such a practice has been shown to save lives in the military setting, the mandatory exploration of all zone II injuries in the civilian experience has exhibited a greater than 50-percent negative exploration rate [5]. This fact has led to trials of observation and selective evaluation of injuries to zone II.

Such a policy mandates careful selection of patients for nonoperative therapy. Patients demonstrating evidence of vascular injury or associated aerophagic tract injury are not suitable for such management. Rather, those patients in stable condition without obvious signs of injury to major anatomic structures are selected. The question then arises as to what modalities are required in this subgroup of patients to rule out significant injury. The approach may include observation, bronchoscopy, esophagoscopy, plain radiologic examination, and angiography. Contrast study of the esophagus may substitute for or supplement endoscopy.

Treatment

In general, injuries to the carotid occurring in zone II may be repaired with standard vascular techniques of end-to-end anastomosis or vein graft interposition. Shunt may be employed according to the preference of the surgeon. Gunshot wounds require resection of adequate margins prior to reconstruction. Proximal internal carotid artery injuries not suitable for arteriorrhaphy may be repaired by means of transposition of the external carotid artery (Fig. 12-2).

High carotid artery injuries, lying within zone III, require special techniques due to the difficulty in obtaining distal control. Exposure of the distal carotid artery may be improved by means of anterior subluxation of the mandible with intermaxillary fixation [6]. This permits access to an additional 2 to 3 cm of the distal carotid. With injuries at the base of the skull, distal control may be impossible even with such maneuvers. In these instances, control of hemorrhage from the intracranial portion of the carotid may be obtained by the inflation of a balloon catheter within the distal vascular lumen. This maneuver is best performed with electroencephalographic (EEG) monitoring; evidence of change in neurologic status may be considered an indication for extracranial to intracranial bypass.

Injuries to the carotid artery at the base of the neck (zone I) present difficulties in the gaining of proximal vascular control. The majority of these injuries will be accessible through the inferior margin of the standard anterior sternocleidomastoid incision. Occasionally, however, an injury to the origin of the carotid artery will require more extensive exposure for management. Techniques of clavicular head resection described for elective vascular procedures are not recommended in the trauma setting. Resection of the medial

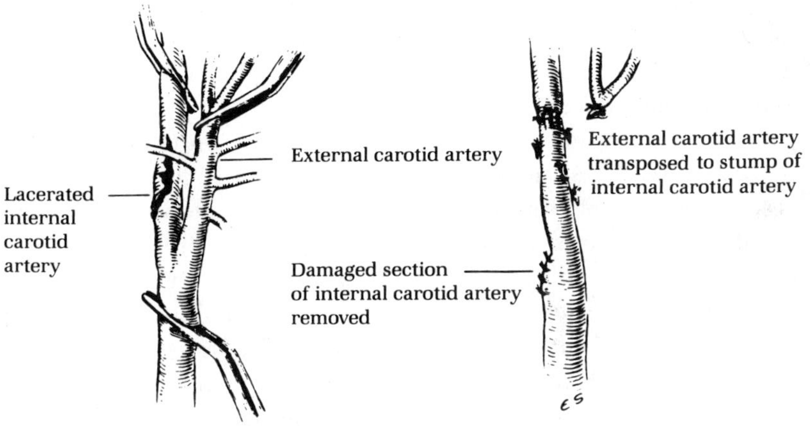

Fig. 12-2. Transposition of the external carotid artery for repair of internal carotid artery injury. (Adapted by permission from F. W. Blaisdell and D. Trunkey, *Cervicothoracic Trauma*. New York: Thieme Medical Publishers, 1986.)

clavicle is time-consuming and affords disappointingly little additional exposure. Further, the replaced clavicular head is prone to nonunion. Rather, it is recommended that if additional exposure of the proximal carotid is required that one proceed directly to median sternotomy. This may be rapidly performed in the trauma setting and affords optimal exposure with a minimum of morbidity. Preoperative angiography in the stable patient allows anticipation of the need for such maneuvers.

Controversy persists regarding the proper management of patients presenting with significant neurologic deficit accompanying cervical vascular injury. Argument surrounds the contention that the neurologic injury of cerebral ischemia secondary to carotid interruption may be aggravated by revascularization with bleeding into what previously was a

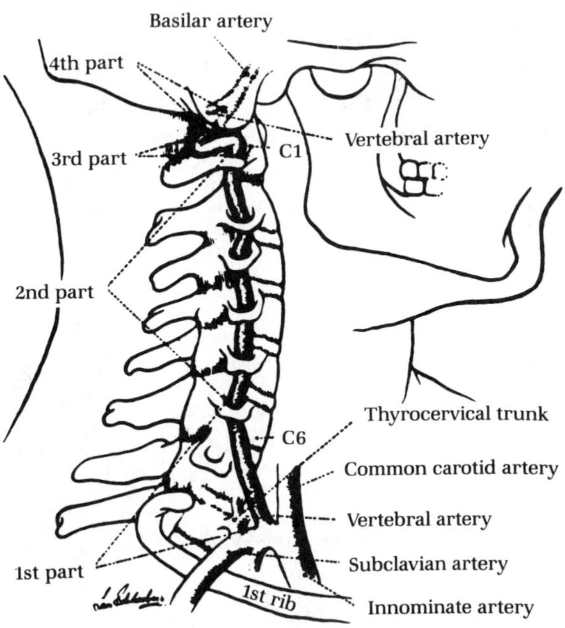

Fig. 12-3. Divisions of the vertebral artery. (Adapted from P. Golueke et al., Vertebral artery injury. *J. Trauma* 27:858, 1987. With permission.)

bland infarct. Little direct evidence exists to substantiate such a claim. There is no doubt, however, that patients with significant preoperative neurologic deficit (coma or hemiparesis) display high mortality and morbidity rates. It is felt that, in general, the carotid artery should be reconstructed whenever possible assuming that distal thrombus may be removed completely.

Once considered a rarity, injury to the vertebral artery is being identified with increasing frequency as a result of the routine use of angiography in the evaluation of cervical trauma. The lack of neurologic sequelae from vertebral artery injury makes clinical diagnosis difficult. Occasionally, posterior cervical triangle hematoma or bruit may indicate the underlying injury. Vertebral artery injuries are most often the result of penetrating injury to the posterior triangle of the neck, although several cases have been reported of injury secondary to severe flexion or rotational forces, as involved in chiropractic manipulation [7].

Clinically, the extracranial vertebral artery is divided into three portions (Fig. 12-3). The first portion extends from its origin at the subclavian artery until the artery enters the vertebral canal within the transverse process of C6. The second portion is that part within the canal of the transverse processes of C6 to C2. Finally, the third portion is the extracranial artery as it leaves the vertebral canal above C2. Again, management is dictated by the level of injury. Injuries in the first portion of the ar-

Fig. 12-4. Surgical approach to the proximal vertebral artery. SCM = sternocleidomastoid muscle. (Adapted by permission from F. W. Blaisdell and D. Trunkey, *Cervicothoracic Trauma*. New York: Thieme Medical Publishers, 1986.)

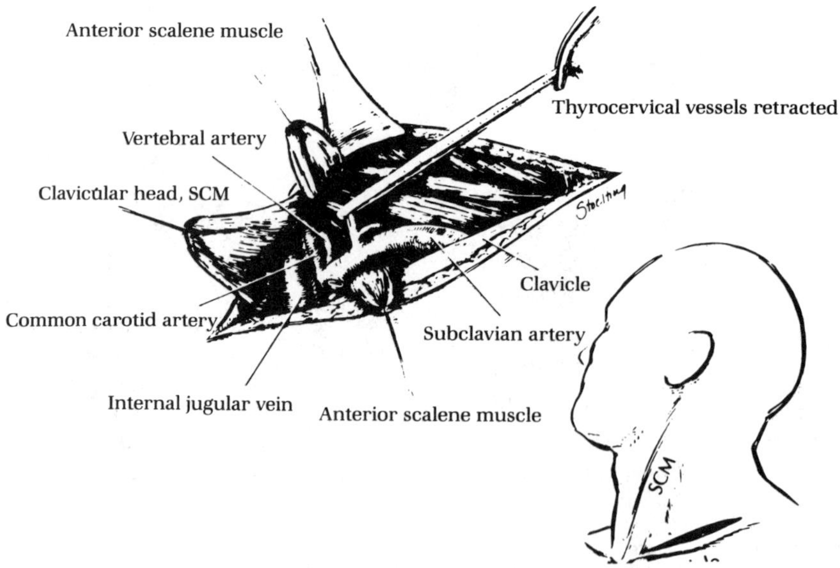

tery are managed by simple ligation by means of the standard anterior approach (Fig. 12-4). This approach utilizes a transverse supraclavicular incision with division of the clavicular head of the sternocleidomastoid muscle. With the internal jugular vein and vagus nerve retracted laterally, the vertebral artery is found lateral and posterior to the proximal common carotid artery. Here the proximal vertebral artery may be easily ligated [8]. While injuries to the second portion of the artery may be approached by surgical methods employing careful resection of the transverse processes of the cervical vertebrae, the difficulty of this procedure is prohibitive. Rather, therapy by way of angiographic catheter embolization of the proximal vessel is preferable [9]. Often the distal vessel as well may be embolized when the catheter can be made to traverse the site of injury. If necessary, the distal portion of the vertebral artery can be approached in its third part for ligation [10] (Fig. 12-5).

Cervical vascular injuries not involving the internal carotid or vertebral arteries are of lesser concern. Because of the extensive collateral circulation of the face and head, the injured external carotid artery may be ligated with impunity. Injury to branches of the external carotid artery can be treated with ligation once adequate exposure is obtained. Similarly, injury to the internal jugular vein can be treated either with lateral venorrhaphy or simple ligation, assuming a patent contralateral internal jugular vein.

Fig. 12-5. Surgical approach to the distal vertebral artery. (From R. Berguer, Distal vertebral artery by-pass. *J. Vasc. Surg.* 2:621, 1985. With permission.)

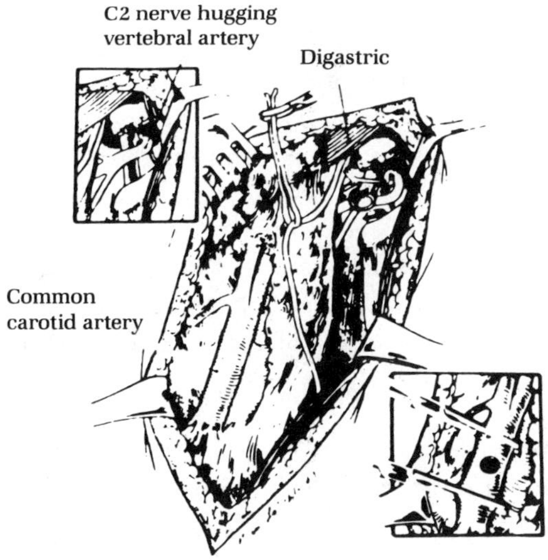

AERODIGESTIVE TRACT INJURIES

While significant cervical trauma most commonly involves the vascular structures of the neck, high morbidity and mortality attend injury to the associated visceral structures in the area. Injuries to the larynx and trachea are usually evident on clinical presentation and amenable to efforts of airway control and primary repair. Repair of the cervical trachea can be accomplished with interrupted nonabsorbable sutures, once adequate mobilization has assured a tension-free anastomosis. Tracheostomy is often a useful adjunct to this repair.

Injuries to the cervical digestive tract may be subtle and escape detection unless a high level of suspicion is maintained. These injuries, left unrecognized, are associated with a high rate of patient mortality and serious morbidity. It is the subtlety and seriousness of injury to the cervical digestive tract that bears witness to mandatory exploration of neck wounds. When discovered promptly, treatment by primary suture repair and drainage is rewarded with great success. Repair is performed in a two-layer technique with the possible addition of a pedicled muscle flap. Delayed diagnosis of esophageal injury demands wide drainage and proximal diversion.

Thoracic Vascular Trauma

Hooshang Bolooki

Diagnosis and management of thoracic vascular trauma are dependent on whether the injury is in the acute or chronic phase. Chronic injuries may have occurred days to years earlier and have gradually developed into symptomatic lesions. Furthermore, in a stable patient, the management of a specific vascular injury may intentionally be delayed to define the extent of damage and to plan the proper surgical approach. This concept has evolved because failure in surgical management of acute intrathoracic major vascular injuries frequently is a result of hasty operative intervention without arteriographic characterization of the site of injury.

THORACIC VASCULAR TRAUMA DURING THE ACUTE PHASE

Incidence

Traumatic injuries to the thoracic vessels account for 15 percent of all civilian vascular injuries [1]. Approximately 90 percent of the wounds that are seen in the emergency room are a result of penetrating trauma (equally divided between high- and low-velocity missiles). The remainder are due to blunt trauma from vehicular accidents or consequent to a fall. The incidence of injury to low-pressure thoracic vessels, such as the superior and inferior vena cavae, the azygous vein, the proximal pulmonary arteries and veins, is small [2–5].

More than 90 percent of patients who receive penetrating wounds of a large intrathoracic high- or low-pressure structure (aorta and its branches, pulmonary artery, and vena cavae) do not reach the hospital alive [1,6]. This is also true for most patients with blunt thoracic trauma when major vessels are involved. These patients die at the scene of the accident or during transport to the emergency room. Little time is available for diagnosis in the other 10 percent of these patients who arrive at the hospital alive and present the opportunity for defining the extent of the lesion prior to surgical management.

Injuries of the descending thoracic aorta due to blunt trauma are more frequently seen than injuries of the ascending aorta. The ratio is about 3 : 1 in our experience. The higher frequency of observation of descending aortic injuries is indicative of the fatal nature of ascending aortic injuries prior to hospital admission, not of a difference in incidence of either injury [1,6].

Pathophysiology

Penetrating vascular injuries are associated with loss of a portion of a vessel wall or total severance of a vessel [6]. This results in a hematoma that gradually expands until the pressure within the surrounding tissue equalizes that of the mean intraluminal blood pressure. Hypotension due to associated injuries and hypovolemia is a natural hemostatic mechanism. Generally, at an arterial blood pressure of 60 mm Hg systolic, bleeding from most 1- to 2-mm arterial vessels ceases. Small-vessel injuries that cause vascular avulsion are associated with more rapid hemostasis (due to retraction of the cut ends) than injuries involving partial disruption of the vessel wall. Communication of a bleeding vessel into a large space such as the thoracic cavity with its physiologically negative pressure enhances blood loss.

The physiologic mechanism of aortic disruption due to blunt trauma is similar to that of an acute aortic dissection, except that traumatic dissection remains localized and does not extend distally. Two areas are susceptible to this injury. In the ascending aorta, the vulnerable area is the segment between the pericardial reflection distally and takeoff of the coronary arteries proximally. A segment of the descending aorta that is most susceptible to rupture is at the aortic isthmus (near the attachment of the ligamentum arteriosus). This area is located between the takeoff of the left subclavian artery proximally and the takeoff of the fourth intercostal artery distally. These two segments are prone to rupture due to blunt trauma because of their minimal fixation (attachment) to the chest wall. Motion of the ascending and the descending aorta in these locations during a cardiac cycle or during rapid deceleration in association with sudden increase in intracardiac and intravascular pressure due to impact of trauma results in a tear (fracture) of the aortic intima and media. Patients with existing conditions such as cystic medial necrosis are predisposed to this injury.

The aortic tear caused by blunt trauma always involves the intima and part of the media. The injury may be limited to a portion of the vessel wall or involve the entire circumference. Descending thoracic aortic injuries are usually associated with more severe and, at times, multiple intimal tears. The ascending aortic injuries usually are singular and involve the medial or lateral wall of the aorta above the sinus of Valsalva. An ascending aortic tear frequently results in instantaneous rupture and death from cardiac tamponade. This is a major mechanism of death in high-speed impacts (plane crash).

Diagnosis

The initial suspicion of intrathoracic vascular injuries may require rapid employment of life-saving measures. As it applies to all patients suffering from multiple trauma, this includes establishment of airway and ventilation followed by maintenance of adequate circulation and volume replacement. Physical examination must be initiated immediately and includes observation, auscultation, percussion, and palpation of the chest. Suspicion of presence of a large quantity of blood and air in the chest cavity requires drainage with chest tubes. The finding of deviation of mediastinal structures (trachea, cardiac impulse and sounds) on physical examination or on chest roentgenogram serves as an important clue to the necessity for urgent thoracostomy with a large-size chest tube. Pericardiocentesis may be needed to confirm the diagnosis of cardiac tamponade.

Thoracic vascular trauma due to penetrating injuries generally results in intrathoracic bleeding (hemothorax) with the resultant hypotension and shock [7]. This is due to volume depletion or to displacement of intrathoracic structures and/or interference with the normal function of the cardiopulmonary system (tension hemothorax). Extensive blood loss may also occur as a result of intrathoracic arterial injuries from total or partial disruption of small vessels such as the internal mammary artery and vein. More frequently, however, the intercostal vessels are involved. These vessels are also injured from blunt trauma and as a result of fractured ribs. A large hemothorax clinically may cause severe shortness of breath with absence of breath sounds and dullness over an entire hemithorax. An associated pulmonary injury ameliorates the clinical condition and may confuse the physical findings by obscuring the extent of dullness.

A rapid physical examination usually suggests intrathoracic vascular injury, although the source of bleeding may remain unknown. Absence of peripheral pulses in the upper extremity, a weak carotid upstroke, and different blood pressure readings in the upper arms are indicative of probable major aortic branch laceration or avulsion. These injuries may also be associated with neurologic findings such as incomplete stroke with waxing and waning mentation or with numbness of extremities. We have seen paraplegia in association with descending aorta transection.

Trauma to the major high-pressure intrathoracic vessels results in intramediastinal bleeding and radiographic evidence of widening of the mediastinum (Fig. 12-6). Excessive bleeding may produce tracheal compression, with shortness of breath and respiratory stridor as the presenting symptoms. Severe associated injuries of the bony thorax such as the upper ribs and clavicle are indicative of the force of impact and require careful evaluation to rule out vascular injuries [8,9,10].

Inferior vena caval disruption from the heart always results in cardiac tamponade [11]. If such a patient is submitted to urgent pericardial exploration, there is a strong possibility that intraoperative exsanguination will ensue. Measures to prevent this catastrophe require meticulous preoperative and intraoperative planning and no panic! Survival from this injury is unprecedented.

Radiographic and Angiographic Findings

The most important test for diagnosis of intrathoracic vascular injuries is a plain upright chest film followed by an angiogram. A poor-quality arteriogram, however, may not reveal the location of the arterial injury in all patients. Clinical suspicion along with a good-quality angiographic study is mandatory for proper localization of the area of vessel damage.

Widening of the mediastinum on an upright chest film is seen in all injuries involving the intrathoracic aorta as well as its major branches [15,16]. Figure 12-7 shows a classic presentation of descending aortic tear due to blunt trauma with its five radiographic characteristics. Injuries of the ascending aorta and the innominate artery also result in widening of the mediastinum (see Fig. 12-6). With these lesions, chest roentgenogram reveals straight-

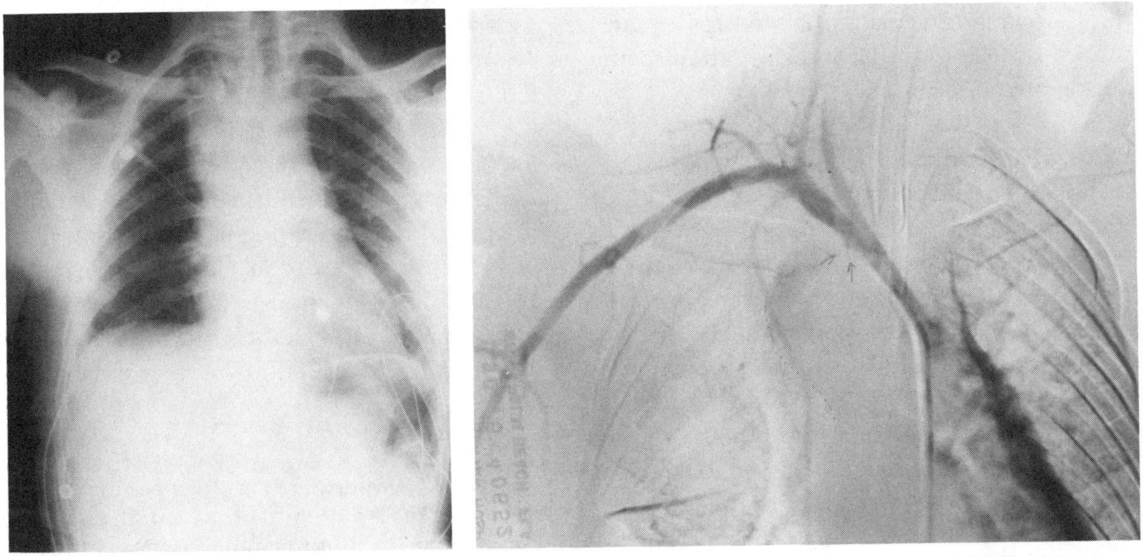

Fig. 12-6. Preoperative posteroanterior (PA) chest film (*left*) of a patient after stab wound of the right second intercostal space. Note widening of the mediastinum and changes of its right border. The selective arteriogram (*right*) shows the site of the innominate artery injury (*arrows*). The extent of hematoma is shown with a faint dotted line. This patient's injury resulted in respiratory difficulty. Repair was accomplished through a trapdoor incision (see Fig. 12-11).

ening of the right side of the mediastinal border without evidence of shift in the mediastinal structures (trachea and esophagus) that is frequently observed with descending thoracic aortic rupture [17] (Fig. 12-7). Other causes of widening of the mediastinum on the chest roentgenogram are thymic vessel injuries, disruption of the intercostal arteries from the descending thoracic aorta, injuries to the proximal parts of major low-pressure intra-

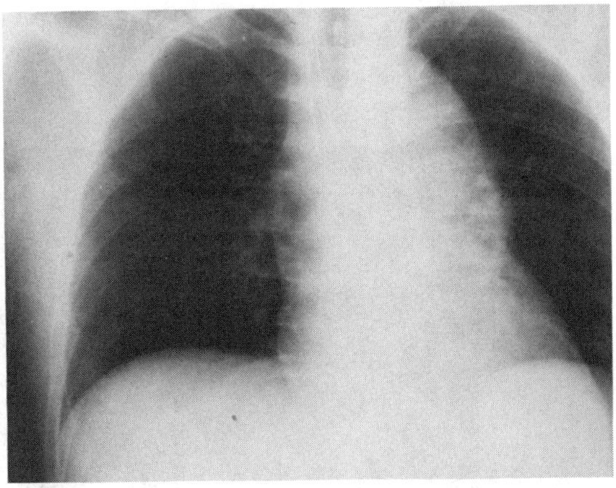

Fig. 12-7. The classic presentation on PA chest film of descending thoracic aortic rupture due to blunt trauma. There are five radiographic signs: mediastinal widening, obscured aortic knob, fullness of aortopulmonary segment, deviation of trachea and nasograstric tube to the right, and blunting of the left apical cap.

thoracic vessels such as vena cavae, pulmonary artery and veins, and fractures of sternum [6,8,18,19]. In all these patients, the aortogram is normal.

Surgical Management

In an ascending aortic injury due to blunt trauma, an aortogram shows an aneurysm in the medial or lateral aspect of the ascending aorta (Fig. 12-8). Since the ascending aorta, in most part, is an intrapericardial structure, these injuries should be treated surgically on an emergency basis to prevent intrapericardial rupture and cardiac tamponade. Acute repair of these lesions requires establishment of cardiopulmonary bypass after median sternotomy. The ascending aorta is then opened, and repair of the site of tear is accomplished frequently by direct suturing or rarely by graft replacement of a portion of the ascending aorta. If there is evidence of a large contained ascending aortic hematoma, such as in the event of survival from a direct stab wound, establishment of cardiopulmonary bypass via the femoral artery and vein prior to opening of the pericardium prevents sudden decompression and rupture. In these patients, to control the ascending aorta for prevention of exsanguination, total circulatory arrest at 10° to 15°C is needed before the pericardial incision is made. A short interval (2 minutes) of intentional induction of ventricular fibril-

Fig. 12-8. Preoperative PA chest roentgenogram (*left*) of a patient with ascending aortic rupture due to blunt trauma. Note position of the nasogastric tube and mediastinal widening. Aortogram (*right*) shows localized false aneurysm of the ascending aorta without aortic valve incompetence. Urgent repair of this lesion with cardiopulmonary bypass resulted in an excellent outcome.

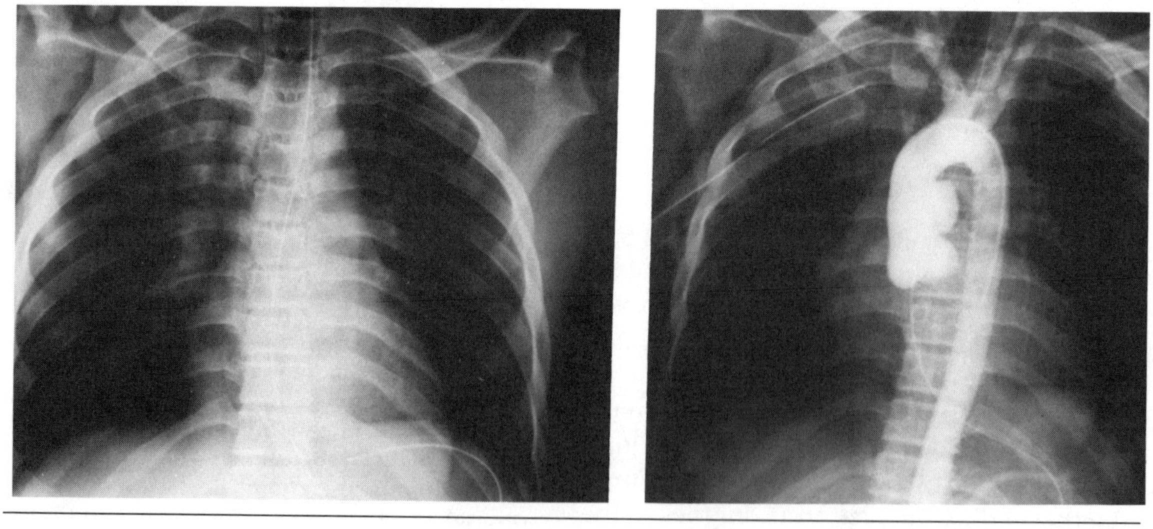

lation with an AC current electrode is another alternative.

Descending thoracic aortic injuries due to blunt trauma present on the aortogram as an aortic disruption or false aneurysm formation (Figs. 12-9 and 12-10). Pathologically, there is a false aneurysm extending medially or laterally. In the absence of hypotension or blood loss, these injuries require immediate control of hematoma by rapid-acting afterload reducing agents of antihypertensive drugs such as propranolol and nitroprusside or trimethaphan. This step is of paramount importance during anesthesia induction. Once the diagnosis of aortic transection is established, if the patient is hemodynamically stable, we have in the past allowed initial surgical care by the general surgeons for associated injuries, especially those of intra-abdominal pathology. During this period, a cardiovascular surgeon is in attendance. After an expeditious abdominal exploration, the patient is repositioned and prepped for standard left lateral thoracotomy.

An important consideration should be given to older patients (>60 years) with thoracic aortic injuries. Frequently, these individuals have associated atherosclerotic lesions of the aorta that pathologically cause multiple aortic tears. Also, because of calcific vessels, cross clamping of the aorta may be associated with complications and technical difficulties. Repair of a diseased, torn aorta requires great surgical skill and experience. A long length of aorta may have to be resected to reach the segments that are free of disease and amenable to suturing. As a consequence, a number of intercostal vessels may have to be ligated, and the prolonged length of the procedure re-

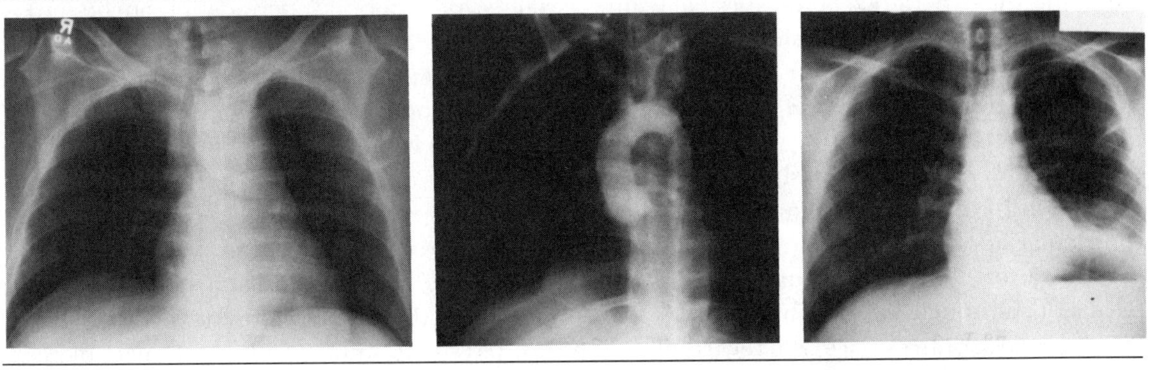

Fig. 12-9. Preoperative anteroposterior (AP) chest film (*left*) of a patient with descending aortic rupture due to a car accident. Note the classic presentation of the chest x-ray, including tracheal deviation. The aortogram (*middle*) shows the "cutoff sign" of contrast column indicating aortic transection due to a (horizontal) intimal tear involving the entire circumference of the aorta. The left subclavian artery did not visualize. Postoperative chest film (*right*) shows normal appearance of the mediastinum with diaphragmatic paresis as a result of surgical repair.

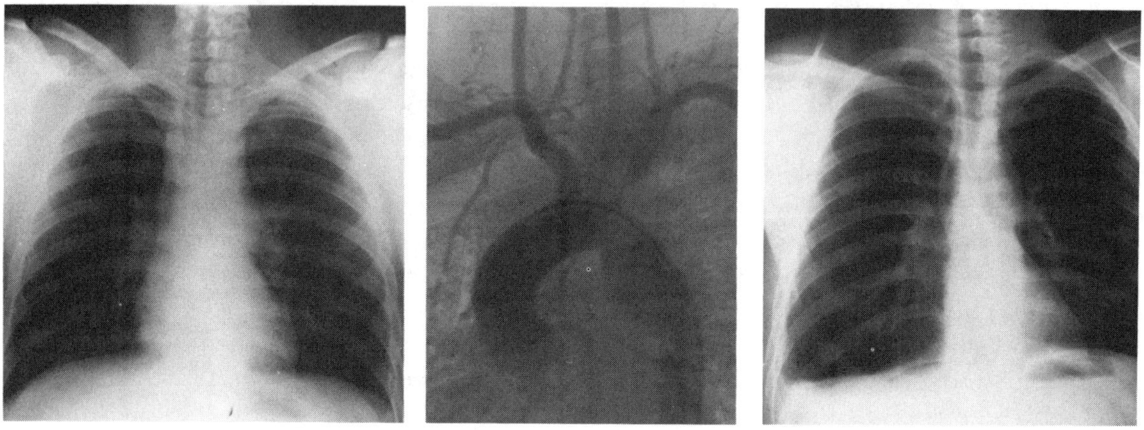

Fig. 12-10. Admission PA chest film (*left*) of a patient after a deceleration injury. The radiographic presentation is classic. There was a 30 mm Hg blood pressure difference between the two arms. The subtraction aortogram (*middle*) shows a large false aneurysm with marked narrowing of the left subclavian artery. The postoperative PA chest film (*right*) shows normal appearance of the mediastinum and tracheobronchial tree.

quires distal perfusion with a bypass technique.

Repair of the descending thoracic aorta frequently is carried out without the use of a heart-lung machine or a vascular shunt. However, alternate methods must be available to establish some type of distal perfusion when the extent of vascular trauma requires longer than 30 to 45 minutes of aortic cross clamping. This decision must be made ahead of time on the basis of gross pathology of the aorta and the experience of the surgical team. The bypass techniques for distal perfusion include temporary shunts and partial cardiopulmonary bypass by femoral vein/artery bypass.

A temporary heparinized shunt (Gott) can be used from the subclavian artery or the left ventricular apex or the proximal aorta to the femoral artery. The shunt maintains distal perfusion, although at lower blood flow rates than normal. Controversy exists regarding the efficacy of distal aortic perfusion with these shunts. In the opinion of some surgeons, presence of a shunt raises the false hope of safety of extended periods of aortic cross clamping. These shunts do not abolish the danger of spinal cord injury. Furthermore, the large size of shunt tubing may cause injury at the site of insertion and may result in reduction of the lumen of the vessel after it is repaired, especially if purse-string sutures are used to secure the shunt in place.

Another method of distal perfusion is by partial cardiopulmonary bypass with or without oxygenation (i.e., with right heart bypass, from femoral vein to femoral artery by using an oxygenator or with left heart bypass from left atrium to femoral artery by using a roller pump only).

To assist with the procedure, to keep the operative field dry, and to prevent excessive blood loss and the need for blood transfusion, we prefer to use a specially designed self-transfusing technique that we have devised [20]. This system allows rapid reinfusion into the saphenous vein of collected blood from the wound during the operation. The device delivers up to 500 ml/min of blood reinfusion. Physiologically, this system is a left (arterial)–to–right (venous) bypass. In my opinion, this system is better for blood saving than other systems because it does not separate the plasma and blood cells and allows immediate reinfusion of the whole blood elements instead of the red cells only. We have used this technique in 35 patients in the past 7 years, and presently it is an adjunct device for all explorations and operations on the descending thoracic aorta and mediastinal vascular injuries and aneurysms. In traumatic aortic injuries, even if a heart-lung machine is needed, we use this device in addition to the support system.

A rapidly expanding descending thoracic aortic hematoma (due to blunt or penetrating trauma) requires immediate surgical care regardless of the clinical status of the patient. If rupture of the descending thoracic aorta into the chest occurs prior to arrival at the surgical suite, prompt exposure and cross clamping of the aorta may be lifesaving. However, such attempts have not always been successful in our hands. This failure is mainly due to the need for a prolonged period of aortic cross clamping. Therefore, all efforts must be directed toward repair of the aortic injury while the periaortic hematoma is contained. Similarly, in other trauma victims when severe cardiovascular collapse is the presenting sign, unless a massive intra-abdominal or intrathoracic arterial hemorrhage is present, intrathoracic cross clamping of the descending thoracic aorta does not result in patient survival. Here again, the main problem lies with hemodynamic instability during the period of declamping of the aorta if this time interval has exceeded 30 minutes.

Disruption of the takeoff of the innominate artery from the aorta due to blunt trauma has been reported sporadically [15,16]. Management of this injury and that of the takeoff of the right subclavian or carotid arteries due to penetrating trauma has been by early or delayed exploration of the area by using a modified trapdoor incision. We begin this incision parallel to and from the superior aspect of the right clavicle (in the neck) and down over the midline to the third costal interspace, where it is extended laterally to the right in a curvilinear fashion (Fig. 12-11). We attempt not to enter the right thoracic cavity, and in fact, the right internal thoracic artery is not ligated. By this technique, the upper portion of the right thoracic wall is lifted off the intrathoracic fascia.

During the acute phase, the trapdoor incision is a valuable approach to the aortic arch branches. However, due to instability of the mediastinal hematoma, it may require additional extension of the incision. An "F incision," composed of incisions over the left supraclavicular area, median sternotomy, and a third or fourth left costal interspace thoracotomy, is needed to achieve access to the prox-

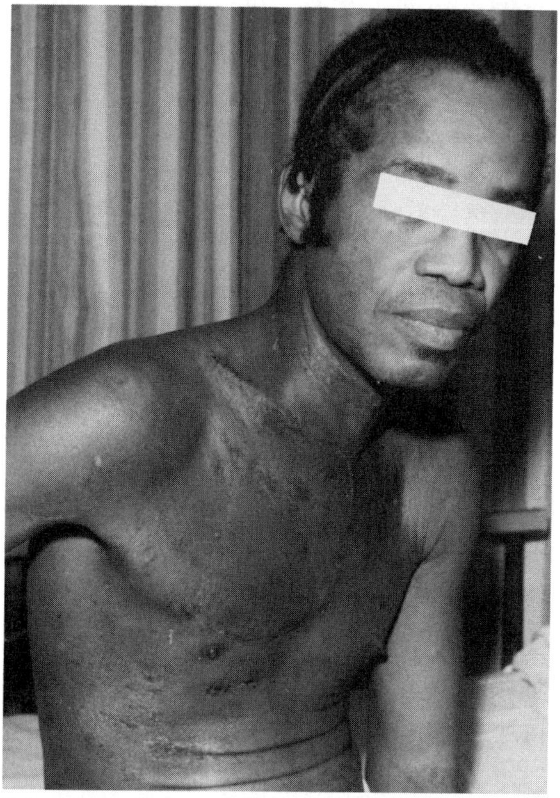

Fig. 12-11. Postoperative appearance of a trapdoor incision modified to avoid entry into the right thoracic cavity and ligation of internal thoracic vessels. Note that the lower part of the incision curves to the right into the third intercostal space and requires incision through medial fibers of the pectoralis major muscle above the nipple. This patient's chest film and the arteriogram are shown in Figure 12-6.

imal aortic arch, distal aorta, left subclavian vessels, and all major aortic branches. A "reversed F" incision allows good exposure of the right subclavian vessels, superior vena cava, and innominate vein as well as the proximal aortic arch. Of course, when the site of injury is known and is limited to the mediastinal vessels, the standard median sternotomy incision gives an excellent exposure of these structures. However, in the absence of an arteriogram and in the presence of a large mediastinal hematoma, a median sternotomy incision in the hands of a nonexperienced surgeon may result in disastrous events because of difficulty with locating the site of the injury and with adequate control of bleeding.

To facilitate exposure of the upper mediastinal structures, I have found no need to cut the clavicles and have followed the doctrine of "control all the entry and exit vessels away from the hematoma before exploring it." Hypotensive anesthesia with nitroprusside infusion, partial cardiopulmonary bypass with a self-transfusing system, and most importantly, a short discussion with the assistants and the anesthesiologist as well as other members of the surgical team prior to exploration of the hematoma allow for a calm and a systematic approach to the problem and may prevent exsanguination. *An arteriographic study must be done, if at all possible, prior to exploration of major thoracic vascular injuries.* In our hands, almost all intraoperative mortalities from thoracic vascular injuries were in patients who had no preoperative arteriographic studies.

Important intraoperative measures include intravenous access for transfusion with multiple large vascular catheters. A reliable central venous line placed away from the site of vascular injury is mandatory. Pulmonary artery pressure monitoring should be done whenever possible. Repair of descending aortic injuries is facilitated by unilateral lung ventilation by a double-lumen endotracheal tube (Carlens).

We routinely use a low-porosity, woven Dacron graft (VeriSoft) for our major vascular surgery. We also routinely use preclotting methods with nonheparinized blood (or by addition of protamine if heparin is already administered). We then autoclave the graft for 3 minutes after it is cleaned of all blood clots. The sutures used are 4-0 polypropylene, and all the anastomoses are done from within the vessel with one row of continuous suturing. The operative site is washed clean. An antibiotic of second- or third-generation cephalosporin type is given routinely every 4 to 5 hours IV during the operation and every 6 hours for 3 days after the operation.

Intra- and postoperative infusion of blood elements may be needed. Chest drainage systems with self-transfusion packages may be used. These will allow reinfusion of blood that is drained into the chest cavity. Early application of this system (in the emergency room) is being practiced routinely. The chest is washed many times and is drained well with multiple large chest tubes. The chest is closed with nonabsorbable suture material by interrupted techniques. The sternum is closed with figure-of-eight wires of No. 5 size [21]. During chest closure, the wound is irrigated numerous times. In our hands, by using this technique, the incidence of wound infection in patients with chest trauma has been equal to elective thoracic and cardiac procedures regardless of the extent of incision.

Vigorous postoperative respiratory care is used similar to all thoracic operations. Diuretics are used to prevent respiratory distress syndrome and to eliminate the excess lung water from the massive crystalloid infusion that invariably is given to these patients during the resuscitation phase from acute trauma. Postoperative electrocardiographic studies and cardiac enzyme measurements are needed to rule out cardiac injury.

THORACIC VASCULAR TRAUMA DURING THE CHRONIC PHASE

We consider the chest trauma is chronic when a time interval of more than a few days has elapsed after the injury. For a variety of reasons, certain intrathoracic vascular injuries are asymptomatic at first and are not diagnosed during the acute phase. These require surgical treatment at a later time when symptoms due to pressure over the adjacent structures begin. Rarely, specific injuries are treated after an intentional delay period that allows for stability of the perivascular hematoma. A frequently missed injury is rupture of the ascending or descending aorta due to blunt trauma (Fig. 12-12).

Penetrating vascular injuries that seem harmless during the acute phase may cause false aneurysms or arteriovenous fistulae that at a later time produce pressure symptoms or cause congestive heart failure, respectively [6]. The delay period from injury to development

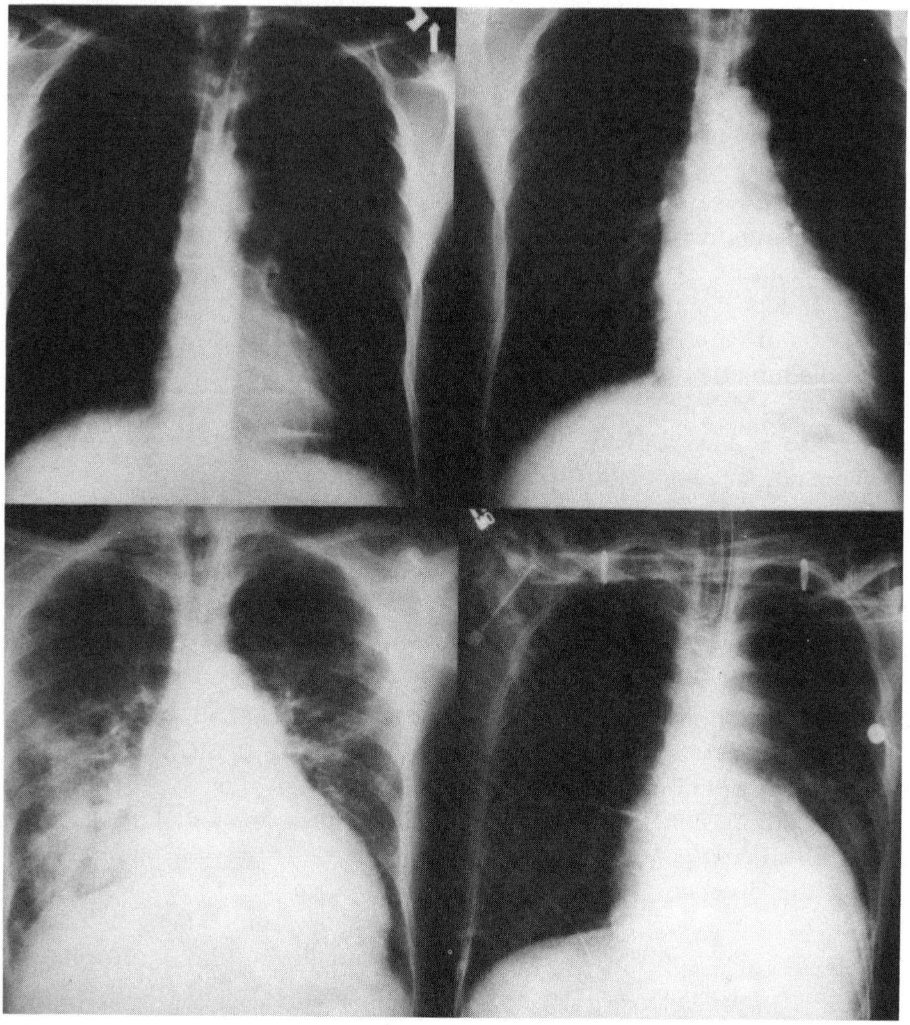

Fig. 12-12. Progressive worsening of cardiac condition in a patient with ascending aortic tear due to deceleration injury. The upper chest films were taken during the emergency room visit (*upper left*) and 1 month later (*upper right*). The lower left film was taken 3 months later during patient admission. Note gradual increase in heart size and eventual development of pulmonary edema. The lower right chest film is an early postoperative AP view. This patient required ascending aortic graft replacement and resuspension of the aortic valve.

of symptoms may vary from a few days to many years.

Some of the old traumatic lesions are found incidentally on a chest roentgenogram. These may not require surgical treatment because of their benign course. For example, a small, well-healed traumatic descending aortic aneurysm that has not resulted in any symptoms and has not enlarged or is surrounded by a calcific periaortic hematoma does not require repair.

Pathophysiology

An expanding hematoma that surrounds a large venous injury is usually made up of extremely friable tissue that is not amenable to surgical repair. Dissection of a venous perivascular hematoma during the acute phase without adequate proximal and distal control frequently leads to uncontrollable hemorrhage [7].

An arterial adventitial hematoma may not stabilize as readily as a venous hematoma. These chronic hematomas are pathologically a false aneurysm with a portion of the expanded wall of the aneurysm made up of blood clots or walls of other structures such as lung, esophagus, trachea, or chest wall [5,6].

Diagnosis and Management

Suspicion of thoracic vascular injuries arises when abnormal thoracic shadows or mediastinal widening develops over time after a penetrating or blunt injury (Fig. 12-13). Scanning images by computed tomography (CT) of the thorax after contrast injection, arteriography, and magnetic resonance imaging (MRI) would be helpful in delineating the relation of the mass to the vascular and other intrathoracic structures. Clinical symptoms may vary from none to severe compression of various organs (trachea, esophagus, superior vena cava, and recurrent laryngeal nerve).

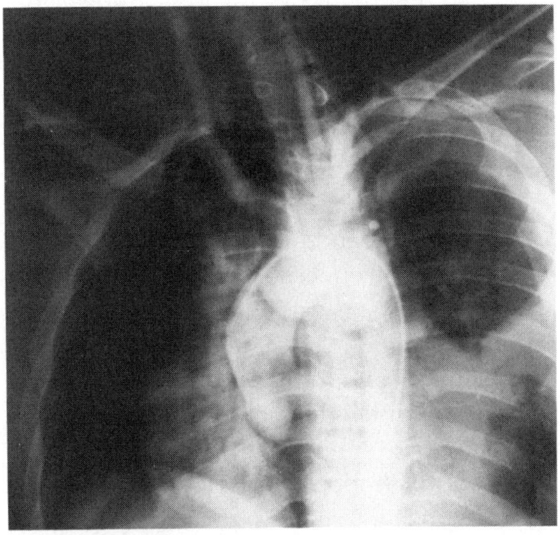

Fig. 12-13. Ascending aortic and arch aortogram from a patient with gunshot wound of the second right interspace. The aortic arch hematoma was explored 48 hours after the incident. It was localized to the midaortic arch and was due to an abrasion of the inferior aspect of the aortic arch. It was repaired through a median sternotomy incision without cardiopulmonary bypass.

Stab wounds of large mediastinal veins (innominate and subclavian) and the aortic arch may result in an arteriovenous (AV) fistula and a loud systolic murmur and thrill, which may be present in the course of hours or days after the initial injury. The murmur is best heard at the upper sternum and the base of the neck. Unexplained tachycardia and congestive heart failure may be the presenting symptoms. Elective surgical repair of these AV fistulae as well as false aneurysms of the takeoff of the innominate and carotid arteries is the suggested approach. With a plan of management established and the exact anatomic location of the lesion delineated by arteriography or CT scan, surgical intervention will result in a high success rate.

Superior vena caval injuries may be treated conservatively initially. Since this structure is in most part extrapericardial, its laceration results in a contained mediastinal hematoma. Furthermore, multiple large veins that lead to this conduit (innominate, right jugular, and subclavian vein branches) make distal control tedious. At times, it is impossible to control all the small and large venous branches that confluent into the superior vena cava and upper mediastinum. In an unstable patient with an expanding mediastinal shadow due to superior vena caval laceration, careful exploration by median sternotomy may be the only sound approach to this injury. However, whenever possible, a conservative approach to this injury is desirable unless acute superior vena caval obstruction is a threat. Lacerations of the innominate vein and the superior vena cava require venous patch grafting with a piece of saphenous vein. This necessitates preparation and sterile draping of the lower legs for procurement of the saphenous veins at the time of mediastinal exploration.

We have seen a few aortic arch injuries due to penetrating wounds with a contained hematoma (Fig. 12-13). These were explored after an initial period of stabilization. All these patients presented with a single wound and hemodynamically were stabilized rapidly after arrival in the emergency room and were studied by aortography. The decision to delay the operative repair for a few hours or days was made during the initial observation while the patients were in the intensive care unit under complete hemodynamic control.

In elective cases (delayed management), the trapdoor incision allows excellent exposure of the innominate artery, the takeoff of the right subclavian artery and of both carotid arteries. It permits good access to a number of major vessels including the innominate vein, the superior vena cava, and the distal ascending aorta. Graft interposition of the takeoff of the innominate or the subclavian artery can be accomplished easily by this method. The graft is taken from the ascending aorta to the carotid artery or to the innominate artery passing below the innominate vein. After establishing the bypass graft, ligation of the false aneurysm completes the procedure. Repair of the innominate artery, during temporary occlusion of this vessel, without graft interposition is possible but may cause right cerebral infarction unless an intravascular shunt is used.

During the chronic phase, arteriovenous fistulae of the innominate artery and innominate vein can be approached through a standard median sternotomy incision. An aorto-innominate fistula and most false aneurysms of major intrathoracic vessels require proximal and distal vascular control. In the case of carotid arteries, the use of an intravascular shunt (JAVID) to maintain the cerebral blood flow is necessary [15]. This will allow leisurely repair of the vascular lesion without fear of cerebral anoxic damage. Intraoperative and postoperative care in these patients is similar to the management described for the injuries during the acute phase of thoracic vascular trauma.

Abdominal Vascular Trauma

David B. Pilcher

ABDOMINAL AORTIC INJURIES

Blunt

Abdominal aortic injuries from blunt trauma are rare but can occur from aortic compression such as with "seat-belt" or "handlebar" trauma or, more rarely, from deceleration injuries similar to traumatic thoracic aortic injuries. With compression injuries, the adventitia may remain intact, with fracture of the intima resulting in thrombosis or more rarely embolization. Such injuries may be related to lumbar spine or pelvic fractures. An aortic aneurysm can rupture, thrombose, or result in emboli secondary to compressive or deceleration trauma.

Penetrating

Major injury to the abdominal aorta usually precludes attempt at salvage due to exsanguination prior to arrival in the emergency room.

More minor penetrating injury to the aorta presents usually as a periaortic (central) hematoma that may be expanding but is confined by the retroperitoneum sufficiently to allow operative intervention if undertaken promptly.

Distal ischemia from penetrating aortic injury associated with embolic distal occlusion or aortic thrombosis is unusual. Distal embolus of a bullet to femoral or distal vessels can occur with aortic injury.

Diagnosis

With blunt trauma, a high index of suspicion is necessary for prompt diagnosis. Transient signs of ischemia, the presence of a bruit, or signs of distal embolization should be searched for. In a young patient, absence of any distal pulses should raise the suspicion of an embolus from suspected blunt aortic injury.

With penetrating trauma, usually hypovolemia will be manifest, and a central (or periaortic hematoma) will be found at urgent laparotomy.

Aortography preoperatively may be possible with blunt trauma if the patient is stable enough to survive a trip to the radiology suite. This will rarely be feasible in penetrating trauma.

Treatment

For purposes of this discussion, the aorta is divided at the renal arteries (Fig. 12-14).

Suprarenal Aortic Injuries

When the patient presents with cardiac arrest following penetrating injury, left anterolateral thoracotomy with open massage and cross clamping of the uninjured thoracic aorta through the thoracotomy incision may be the requisite first step. Intravenous access must simultaneously be obtained by other members of the trauma team.

Assuming injury not producing cardiac ar-

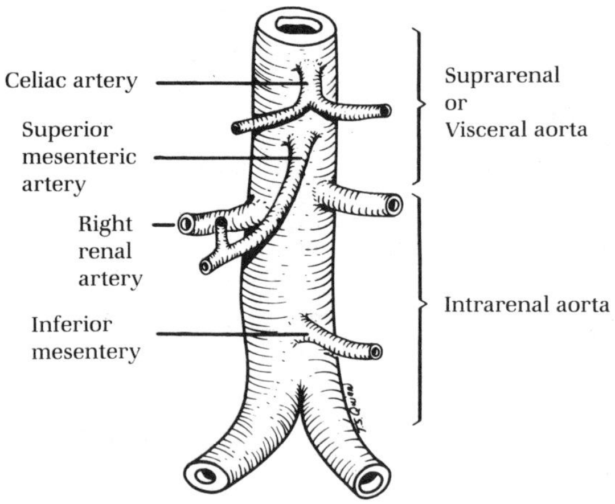

Fig. 12-14. Division of abdominal aorta into supra- and infrarenal segments.

rest, the abdomen should be entered with a long midline incision. If a midline or left or right central hematoma suggests suprarenal aortic injury, the aorta should be compressed manually against the vertebral column at the hiatus. Veith and coworkers [1] describe retracting the liver upward and bluntly dissecting to the right of the gastroesophageal junction to allow placement of an occluding clamp on the aorta at this level. The vena cava and aorta are widely separated at this level, making chances of vena caval injury much less than when clamping the aorta at a lower level. Although Veith and coworkers [1] reported no renal or visceral "impairment" with 8 to 67 minutes of supraceliac aortic clamping, reestablishment of visceral and renal perfusion should be a priority, with clamping at a lower level as soon as feasible.

With central or left central hematoma suggesting suprarenal aortic injury, the viscera including stomach, colon, pancreas, spleen, and kidney should be rotated medially, as popularized by Mattox and colleagues [2] (Fig. 12-15A). The viscera can also be rotated medially anterior to the kidney, as suggested by Buscaglia and associates [3].

When there is a right central hematoma or associated vena caval injury, exposure of the aorta may be gained by a Cattel maneuver, rotating the viscera medially from the right side [3] (Fig. 12-15B).

Occasionally, additional exposure may be required and can be gained by extending the midline incision into the right or left thorax or as a median sternotomy extension.

Lateral repair of the aorta is usually possible. If a graft is required, autogenous material may have advantages [3], but synthetic grafts may be more practical, and Mattox and colleagues [2] have reported no infection in seven cases of aortic injury using Dacron grafts.

Bullet emboli may result from aortic penetration, and aortic injury should raise this suspicion, as should distal bullets or unilateral ischemia after abdominal gunshot wounds.

RESULTS

Mortality has ranged from 50 to 80 percent in reported series of patients with suprarenal aortic injuries who survived to reach the hospital. Eighty percent of such injured patients died before arrival at the hospital [2].

Associated injuries are frequent, and vena caval injury is present in one-third of such patients.

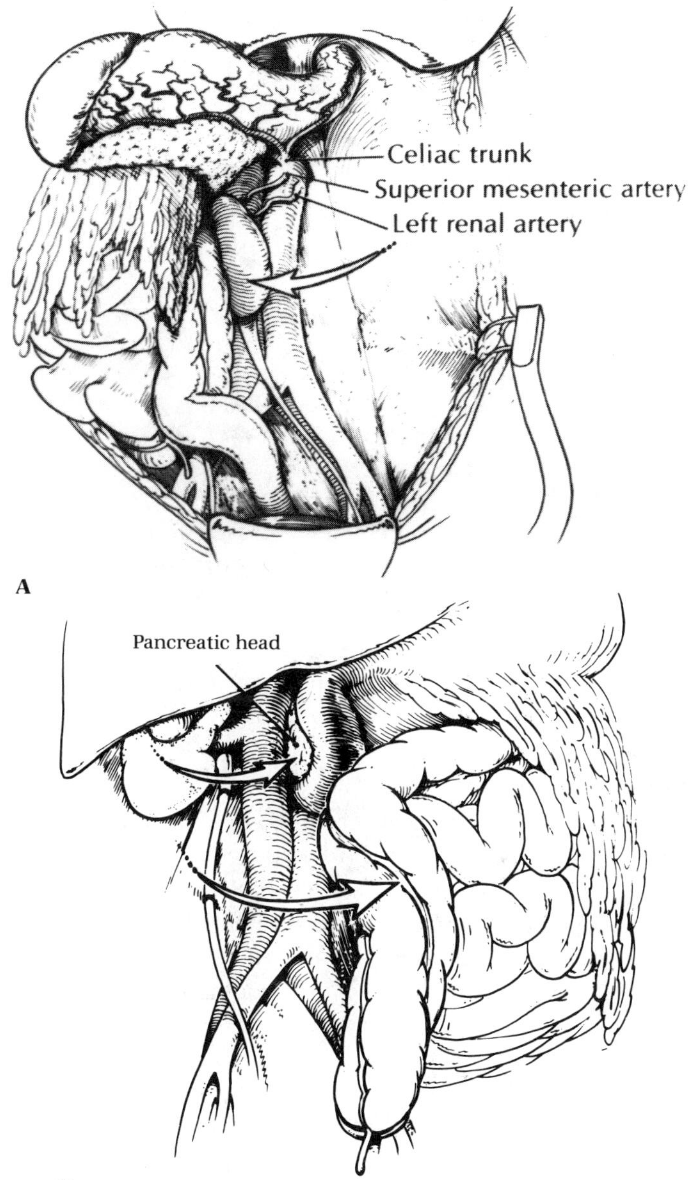

Fig. 12-15. Medial rotation of the viscera from (*A*) the left ("Mattox maneuver") or from (*B*) the right ("Cattel maneuver") to expose major vessels. (Reproduced by permission from K. L. Mattox and D. V. Feliciano, *Visceral Vascular Trauma*. In E. E. Moore, B. Eiseman, and C. W. Van Way III, *Critical Decisions in Trauma*. St. Louis: Mosby, 1984. Artwork © Baylor College of Medicine.)

Infrarenal Aortic Injuries

Blunt intimal injury ("seat-belt aorta") may have a delayed presentation or recognition.

When the level of suspected aortic injury appears to be below the renal arteries, temporary aortic occlusion may rarely be required above the visceral arteries, as with suprarenal injuries. The usual approach to the aorta of rotating the small intestine and duodenum upward and to the right will allow expeditious placement of an infrarenal aortic clamp.

Balloon aortic occluders inserted through the femoral artery either by cutdown or percutaneously may be possible prior to opening an infrarenal central hematoma.

As with suprarenal aortic injuries, lateral repair will usually be possible. Through-and-through aortic penetrating injuries can usually be managed by dividing lumbar arteries and rotating the infrarenal aorta. With proximal and distal clamping, holes in the posterior aorta (or aortocaval fistulae) can be managed by suturing the posterior aorta from within the opened aortic lumen (as shown in Fig. 12-19 for vena cava).

Aortic interposition tube graft may be appropriate. With delayed presentation or, as in one of the author's cases, endarterectomy (intimectomy) and patch grafting may be possible (Fig. 12-16).

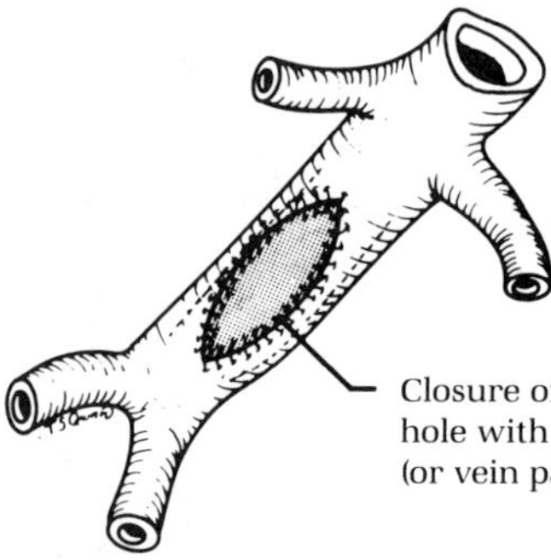

Fig. 12-16. Patch graft closure may be necessary to avoid narrowing of aortic "lateral" repair.

RESULTS

Soldano and coworkers [4] have shown that atherosclerotic plaques have developed at the site of lateral aortic repairs with late follow-up. This may suggest the need for debridement of injured vessels or a place for patch grafting to avoid turbulence.

ILIAC ARTERIAL INJURIES

Iliac arterial injuries from blunt trauma or minor injuries from penetrating trauma may result in intimal disruption with occlusion or, more unusually, embolization with distal ischemia and contained hematoma. Prompt recognition of decreased pulses and signs of ischemia is the key step. Intermittent ischemia from an intimal flap may precede thrombosis and will be diagnosed only if a high index of suspicion is maintained (see Fig. 12-17).

Disruption of an iliac artery or major injury produces rapid exsanguination poorly responsive to volume resuscitation.

A less frequent circumstance occurs with penetrating trauma, with arterial and venous injury producing an acute arteriovenous (AV) fistula that may be associated with exsanguination or ischemic symptoms.

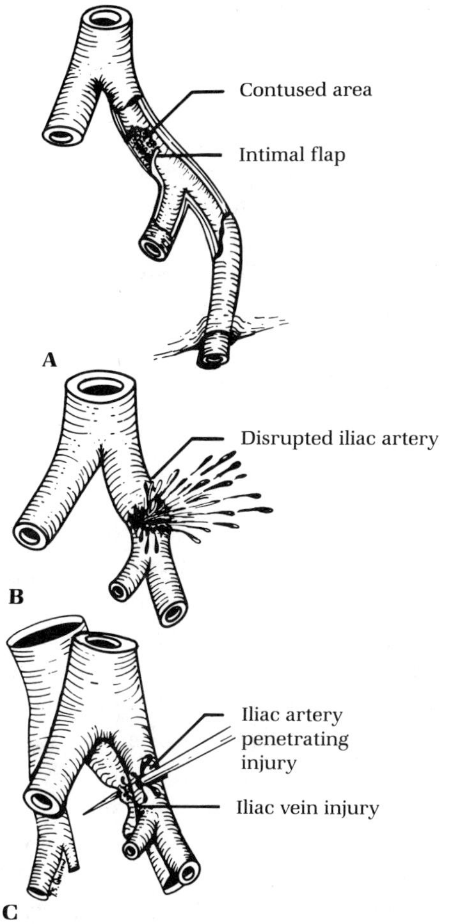

Fig. 12-17. Types of iliac artery injuries. *A.* Intimal flap. *B.* Disruption. *C.* Traumatic AV fistula.

fistula that may be associated with exsanguination or ischemic symptoms.

Diagnosis

Even with contusion and intimal injuries, the magnitude of trauma will usually have other associated injuries and urgent indications of hypovolemia mandating emergent laparotomy. Rarely will circumstances permit the luxury of a preoperative angiogram.

Treatment

Contusion of an iliac artery from blunt trauma may be managed by intimectomy and thrombectomy, preserving the native artery (Fig. 12-17A). Penetrating trauma will usually require interposition grafting, as in Figure 12-17B. The large size of the iliac arteries usually mandate synthetic grafts. Occasionally repairs can be effected by suturing two segments of saphenous vein longitudinally ("panel graft").

Since the iliac veins are intimately associated with the arteries, acute AV fistulae should be searched for carefully and the vein also repaired (Fig. 12-17C).

RENAL ARTERIAL INJURIES

Proximal renal arterial injuries (termed renal pedicle injuries) are usually caused by penetrating trauma (gunshot wounds) and are frequently associated with relatively confined hematoma due to the retroperitoneal location of the renal artery. Blunt trauma produces thrombosis in almost half of the recognized pedicle injuries (due to intimal injury/dissection) without disrsuption of the adventitia. Complete avulsion of the renal artery is also rarely seen with blunt trauma.

Hematuria may be absent (one-fourth of patients with blunt trauma), but nonvisualization on intravenous pyelogram (IVP) is usual. There may be sufficient time for angiography. Delay in diagnosis is frequent and is reported in half of the patients with blunt renal artery injury reported by Clark and associates [5]. Renal pedicle injuries may also be noted on CT scan. Goldstein and colleagues [6] have suggested that CT scan may be more sensitive and specific than IVP and tap and lavage in such patients.

Morton and Crawford [7] reported successful return of function in bilateral injury with repair after 18 hours. Clark and associates [5] reported 12 successful repairs for blunt trauma done 3 to 18 hours after injury. If injury is unilateral and severe warm ischemia has persisted more than 90 minutes, nephrectomy may be indicated; however, as Clark and associates [5] have emphasized, only about one-third of unsuccessful repairs or nonrepairs of the renal artery subsequently develop hypertension and require later nephrectomy.

VISCERAL ARTERIAL INJURIES

Major visceral arterial injuries usually are discovered acutely when penetrating trauma victims are explored for hemorrhage. Treatment depends on recognition of degree of ischemia and therefore may entail ligation with or without resection of the intestine or spleen, for example.

Ligation, lateral repair, and synthetic or autologous vein graft repair have all been successful, as well as replantation of vessels into the aorta. Late complications are usually related to infection and are frequently related to associated injuries. Adjacent veins are frequently injured and should be repaired.

Graham and coworkers [8] report a mortality of 40 percent with celiac or superior mesenteric artery (SMA) injuries and suggest ligation of the celiac axis is better tolerated than ligation of the superior mesenteric artery.

Sirinek and Levine [9] suggest that proximal superior mesenteric exposure can be obtained through the lesser sac or root of the mesentery. They state that medial rotation of the viscera as recommended for suprarenal aortic injuries results in unwarranted delay. Intestinal viability after vascular repair can be assessed by Doppler or fluorescein testing. Mortality in Sirinek and Levine's series [9] was 19 percent among 21 patients with proximal SMA injuries.

HEPATIC ARTERY INJURIES

If hepatic artery injury occurs without portal vein injury, ligation is frequently the most appropriate therapy. Minor injuries may be appropriately repaired. The occurrence of hepatic necrosis in humans after hepatic artery ligation is a very rare event [10].

If the portal vein is injured simultaneously with the hepatic artery, repair of one or both vascular structures is mandatory. Sheldon and colleagues [11] found hepatic artery injuries in only 4 of 31 portal vein injuries.

PORTAL VEIN INJURIES

Most portal vein injuries are accompanied by other major injuries and are associated with a 54- to 71-percent mortality rate [11]. Exposure of the retropancreatic portion of the portal vein may require an extended Kocher maneuver (medial rotation of the colon and duodenum).

Pachter and associates [12] state that acute portal vein ligation is tolerated by 80 percent of patients. Sheldon and colleagues [11] recommend repair when possible, with a second-look procedure to ensure intestinal viability if portal vein ligation is required. They suggest that performance of a portosystemic shunt is unnecessary and inadvisable in the unstable patient. Portal venous injuries have usually been repaired by lateral venorrhaphy.

VENA CAVAL INJURIES

The vena cava may be injured with blunt or penetrating trauma, almost always with other major intra-abdominal injuries mandating emergent exploration. It is generally felt that the consequences of not repairing a "missed" vena caval injury are not severe, but there is little evidence to support this. Ligation of the infrarenal vena cava is usually well tolerated *if* there are no distal venous thrombi. Late pulmonary embolism from missed vena caval injuries has not been recognized.

Control of infrahepatic venous injuries can usually be obtained by direct pressure above and below and clamping. Intraluminal Fogarty embolectomy catheters occasionally are helpful (Fig. 12-18). Larger vena caval injuries may require clamping above and below the injury for repair (Fig. 12-19).

RETROHEPATIC VENA CAVAL INJURY

Injury to the retrohepatic vena cava is almost always associated with significant blunt or penetrating hepatic trauma and with massive blood loss.

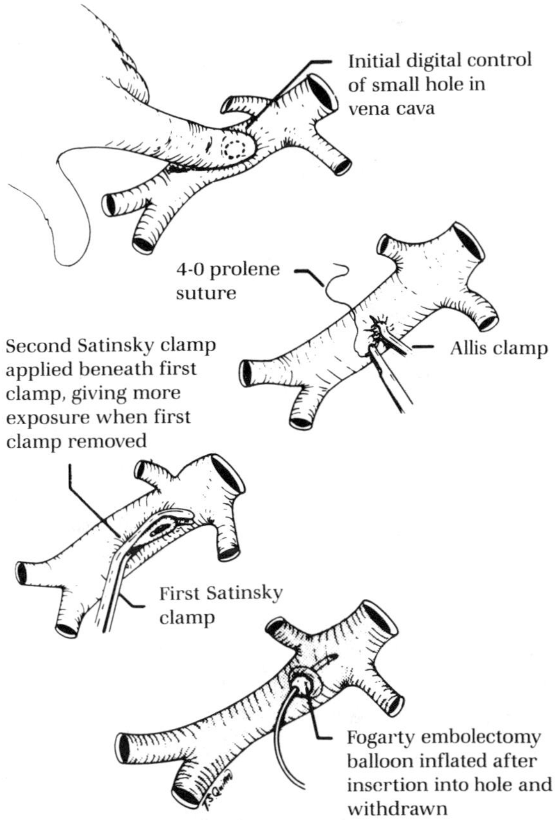

Fig. 12-18. Techniques of gaining control of infrahepatic vena caval injuries.

Diagnosis

During laparotomy and exploration of a deep anterior or posterior liver laceration, bleeding can usually be controlled by direct manual pressure. To control bleeding while exploring and repairing the liver injury, the portohepatic structures are manually compressed (the "Pringle maneuver"). Common bile duct, hepatic artery, and portal vein are all com-

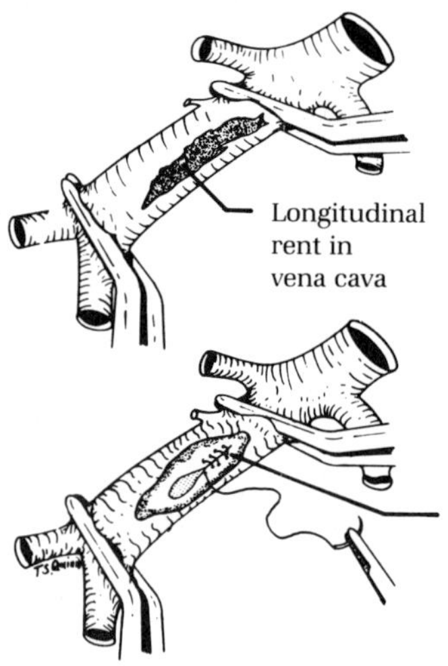

Fig. 12-19. Techniques of control and repair of larger vena caval injuries below liver.

pressed without dissecting out individual structures. If, despite the Pringle maneuver, one is greeted with massive dark blood obscuring the field, one should presume injury to the retrohepatic vena cava or hepatic veins.

Direct pressure will usually control hepatic vein bleeding while further exposure is gained. A midline abdominal incision may allow adequate exposure by mobilizing the right lobe of the liver from its diaphragmatic attachments, allowing exposure of the vena cava–hepatic vein junction from above. Further exposure can be obtained by extending the incision as a median sternotomy or with a right ninth interspace anterolateral thoracotomy excision.

If major vena cava–hepatic vein injury precludes exposure for repair, an internal caval shunt combined with a Pringle maneuver can provide a bloodless field to permit repair of the injury. The hypovolemic patient does not tolerate clamping the vena cava at the diaphragm, so several techniques of internal shunting to preserve venous return to the heart have been used. These include

1. A right atrial–caval shunt with tourniquet above the liver and between the liver and renal veins, as advocated by Shrock and coworkers [13] (Fig. 12-20)
2. A balloon-caval shunt introduced through the femoral vein into the groin, as advocated by Pilcher and colleagues [14] (Fig. 12-21)
3. Shunts introduced through the inferior vena cava with and without balloons

Pachter and associates [15] reviewed the reported experience with atriocaval shunts and found a 77-percent mortality in the past 15 years. They advocated steroids and topical hypothermia with a Pringle maneuver and finger fracture through the liver to the site of vascular injury for repair of the vena cava and hepatic veins. A mean portal triad occlusion time of 46 minutes was associated with survival of five consecutive patients with juxtahepatic venous injuries. In four of five patients with hepatic vein injuries, the hepatic veins were ligated.

With retrohepatic inferior vena caval or hepatic vein injury, temporary packing may be the appropriate treatment if the surgeon is not prepared to treat the injury definitively. In severe liver injuries involving such vessels, closure of the abdomen with such packs in place has been successful as definitive therapy, with removal of the packs several days later (5 days).

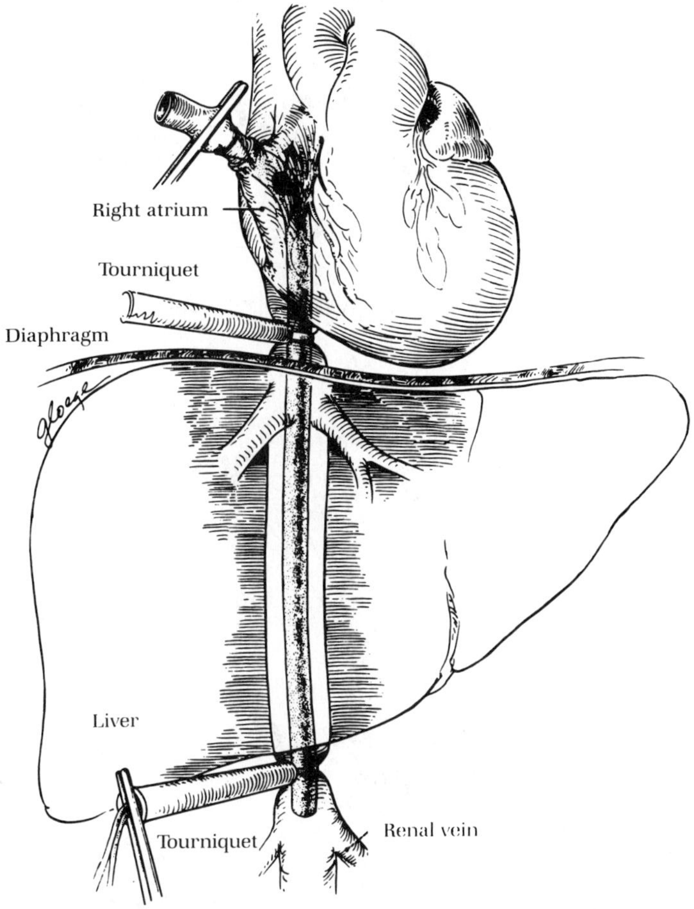

Fig. 12-20. A right atrial–vena caval shunt allows venous return while a retrohepatic vena caval laceration is isolated (together with occlusion of the portal vein and hepatic artery in the portal triad by a Pringle maneuver).

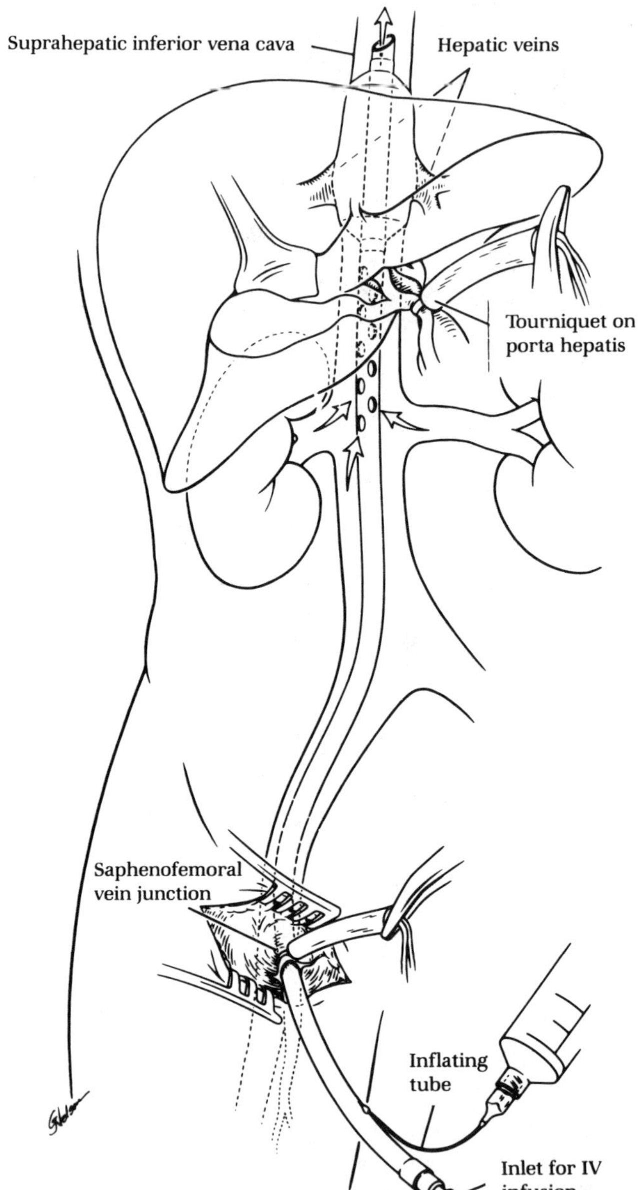

Fig. 12-21. A balloon-caval shunt introduced through the groin has benefits of the "Shrock shunt" from the groin without requiring opening the heart.

Vascular Trauma of the Extremities

Gerardo A. Gomez and Larry C. Martin

Despite the first reported arterial repair occurring in the eighteenth century, the technique of repair and use of autografts and homografts awaited the work of Carrel and Guthrie in the early twentieth century [1]. Military experience provided the bulk of published reports. Initially ligation and later amputation were the preferred treatment, with amputation rates of approximately 50 percent in World War II [2]. With more effective transportation, resuscitation, and antibiotics used during the Korean War, vascular repair and reconstruction became more feasible, and amputation rates were reduced to 13 percent [3]. More recent experience in Vietnam and in civilian practice has further reduced rates of amputations and subsequent functional limb salvage [4–6].

ARTERIAL INJURIES

Mechanism of Injury

Vascular injuries may occur from a variety of sources, including blunt and penetrating trauma. Blunt trauma usually results from crush injuries involving fractures and soft tissue damage, which complicates repair and recovery considerably. High-velocity gunshot wounds and shotgun blasts may also cause similar injuries. Penetrating trauma accounts for approximately 90 percent of vascular injuries, with gunshot wounds responsible for 55 to 75 percent in civilian series. Blunt trauma accounts for the remaining 10 percent [7,8].

Stab wounds often produce distinct localized arterial trauma, while gunshot wounds frequently cause widespread tissue destruction and neurovascular compromise most often due to blast effect or energy disposition. Shotgun wounds may be particularly destructive because the multiplicity of pellets present causes a wider area of injury. Often necrotic debris, clothing, and skin are carried deep into the tissues, which requires diligent debridement to prevent infection. Blunt trauma may cause vascular injury by traction, crushing blow, fractures, or dislocations.

The relative frequency of these injuries is shown in Table 12-1. The extent and location of the injury are the most important factors in determining the surgical approach to vascular injuries.

Initial Management and Diagnosis

Priority in management should always involve airway control and restoration of circulatory blood volume. Once this is accomplished, attention can be turned to any potential vascular injury. Bleeding is best controlled by direct pressure, as blind probing and clamping may cause further damage to neurovascular structures and dislodge clots, causing further bleeding. Once a vascular injury is documented, it should be repaired as soon as other more life-threatening problems have been dealt with (i.e., chest or abdominal injuries).

The majority of vascular injuries can be detected by an accurate history and physical examination [9]. The mechanism of injury can

Table 12-1. Anatomic Location of Vascular Injuries of the Extremities (percent)

Vessels	Drapanas [4]	Kelly [25]	Perry [8]	Feliciano [5]	Total
Axillary	7.7	2.3	10.7	8.6	7.3
Brachial	25.0	42.0	22.0	32.5	30.4
Forearm	29.5	14.8	27.4	12.5	21.1
Common femoral	4.5	19.3	3.1	6.7	8.4
Superficial femoral	19.9	8.0	26.3	19.2	18.4
Profunda femoris	—	3.4	2.3	6.7	4.1
Popliteal	9.0	6.8	4.8	11.7	8.1
Tibioperoneal	4.5	3.4	3.4	2.5	3.5

be very helpful, especially with blunt injuries. Physical examination is the best initial method of assessing the adequacy of distal perfusion. Pulses should be assessed for their presence and character and always compared with an uninjured extremity for any pulse deficit. Capillary refilling, extremity color, temperature, and neurologic status are helpful in assessing the degree of ischemia, as a loss of sensory function distally may be the first indicator that arterial flow is not adequate and that a significant degree of ischemia is present. The presence of an expanding hematoma, arterial bleeding, thrills, bruits, or proximity injury to a large vessel is suggestive of possible injury.

The presence of palpable distal pulses may be a misleading finding, as Drapanas and coworkers [4] found that 27.3 percent of 120 patients had pulses distal to a vascular injury. These findings in general were similar for both the upper and lower extremities, at 25 and 29 percent respectively. More than likely, this is a result of good collateral flow or an injury that has not resulted in complete occlusion of the vessel in question, such as intimal flaps or pseudoaneurysms. The fact that collateral circulation can provide adequate flow is demonstrated by a comparison of subclavian injuries where collateral circulation is good and popliteal injuries where there is little collateralization. Normal pulses could be found in 55 percent of subclavian injuries but only in 16 percent of popliteal injuries [10,11]. Physical findings alone have been found to be falsely positive in 42 percent and falsely negative in 20 percent [12]. Doppler studies may be useful in demonstrating the presence of flow distal to an injury, but again this may be due to the presence of collateral circulation. The involved as well as noninvolved extremities should be examined and Doppler pressures obtained. A systolic pressure above 30 to 50 mm Hg is usually adequate to maintain some degree of viability, and other major injuries may be addressed before revascularization. A pressure differential between the involved and noninvolved extremities of greater than 20 mm Hg has been used as an indication for arteriography [13]. While other noninvasive studies such as Duplex scans may be useful, to date arteriography continues to be the diagnostic procedure of choice to evaluate an extremity for potential vascular injury.

Arteriography

The overall value of arteriography lies not only in its accuracy in documenting the location and extent of a detected injury, but also in ruling out serious vascular injury with a normal study. In patients with obvious evidences of vascular injury, that is, expanding hematoma, bruit, thrill, or pulse deficit, arteriography is not usually necessary. However, in patients with equivocal physical findings, it has been shown to be accurate. Snyder and colleagues [14], in a landmark study on 183 penetrating extremity wounds using both arteriography and surgical exploration regardless of angiographic findings, reported 31 true-positive, 132 true-negative, 14 false-positive, and 1 false-negative arteriograms. The accuracy rate for angiography in detecting vascular injuries was 92 percent. Although there was a false-positive rate of 7.6 percent, it was significantly less than the 64-percent negative rate of Sirinek and associates [15] when routine exploration was employed.

Arteriography can be accomplished safely with minimal morbidity (approximately 0.4 percent) and no mortality, according to several large series [16–18]. However, the procedure may require considerable time, often in a remote area of the hospital, which may compromise the care of a critically injured patient. An alternative, using emergency department arteriography, has been described by O'Gorman and coworkers [19]. Using a technique of arterial puncture, dye injection, and anteroposterior radiography in the emergency department, excellent results have been reported. Routine use of this technique has resulted in detection of approximately 17 percent of injuries in arteriograms done for proximity injuries alone, with 13 percent requiring surgical correction. The use of arteriography for proximity injuries alone was evaluated by Gomez and colleagues [9]. They found that when studies were done for proximity, only without further evidence of vascular injury, the arteriogram was normal in 76 percent, 24 percent had arteriographic abnormalities that did not require surgery, and the one patient with a positive arteriogram actually had a negative exploration. The patients were hospitalized for 24 hours, and none developed evidence of vascular injury during this time; however, long-term follow-up was not provided. Based on these conflicting reports, routine arteriography should probably be done based on clinical judgment. Intraoperative arteriograms may be useful in patients requiring emergent surgery for other injuries and are certainly useful in the evaluation of vascular repairs and distal flow at the conclusion of vascular reconstruction [20].

A newer imaging technique, namely digital subtraction angiography (DSA), has been used recently [21,22]. Intra-arterial DSA is preferred because it decreases contrast loads and increases resolution and definition of suspected areas. Intravenous DSA has also been used in trauma; however, larger loads of contrast are required, and the definition may not be adequate to assess injuries accurately.

Arteriographic findings indicative of vascular injury include complete vessel occlusion, irregularity of the vessel wall, filling defects, premature venous filling, extravasation of contrast, or psuedoaneurysm.

Completion arteriography should be obtained to evaluate vascular reconstruction. In one particular study, 23 percent of reconstruction procedures revealed unsuspected technical errors; 79 percent of these were successfully revised prior to completion of the case [23].

The injection of contrast material should be just above the area in question if possible, and inflow occlusion with a vascular clamp or digital pressure will give better opacification on a single exposure. The volume of contrasts required will vary with the arterial bed being studied, approximately 20 ml in the axillary artery for adequate visualization of the brachial artery and 30 ml in the femoral artery for adequate visualization of the popliteal vessel to the ankle.

Management of Arterial Injuries

The type of arterial injury will depend on the mechanism of injury, and the specific type of injury will dictate the required repair or reconstruction. Lacerations and transections account for 50 and 40 percent of injuries, respectively, in both military [6,24] and civilian series [4,5,7,8,25]. The remainder are puncture wounds, AV fistulae, and contusions due to crush injury and blast effect of gunshot wounds, which may result in flaps and thrombosis.

The operative choices available include lateral suture, patch angioplasty, resection of the injured segment with either primary anastomosis or bypass graft, extra-anatomic bypass, or primary ligation. Each technique is useful in specific situations (Fig. 12-22).

Once adequately debrided, most repairs of peripheral arteries can be done using polypropylene suture in a continuous manner, although small vessels may need interrupted sutures to avoid narrowing of the lumen. Injuries requiring resection can be repaired primarily if adequate mobilization of both proximal and distal ends is adequate, which can be gained by division of small branches and provided that there is no tension on the anastomosis. Also, it is important to note that bony alignment has been obtained or taken into account to avoid change in tension once orthopedic injuries are addressed.

Small, low-velocity wounds may only require resection of a few millimeters of normal-appearing vessel, while those from high-velocity gunshot wounds or shotgun blast may require removal of 1 cm or more of vessel. Once this is accomplished, the interior at the proximal and distal ends should be closely inspected to ensure that no intimal injury is present that may promote platelet adherence and subsequent thrombosis.

The appropriate sequence of repair of venous, arterial, and bony injuries is of utmost importance. If there is adequate collateral flow to prevent severe ischemia, the sequence is of less importance, and probably the vein should be repaired first, but in the ischemic extremity, where arterial flow is inadequate, the highest priority should be paid to providing flow either by immediate arterial repair or, if not possible or convenient, by the use of a Silastic shunt [26]. This may allow time for repair of venous injuries or even stabilization of skeletal injuries before the final arterial repair

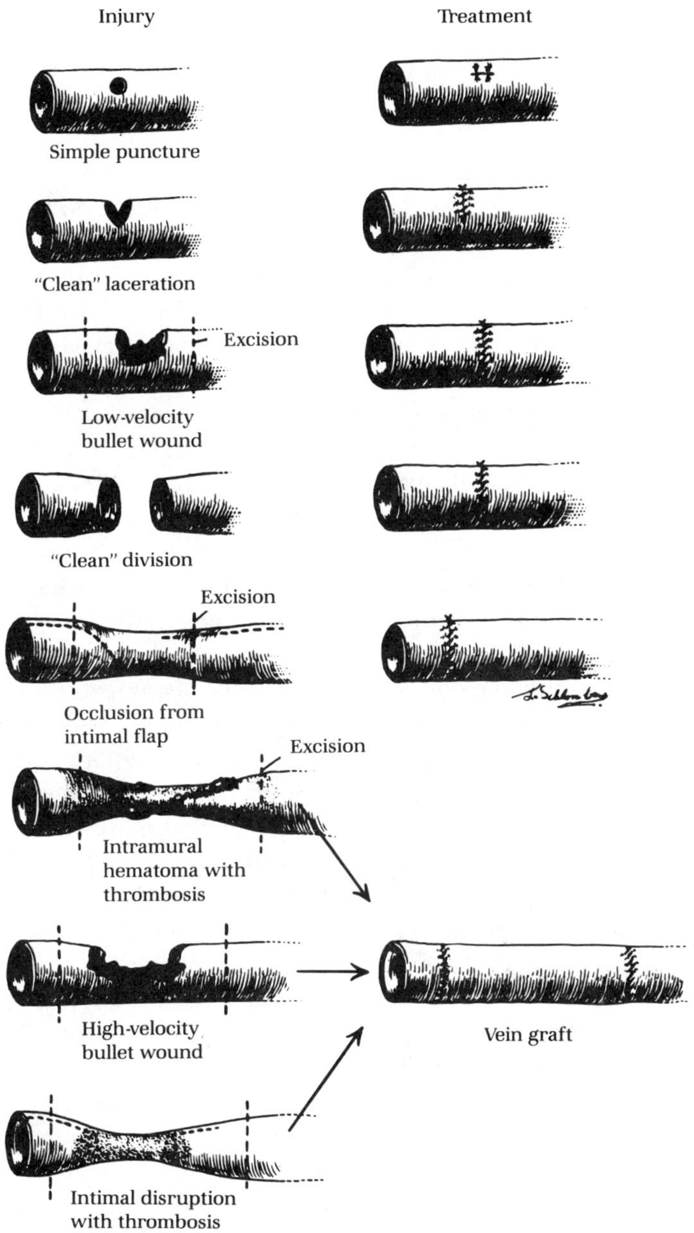

Fig. 12-22. Types of injuries and suggested repair. (From G.D. Zuidema, R.B. Rutherford, and W.F. Ballinger, *The Management of Trauma* [4th ed.]. Philadelphia: Saunders, 1985.)

is performed. It is important to prevent prolonged ischemia, as histologic changes appear by 4 to 6 hours and, by 12 hours, 90 percent of muscle fibers have lost contractility. This has been shown to affect the incidence of amputations directly [27]. If there is an associated venous injury and this is the sole source for venous outflow, resulting in significant venous hypertension, the venous repair should be accomplished prior to definitive arterial repairs. This will enhance outflow and success of arterial repair.

Stabilization of fractures should take secondary importance in the ischemic extremity, although the final alignment must be taken into account to prevent undue tension or kinking of the repaired vessel. In the nonischemic extremity with adequate collateral flow, it may be best to allow bony stabilization first if this does not interfere with the needed exposure for repair, as the concern is that an anastomosis done prior to stabilization may be disrupted during orthopedic manipulation. The best way to handle this problem is for the trauma surgeon to remain in attendance during manipulation of the extremity to prevent excessive movement and injury [11].

Following repair, adequate debridement must be accomplished to prevent necrotizing infection and subsequent disruption of vascular anastomosis. Large amounts of skin and muscle may need to be resected, resulting in lack of coverage of vascular repair, which may lead to disruption. In these patients, it is extremely important to use rotation muscle flaps to cover vascular grafts because a delay in coverage inevitably will lead to occlusion or delayed blowout of suture lines [7].

Technique of Repair

The type of injury and amount of required debridement will determine the repair. Small, clean lacerations from stab wounds or small puncture wounds are ideally suited for primary lateral repair. When narrowing of the lumen is anticipated, a vein patch can be used. In firearm wounds, the amount of tissue destruction often requires extensive debridement of injured vessels. When primary repair is not possible, an adequate vascular conduit is required. Saphenous vein continues to be the graft of choice. More recently, polytetrafluoroethylene (PTFE) grafts have been used, but not without some controversy.

The use of autogenous tissue in reconstruction of traumatic vascular injuries has gained widespread acceptance since it has been reported that approximately 77 percent of patients in whom prosthetic grafts were employed had graft failure due to infections and thrombosis, with 31 percent requiring subsequent amputation [28,29]. However, more recent experience has documented improved results using PTFE for reconstruction, even in contaminated wounds.

The most extensive study of PTFE in traumatic arterial injuries is that of Feliciano and coworkers [7]. They reported 206 arterial injuries over a 5-year period treated with PTFE interposition grafts. Major complications encountered included early occlusions in 12 patients, most commonly in the brachial artery where 4-mm grafts were used. Decreased flow through small grafts and through the collateral circulation was probably the cause of failure, leading to subsequent thrombosis; otherwise early occlusion was unusual. Blowout occurred in four grafts, related to exposure or infection in the area. Exposed grafts failed uniformly despite the use of porcine xenograft for coverage when soft tissue was not available. Unfortunately, only 18 percent of patients were available for long-term follow-up (25 months), and 29 percent of these had evidence of graft occlusion. However, this figure may represent a realistic approximation of late occlusion, as a major disadvantage of PTFE has been poor long-term patency, perhaps due to initial hyperplasia at the anastomosis, and lack of endothelialization. The benefits of using antiplatelet agents to prevent late occlusion is not clear as yet, with numerous reports both for and against their efficacy [30–33].

In conclusion, the saphenous vein seems to be the ideal substitute at the present time and should be used whenever possible, as both short-term and long-term results are better. However, there are specific circumstances in which prosthetic material may be indicated, and PTFE appears to be the best at present. These include absence of or an inadequate sized vein (not dilatable to >4 mm), a severely diseased vein, or a severely injured extremity where time for harvesting and utilization of a vein may cause unwarranted delays in other operative intervention. In these cases PTFE is an acceptable alternative with adequate results.

Once a material is selected for reconstruction or a vein harvested, preferably from the noninjured extremity to preserve venous outflow if a venous injury is also present and the vessel debrided adequately, preparation is made for repair. A Fogarty catheter should be passed distally to clear the vessel of any debris or clot and to irrigate with heparinized saline solution to prevent thrombosis during the repair. Systemic heparinization can be used in selected circumstances, but most surgeons are reluctant to anticoagulate a patient with extensive soft tissue injuries and potential for blood loss. If there is a size discrepancy between the graft and artery, then one or both can be spatulated to enlarge the anastomosis and prevent stenosis. The graft should be of appropriate length and sutured using 5-0 or 6-0 polypropylene suture in a continuous fashion (interrupted sutures may be necessary for smaller vessels). Prior to completion of the anastomosis, the graft is flushed to remove any debris to prevent distal embolization, and the distal clamp is taken off just to flush any air out of the system. Once this is accomplished, the sutures tied, and the proximal clamp removed, any anastomotic bleeding can usually be controlled with hemostasis agents, Gelfoam with thrombin or Avitene.

The distal circulation should be assessed immediately through a plastic bag used to exclude the hand or foot at the time of draping to see a return of peripheral pulse and color to the ischemic extremity. The adequacy of repair should be assessed by completion arteriogram intraoperatively on a routine basis and any inadequacy corrected at that time. The wound is irrigated with antibiotic solution and closed in layers. If covering of the graft is not feasible due to extensive tissue loss, a myocutaneous flap may be necessary to prevent graft exposure and subsequent complications. Patients are not usually kept on systematic anticoagulant following surgery, but the use of aspirin may be useful during the first postoperative month [33,34].

Upper Extremity Injuries

Upper extremity injuries include the axillary, brachial, radial, and ulnar arteries, making up approximately 40 percent of vascular injuries [4,6–9,25]. Penetrating trauma is the most common cause; less than 5 percent are the result of blunt trauma [35].

The incidence of amputation following arterial injury to the upper extremity varies according to which vessel is involved. During World War II, in which ligation was carried out in the majority of patients, the ratio was highest for axillary injuries (43 percent) and lowest for brachial injuries (26 percent), with forearm injuries responsible for approximately a 40-percent amputation rate [4]. By the time of the Vietnam War, the amputation rate for both brachial and axillary arterial injuries was reduced to approximately 5 percent due to improved casualty evacuation systems and more aggressive attempts at vascular repair [36]. This is consistent with recent reports of civilian experiences as well [4,8]. Long-term disability with these injuries is not uncommon, even after successful vascular reconstitution, due to the close proximity of major nerves of the brachial plexus and also the degree of soft tissue injury. Concomitant venous injury and subsequent ligation have little effect on the outcome because of the rich collateral pathways present.

Approximately 20 percent of patients with documented vascular injury will have normal pulses due to the extensive collateral network present in the upper extremity. In these patients, Doppler pressure examination of both extremities with a 20 mm Hg difference or greater may indicate the presence of a vascular injury [37]. If doubt exists, arteriography should be obtained.

Axillary Artery Injuries

The axillary artery begins as the subclavian artery passes beneath the first rib and continues to the inferior margin of the teres major muscle, where it becomes the brachial artery. It is divided into three portions by the pectoralis minor muscle and has several branches that form an extensive anastomotic network around the shoulder. The brachial plexus is in very close proximity to the artery, which explains the frequency of peripheral nerve injuries in association with axillary artery injuries.

DIAGNOSIS

The findings on physical examination in patients with axillary artery injuries are those of any other vascular injury, such as expanding hematoma or distal pulse deficit, but due to the rich collateral network around the shoulder, profound ischemia is rare and distal pulses may remain intact despite complete transactions of the vessel. Since the brachial plexus surrounds the axillary artery as it passes through the axilla, the presence of nerve deficit should be an indication for angiography. Digital subtraction angiography is useful in eliminating overlying bony structures that may obscure minor defects.

OPERATIVE MANAGEMENT

Repair of axillary artery injuries in general produces optimal results, although ligation can be performed in selected patients if repair is not possible or the patient's condition does not allow time for repair. The entire chest and arm should be included in the field, as well as provision made for harvesting a saphenous vein, as an interposition graft may be necessary.

The approach is through an axillary incision beginning below the midportion of the clavicle, through the axilla, and down the arm along the course of the artery (Fig. 12-23). It is best to have the arm in an abducted position and externally rotated to provide the best exposure. To gain adequate exposure, it may be necessary to divide the pectoral muscles near their insertions and reapproximate them later. If more proximal control is required, re-

Fig. 12-23. Surgical exposure of the axillary artery with subclavian artery exposure via resection of the clavicle. (From H. Haimovici, *Vascular Surgery* [2nd ed.]. Norwalk, Conn.: Appleton-Century-Crofts, 1984.)

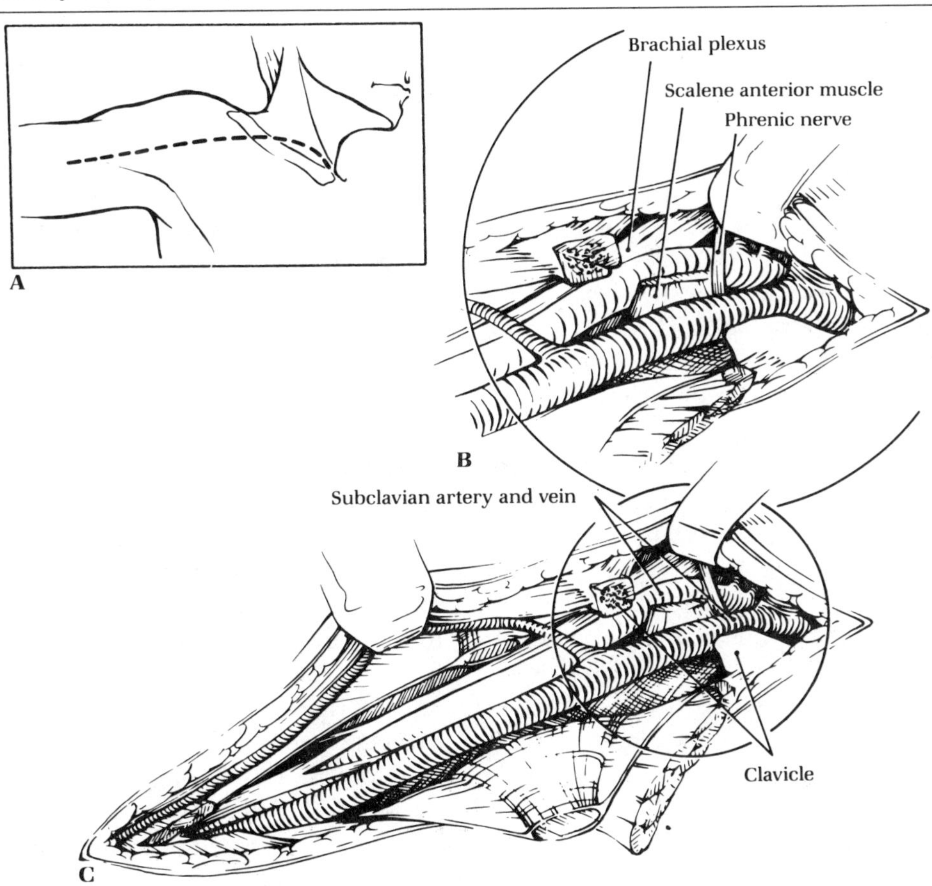

section of the clavicle and exposure of the subclavian artery may be necessary. The type of repair is dictated by the extent of injury, as previously described. If an interposition graft is required, either the saphenous vein or a 6-mm PTFE graft can be used as a conduit in this location. Once the repair is completed, distal pulses should be regained, and completion arteriography should be used liberally. Early and late results have been excellent [38]. Fasciotomy may occasionally be necessary in patients with severe combined arterial and venous injuries or, in rare cases, with prolonged ischemia.

Brachial Artery Injuries

The brachial artery is a continuation of the axillary artery, beginning at the teres major and extending distally to the bifurcation into the radial and ulnar arteries. The major branches include the deep brachial and superior and inferior ulnar collateral vessels. This is of importance in that occlusion of the brachial artery above the origin of the deep brachial doubles the amputation rate, as shown in World War II data when ligation proximal to this branch resulted in a 51-percent amputation rate as compared with 26 percent if ligation was distal to the deep brachial [24]. These amputation rates were similar for the Vietnam War if the vessels were ligated, but if repaired, the amputation rate fell to 5.7 percent [6]. These high rates of amputation in both wars were most likely due to the extent of soft tissue damage associated with bony involvement in the presence of a brachial arterial injury.

DIAGNOSIS

Diagnosis is usually made on the basis of physical examination, especially with more proximal injuries, as the extent of collateral circulation is less, leading to greater pulse difficulty. In questionable cases, Doppler pressure may be useful, as a 20 mm Hg or higher difference compared with the uninjured extremity may indicate the presence of an injury [37]. Arteriography is helpful in questionable cases and should be used aggressively.

OPERATIVE APPROACH

The brachial artery can be exposed by an incision along the medial aspect of the arm between the muscle bellies of the biceps and triceps. Distal control can be attained by directing this incision more laterally toward the midpart of the arm of the antecubital crease. Exposure of the vessel is not difficult, but care must be taken to protect the median nerve as it crosses the brachial artery from lateral to medial. Once adequate control is obtained, the same principles of vascular repair apply to the brachial artery as previously described. If an interposition graft is required, the autogenous vein is the conduit of choice, as PTFE used in this location has a high incidence of occlusion probably related to the size and extensive collateral flow that decreases flow through the graft [7]. If the vein is of small size, it can be spatulated to accommodate a longer artery. Prior to completion of the anastomosis, catheter thrombectomy distally is often beneficial to remove distal clots that may have formed during the repair. When carefully managed, excellent results can often be achieved, with amputation being an infrequent event [2].

Radial and Ulnar Arterial Injuries

Vascular injury in the forearm accounts for approximately 40 percent of upper extremity vascular injury and 20 percent of peripheral arterial injuries, most due to penetrating trauma [4,8].

During World War II, ligation of isolated radial or ulnar injuries resulted in amputation rates of 5.1 and 1.5 percent, respectively, but for combined injuries, this rose to almost 40 percent [24]. In a recent series of combat injuries to the upper extremity, the location most often associated with amputation was at the bifurcation of the brachial artery, which resulted in a 50-percent amputation rate (three of six patients) [38].

DIAGNOSIS

Due to extensive collateral flow through the palmar arch, distal pulses are often maintained after injury to only one of the forearm vessels. In the palmar arch the superficial and deep components are patent in 80 and 97 percent of extremities, respectively. Gelberman and associates [39] found that occlusion of one forearm vessel resulted in moderate ischemia but usually produced no symptoms. However, since the conditions of the palmar arch may not be known preoperatively, they recommend repair of these injuries to prevent potential sequelae. Due to the difficulty in making an accurate diagnosis by physical examination alone, arteriography is useful and should be used liberally to exclude pseudoaneurysm, AV fistulae, and intimal injuries that may result in late complications.

OPERATIVE MANAGEMENT

Exposure of the radial and ulnar vessels is by incision over the course of the vessel, usually not requiring extensive dissection, as they are located in a somewhat superficial position. In patients with adequate collateral flow with a patent palmar arch, a single vessel can often be ligated with little consequence. However, if the condition of the arch is unknown or there is extensive soft tissue damage that may cause interruption of collateral flow, then repair should be undertaken. This requires meticulous attention to detail to repair these small vessels successfully. The use of magnification, dilatation of the vessels, interrupted sutures, and spatulation of the anastomosis are helpful. In severe injuries, fasciotomy may be needed to prevent compartment syndrome and Volkmann's ischemic contracture. The results of one-vessel injuries are excellent, but when there is extensive soft tissue damage and both vessels are injured, the amputation rate as well as long-term morbidity can be substantial [38].

Lower Extremity Injuries

Lower extremity injuries are distal to the inguinal ligament and include the common femoral, superficial femoral, profunda femoris, popliteal, and distal tibioperoneal vessels. The majority of these injuries result from penetrating trauma, but approximately 15 percent are due to blunt trauma often associated with fractures or dislocations. Injuries to these vessels account for approximately one-half of peripheral vascular injuries [4,5,7,8,24,40].

Distal ischemia following injury to these vessels is the most pressing problem, with delays in therapy directly correlating with a poor outcome [26]. The signs and symptoms of vascular injury here are no different from elsewhere, and again arteriography can be helpful to exclude the presence of an injury in equivocal cases, particularly in finding minor abnormalities, such as intimal flaps, that may result in late morbidity, especially after blunt trauma, where injury is relatively common but initial findings may be minimal [41].

Overall, these injuries should be repaired, as experience with ligation has shown that overall amputation rates can be 70 to 80 percent for common femoral and popliteal wounds [24], but when repaired, this can be reduced significantly [42]. For vessels below the popliteal, this may not apply, and often repair of these vessels is not necessary if a single vessel remains intact to the foot.

Femoral Vessels

Injuries to the common femoral, superficial femoral, and profunda femoris vessels account for approximately 25 percent of all peripheral arterial injuries [4]. During World War II, most injuries were ligated, and amputation rates of 81 percent for common femoral and 55 percent for superficial femoral were reported [24]. However, when repair became the treatment of choice, amputation was reduced to approximately 15 percent [6] and in civilian series has been reduced to negligible levels [4,8]. Therefore, an aggressive approach to operative repair of these injuries should be attempted as the rule. The significance of profunda femoris injury has yet to be determined, but it seems that in patients with a normal superficial femoral artery and isolated injury to the profunda, ligation would be an acceptable alternative if the injury is complex or the patient has other more significant associated injuries.

DIAGNOSIS

With absent distal pulses and expanding hematoma or active arterial bleeding from a wound, the diagnosis is obvious. Arteriography, again, can be used for equivocal cases or where there have been changes in pulses distally before or after orthopedic manipulation, but arteriography should not delay surgery when there are signs of obvious ischemia.

OPERATIVE MANAGEMENT

Both lower extremities are exposed down to the feet, which should be covered with plastic bags to allow visual inspection and palpation of pulses. The contralateral leg is exposed to allow the saphenous vein to be available for potential harvest as a vein taken from the ipsilateral leg may compromise venous flow if there has been a concomitant venous injury.

The incisions are planned such that proximal and distal control can be obtained without entering the hematoma surrounding the injured vessel. This may involve a groin incision extending above the inguinal ligament, which can be divided and later reconstructed if necessary, or extension superiorly to the retroperitoneal iliac artery. The more distal superficial femoral artery can be exposed through a medial incision. Care should be taken to avoid injury to the saphenous vein and saphenous nerve. Control at the level of the femoral bifurcation requires control of the profunda femoris artery, which is deep to the superficial femoral artery. If control is difficult due to the extent of the injury, this can be obtained with balloon-tipped catheters placed proximally and distally. These injuries are repaired as previously described. If an interposition graft is required, the saphenous vein or PTFE graft can be used. It is best to perform a balloon thrombectomy prior to repair to remove any distal clots and to inject local heparin distally to maintain vessel patency while repair is in progress. Once repair is complete and flow reestablished, the distal pulses should be palpated, and completion arteriography should be performed. Any abnormality concerning the reconstruction should be corrected at this time.

It is best to assess the need for fasciotomy at the time of the initial procedure. Prolonged ischemia (>6–8 hours) or combined arterial and venous injury and extensive crushing injuries are obvious indications for fasciotomy. It is of utmost importance that these vascular wounds be covered with viable soft tissue, and all necrotic material should be adequately debrided prior to closure, as open exposed vascular grafts notoriously fail [7].

Popliteal Arterial Injuries

Popliteal arterial injuries account for 10 to 20 percent of vascular wounds in military and civilian series [6,24,36,43,44] with most injuries due to penetrating trauma, although in some series blunt trauma accounts for 50 percent of patients [45]. Amputation rates during World War II, when ligation was the most common approach, were as high as 72.5 percent [24]. During the Korean and Vietnam conflicts, when more aggressive attempts to repair were utilized, the amputation rate was 32.4 [3] and 29.5 percent [6], respectively. The amputation rate in civilian experience has been reported from 0 [42] to 40 percent [4,45], with a more recent series reporting 12.7 percent [44]. In almost all series, the amputation rate was directly related to the mechanism of injury, the lowest for stab wounds and the highest for those injuries secondary to blunt trauma [11,44,45]. Improved results have been reported for blunt injuries utilizing an aggressive approach to diagnosis and therapy. The incidence of popliteal injury in dislocation of the knee is approximately 30 percent [41], although incidence as high as 80 percent has been reported [4]. This is an especially challenging injury that requires a high index of suspicion and requires aggressive use of diagnostic arteriography followed by operative intervention, if indicated [46].

The major problems resulting from popliteal injury are the incidences of associated soft tissue skeletal and neurologic injury. The collateral flow around the knee may be interrupted or inadequate following injury, which leads to a high degree of ischemia and distal thrombosis. Early revascularization will prevent some of these sequelae, and fasciotomy prior to repair to facilitate collateral flow and flow after revascularization has been found to be beneficial in a series by Lim and colleagues [42] and Daugherty and associates [43]. In experimental animal studies where popliteal artery interruption was performed, extremity salvage was directly related to the ischemic time, being 96 percent after 6 hours but only 24 percent by 24 hours [47]. As Lim and colleagues [42] have shown, attention to detail and an aggressive approach can reduce the incidence of amputation associated with these injuries to an acceptable rate.

DIAGNOSIS

The signs and symptoms of injury to the popliteal artery are no different than those found for other arterial injuries. The extremity should be examined carefully, and in addition to the mechanism of injury, the findings will often lead to the correct diagnosis without elaborate tests or arteriography [44]. However, when these findings are equivocal, arteriography is very useful and may facilitate repair of injuries by allowing a preoperative plan of the surgical approach.

Diagnosis of vascular injury in patients with lower extremity fractures and dislocations may be difficult. Arteriography should be performed, especially with knee dislocation, where the incidence of vascular injury is in the range of 30 percent [46]. Arteriography is recommended for all patients with knee dislocation, in patients with displaced fractures in the knee area with circulatory deficits, even if normal pulses return after orthopedic reduction, and in patients with equivocal findings.

OPERATIVE MANAGEMENT

Both lower extremities should be included in the operative field for optimal exposure and to have the saphenous vein readily available from the contralateral limb. Popliteal exploration is best conducted through a medial incision, as this can be extended superiorly or inferiorly for additional exposure of the superficial femoral artery or tibioperoneal trunk.

Through the medial approach, proximal and distal control is obtained prior to entering the area of injury if possible (Fig. 12-24). Dissection of the popliteal artery is accomplished by displacing the semimembranosus posteriorly and dissecting between it and the adductor magnus muscle. The popliteal artery is usually the most medial structure, with the nerve and vein posterior and lateral. Distal exposure may require division of the medial head of the gastrocnemius and tendons of the semimembranosus and semitendinosus muscles. Care should be taken during the dissection to avoid injury to the saphenous nerve and vein as well as the delicate collateral vessels around the knee.

Once vascular control is obtained and the injury assessed, it is usually wise to proceed with distal thrombectomy to remove any distal clot that may have formed during the period of low flow. Systemic heparinization may be used, but with extensive soft tissue injury, this can result in increased bleeding. Rather, local heparinization can be used by injecting heparinized normal saline distally following thrombectomy. The injured vessel should be resected if there is any doubt as to the viability of the arterial wall. A primary anastomosis should be performed if it can be done without tension. When an interposition graft is required the saphenous vein should be used preferentially; however, PTFE of 6 mm size may be adequate. Completion arteriography should be performed to detect any technical defects at the anastomosis, distal thrombosis, or missed injuries. Patency of at least one tibial vessel will provide adequate perfusion in most patients.

At the conclusion of the procedure, consideration must be given to the need for fasciotomy if not already performed, since in up to half of the cases, fasciotomy has been found to be indicated [11].

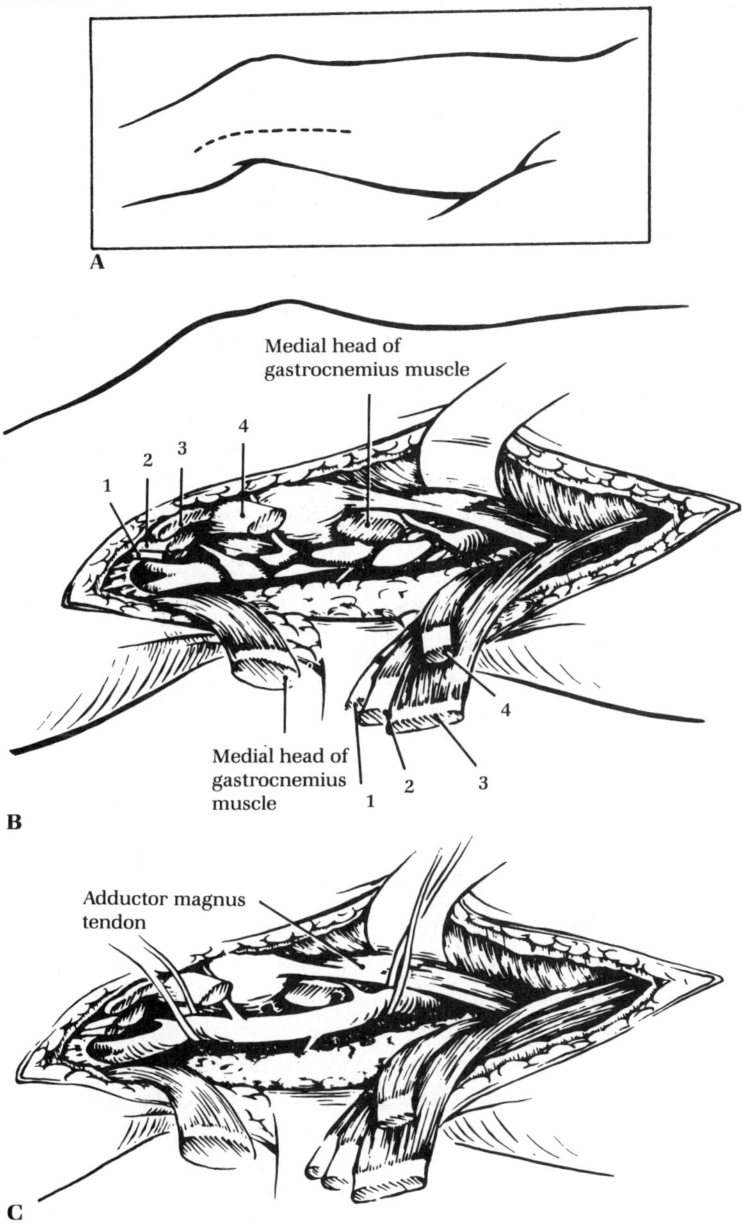

Fig. 12-24. Medial exposure of the popliteal artery. (From H. Haimovici, *Vascular Surgery* [2nd ed.]. Norwalk, Conn.: Appleton-Century-Crofts, 1984.)

In patients who have an associated skeletal injury, a decision must be made as to whether to stabilize the orthopedic injury or repair the arterial tree first. In general, it is best to proceed with arterial repair first if there is evidence of distal ischemia unless the skeleton is so unstable that adequate repair cannot be accomplished. In these patients, the use of an intraluminal shunt will provide distal flow while stabilization is obtained [26]. When vascular reconstruction is performed first, it is important for the surgeon to remain in attendance while orthopedic manipulation is done to ensure that there is no disruption of the repair. Recent experience with these difficult injuries has shown that attention to detail and meticulous technique with early revascularization can produce excellent results [46].

Injuries Below the Knee

Injuries below the knee are distal to the popliteal artery and involve the tibial vessels or peroneal artery, including injuries to the tibioperoneal trunk. They account for approximately 5 percent or less of civilian vascular injuries, although have been documented in up to 20 percent of military injuries [4,6,8,24,25,40]. The amputation rate following ligation of these vessels after injury is reported to be 13.5 percent for posterior tibial, 8.5 percent for anterior tibial, and 69 percent for combined injuries [24]. Despite the fact that soft tissue and bony injuries may have contributed a great deal to these results, this stresses the importance of diagnosis and therapy for these injuries.

DIAGNOSIS

Indications for arteriography and operative intervention in injuries below the knee are no different than for those in other locations, that is, distal ischemia, expanding hematoma, or arterial bleeding. Controversy has arisen in regard to how aggressively these injuries should be repaired when a single vessel is injured. In general, patency of at least one tibial vessel should be acceptable unless there is evidence of ischemia. When there are injuries to both tibial vessels, operative repair should be undertaken.

OPERATIVE APPROACH

Both lower extremities again should be included in the operative field for access to the saphenous vein from the contralateral leg. The proximal tibial vessels can be exposed through a medial vertical incision below the knee (Fig. 12-25) and the midportion of the tibial vessels exposed through a laterally placed incision at midleg and resection of a segment of the fibula (Fig. 12-26). If distal exposure is required, the posterior tibial can be found through a medially placed incision and the anterior tibial approached through a lateral incision between the distal tibial and extensor hallucis longus muscles. These repairs can be technically difficult due to the small size of the vessels, but in general repair in this location is performed as previously described. As with popliteal injuries, thrombectomy, local heparinization, and completion arteriography are recommended. Fasciotomy should be considered, especially with blunt crush injuries and in injuries where there is a de-

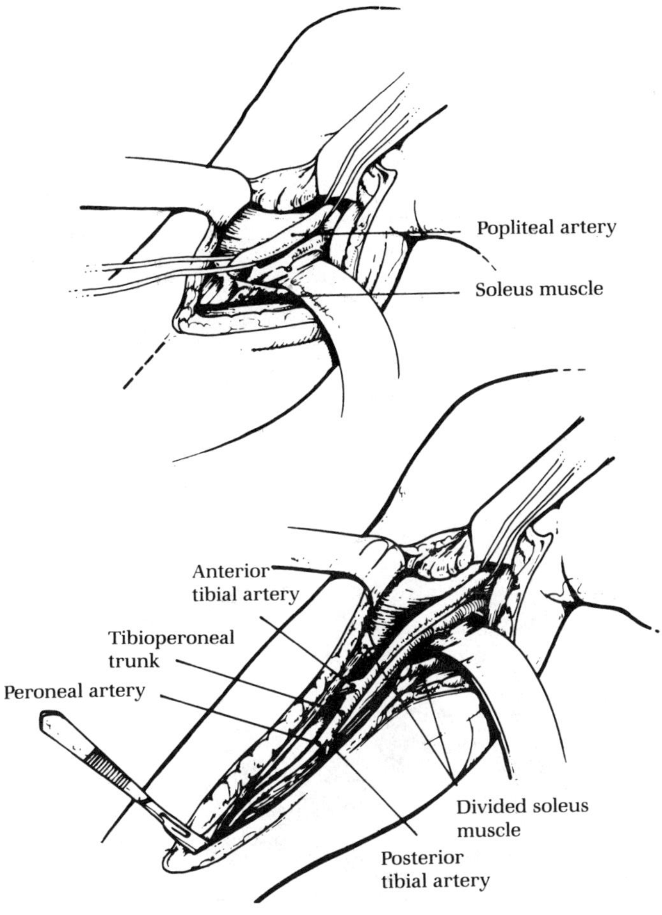

Fig. 12-25. Exposure of proximal tibial vessels. (From H. Haimovici, *Vascular Surgery* [2nd ed.]. Norwalk, Conn.: Appleton-Century-Crofts, 1984.)

lay in revascularization or intracompartmental bleeding. Skeletal stabilization and soft tissue coverage can often be a significant problem in this location but should be dealt with in a similar fashion as described for popliteal injuries.

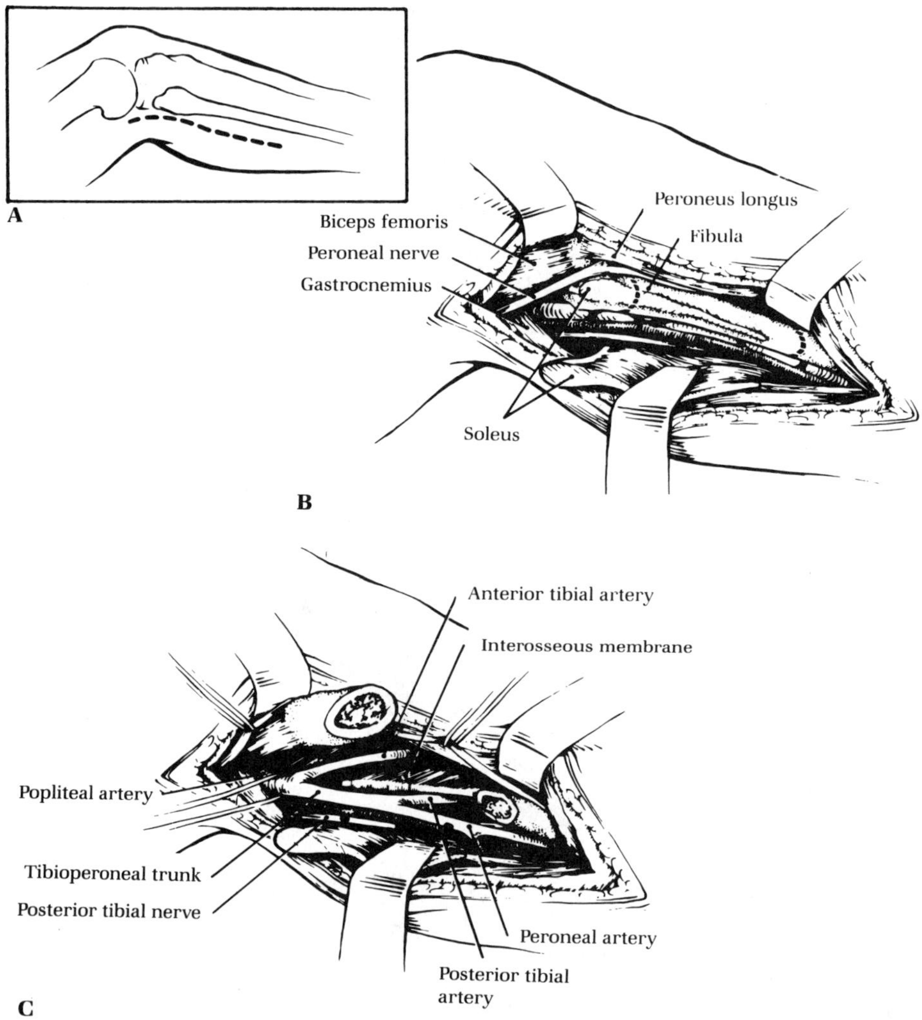

Fig. 12-26. Exposure of midposition of the tibial vessel via lateral incision. (From H. Haimovici, *Vascular Surgery* [2nd ed.]. Norwalk, Conn.: Appleton-Century-Crofts, 1984.)

VENOUS INJURIES

Schefa in 1882 first successfully repaired a venous laceration in a human by lateral repair, and Travers and Guthrie are credited with closing a small laceration of a vein in the nineteenth century [48]. However, routine venous repair was not common; in fact during World War I, ligation was the proposed treatment even if the vein was not injured. It was proposed that the vein be ligated if an injured artery required ligation [24]. This practice continued until World War II with poor results [24]. Repair of injured veins was more common during the Korean War, but it was not until the Vietnam War that repair of venous injuries was advocated [49].

The incidence of venous injury in victims in Vietnam was between 27 [50] and 38 percent [6], with repair in approximately one-third of patients. Presently repair of venous disruption is advocated in most locations if the patient is stable and without more significant associated injuries.

Incidence

Interest in venous injuries is relatively recent compared with that of arterial injuries. The first large series was reported in 1960 [51]. In this series, 22 percent of 228 patients with arterial injuries had associated venous injuries, the superficial femoral vein being the most frequently involved. The incidence of arterial injury associated with venous injury ranges from 93 percent with the superficial femoral vein to only 29 percent with the common femoral vein and in general occurs approximately 80 percent of the time [52]. The most common mechanisms of injury are gunshot wounds in 52 percent, stab wounds in 36 percent, blunt trauma in 7 percent, and shotgun wounds in 5 percent.

Diagnosis

Arterial injury will usually produce sufficient clinical findings to warrant further evaluation. The fact that arterial and venous injury occur concomitantly often allows detection of the venous problem. However, in the case of isolated venous injuries, noted to occur in 11 percent of cases by Perry and coworkers [8], diagnosis remains a problem and they may go undetected. As arteriography is used in detecting arterial injury, venography can be used in a similar fashion to document venous abnormalities [53]. Other noninvasive measures, such as venous Doppler studies [54] or Duplex scanning [55], may eventually be useful but at present have not been used widely for detection of venous injuries. Radionuclide scans offer no advantage over venography in detection of abnormalities. At present, only a high index of suspicion and frequent use of venography will result in detection and repair of the isolated venous injury, which fortunately is not a frequent occurrence.

Management of Venous Injuries

Initial management of venous injuries requires control of hemorrhage. Digital pressure or compression dressings will usually control venous bleeding and prevent air entry into the venous system with subsequent air embolism.

As arterial injuries are often present, some controversy may arise as to which injury should be repaired first. When the limb is not ischemic, early repair of the venous injury facilitates the arterial repair, or if the venous repair is easily accomplished, as with lateral suture, this should probably be done first. However, if there is any evidence of ischemia or that a prolonged repair would be necessary, then arterial repair should definitely be done prior to venous repair. Once adequately exposed, venous bleeding can be controlled with a proximal tourniquet, digital pressure, or atraumatic vascular clamps. Often partial occluding clamps can be used for lateral suture repairs.

Prior to attempting repair, all clots proximal and distal to the injury must be evacuated, which frequently can be done by milking the clot through the injured area. Debridement of any devitalization vessel as well as nonviable soft tissue should be done prior to any attempt at reconstruction.

Surgical options for control of venous injury are many, including ligation, lateral suture, primary resection and anastomosis, vein patches, venous autograft, and prosthetic graft to replace an injured venous segment. Very little controversy exists regarding the benefits of lateral suture over ligation, as most surgeons would recommend repair in this setting regardless of the location of the injury. However, venous repair can be very challenging and technically difficult, requiring great attention to detail [56]. More extensive repair and reconstructions should only be attempted if they will not jeopardize the patient's life or limb in the process.

For upper extremity veins, axillary or brachial ligation will very rarely result in compromised venous flow due to the extensive collateral network present [57]. The lower extremity presents a more complex problem. In a series by Mullins and colleagues [58], the incidence of postligation edema was low if a strict regimen of bed rest and elevation was followed. However, in a series by Rich and associates [59] involving popliteal injuries, the incidence of edema was reduced from 51 percent after ligation to 13 percent following repair. The previously alluded increased incidence of thrombophlebitis and pulmonary embolism has not been a major problem in those undergoing repair [57,59]. The stated objection to repair based on the premise that all eventually thrombosed has been somewhat refuted by Phifa [28], who showed patency of venous repairs by venography.

Feliciano and colleagues [7] have even used prostatic grafts in lower extremity venous injuries, since they seemed to diminish bleeding from soft tissue wounds and fasciotomy sites despite eventual occlusion. These grafts may allow time for collateralization and may contribute to increased arterial repair patency, as it has been shown that acute occlusion of the common femoral vein will reduce arterial flow by 50 to 75 percent [5,60].

Summary of Management

1. Upper extremity venous injury should be repaired if possible, but ligation usually will not result in long-term morbidity.
2. Lower extremity venous injuries should be repaired when possible, particularly superficial femoral and popliteal injuries.
3. Despite eventual thrombosis of some repairs, the time period of patency may reduce acute edema, decrease bleeding distally, and improve arterial patency, although many do appear to remain patent.
4. If ligation is necessary, a regimen of strict bed rest/elevation may prove beneficial and significantly reduce morbidity.
5. There does not seem to be any increased incidence of thrombophlebitis or pulmonary embolism following repair of venous injuries.

EXTREMITY COMPARTMENT SYNDROME AND FASCIOTOMY

Compartment syndrome is a condition in which high pressure within a closed fascial space reduces capillary blood perfusion below a line necessary for tissue viability [61]. In relation to the injured extremity, compartment syndrome can result from prolonged ischemia due to arterial injury and reperfusion, extensive soft tissue injury, or fractures with resultant hemorrhage.

Regardless of the type of injury, the pathophysiology and common outcome are the same, involving increased interstitial edema and ultimate disruption of the microcirculation, which may compromise tissue perfusion sufficiently to cause muscle ischemia and possible infarction.

Etiology and Diagnosis

The most frequent causes of compartment syndrome are fractures (the majority being fractures of the tibia), acute arterial occlusion, and soft tissue injuries. Compartment syndrome in these circumstances may result from constructive dressings and casts in which elevation of the extremity may further compound the ischemic changes by reducing arterial flow.

The diagnosis of compartment syndrome is often dependent on the demonstrations of functional and sensory loss, although pain is usually the first noted symptom. Often the only physical finding present is a swollen and tense compartment. The presence of pulses distal to the area of involvement is the *usual finding*, since this syndrome affects the microcirculation rather than the macrocirculation.

Further diagnostic maneuvers include measurement of intracompartmental pressures. The methods employed include the infusion technique, Wick catheters, and the solid-state transducer catheter. Although most compartment syndromes can be diagnosed clinically, these techniques are particularly useful when dealing with unresponsive or uncooperative patients. The internal pressure at which muscle ischemia necrosis may occur is controversial, but levels of 30 to 40 mm Hg are considered indications for fasciotomy [61]. At this point, any other therapy, such as elevation, may actively diminish capillary blood flow to the extremity.

Fasciotomy

Upper Extremity

The forearm consists of two major compartments—volar and dorsal. The median nerve is found in the volar compartment, as is the ulnar nerve, artery, and vein as well as the radial nerve, artery, and vein. The dorsal compartment contains the posterior interosseous nerve, a branch of the radial nerve.

The volar compartment can be opened by a single long incision from the area just proximal to the antecubital fossa, extending distally to the midpalm, including release of the carpal tunnel at the wrist. The dorsal compartment is usually opened through a long incision the length of the forearm and subsequently through the dorsal fascia. Once the fascia compartments are opened, nonviable muscle should be debrided, although questioned tissue should be left intact, as some reperfusion may salvage this tissue. However, the wounds must be inspected on a regular basis and debrided postoperatively and left open with a bulky dressing applied as necessary. These wounds may be able to be closed secondarily at a later time or skin grafted.

Lower Extremity

There are four compartments of the leg, consisting of the anterior and lateral compartments—anterior to the interosseous membrane—and the superficial and deep posterior compartments—posterior to the interosseous membrane. The nerves run through each compartment, including the deep peroneal nerve in the anterior compartment, the superficial peroneal in the lateral compartment, the tibial in the deep posterior compartment, and the sural nerve in the superficial posterior compartment. Sensory deficits along any of these nerves may give some indication as to which compartment is involved.

The anterior and lateral compartments are best exposed through a lateral incision, avoiding injury to the superficial peroneal nerve. The incision is begun distal to the fibula head extending to just above the ankle. The anterior and lateral fascia must be opened separately through the length of the incision for adequate decompression. The superficial and deep posterior compartments are decompressed using a medial incision, just posterior to the tibia. By incising the fascia of the soleus, the deep posterior compartment is exposed, and in so doing this fascia is likewise incised along the course of the incision. Once four-compartment decompression is accomplished, any necrotic muscle is debrided, wounds left open with packing. Any questionable muscle should be left intact and may recover following establishment of blood flow. Other techniques of lower extremity decompression involve single lateral incisions and fibulectomy, but these are probably no more effective than the medial and lateral incisions with direct division of the fascia that are described.

The concept of prophylactic fasciotomy has decreased in importance somewhat due to the frequent use of measured compartment pressures to assess the presence of a compartment syndrome. However, this should be considered when the ischemic time has been prolonged, exceeding 6 hours, or when there are combined arterial and venous injuries.

Following completion of fasciotomy, reperfusion of the extremity may result in myoglobinemia and subsequent renal insufficiency. It is imperative to maintain adequate hydration, perhaps with the use of mannitol to maintain adequate blood flow to the kidneys. Inspection of the fasciotomy sites on a routine basis is also imperative to be sure that all necrotic muscle is debrided and infection has not become a problem.

REFERENCES

Cervical Vascular Trauma

1. Garrison, E. H. *History of Medicine*. Philadelphia: Saunders, 1929.
2. Rich, N., and Spencer, F. C. Carotid and Vertebral Artery Injuries. In N. Rich and F. C. Spencer (eds.), *Vascular Trauma*. Philadelphia: Saunders, 1978.
3. Fogelman, J. J., and Stewart, R. D. Penetrating wounds of the neck. *Am. J. Surg.* 91:581, 1956.
4. Yamada, S., Kindt, G. W., and Youmans, J. R. J. Carotid artery occlusion due to nonpenetrating injury. *J. Trauma* 7:333, 1967.
5. Saletta, J. D., Lowe, R. J., Lim, L. T., et al. Pene-

trating trauma of the neck. *J. Trauma* 16:579, 1976.
6. Fry, R. E., and Fry, W. F. Extracranial carotid artery injuries. *Surgery* 88:581, 1980.
7. Davidson, K. C., Welford, E. D., and Dixon, G. D. Traumatic vertebral artery pseudoaneurysm following chiropractic manipulation. *Radiology* 115:651, 1975.
8. Edwards, W. H., and Mulherin, J. L. The surgical approach to significant stenosis of vertebral and subclavian arteries. *Surgery* 87:20, 1980.
9. Golueke, P., Sclafanis, Phillips T., et al. Vertebral artery injury: Diagnosis and management. *J. Trauma* 27:856, 1987.
10. Berguer, R. Distal vertebral artery bypass: Technique, "the occipital connection," and potential uses. *J. Vasc. Surg.* 2:621, 1985.

Thoracic Vascular Trauma

1. Feliciano, D. V., Bitondo, C. G., Mattox, K. L., et al. Civilian trauma in the 1980s: A one-year experience with 456 vascular and cardiac injuries. *Ann. Surg.* 199:717, 1984.
2. Baldwin, J. C., Oyer, P. E., Guthaner, D. F., and Stinson, E. B. Combined azygous vein and subclavian artery injury in blunt chest trauma. *J. Trauma* 24:170, 1984.
3. Sherani, T. M., Fitzpatrick, G. J., Phelan, D. M., et al. Ruptured azygous vein due to blunt chest trauma. *Br. J. Surg.* 73:885, 1986.
4. DiMarco, R. F., Layton, T. R., Manzetti, G. W., and Pellegrini, R. V. Blunt traumatic rupture of the right atrium and the right superior pulmonary vein. *J. Trauma* 23:353, 1983.
5. Dillon, W. P., Taylor, A. T., Mineau, D. E., and Datz, F. L. Traumatic pulmonary artery pseudoaneurysm simulating pulmonary embolism. *A.J.R.* 139:818, 1982.
6. Rosen, P., and Murphy, M. F. Thoracic vascular pathologies. *Emerg. Med. Clin. North Am.* 1:417, 1983.
7. Richardson, J. D., Flint, L. M., Snow, N. J., et al. Management of transmediastinal gun-shot wounds. *Surgery* 90:671, 1981.
8. Gundry, S. R., Williams, S., Burney, R. E., et al. Indications for aortography in blunt thoracic trauma: A reassessment. *J. Trauma* 22:664, 1982.
9. Albers, J. E., Rath, R. K., Glaser, R. S., and Poddar, P. K. Severity of intra-thoracic injuries associated with first rib fractures. *Ann. Thorac. Surg.* 33:614, 1982.
10. Gardner, M. A., and Bidstrup, B. P. Intra-thoracic great vessel injury resulting from blunt chest trauma associated with posterior dislocation of the sternoclavicular joint. *Aust. N.Z. J. Surg.* 53:427, 1983.
11. Gaines, T., Cavanaugh, D. G., and Butler, J. Traumatic avulsion of the inferior vena cava from the right atrium: Case report. *Milit. Med.* 148:48, 1983.
12. Schwab, C. W., Lawson, R. B., Lind, J. F., and Garland, L. W. Aortic injury: Comparison of supine and upright portable chest films to evaluate the widened mediastinum. *Ann. Emerg. Med* 13:896, 1984.
13. Marnocha, K. E., and Maglinte, D. D. Plain-film criteria for excluding aortic rupture in blunt chest trauma. *A.J.R.* 144:19, 1985.
14. Barcia, T. C., and Livoni, J. P. Indications for angiography in blunt thoracic trauma. *Radiology* 147:15, 1983.
15. Faro, R. S., Monson, D. O., Weinberg, M., and Javid, H. Disruption of aortic arch branches due to non-penetrating chest trauma. *Arch. Surg.* 118:1333, 1986.
16. Dula, D. J., Hughes, H. G., and Majernick, T. Traumatic disruption of the brachiocephalic artery. *Ann. Emerg. Med.* 12:639, 1983.
17. Cole, D. C., Knopp, R., Wales, L. R., and Morishima, M. S. Nasogastric tube displacement to the right as a sign of acute traumatic rupture of the thoracic aorta. *Ann. Emerg. Med.* 10:623, 1981.
18. Richardson, J. D., and Flint, L. M. Cervicomediastinal injuries following blunt trauma. *Am. Surg.* 48:141, 1982.
19. Harley, D. P., and Mena, I. Cardiac and vascular sequelae of sternal fractures. *J. Trauma* 26:553, 1986.
20. Galbut, D. L., and Bolooki, H. Surgery of descending aorta: A method of autotransfusion and intercostal artery preservation. *Chest* 82:590, 1982.
21. Goodman, G., Palatianos, G. M., and Bolooki, H. Technique of closure of median sternotomy with trans-sternal figure-of-eight wires. *J. Cardiovasc. Surg.* (Torino) 27:512, 1986.

Abdominal Vascular Trauma

1. Veith, F. J., Gupta, S., and Daley, V. Technique for occluding the supraceliac aorta through the abdomen. *Surg. Gynecol. Obstet.* 151:426, 1980.
2. Mattox, K. L., McCollum, W. B., Beall, A. C., Jr., et al. Management of penetrating injuries of the suprarenal aorta. *J. Trauma* 15:808, 1975.
3. Buscaglia, L. C., Blaisdell, F. W., and Lim, R. C., Jr. Penetrating abdominal vascular injuries. *Arch. Surg.* 99:764, 1969.
4. Soldano, S. L., Rich, N. M., Collins, G. J., et al. Long-term follow-up of penetrating abdominal aortic injuries. *J. Trauma,* in press.
5. Clark, D. E., Georgitis, J. W., and Ray, F. S. Renal arterial injuries caused by blunt trauma. *Surgery* 90:87, 1981.
6. Goldstein, A. S., Sclafani, S. J. A., Kupferstein, N. H., et al. The diagnostic superiority of computerized tomography. *J. Trauma* 25:938, 1985.
7. Morton, J. R., and Crawford, E. S. Bilateral traumatic renal artery thrombosis. *Ann. Surg.* 176:62, 1972.
8. Graham, J. M., Mattox, K. L., Beall, A. C., et al. Injuries to the visceral arteries. *Surgery* 84:835, 1978.
9. Sirinek, K. R., and Levine, B. A. Traumatic injury to the proximal superior mesenteric vessels. *Surgery* 98:831, 1985.
10. Lucas, C. E., and Ledgerwood, A. M. Liver necrosis following hepatic artery transsection due to trauma. *Arch. Surg.* 113:1107, 1978.
11. Sheldon, G. F., Lim, R. C., Yee, E. S., and Petersen, S. R. Management of injuries to the porta hepatics. *Ann. Surg.* 202:539, 1985.
12. Pachter, H. L., Drager, S., Godfreg, N., and LeFleur, R. Traumatic injuries of the portal vein: The role of acute ligation. *Ann. Surg.* 189:383, 1979.
13. Shrock, T., Blaisdell, F. W., and Mathewson, C. Management of blunt trauma to the liver and hepatic veins. *Arch. Surg.* 96:698, 1968.
14. Pilcher, D. B., Harman, P. K., and Moore, E. E., Jr. Retrohepatic vena cava balloon shunt introduced via the saphenofemoral junction. *J. Trauma* 17:837, 1977.
15. Pachter, H. L., Spencer, F. C., Hofstetter, S. R., et al. The management of juxtahepatic venous injuries without an atriocaval shunt: Preliminary clinical observations. *Surgery* 99:569, 1985.

Vascular Trauma of the Extremities

1. Rich, N. M., and Hughes, C. W. The fate of prosthetic material used to repair vascular injuries in contaminated wounds. *J. Trauma* 12:459, 1979.
2. Borman, K. R., Snyder, W. H., and Weigelt, J. A. Civilian arterial trauma of the upper extremity: An 11 year experience with 267 patients. *Am. J. Surg.* 148:796, 1984.
3. Hughes, C. W. Arterial repair during the Korean War. *Ann. Surg.* 147:555, 1958.
4. Drapanas, T., Hewitt, R. L., Weichert, R. F., and Smith, A. D. Civilian vascular injuries: A critical appraisal of three decades of management. *Ann. Surg.* 172:351, 1970.
5. Feliciano, D. V., Bitondo, C. G., Mattox, K. L., et al. Civilian trauma in the 1980's. *Ann. Surg.* 199:717, 1984.
6. Rich, N. M., Baugh, J. H., and Hughes, C. W. Acute arterial injuries in Vietnam: 1,000 cases. *J. Trauma* 10:359, 1970.
7. Feliciano, D. V., Mattox, K. L., Graham, J. M., and Bitondo, C. G. Five-year experience with PTFE grafts in vascular wounds. *J. Trauma* 25:71, 1985.
8. Perry, M. O., Thal, E. R., and Shires, T. G. Management of arterial injuries. *Ann. Surg.* 173:403, 1971.
9. Gomez, G. A., Kreis, D. J., Jr., Ratner, L., et al. Suspected vascular trauma of the extremities: The role of angiography in proximity injuries. *J. Trauma* 26:1005, 1986.
10. Flint, L. M., Snyder, W. H., Perry, M. O., and Shires, G. T. Management of major vascular injuries in the base of the neck: An 11 year experience with 146 cases. *Arch. Surg.* 106:407, 1973.
11. Snyder, W. H., III, Watkins, W. L., Whiddon, L. L., and Bone, G. E. Civilian popliteal artery trauma: An eleven year experience with 83 injuries. *Surgery* 85:101, 1979.
12. McCormick, T. M., and Burch, B. H. Routine angiographic evaluation of neck and extremity injuries. *J. Trauma* 19:384, 1979.
13. Bergan, J. J., and Yao, J. S. T. *Vascular Surgical Emergencies.* Orlando, Florida: Grune & Stratton, 1987. Pp. 103–111.
14. Snyder, W. H., Thal, E. R., Bridges, R. A., et al. The validity of normal arteriography in penetrating trauma. *Arch. Surg.* 113:424, 1978.
15. Sirinek, K. R., Levine, B. A., Gaskill, H. V., and

Root, H. D. Reassessment of the role of routine operative exploration in vascular trauma. *J. Trauma* 21:339, 1981.
16. Geuder, J. W., Hobson, R. W., Padberg, F. T., et al. The role of contrast arteriography in suspected arterial injuries of the extremities. *Am. Surg.* 51:89, 1985.
17. Lang, E. K. Prevention and treatment of complications following arteriography. *Radiology* 88:950, 1968.
18. Smith, R. F., Elliott, J. P., Hageman, W. H., et al. Acute penetrating arterial injuries of the neck and limbs. *Arch. Surg.* 109:198, 1974.
19. O'Gorman, R. B., Felician, D. V., Bitondo, C. G., et al. Emergency center arteriography in the evaluation of suspected peripheral vascular injuries. *Arch. Surg.* 119:568, 1984.
20. Lumpkin, M. B., Logan, W. D., Couves, L. M., and Howard, J. M. Arteriography as an aid in the diagnosis and localization of acute arterial injuries. *Ann. Surg.* 147:353, 1958.
21. Davis, P. C., and Hoffman, J. C. Work in progress. Intraarterial digital subtraction angiography: Evaluation of 150 patients. *Radiology* 148:9, 1983.
22. Weinstein, M. A., Pavlicek, W. A., Modic, M. T., et al. Intra-arterial digital subtraction angiography of the head and neck. *Radiology* 147:717, 1983.
23. Plecha, F. R., and Pories, W. J. Intraoperative angiography in the immediate assessment of arterial reconstruction. *Arch. Surg.* 105:902, 1972.
24. DeBakey, M. E., and Simeone, F. A. Battle injuries of the arteries in World War II. *Ann. Surg.* 123:534, 1946.
25. Kelly, G. L., and Eiseman, B. Civilian vascular injuries. *J. Trauma* 15:507, 1975.
26. Eger, M., Goldman, L., Goldstein, A., and Hirsh, M. The use of temporary shunt in the management of arterial vascular injuries. *Surg. Gynecol. Obstet.* 132:67, 1971.
27. Cohen, A., Baldwin, J. N., and Grant, R. N. Problems in the management of battlefield vascular injuries. *Am. J. Surg.* 118:526, 1969.
28. Bergan, J. J., and Yao, J. S. T. *Vascular Surgical Emergencies.* Orlando, Florida: Grune & Stratton, 1987. Pp. 179–189.
29. Bergan, J. J., and Yao, J. S. T. *Vascular Surgical Emergencies.* Orlando, Florida: Grune & Stratton, 1987. Pp. 191–202.
30. Carson, S., Demling, R., Esquivel, C., et al. Testing and treatment of arterial graft thrombosis. *Am. J. Surg.* 142:137, 1981.
31. Claus, P. L., Gloviczki, P., Hollier, L. H., et al. Patency of polytetrafluoroethylene microarterial prostheses improved by ibuprofen. *Am. J. Surg.* 144:180, 1982.
32. Hagen, P. O., Wang, Z. G., Mikat, E. M., et al. Antiplatelet therapy reduces aortic intimal hyperplasia distal to small diameter vascular prostheses (PTFE) in nonhuman primates. *Ann. Surg.* 195:328, 1982.
33. Oblath, R. W., Buckley, F. O., Jr., Green, R. M., et al. Prevention of platelet aggregation and adherence to prosthetic vascular grafts by aspirin and dipyridamole. *Surgery* 84:37, 1978.
34. Richter, R. C. Antiplatelet therapy in surgery. *Infect. Surg.* 3:137, 1984.
35. Sitzman, J. V., and Ernst, C. B. Management of arm arterial injuries. *Surgery* 96:895, 1984.
36. Rich, N. M., Baugh, J. H., and Hughes, C. W. Popliteal artery injury in Vietnam. *Am. J. Surg.* 118:531, 1969.
37. Tuzzeo, S., Saad, S. A., Hastings, O. M., et al. Management of brachial artery injuries. *Surg. Gynecol. Obstet.* 146:21, 1978.
38. Adar, R., Schramek, A., Khodadadi, J., et al. Arterial combat injuries of the upper extremity. *J. Trauma* 20:297, 1980.
39. Gelberman, R. H., Blasingame, J. P., Fronck, A., and Dimick, M. P. Forearm arterial injuries. *J. Hand Surg.* 4:401, 1979.
40. Rich, N. M. Vascular trauma. *Surg. Clin. North Am.* 53:1367, 1973.
41. Welling, R. E., Kakkasseril, J., and Cranley, J. J. Complete dislocation of the knee with popliteal vascular injury. *J. Trauma* 21:450, 1981.
42. Lim, L. T., Michuda, M. S., Flanigan, D. P., and Pankovich, A. Popliteal artery trauma. *Arch. Surg.* 115:1307, 1980.
43. Daugherty, M. E., Sachatello, C. R., and Ernst, C. B. Improved treatment of popliteal arterial injuries. *Arch. Surg.* 113:1317, 1978.
44. Snyder, W. H. Vascular injuries near the knee: An updated series and overview of the problem. *Surgery* 91:502, 1982.
45. Conkle, D. M., Richie, R. E., Sawyer, J. L., and Scott, H. W. Surgical treatment of popliteal artery injuries. *Arch. Surg.* 110:1351, 1975.
46. Shah, D. M., Naraynsingh, V., Leather, R. P., et al.

Advances in the management of acute popliteal vascular blunt injuries. *J. Trauma* 25:793, 1985.
47. Milier, H. H., and Welch, C. S. Quantitative studies on the time factor in arterial injuries. *Ann. Surg.* 130:428, 1949.
48. Bergan, J. J., and Yao, J. S. T. *Vascular Surgical Emergencies.* Orlando, Florida: Grune & Stratton, 1987. Pp. 441–449.
49. Rich, N. M., Hobson, R. W., and Wright, C. B. Repair of lower extremity venous trauma: A more aggressive approach required. *J. Trauma* 14:639, 1974.
50. Rich, N. M., and Hughes, C. W. Vietnam vascular registry: A preliminary report. *Surgery* 62:218, 1969.
51. Gaspar, M. R., Treiman, R. L., Payne, J. H., et al. Principles of treatment and special problems in vascular trauma. *Surg. Clin. North Am.* 48:1355, 1968.
52. Agarwal, N., Shah, P. M., Clauss, R. H., et al. Experience with 115 civilian venous injuries. *J. Trauma* 22:827, 1982.
53. Gerlock, A. J., Thal, E. R., Snyder, W. H., III. Venography in penetrating injuries of the extremities. *Am. J. Roentgenol.* 126:1023, 1976.
54. Strandness, D. E., Jr. Echo-Doppler (duplex) ultrasonic scanning. *J. Vasc. Surg.* 2:341, 1985.
55. Sumner, D. S. Doppler Evaluation of the Venous Circulation. In R. B. Rutherford (ed.), *Vascular Surgery* (2nd ed.). Philadelphia: Saunders, 1985. P. 185.
56. Hobson, R. W., II, Reynolds, D. G., and Swan, K. G. (eds.). *Venous Surgery in the Lower Extremities.* St. Louis: Warren H. Green, 1975.
57. Rich, N. M., Hughes, C. S., and Baugh, J. H. Management of venous injuries. *Ann. Surg.* 171:724, 1970.
58. Mullins, R. J., Lucas, C. E., and Ledgerwood, A. M. The natural history following venous ligation for civilian injuries. *J. Trauma* 20:737, 1980.
59. Rich, N. M., Hobson, R. W., Collins, G. J., Jr., and Anderson, C. A. The effect of acute popliteal venous interruption. *Ann. Surg.* 183:365, 1976.
60. Barcia, P. J., Nelson, T. G., and Whelan, T. J., Jr. Importance of venous occlusion in arterial repair failure: An experimental study. *Ann. Surg.* 175:223, 1972.
61. Mubarek, S. T., and Hargens, A. R. Acute compartment syndrome. *Surg. Clin. North Am.* 63:539, 1983.

13
Orthopedic Trauma

Gregory A. Zych

It has been estimated that annually 25 percent of the population of the United States sustain significant musculoskeletal injuries, accounting for $22.2 billion in direct costs and $5.2 billion in indirect costs [1]. Most of these patients will receive initial treatment in the hospital emergency department and be referred for continued outpatient care. The remainder represent more severe injuries and will require hospital admission for definitive care. Due to the increase in high-energy motor vehicle accidents, more patients are being seen with injuries to multiple body systems. Traditionally, it was felt that extremity and pelvic fractures were low on the list of treatment priorities when compared to head, chest, and abdominal injuries. Recently evidence has accumulated that victims of multiple trauma with pelvic or long-bone fractures may fare significantly worse if the fractures are not treated aggressively by early operative stabilization [2,3]. The physician involved in the treatment of trauma victims should therefore have a working knowledge of the common mechanisms, diagnosis, and proper early management of musculoskeletal injuries.

DIAGNOSIS OF MUSCULOSKELETAL INJURY

History

The two most important aspects of the clinical history are the injury mechanism and the subjective complaints. The severity and extent of musculoskeletal damage are roughly correlated with the level of energy of the causative trauma. For example, a person who falls from a standing position could be anticipated to have an isolated injury to perhaps the wrist, whereas the construction worker who falls from a height of three stories might have multiple upper and lower limb fractures. The direction of the traumatic force is also valuable. These points are illustrated in Table 13-1, which lists various mechanisms of musculoskeletal injuries and their typical fractures.

The most common subjective complaint is pain. Often this will localize the site of injury in the extremities or pelvis. Pain secondary to a fracture is sharp, intense, and well localized to the fracture site. Inability to use an extremity or to walk, so-called pseudoparalysis, is an associated complaint. Neurovascular deficit may lead to complaints of numbness or tingling distal to the suspected injury. All of these complaints can be an important aspect of the history, depending on the patient's mental status.

Table 13-1. Patterns of Musculoskeletal Injury

Mechanism of injury	Injury pattern
Fall from height	Distal radius fracture or lumbar spinal compression fracture, calcaneal fracture
Pedestrian-auto	Pelvic fracture, proximal tibia fracture
Auto driver in frontal collision	Patellar fracture or ligamentous knee injury, posterior hip dislocation
Auto driver in lateral collision	Pelvic or acetabular fracture, forearm fracture, knee injury

Physical Examination

In the multiply injured patient, the physical examination should proceed in an orderly and sequential manner according to established protocols. However, it should be stressed that simultaneously with the evaluation of the head, chest, and abdomen, a rapid but thorough examination of the extremities and pelvis should be performed. This is essential for two reasons: (1) to recognize potential injuries and avoid further tissue damage by applying early immobilization and (2) to identify those injuries that can have a profound effect on the early care of the patient, such as the unstable pelvic fracture or femoral shaft fracture.

All extremities should have a gross assessment of the vascular status by palpation of the peripheral pulses and observation of the skin color and temperature. Next, distal sensory and motor function are best evaluated by light touch sensation and asking the patient to move the distal extremity or observing involuntary movement. Any suspected deficit must be documented.

Palpation of the extremities and pelvis may reveal tenderness, crepitus, or false motion secondary to a fracture or dislocation. All joints that are not obviously injured should be put through a passive range of motion. Any skin wound on the extremities or pelvis should be regarded as a possible open fracture or open joint and should be dressed with sterile gauze.

Extremities with either obvious or suspected fracture or dislocation must be splinted, generally for the entire extremity length, immediately upon recognition. This must be accomplished prior to transporting the patient for further diagnostic studies. Correct immobilization will decrease pain and blood loss and prevent further tissue damage.

The orthopedic surgeon should be notified when a musculoskeletal injury is diagnosed, and it is most appropriate to do this prior to sending the patient for initial radiographic examination, since the orthopedic surgeon can suggest the types of radiographs that would be most helpful in assessing the injury. For example, a patient with a suspected fracture of the midshaft of the tibia should have radiographs in two planes of the entire tibia, including the knee and ankle joints. Acetabular and pelvic injuries require specific radiographic studies to arrive at a proper diagnosis.

CLAVICLE FRACTURES

The clavicle is an S-shaped bone that lies between the acromion process of the scapula and the sternum. The proximal articulation is the sternoclavicular joint, and the distal is the acromioclavicular joint complex, including the coracoclavicular ligaments. The function of the clavicle is twofold: to connect the axial and appendicular parts of the skeleton and to protect the lungs and deeper neurovascular structures. Fractures of the clavicle are produced by both indirect and direct trauma. The clavicle is somewhat superficial and prone to direct injury. Indirectly, fractures can result from either a blow on the shoulder or a fall on the extremity.

Diagnosis

The diagnosis of a clavicle fracture can usually be made by palpating the clavicle for crepitus, local tenderness, and false motion. The patient will complain of inability to move the involved extremity. The skin must be carefully inspected for puncture wounds or lacerations indicating an open fracture. A thorough neurovascular examination is indicated, as there may be brachial plexus or axillary artery injury. Radiographs of the clavicle should be obtained in two planes, a standard anteroposterior (AP) and 20 degrees cephalad. Special views of the associated joints may be required if these are suspicious for injury.

Treatment

The majority of clavicle fractures can be satisfactorily treated with application of a clavicle or figure-of-eight strap. Fracture healing will be complete in 6 weeks. Indications for open reduction and internal fixation are limited to (1) neurovascular compromise secondary to pressure from displaced fracture fragments or (2) unacceptable fracture position with tenting of the skin.

SCAPULAR FRACTURES

Fractures of the scapula can involve the body of the scapula or the glenoid portion that articulates with the humerus. Most of the scapula is covered by the muscles that control shoulder movement. Direct trauma is most often the mechanism of injury. Due to the anatomic location on the upper posterior thorax, scapula body fractures are commonly associated with underlying rib fractures or pneumothorax.

Diagnosis
Direct palpation will reveal local tenderness and possibly crepitus. Shoulder motion will be restricted, especially if the glenoid is involved. Swelling is commonly seen.

Radiographs should include an AP view and a transscapular lateral. Most patients with direct trauma also require a chest film to rule out pneumothorax.

Treatment
Fractures of the scapular body can be immobilized with an arm sling for symptomatic relief. Within a few days, passive motion of the shoulder should be instituted to avoid intracapsular adhesions. These fractures will be healed in 4 to 6 weeks.

Many glenoid fractures will have excellent functional results if treated in a similar manner as for body fractures. Large displaced glenoid fragments in the shoulder joint may, however, necessitate open reduction and internal fixation.

PROXIMAL HUMERAL FRACTURES

The proximal humerus can be divided into four anatomic areas: the greater and lesser tuberosities, the articular surface, and the surgical neck or proximal shaft. The tuberosities serve as the insertion points for the rotator cuff muscles and are the pathway for the major blood supply to the humeral head. The proximal shaft region immediately inferior to the tuberosities is called the surgical neck, since it is often the site of fractures.

The brachial plexus of nerves and the axillary and brachial vessels are in close proximity to the proximal humerus, and potential injury to these structures must be remembered.

There appear to be two basic injury mechanisms that cause these fractures. The elderly patient may simply fall from a standing height and, due in part to osteopenic bone, sustain a fracture, this being a low-energy injury. On the other hand, high-energy trauma is typically required in the younger patient to produce this fracture.

Diagnosis
Patients with proximal humeral fractures complain of inability to move the limb and severe pain. Extensive local hematoma is common, and this may actually involve the entire distal limb. At least two radiographs are needed for proper diagnosis: a true AP and a transscapular lateral. These views do not require painful positioning and should be obtained in all suspected cases of shoulder trauma.

Treatment
A classification system has been developed to describe these fractures and provide a prognosis [4]. The proximal humerus can be divided into four parts: the humeral head, greater tuberosity, lesser tuberosity, and proximal shaft. Fractures (or fracture-dislocations) can involve two of these parts or any combination. A major complication of the three- and four-part fractures is avascular necrosis of the humeral head, often resulting in severe functional loss. Most fractures are treated nonoperatively with brief periods of immobilization in an arm sling followed by early motion. This is done to prevent shoulder stiff-

ness, which invariably accompanies these fractures.

Surgical treatment is usually reserved for the more complicated fractures or fracture-dislocations. Younger patients with multiple trauma or severely displaced fractures are best treated by open reduction and internal fixation. Elderly patients who have fractures with a poor prognosis may be treated with prosthetic replacement of the humeral head.

SHOULDER DISLOCATIONS

The shoulder joint consists of the humeral head articulating with the scapular glenoid, surrounded by a fibrous capsule and musculotendinous cuff. Stability of the shoulder is provided by these soft tissues, as there is no intrinsic stability in the geometry of the joint. The arrangement allows the superb range of motion that is possible in the shoulder joint. Shoulder dislocations occur when the humeral head is forced, usually anteriorly away from the glenoid. This typically happens during athletic activity, especially when the arm is abducted and externally rotated, such as in pitching a ball or making a tackle. Any violent trauma can cause this as well. Patients with recurrent dislocation can have very minor trauma produce the dislocation. After the dislocation, the humeral head will lie in front of the scapula.

Diagnosis

The patient with a shoulder dislocation will present with severe pain and inability to move the arm. Recurrent dislocation, particularly in the younger age group, is not uncommon, and the patient may give a clear history of previous dislocations. If a patient has a seizure disorder, then a posterior dislocation must be strongly suspected. Some patients can voluntarily dislocate their shoulders and may do this to receive narcotic analgesics surreptitiously.

Examination will reveal the arm to be rather fixed in position and tender with any motion. The humeral head may be palpated anterior to the scapula, and the normal fullness of the shoulder laterally will be absent. If the arm is in marked internal rotation, then posterior dislocation must be considered. There can be loss of sensation in the proximal lateral upper arm secondary to axillary nerve injury. Two basic radiographs should be obtained in all patients with shoulder dislocations. A true AP of the shoulder and a transscapular lateral view can be taken in any patient without causing pain or further damage. The absolute position of the humeral head will most frequently be superimposed on the scapula inferior to the coracoid process. The radiographic signs of a posterior dislocation might be quite subtle.

Treatment

After diagnosis, shoulder dislocations should be promptly reduced to decrease pain and swelling and prevent neurovascular embarrassment. Several methods of closed reduction have been developed to accomplish this, and adequate muscle relaxation is necessary [5]. All of these maneuvers have in common initial longitudinal traction in line with the deformity. During reduction, the elbow should be flexed and the patient's head either turned toward the side of dislocation or in neutral rotation to avoid stretching the brachial plexus. It behooves the physician to determine the neurovascular status accurately both before and after reduction. Reduction of the humerus is usually accompanied by an audible and palpable "clunk." The patient will then be able to move the shoulder actively and experiences almost complete relief of pain.

After reduction, the arm can be maintained in a sling to prevent redislocation. Treatment beyond this point is controversial and dependent on the patient's age, activity level, and whether the dislocation was primary or recurrent.

In a few patients, closed reduction may be unsuccessful due to impalement of the humeral head on the anterior glenoid or some other reason. Surgical reduction is then indicated and may be a formidable procedure.

HUMERAL SHAFT FRACTURES

The humeral shaft is that area that lies between the surgical neck and the supracondylar region. The brachial vessels and the median, radial, and ulnar nerves are in close proximity and may be injured with shaft fractures. High-energy trauma often produces transverse or comminuted fractures, whereas torsional fractures are commonly secondary to low-energy forces. Bilateral humeral shaft fractures are seen frequently in sudden deceleration, along with thoracic injury.

Diagnosis

Humeral shaft fractures present with local swelling, tenderness, and false motion. Muscle action yields obvious deformity at the fracture site. Any motion of the extremity is quite painful. AP and lateral radiographs should be obtained of the entire humerus. Caution must be exercised, however, when the lateral radiograph is taken, as inexperienced personnel will rotate the patient's injured arm through the humeral fracture site, in the belief that they are actually rotating the whole arm.

Treatment

The vast majority of humeral shaft fractures will have excellent functional and anatomic results if treated nonoperatively. A number of methods are used, ranging from a simple arm sling to plaster casts. State of the art treatment utilizes a plastic fracture brace, which may even be applied the day of injury and allows almost immediate function of the injured extremity. Shoulder and elbow stiffness are thus eliminated, and muscle atrophy is minimized. Fracture healing is complete in approximately 10 weeks. There are several indications for operative stabilization of humeral shaft fractures. Patients with both upper and lower limb or chest injuries, bilateral shaft fractures, open fractures, ipsilateral upper extremity fractures, or brachial artery injury are good surgical candidates. With surgery, these patients can be mobilized quicker, nursing care is facilitated, and rehabilitation can be started much sooner.

ELBOW INJURIES

The elbow is a complex joint and actually consists of three separate articulations; the humeroulnar, humeroradial, and proximal radioulnar. Both elbow flexion/extension and forearm supination/pronation are made possible by this interrelationship of joints.

Fractures or dislocations may be caused by a fall on the elbow with low-energy trauma. Usually the most severe injuries are secondary to high-energy forces such as sideswiping a vehicle with the elbow exposed or a fall from a great height. Not infrequently these severe injuries are open fractures of joints.

Swelling is a particular problem relating to elbow trauma. Any elbow fracture or dislocation can have a large hematoma develop underneath the deep fascia of the elbow or forearm. This hematoma can therefore cause vascular compression or tissue ischemia. This may produce a compartment syndrome, which if unrecognized and untreated will lead to Volkmann's contracture and a useless extremity. In the author's center, all patients with elbow fracture or dislocation are admitted for at least a 24-hour observation period to eliminate this complication.

Diagnosis

Unless seen early, the majority of patients with elbow trauma will have significant swelling. Point tenderness over the injured structure may be the only clue to localize the injury. Severe limitation of motion is the rule. It is mandatory to examine the distal neural and vascular status of the extremity.

Good quality AP and lateral radiographs of the elbow are essential. Forearm views are also often indicated, since elbow and forearm injuries frequently coexist.

Treatment

Elbow dislocations require prompt closed or open reduction to restore the anatomy and prevent neurovascular compromise. After reduction, most are stable and will be treated with progressive motion with good functional results.

Fractures can occur in the distal humerus, proximal radius, ulna, or any combination. Since most of these fractures are intra-articular, the goal of treatment is to obtain anatomic reduction and restore early function. Therefore, open reduction and internal fixation are indicated in these cases. Cast immobilization may be utilized in nondisplaced fractures or some elderly patients.

Compartment syndrome in elbow injuries can be diagnosed early and is for the most part wholly preventable. Circumferential casts should not be used acutely, and all patients require close observation within the first 24 to 48 hours after injury.

FOREARM INJURIES

The forearm comprises two long bones, the radius and ulna, joined together by a dense interosseous membrane. The deep fascia of the forearm is circumferential and continuous with the distal brachial fascia proximally and the carpal tunnel distally. This fascial arrangement makes forearm injuries susceptible to compartment syndrome.

Displaced fractures of the forearm are typically due to either direct or violent torsional trauma. A substantial number may also be caused by penetrating knife or gunshot trauma. It can be said that the greater the displacement of the fracture, the greater the soft tissue damage.

Diagnosis

Many forearm fractures will present with obvious deformity secondary to fracture displacement. Forearm rotation is impossible. A careful search must be made for any small puncture wound, as it may indicate an open fracture. Standard AP and lateral radiographs are necessary. If there is swelling in either the elbow or wrist, then views of these joints are also warranted. A baseline motor and sensory examination is mandatory and must be documented.

Treatment

Generally, displaced forearm fractures are treated operatively because of the excellent, consistent results reported with this method. Isolated fractures of the ulna, the "nightstick injury," may be treated nonoperatively and successfully with a fracture brace and early function.

Special attention must be devoted to diagnosing a compartment syndrome early, as the forearm is one of the two most common sites for this complication [6]. Immediate fasciotomy is the only correct treatment.

WRIST AND HAND INJURIES

The wrist and hand include the distal radius, ulna, multiple carpal bones, and multiple small bones of the hand. Due to the exposed, peripheral location, many patients with multiple trauma often have wrist and hand injuries. Also because of the complex radiographic anatomy, injuries are often missed, since only minor changes may be noted on the radiograph. Open injuries are common, along with associated nerve injury. Trauma to this region may not be important to the life of a patient but is of maximum functional significance and can profoundly affect rehabilitation.

Diagnosis

Local point tenderness and deformity are the best clues to localizing a wrist or hand injury. A complete distal motor and sensory examination is essential. Function will be impaired according to the magnitude of injury.

For the wrist, AP and lateral radiographs are required. Special views may be necessary to assist in the diagnosis of the more occult injuries. In general, for hand trauma, the involved digit should be individually radiographed if distal to the metacarpophalangeal joint. Metacarpal fractures can readily be seen on AP and lateral views of the hand.

Treatment

Fractures of the distal radius are most often treated with closed reduction and cast immobilization, with a lesser number, especially in younger patients, having either external or internal fixation. The majority will have acceptable results.

Carpal injuries often need operative stabilization, since ligament damage is common and must be reconstructed. Many isolated fractures of the scaphoid are preferably treated with cast immobilization. Hand injuries have a broad spectrum of treatment possibilities, depending on the treating surgeon's philosophy and the exact location of fracture. There is a definite trend toward operative treatment, since early restoration of function is the goal.

PELVIC INJURIES

Pelvic injury is being seen with increasing regularity in most trauma centers, largely due to the increase in motor vehicle accidents. Most pelvic injuries are stable, require only symptomatic treatment and early mobilization, and have minimal future sequelae. The unstable pelvic injury, however, is associated with significant morbidity and mortality and demands aggressive treatment. The challenge, therefore, is to identify the unstable injury and manage it properly.

Anatomy

Some basic anatomic points are necessary to understand pelvic trauma. The bony skeleton of the pelvis can be regarded as a ring divided into anterior and posterior parts. The anterior parts, the ischiopubic rami and pubic symphysis, serve to protect the pelvic viscera and act as attachment sites for muscles. The posterior portion comprises the sacroiliac joints, adjacent sacrum, and ilium and functions to connect the axial and lower appendicular skeletons and to transmit body weight from the spine to the lower extremities. The normal forces applied to the posterior pelvis are much greater in magnitude than anteriorly, and of necessity, the posterior ligamentous complex is quite strong. On the other hand, the anterior pelvis is not stressed heavily and possesses a relatively weak ligament support. This is clinically relevant in that it has been known that posterior pelvic fracture or dislocation generally is indicative of high-energy trauma with greater hemorrhage, soft tissue damage, and multiple systemic injuries.

Another important aspect relates to the "ring" concept of the pelvis. Intuitively, it is difficult to apply a disruptive force to a ring structure and expect only one break in the ring. This is clinically observed in most patients with "only" anterior pelvic injury. Some type of posterior injury can often be demonstrated, either on standard radiographs, computed tomography (CT) scan, or bone scan.

Diagnosis

The physical examination of patients with pelvic trauma is important to localize the injuries and assist in the determination of stability [7]. Observation may show localized swelling of the pelvis. Rotational deformities or shortening of the lower limbs can be a clue to the type of pelvic injury and the hemipelvis involved. Palpation must include all accessible portions of the anterior and posterior pelvis, especially the posterior sacroiliac areas. Direct lateral compression of the iliac wings toward each other and anterior to posterior compression will usually elicit pain in the individual sites of fracture or joint injury. Clinical signs suggestive of severe injury are limb shortening or rotational deformity, particularly external rotation; large posterior hematoma; and detection of "sloppiness" or "loose jointedness" in the pelvis with iliac compression. Perineal wounds, especially in the vagina or rectum, may communicate with the site of pelvic injury, thus indicating an open fracture.

An AP radiograph of the pelvis is the essential minimum to visualize the injured structures. Additional tangential views, pelvic inlet and outlet, are most helpful and should be done when posterior injury is suspected [7]. The definitive procedure for exact analysis of the posterior pelvis is the CT scan at 5-mm intervals. With this study, a cross section of the sacroiliac complex is obtained, and even subtle pathology can be found.

Most high-energy pelvic trauma can be divided among three categories. The most common, lateral compression, is caused by a direct blow to the side of the pelvis. This type is often observed in the driver of an automobile or a pedestrian struck by an automobile. The anterior component has fractures of the superior and inferior pubic rami (rarely bilateral) with contralateral or ipsilateral sacral or iliac fracture. The sacral fracture is usually impacted, and the hemipelvis is internally rotated a variable degree.

The second pattern of pelvic injury, anterior compression, is typically caused by a force directed from anterior to posterior or vice versa. This is the mechanism in frontal collisions or crushing trauma, such as a horse falling on top of the rider. The anterior injury may be bilateral pubic rami fractures (straddle fracture) or a disruption of the pubic symphysis. If the force was sufficient, there may be sacroiliac joint disruption. There is a significant incidence of genitourinary injury in this pattern. The anterior compression injury is considered stable if the pubic diastasis is less than 2.5 cm or the posterior component is minimal.

If the pubic diastasis is 2.5 cm or greater, then potential instability exists because the sacrospinous ligaments are disrupted. As the diastasis becomes greater, the sacroiliac ligaments can, in rare cases, be torn. It should be apparent that a tremendous force is needed to disrupt the pelvis in this manner, and significant hemorrhage may be encountered.

The third type of pelvic injury, the vertical shear, is the most devastating and has the highest morbidity and mortality of all basic categories. The mechanism of injury can best be described as if some force were applied to the lower extremity and an attempt was made to avulse the extremity and the pelvis from the rest of the body. This requires an extremely strong vertically directed force that shears the affected hemipelvis from the axial skeleton. A reasonably accurate description would be an incomplete traumatic hemipelvectomy! Approximately 40 percent of patients with this trauma will require laparotomy for associated abdominal injuries [8].

Anteriorly, there may be pubic symphysis disruption or fractures of the pubic rami. This is the break in the anterior ring. In the posterior ring, there will be either sacral or iliac fracture adjacent to the sacroiliac joint or disruption through the joint. A clue to the vertical shear type is an ipsilateral fracture of the L5 transverse process, a sign of posterior instability. The affected hemipelvis will be displaced superiorly and posteriorly, the amount dependent on the degree of ligament damage.

On examination, the patient will have significant tenderness over the anterior and especially posterior pelvis. A large hematoma may form posteriorly as well. The affected side may show limb shortening and an external rotation deformity, possibly with ipsilateral limb fractures. Anterior pressure over the iliac crests may elicit crepitus or abnormal movement of the hemipelvis, denoting instability.

Treatment

Algorithms have been developed to assist in the management of the patient with severe pelvic injury [9]. In the case of significant hemorrhage, in addition to proper fluid resuscitation, various methods have been proposed: pneumatic anti-shock garment (PASG) [10], external fixation [11], and pelvic angiography with selective embolization [12]. Each of these treatment modalities has had reasonable success. From recent reports, it does appear that early (within 24 hours) stabilization of the bleeding pelvis with an external fixator can substantially reduce blood loss in most patients and decrease their transfusion requirements. External fixation has thus been suggested as the first line of treatment, and this is the current practice in many trauma centers. In fact, some centers apply the external fixator as soon as the patient is seen in the emergency care setting [7].

Definitive treatment of the severe pelvic injury will generally necessitate either continued external fixation, internal fixation, or a combination of both. This aggressive approach is justified by the early and long-term results of surgical management of this complex injury [13].

Predominately, the lateral compression injury is regarded as stable due to the impacted posterior fracture and, as such, does not indicate the need for external or internal fixation. Patients with this injury may be safely logrolled in bed and may be allowed to sit in a chair. When the pain is diminished in a few days, protected ambulation may begin. In rare instances, the internal rotation deformity of the pelvis may be excessive, and this is an indication for surgical stabilization, as the correction of the deformity will destabilize the pelvic ring.

The stable anterior compression injury can be treated as for the stable lateral compression type. If the pubic diastasis is 2.5 cm or greater, the anterior compression injury is a prime indication for surgical stabilization. This may be accomplished by a closed reduction under anesthesia and either application of an external fixator to the iliac crests or plate fixation of the pubic symphysis.

Treatment of the patient with a vertical shear injury should be directed at stabilizing the pelvis to reduce bleeding, diminish pain, and prevent further soft tissue damage. As soon as possible, an external fixator should be applied, and this can even be performed in the emergency room setting. A less suitable alternative is to apply skeletal traction to the affected extremity with a femoral pin. An anatomic reduction is not as important as providing compression to the unstable pelvis and producing a tamponade effect to the large area of bleeding cancellous bone at the multiple fracture sites.

External Fixation

External fixation of the pelvis consists of the insertion of pins percutaneously into the anterior iliac crests. These pins are then connected to an external mechanical frame, which couples the two sides of the pelvis together. When the frame is appropriately tightened, a compressive force is applied to the pelvis, producing stabilization of fracture surfaces and dislocated joints. Most types of pelvic external fixators will allow ready access to the abdomen for surgery or observation of suspected intra-abdominal injury. Limited mobilization of the patient is permitted with the fixator in place for diagnostic or therapeutic procedures.

CASE 1

A 34-year-old man was riding a motorcycle when he was struck by an automobile. He sustained multiple injuries, including a pelvic injury. The initial AP radiograph (Fig. 13-1A) revealed a large sacroiliac joint diastasis with an external rotation deformity of the right hemipelvis. CT scan (Fig. 13-1B) clearly demonstrated complete disruption of the posterior sacroiliac complex with posterior displacement of the hemipelvis. Because of the radiographic findings and continued drop in hematocrit despite adequate fluid resuscitation, surgical stabilization was thought to be indicated. Under general anesthesia, a closed reduction of the pelvis was done and external fixator applied within the first 24 hours (Fig. 13-2). Postoperatively, the hematocrit stabilized, and the patient had minimal pain from

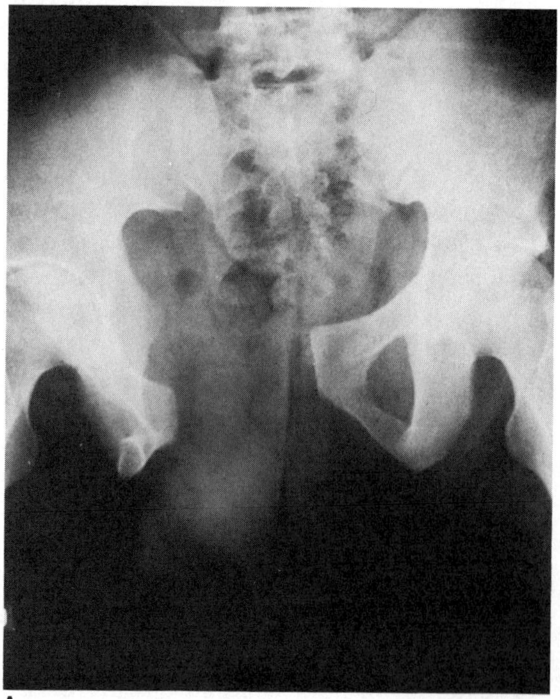

A

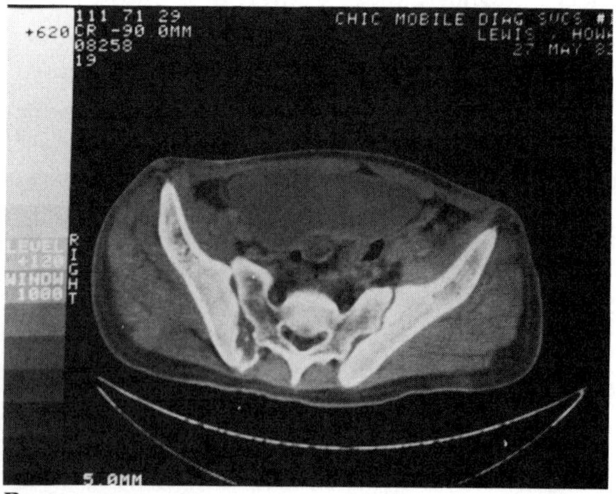

B

Fig. 13-1. ***A.*** **Anteroposterior radiograph showing severe pubic symphysis diastasis and widening of the right sacroiliac joint. There is external rotation of the hemipelvis.** ***B.*** **CT scan of the upper pelvis delineates the posterior sacroiliac disruption with posterior displacement of the hemipelvis, consistent with a vertical shear injury.**

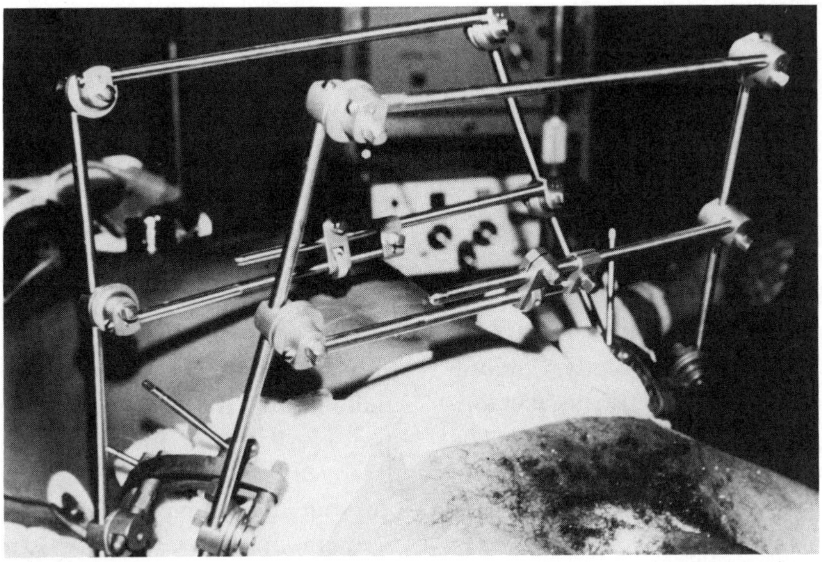

A

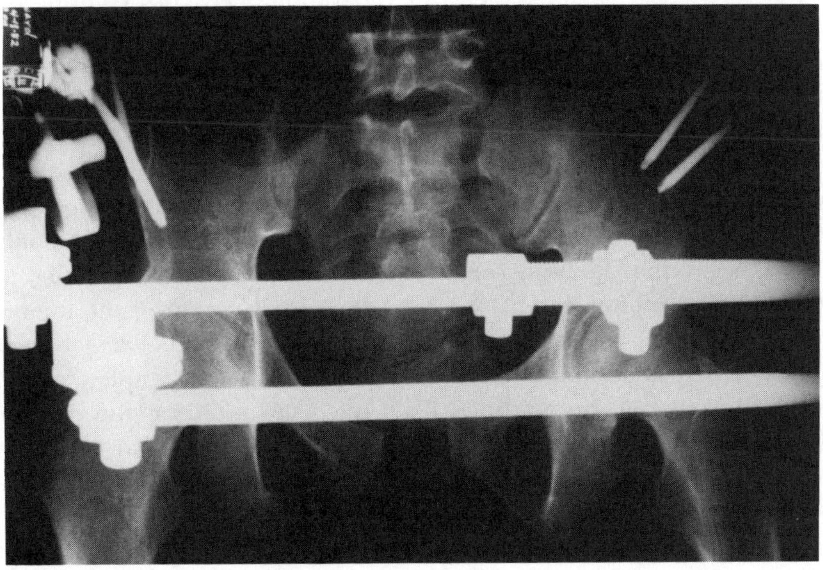

B

Fig. 13-2. ***A.*** **The external fixator applied to the iliac crests by percutaneous pins.** ***B.*** **Postoperative radiograph shows a significant reduction of the pelvic diastasis and correction of the external rotational deformity.**

the injured pelvis, such that he was sitting in a chair by the third postinjury day.

HIP DISLOCATIONS AND ACETABULAR FRACTURES

The hip joint is composed of the femoral head, which is in contact with the acetabulum, thus forming a ball-and-socket joint. The capsule of the hip is extremely strong and said to be one factor for the rarity of hip dislocations. The sciatic nerve is in close proximity to the hip posteriorly as it exits from the inner pelvis.

Most hip dislocations and many acetabular fractures occur in occupants of motor vehicles. In the sitting position, the lower extremities are flexed at the hips and knees. In frontal collisions, the knee may strike the dashboard and transmit the force to the hip, driving it out posteriorly. Because this force is applied at the knee, there may be an associated patellar fracture or ligament injury. More uncommonly, the hip can be dislocated anteriorly if the hip is widely abducted. A force applied to the lateral aspect of the proximal thigh will likely result in an acetabular fracture.

Diagnosis

Patients with hip dislocations have dramatic presentations with gross deformity and inability to walk. Generally, severe pain is produced with any attempt at motion of the involved hip. Posterior hip dislocation has a classic deformity of lower extremity shortening, hip adduction, and internal rotation. Anterior hip dislocation may have the opposite of this, with hip abduction and external rotation. Thorough neurovascular examination is indicated, as approximately 15 percent of posterior dislocations will have a sciatic nerve injury.

Many acetabular fractures have a benign external appearance with perhaps only some shortening of the extremity. Hip motion is painful, and this is usually in proportion to the severity of the fracture. Percussion of the lateral thigh will elicit pain. For initial radiographic diagnosis, a high-quality AP pelvis film is mandatory. With this study, the exact dislocation or fracture can be determined. Radiographic signs of posterior dislocation include a smaller femoral head size, loss of the normal relationship of the femoral head and the superior acetabulum, and malposition of the proximal femur corresponding to the lower extremity deformity. Anterior dislocation is recognized by the location of the femoral head. Hip dislocation is often associated with some type of acetabular wall fracture. Central dislocation of the femoral head with fracture of the medial acetabular wall can also occur (Fig. 13-3). Complete evaluation of fracture dislocation of the hip requires that oblique views, internal and external, be obtained [14].

Treatment

Dislocation of the hip is a true orthopedic emergency, and there are several reasons for this. The gross distortion of anatomy that accompanies this injury may compromise the sciatic nerve and even the major femoral vessels. The longer the hip remains dislocated, the greater the incidence of avascular necrosis of the femoral head, a disabling condition without effective treatment. Finally, reduction

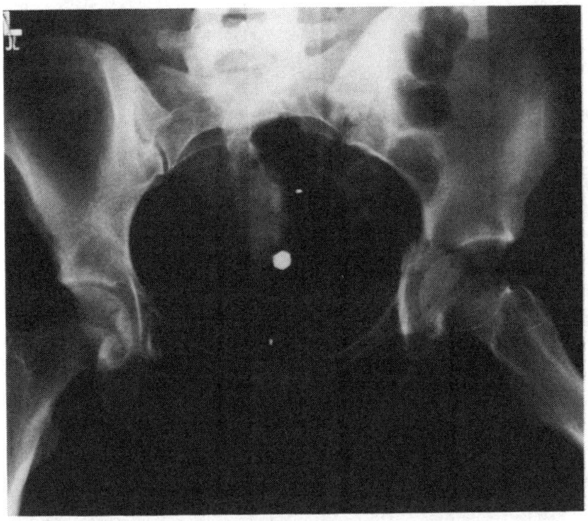

Fig. 13-3. Pelvic radiograph of a displaced fracture through both columns of the left acetabulum with central dislocation of the femoral head. Note the loss of position of the femoral head from beneath the superior acetabular roof.

of the hip becomes much more difficult with increasing time from injury. The majority of hip dislocations can be relocated with closed reduction if done promptly. This maneuver requires adequate anesthesia, longitudinal traction, hip flexion, and various other movements. It has been well described previously [15]. After reduction, the AP pelvis radiograph is repeated to confirm reduction. In a small percentage of patients, open reduction may be required. Definitive treatment will depend on the orthopedic surgeon.

Acetabular fractures that are minimally displaced may be treated with bed rest alone. Displaced fractures are usually managed in traction or surgically reduced, especially if the patient is younger [14].

FEMORAL FRACTURES

The femur can be divided into three separate anatomic areas: proximal, shaft, and distal. The proximal and distal regions are composed of cancellous bone, and fractures in these areas are associated with involvement of the hip or knee joints. The shaft lies between the proximal and distal areas and is essentially a tubular structure of thick, dense cortical bone. Although shaft fractures may be caused by a relatively low level of force, such as indirect twisting, it is far more common to have a high level of energy applied directly to the thigh, producing the typical transverse midshaft fracture. Laboratory measurements have shown that a minimum force equal approximately to 800 kg (1800 lb) or five times the body weight is required to produce a midshaft femoral fracture [16]! With such enormous forces, it is not surprising that patients with femoral fractures also often have related systemic or other musculoskeletal injuries.

Special mention should be made of two specific problems in patients with femoral fractures—hemorrhage and hypoxemia. A single fracture of the femoral shaft may produce blood loss in the range of 1.0 to 2.5 liters, depending on the mechanism of injury. Open fractures may have substantially greater blood loss. Serial blood count determinations are essential in all patients with femoral fractures, and appropriate fluid resuscitation is mandatory. It has been observed that a number of patients with femoral shaft fractures, on the day of injury, have arterial hypoxemia, with PO_2 values as low as 60 mm Hg [3]. This has occurred in the absence of pulmonary trauma or other causes of arterial hypoxemia. Subclinical fat embolism from the femoral fracture has been suggested as the pathophysiology for this pulmonary dysfunction, and this appears likely. For this reason, all patients with femoral fractures, even those with isolated fractures, should have a baseline arterial blood gas determination on admission and thereafter as needed.

Diagnosis

Patients with femoral shaft fractures will usually arrive in the emergency care setting having had application of a traction splint in the field, with the diagnosis made or suspected. Rarely patients may present with unsplinted fractures, and it is imperative that proper immobilization be applied immediately. A search should be carried out for any skin wounds of the thigh, which may indicate an open fracture. Radiographs of the entire femur in two planes including the hip and knee are necessary. There is a definite incidence of ipsilateral femoral shaft and femoral neck fractures [17]. The hip views must be scrutinized carefully, since often the femoral neck fracture is minimally displaced and easily missed. In our center, an AP radiograph of the pelvis is also routinely obtained to examine the acetabulum and pelvis.

Treatment

As soon as possible, the patient with a femoral shaft fracture should be placed in skeletal traction, usually with a proximal tibial pin, and an appropriate traction splint applied. This will reduce pain and muscle spasm, prevent further soft tissue damage, and maintain fracture position. "Field" traction with an ankle and foot hitch is not effective for this purpose. After skeletal traction has been instituted, the patient can be transported as required. The average amount of traction weight for an adult is one-fifth of body weight or 30 pounds.

Definitive management of the femoral shaft fracture is dependent on several variables: associated systemic or musculoskeletal injuries, fracture pattern and type, and the treating surgeon's clinical experience and technical expertise.

Nonsurgical treatment consists of skeletal traction for a variable period, ranging from several days to several weeks, followed by immobilization in either a fracture brace or cast. Traction is mainly indicated for patients with isolated femoral shaft fractures who are capable of tolerating the prolonged bed rest inherent in this method. Nevertheless, it is a time-honored technique that has been proved to result in a high rate of fracture union and acceptable functional results.

Clearly, surgical stabilization has become the treatment of choice for adult femoral shaft fractures. Several types of internal fixation devices are available, with the two basic groups being intramedullary nails and compression plates. Of these, intramedullary nails inserted with "closed" technique have yielded fracture union rates of 98 percent, infection in less than 1 percent, and excellent functional results in the vast majority [17]. In addition to being an excellent method for management of the fracture itself, operative stabilization probably has important physiologic advantages. Johnson and associates [2] studied multiply injured patients with fractures of the spine, pelvis, or femur. In those patients with early (within 24 hours after injury) operative stabilization of these fractures, the incidence of

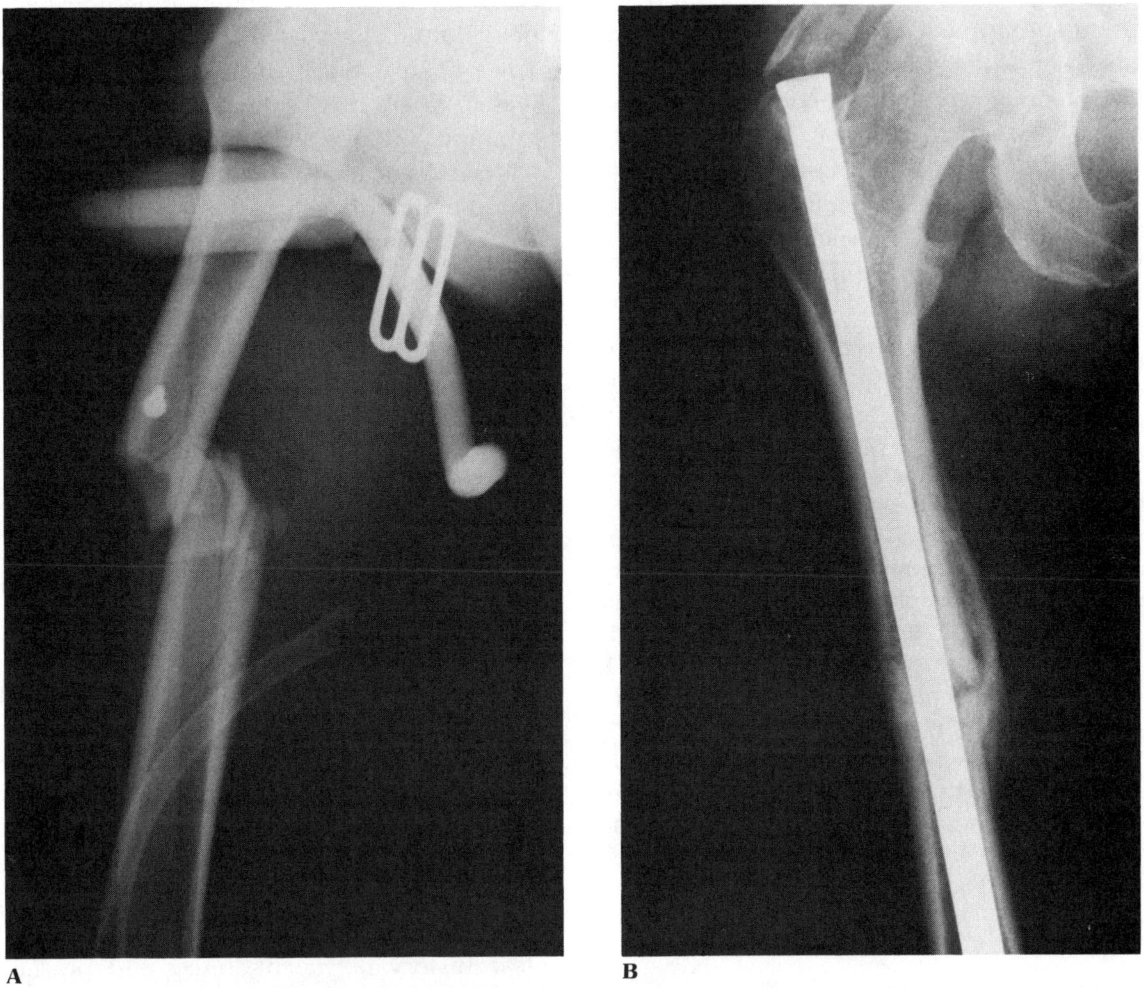

Fig. 13-4. *A.* A displaced and comminuted fracture of the femoral shaft. *B.* The femur has been stabilized by closed intramedullary nailing with complete fracture consolidation, as seen at long-term follow-up.

adult respiratory distress syndrome and pulmonary complications was decreased to one-fifth of that in a comparable patient group not operated on early. This effect was most notable in the more severely injured patient. Other authors [3,18] have presented data to support this concept. While the exact mechanism is unknown, the beneficial effect of fracture fixation surely relates to the avoidance of the supine position and subsequent orthostatic pneumonia or pulmonary complications. Additionally, some alteration in the patient's metabolic response to trauma may occur. It could conceivably be a combination of these or factors not yet delineated.

CASE 2

An 18-year-old man was a pedestrian when he was struck by an automobile. On presentation to the emergency room, he had an obvious closed fracture of the right femoral shaft (Fig. 13-4A). The initial hematocrit was 38 percent, and arterial blood gases showed a PO_2 of 60 mm Hg. A chest radiograph and electrocardiogram were normal. The medical history was negative for previous cardiopulmonary disease, and the patient was asymptomatic without respiratory difficulty. The low PO_2 value was felt to be due to subclinical fat embolism. On the fourth day after injury, the PO_2 was 85 mm Hg without any specific treatment, and a closed intramedullary nailing of the femur fracture was performed (Fig. 13-4B). The postoperative course was uneventful, and the patient was discharged 1 week after injury.

KNEE DISLOCATIONS

The knee joint is composed of the distal femur and the proximal tibia. These surfaces are not very conforming and necessitate a strong joint capsule and ligamentous complex to provide primary stability and allow proper function and weight transmission. Posterior to the knee lies the major neurovascular conduit to the lower leg. The sciatic nerve divides into the common peroneal and posterior tibial nerves near the popliteal fossa. The popliteal artery begins at the adductor hiatus, where it is firmly fixed against the femur and continues distally to the trifurcation.

Knee dislocation is a complete loss of anatomic contact between the femur and tibia. Due to the strong soft tissue restraints, a violent force is usually necessary to produce the dislocation [19]. Generally, one side of the knee joint is fixed, and the other side has the applied force. Most of the major ligaments of the knee are disrupted. The joint may dislocate in any direction, and this is named by the displacement of the tibia on the femur. Anterior and posterior dislocations are encountered often. Motor vehicle accidents and contact sports are common mechanisms [20].

The severe trauma and peculiar anatomy account for a high percentage of knee dislocations with neurovascular injuries. Popliteal artery rupture is the most dreaded complication and often results in amputation of the leg [21]. Late thrombosis secondary to an intimal injury is also possible.

Diagnosis

Most patients with knee dislocations have a clear history of violent injury and present with severe pain and gross deformity. The knee is usually flexed to some degree and cannot be moved. There can be much swelling about the knee. Distal pulses should be checked, and a neurologic examination must be performed.

Immediate AP and lateral radiographs of the knee are done to confirm the diagnosis and search for associated fractures. This is a true surgical emergency and should be recognized as such. A closed reduction is carried out by longitudinal traction and appropriate maneuvering depending on the type of dislocation. After reduction, the distal neurovascular status should be reassessed and repeat radiographs done. In our center, all patients without obvious signs of vascular embarrassment then have arteriography of the lower extremity, due to the high incidence of accompanying vascular injury. If there is vascular insufficiency after the joint is reduced, then operative exploration of the vessels is done. Some injuries cannot be reduced and may need surgical reduction. Definitive treatment of the knee dislocation varies according to the vascular status, type of dislocation, patient's age, and surgeon's preference.

CASE 3

A 48-year-old woman was the driver of an automobile that was involved in a multiple automobile collision. At the accident scene, she was noted to have a gross deformity of the knee, and there were no distal pulses palpable. The limb was gently realigned and splinted, and the patient was then transported to the hospital.

Subsequent radiographs of the knee revealed a posterolateral dislocation of the knee (Figs. 13-5A and B). An immediate closed reduction was done, and the distal pulses were still absent by palpation but could be detected by Doppler examination. An emergency arteriogram demonstrated complete occlusion of the popliteal artery with minimal distal runoff (Fig. 13-5C). At vascular exploration, there was a severe intimal injury, and the damaged segment was resected and a reversed saphenous vein graft was interposed. Excellent flow and pulses were restored, and the limb was salvaged. Because of the patient's age and functional demands, the knee injury was treated nonsurgically with cast immobilization.

TIBIAL SHAFT FRACTURES

Fractures of the tibial shaft are caused by both indirect and direct trauma [22]. The direct trauma is usually a result of motor vehicle accidents involving either occupants or pedestrians. These are high-energy injuries, and open fractures are commonly seen. The tibia is particularly susceptible to open fractures, since it is a vulnerable part of the body and the bone is subcutaneous throughout its length. Invariably, high-energy tibial fractures have severe soft tissue damage and neurovascular injury. Many of these fractures are caused by crushing forces with much more tissue injury than can be appreciated by merely looking at the leg or the fracture on the radiographs. It is this extensive damage that very often leads to compartment syndrome [23].

Diagnosis

Patients with tibial shaft fractures typically have the symptoms and signs of acute fractures. If the fracture is displaced, deformity and angulation may be present. Any violation of the skin must be considered an open fracture, regardless of the location, until proved otherwise. Adequate assessment of neurovascular status of the leg includes pulses and motor and sensory function. High-quality ra-

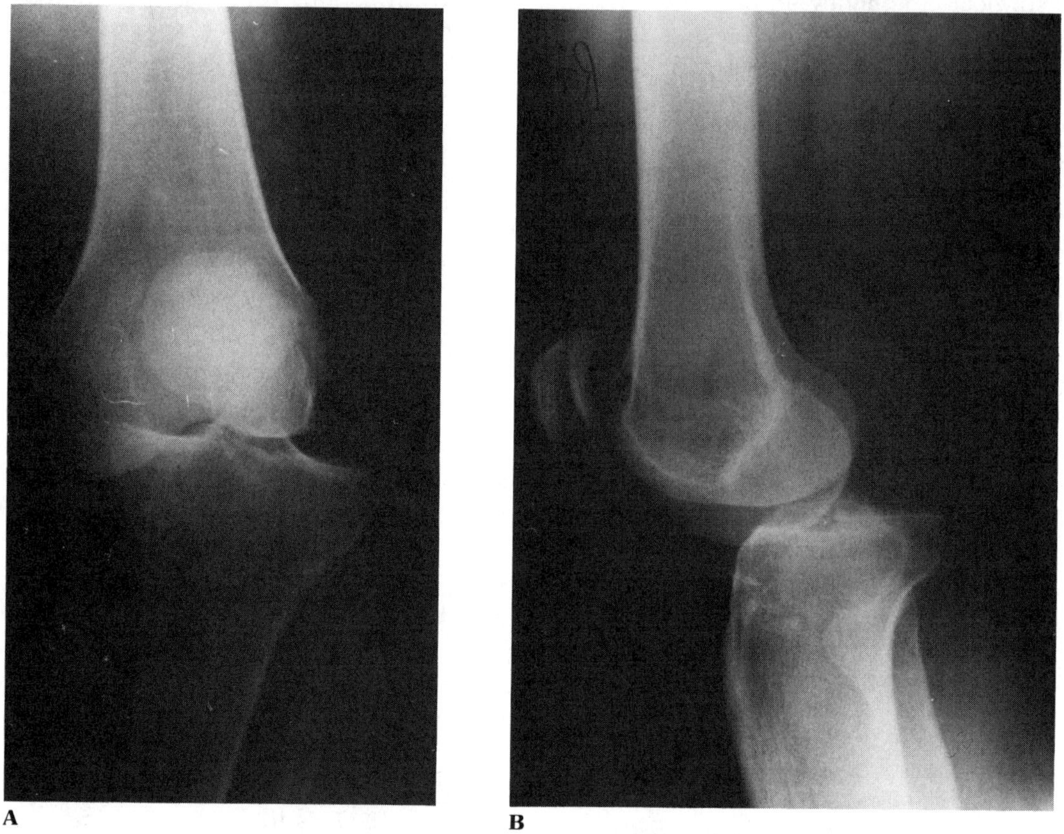

A B

Fig. 13-5. ***A and B.*** **Radiographs of the knee with the tibia dislocated posterolaterally.**

diographs of the entire tibia in both AP and lateral views are standard. The adjacent knee and ankle joints should also be included.

A few words about compartment syndrome. The earliest symptom is progressive pain out of proportion to the injury, and the earliest sign is hypesthesia in the distribution of the nerve in the affected compartment(s) [24]. Related findings are tenseness of the compartment, pain with passive stretching of the toes, and very late, vascular deficit. It is helpful to measure intracompartmental pressures to assist in the diagnosis, and these techniques have been described [6,23,24]. The time of ischemia is crucial to the eventual outcome, and therefore, this condition must be considered a surgical emergency, with immediate decompression by fasciotomy done as soon as the diagnosis is made.

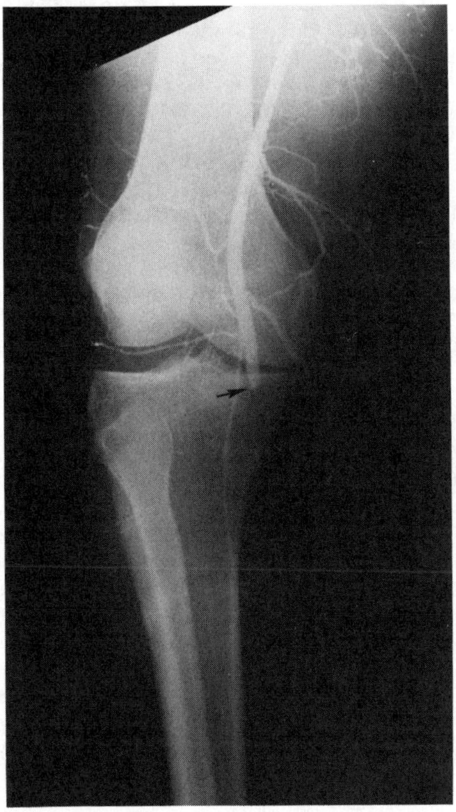

C

Fig. 13-5. (continued). *C.* Arteriogram showing complete occlusion of the popliteal artery at the level of the knee joint (*black arrow*).

Treatment

Early treatment of the tibial shaft fracture should include prompt reduction and appropriate immobilization. The metal and plastic splints applied in the field are not effective and need to be changed to some type of long leg plaster splint or cast. Elevation of the leg is also desirable. Definitive treatment is predicated on many factors.

Open fractures follow the same basic principles as above. Additionally, the open fracture wound should be cultured, irrigated with sterile saline, and dressed, and the patient started on intravenous antibiotic with proper tetanus prophylaxis. Surgical debridement is preferably done as soon as the patient can be transported to the operating suite.

REFERENCES

1. Grazier, K. L., Holbrook, T. L., Kelsey, J. L., and Stauffer, R. N. The Frequency of Occurrence, Impact and Cost of Musculoskeletal Conditions in the United States. Presented to the American Academy of Orthopedic Surgeons Annual Meeting, 1984.
2. Johnson, K. D., Cadambi, A., Seibert, G. B. Incidence of adult respiratory distress syndrome in patients with multiple musculoskeletal injuries: Effect of early operative stabilization of fractures. *J. Trauma* 25:375, 1965.
3. Riska, E., Von Donsdorff, H., Hakkinen, S., et al. Prevention of fat embolism by early internal fixation of fractures in patients with multiple injuries. *Injury* 8:110, 1976.
4. Neer, C. S. Fractures about the shoulder. Part I in Chapter 11, Fractures and Dislocations of the Shoulder. In C. A. Rockwood and D. P. Green (eds.), *Fractures in Adults*. Philadelphia: Lippincott, 1984. Vol. I, pp. 675–721.
5. Rockwood, C. A. Subluxations and dislocations about the shoulder. Part II in Chapter 11, Fractures and Dislocations of the Shoulder. In C. A. Rockwood and D. P. Green (eds.), *Fractures in Adults*. Philadelphia: Lippincott, 1984. Vol. I, pp. 743–747.
6. Gelberman, R. H., Garfin, S. R., Hergenroeder, P. T., et al. Compartment syndromes of the forearm: Diagnosis and treatment. *Clin. Orthop.* 161:252, 1981.
7. Tile, M. *Fractures of the Pelvis and Acetabulum*. Baltimore: Williams & Wilkins, 1984.

8. Murr, P. C., Moore, E. E., Lipscomb, R., and Johnston, R. I. Abdominal trauma associated with pelvic fracture. *J. Trauma* 20:919, 1980.
9. McMurtry, R., Walton, D., Dickinson, D., et al. Pelvic disruption in the polytraumatized patient: A management protocol. *Clin. Orthop.* 151:22, 1980.
10. Flint, L. M., Brown, A., Richardson, J. D., and Polk, H. C. Definitive control of bleeding from severe pelvic fractures. *Ann. Surg.* 169:709, 1979.
11. Slatis, R., and Karaharju, E. D. External fixation of unstable pelvic fractures: Experiences in 22 patients treated with a trapezoid compression frame. *Clin. Orthop.* 151:73, 1980.
12. Stock, J. R., Harris, W. H., and Athanasoulis, C. A. The role of diagnostic and therapeutic angiography in trauma to the pelvis. *Clin. Orthop.* 151:31, 1980.
13. Letournel, E. Surgical fixation of displaced pelvic fractures and dislocations of the symphysis. *Rev. Chir. Orthop.* 67:771, 1981.
14. Letournel, E., and Judet, R. Fractures of the acetabulum. *Rev. Chir. Orthop.* 67:771, 1981.
15. Epstein, H. C. Traumatic dislocations of the hip. *Clin. Orthop.* 136:56, 1979.
16. Latta, L. Unpublished data, 1986.
17. Hansen, S. T., and Winquist, R. A. Closed intramedullary nailing of the femur: Kuntscher technique with reaming. *Clin. Orthop.* 136:56, 1979.
18. Hansen, S. Concomitant Fractures of the Long Bones. In M. Meyers (ed.), *The Multiply Injured Patient with Complex Fractures.* Philadelphia: Lea & Febiger, 1964. Pp. 401–411.
19. Kennedy, J. C. Complete dislocation of the knee joint. *J. Bone Joint Surg.* [Am.] 45A:889, 1963.
20. Larson, R. L., and Jones, D. C. Dislocations and ligamentous injuries of the knee. Part II in Chapter 16, Fractures and Dislocations of the Knee. In C. A. Rockwood and D. P. Green (eds.), *Fractures in Adults.* Philadelphia: Lippincott, 1984. Vol. II, pp. 1502–1506.
21. Green, N. E., and Allen, B. L. Vascular injuries associated with dislocation of the knee. *J. Bone Joint Surg.* [Am.] 59A:236, 1977.
22. Leach, R. E. Fractures of the Tibia and Fibula. In C. A. Rockwood and D. P. Green (eds.), *Fractures in Adults.* Philadelphia: Lippincott, 1984. Vol. II, pp. 1593–1657.
23. Matsen, F. A., Winquist, R. A., and Krugsmire, R. B. Diagnosis and management of compartmental syndrome. *J. Bone Joint Surg.* [Am.] 62A:266, 1980.
24. Mubarak, S. J., Owen, C. A., Hargens, A. R., et al. Acute compartment syndrome: Diagnosis and treatment with aid of the wick catheter. *J. Bone Joint Surg.* [Am.] 60A:1091, 1976.

14

Burns

C. Gillon Ward
Jeffrey S. Hammond

Burn injury represents a formidable public health problem. Each year in the United States, 2 million people are burned, and 300,000 cases are serious enough to require hospitalization of the patient. Of these, approximately 10,000 patients die [1,2]. Burns represent the third leading cause of accidental death in the United States. One-third of these deaths are in children under 15 years of age. For each death caused by burns, three serious disabilities result.

EMERGENCY CARE AND GENERAL APPROACH

The initial approach to the burn patient sets the tone for further care. One must consider that the burn victim has been subjected to trauma, albeit a special form of trauma. The victim may have associated injuries other than burns (e.g., from an explosion, automobile accident). The ABCs of emergency care should be followed beginning when the patient is first seen at the site of the accident. Burn injuries do not bleed in the acute phase, and therefore evidence of hemorrhage indicates an associated injury.

Once integrity of the airway is ensured and adequate cardiopulmonary function is achieved, the burn wound must be assessed. Management decisions depend on the size (percent total body surface area [TBSA]) and depth of the burn. Rapid evaluation of burn size is made using the "rule of nines"; however, the estimate of size must be confirmed and documented using the Lund and Browder body surface area chart (Fig. 14-1) [3,4]. In infants and small children, the head accounts for a larger percentage and the limbs a smaller percentage of the body surface area than in an adult. Adult proportions are acquired at the age of 10 to 12 [5]. For burns that are highly irregular in shape, such as tar injuries,

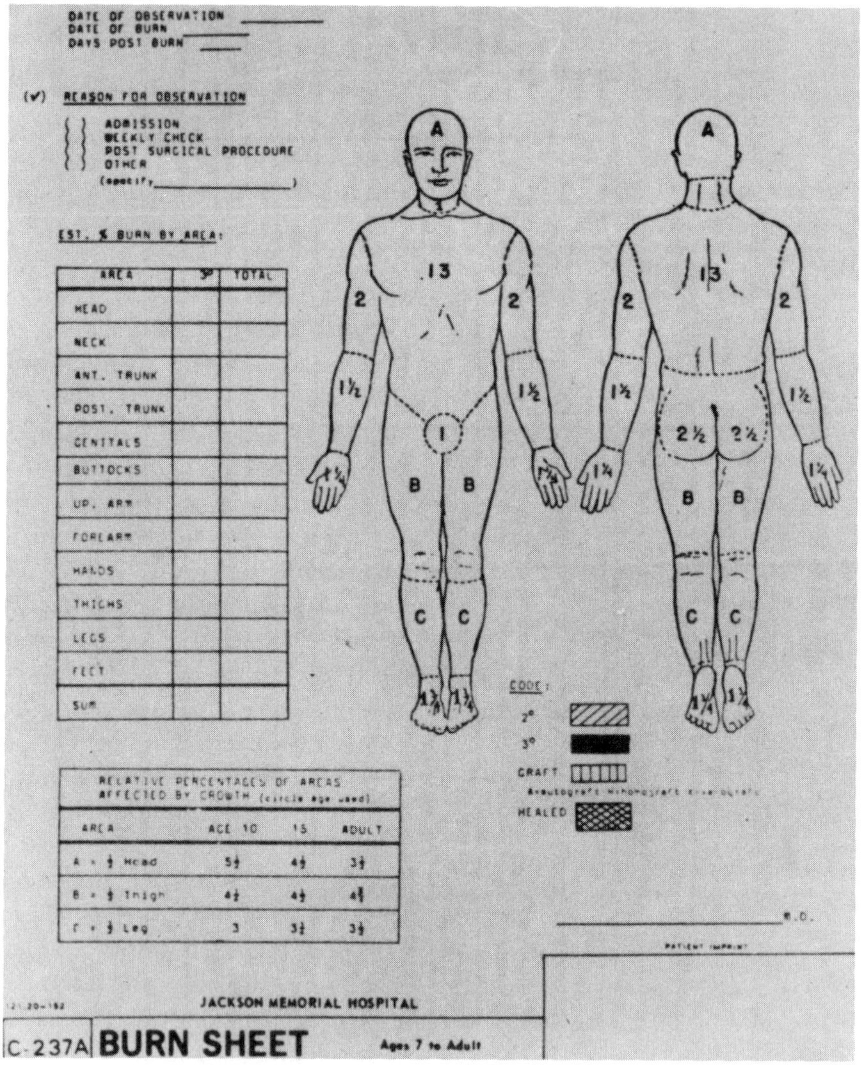
DATE OF OBSERVATION ________
DATE OF BURN ________
DAYS POST BURN ____

(✔) REASON FOR OBSERVATION

( ) ADMISSION
( ) WEEKLY CHECK
( ) POST SURGICAL PROCEDURE
( ) OTHER
(specify ______________)

EST. % BURN BY AREA:

AREA	3°	TOTAL
HEAD		
NECK		
ANT. TRUNK		
POST. TRUNK		
GENITALS		
BUTTOCKS		
UP. ARM		
FOREARM		
HANDS		
THIGHS		
LEGS		
FEET		
SUM		

RELATIVE PERCENTAGES OF AREAS AFFECTED BY GROWTH (circle age used)			
AREA	AGE 10	15	ADULT
A = ½ Head	5½	4½	3½
B = ½ Thigh	4¼	4½	4¾
C = ½ Leg	3	3¼	3½

CODE:
2°
3°
GRAFT
Autograft Homograft Heterograft
HEALED

______________ M.D.

PATIENT IMPRINT

JACKSON MEMORIAL HOSPITAL

C-237A BURN SHEET Ages 7 to Adult

Fig. 14-1. Worksheet illustrating the Lund-Browder chart.

Table 14-1. Clinical Assessment of Burn Depth

Degree	Color	Surface	Pain
First	Red	Intact	+
Second	Red	Blisters, weepy	+ + (but ↓ in deep second-degree)
Third	Blanched, white	Leathery	Dull or absent

a hand count may be beneficial in assessing burn size. Each individual's hand is approximately 1.25 percent of their TBSA.

Assessment of burn depth is a clinical decision based on the presence or absence of hair follicles, pain, bullae, and general wound appearance (Table 14-1). The criteria are crucial in deciding whether hospitalization is necessary and if transfer to a specialized burn center is warranted. The differentiation of second-degree from third-degree is not as important in the emergency setting as the recognition that burns of second-degree or greater exist. First-degree injuries have no physiologic significance and are not counted.

Other significant factors are the location of the wounds, the presence or absence of respiratory involvement, the nature of the burning agent, the age of the patient, and the patient's preburn medical history (Table 14-2). These factors, singly or in combination, determine need for hospitalization. The burning agent is important in estimating the depth of the wound. Hot water scalds are usually second-degree burns; flame burns are generally deeper. Immersion burns are deeper than splashes; food and soup deeper than hot water burns. Grease and tar burns are deceptively deep and are usually deep second-degree injuries or greater.

Table 14-2. Admissions Criteria

- Significant injury
  - Adult: >20% TBSA
  - Child: >15% TBSA
  - Extent: >2% TBSA third-degree
- Age: elderly (60 years)
- Inhalation injury
- Suspicion of child abuse
- Circumferential limb injury
- Electrical injury
  - High voltage: ≥1000 volts
  - Arrhythmias; loss of consciousness
- Chemical injuries
- Infected burns
- Special locations
  - Face, neck, eyes, ears
  - Hands, feet
  - Flexor creases, joints
  - Perineum, genitalia
- Medical history
  - Cardiac, chronic obstructive pulmonary disease
  - Renal, hepatic
  - Diabetes, sickle cell disease
- Unable to care for self

TBSA = total body surface area.

Inhalation Injury

A major concern in the early management of burns is the possibility of an inhalation injury. The presence or absence of pulmonary injury is a major determinant of survival. Inhalation injury is associated with a reported mortality of 45 to 78 percent [6].

True respiratory burns of the lower pulmonary tree are rare, generally occurring only with inhalation of superheated steam [7]. Moist air has 4000 times the heat-carrying capacity of dry air and interferes with the upper respiratory tract mucosa's ability to dissipate heat efficiently. What is commonly thought of as an inhalation injury is, in truth, either carbon monoxide poisoning or smoke inhalation, or both, leading to hypoxemia associated with bronchospasm and bronchorrhea. Either syndrome will increase the patient's potential for morbidity and mortality. Carbon monoxide, with an affinity for oxygen 200 times that of hemoglobin, will seriously impair oxygen delivery to the tissues. Incomplete products of combustion, such as aldehydes, nitrogen dioxide, and hydrochloric acid, cause direct parenchymal lung damage.

Early diagnosis of an inhalation injury can be difficult. Classic signs and symptoms, such as air hunger, shortness of breath, dysphonia, singed nasal hairs, and carbonaceous sputum, may be absent; they serve only as rough indicators of an inhalation injury. The history of being burned in an enclosed space in the presence of one or more "classic" signs serves to increase one's index of suspicion. The strongest correlation for a pulmonary injury is a history of the burn occurring in an enclosed space coupled either with facial burns or a history of a patient unconscious from alcohol or drugs [6,8].

The arterial blood gas determination and chest x-ray examination are often normal on admission to the emergency department. The serum carbon monoxide level may or may not be elevated, depending on time elapsed. The prognostic significance of a serum carbon monoxide level is debatable, especially if obtained after the patient has had supplemental oxygen [9]. Measured arterial oxygen saturation (not calculated from PaO_2) more accurately reflects hypoxemia. The concentration of carboxyhemoglobin is reduced by 50 percent for each 40-minute period of treatment with high-flow oxygen [10]. The half-life of carbon monoxide on the hemoglobin molecule is approximately 4 hours but drops to 30 minutes with administration of 100% oxygen.

Clinical or laboratory changes consistent with worsening pulmonary function and pulmonary edema may not become apparent until 18 to 36 hours after the respiratory insult [11]. Bronchoscopy and xenon scan studies of the lung may be helpful in the early diagnosis of respiratory injury [12,13] but are generally impractical. These tests are not universally available, nor are they easily done in the immediate postburn period. By themselves, they do not improve the accuracy of diagnosis; together the 85-percent accuracy is similar to assessment based on use of history and physical examination alone. As an alternative to bronchoscopy, direct laryngoscopy allows investigation for upper airway edema by visualization of the upper trachea and vocal cords. What remains, therefore, is a dependence on clinical judgment and index of suspicion.

If there is a question of possible inhalation injury, the patient should be admitted for 24 hours of observation. Use of prophylactic antibiotics will select out resistant organisms and is not recommended. Steroid therapy is not beneficial [14]; however, aggressive bronchodilator therapy and chest physiotherapy are advantageous. Fluid resuscitation should not be restricted but must be given in accordance with the patient's physiologic needs. In severe cases, ventilatory support with positive end-expiratory pressure (PEEP) is needed.

A burn patient arriving in an emergency department may be greeted by medical personnel superficially familiar with the principles of burn care. Mistakes of commission and omission begin to occur when the patient becomes combative and uncooperative. Hypoxia may be mistaken for pain. Fluid and oxygen are the treatment of choice rather than narcotics until it can be established that the patient is not hypovolemic or hypoxic. Narcotics are given intravenously rather than intramuscularly to avoid deposition into a nonperfused area. Pain medication delivered subcutaneously or intramuscularly during this early period will be ineffective, leading to repeated doses that may accumulate to be absorbed rapidly once this depot is mobilized. Immediate effects of intravenously administered morphine can be observed and reversed with naloxone (Narcan) if necessary.

Ventilatory support is essential for patients who present in acute respiratory distress or who later develop the adult (acute) respiratory distress syndrome secondary to smoke inhalation or sepsis. Indications for intubation include need to protect the airway, pulmonary toilet due to bronchorrhea, increased respiratory effort as evidenced by patient fatigue or carbon dioxide retention, and hypoxemia. Endotracheal or nasotracheal intubation is the preferred route for airway maintenance rather than early tracheostomy. Early tracheostomy is associated with increased morbidity and mortality [15]. A tracheostomy is indicated only when associated facial trauma prohibits intubation by the conventional approach or after a patient fails weaning from the ventilator.

Fluid Resuscitation

The purpose of fluid resuscitation in the early postburn period is reexpansion of plasma volume within the extracellular space. The pathophysiology of the vascular shift involves three processes: (1) loss of microvascular integrity, (2) impairment of the cell membrane, and (3) hypoproteinemia coupled with increased osmotic pressure in burned tissue [16]. Thus, the essential requirement in acute fluid resuscitation is a delivery of adequate amounts of sodium ion into the extracellular space, resulting in cellular transmembrane potentials returning to normal [17].

A variety of fluid resuscitation formulas exist [18–20]. Controversy over the early use of crystalloid versus colloids continues; however, all agree that adequate fluid resuscitation and repletion of plasma volume are essential in preventing complications of renal failure and "burn shock" [21]. The standard approach is to use the Parkland formula (4 ml × weight (kg) × percentage TBSA burned). The hourly rate is derived by dividing the calculated daily total by 24. Our philosophy is to withhold the use of colloids during the first 24 hours or until capillary leakage has ceased.

The quantitative measure of successful resuscitation is adequate urine output. This is based on the formula of 600 to 800 ml of urine/m^2 TBSA/day. Other nonrenal indicators of successful perfusion, such as pulse, blood pressure, mental status, and skin color, are inaccurate or unreliable. The use of right heart pressure measurements by Swan-Ganz catheterization during the acute phase to determine fluid resuscitation needs is ill-advised. One cannot assume that the Swan-Ganz values will be "normal" during resuscitation [21], there is a risk of fluid overload if one attempts to reach a preconceived "optimal" level, and filling pressures do not reflect adequate perfusion. Immediately after a burn, cardiac output decreases even with "good" filling pressures. Later cardiac output is high. Urine output continues to be the safest standard for monitoring visceral perfusion and is the most important resuscitation parameter. Because of this, the use of diuretics is a relative contraindication. If a respirator is required because of an inhalation injury however, a Swan-Ganz catheter may be appropriate to measure cardiac output and the effects of increasing PEEP.

All fluid resuscitation formulas are guidelines, and hourly adjustments may be necessary. Remember, "the patient is the formula." When the volume required exceeds that calculated by more than 20 percent to maintain urine output, look for errors in the assessment of the extent of the burn or the estimation of body weight. When all arithmetic errors are eliminated and the required resuscitation volume exceeds the calculated volume by more than 25 percent, the presence of an inhalation injury should be strongly suspected [22]. In this case, the injured lung requires additional fluid not accounted for in the resuscitation formula.

The use of hypertonic sodium solution allows successful resuscitation and reduces attendant edema [23,24]. Hypertonic resuscitation minimizes potential complications of edema, thus avoiding laryngeal obstruction requiring intubation, limb edema requiring escharotomies to relieve ischemia, or prolonged ileus [25]. The use of hypertonic resuscitation is based on the fact that much of the fluid "losses" early postburn represent an intracellular shift of sodium and that sodium replacement is the effective component of resuscitation [17]. It can be replaced by giving the required amount of sodium in a variable amount of fluid, either less volume (hypertonic) or greater volume (isotonic).

Complications of hypertonic saline resuscitation include hyperosmolarity, hypernatremia, and hyperchloremic acidosis. We advocate the use of a hypertonic sodium solution low in chloride to avoid these complications. The solution used at the University of Miami/Jackson Memorial Burn Center is 1 liter of lactated Ringer's solution to which 100 mEq of sodium acetate has been added. This is administered at the rate to deliver 0.52 mEq of sodium/kg/percentage TBSA burned over 24 hours. Hypertonic resuscitation should be closely monitored and overhydration avoided. Free water may be required if the serum sodium level exceeds 155 mEq/L or sodium osmolarity is greater than 320 mOsm/L.

Fear that seemingly large volumes of correctly calculated resuscitation fluid will lead to pulmonary edema is unjustified. However, the overzealous infusion of fluids must also be avoided. Large volumes given initially in the field or emergency room are not retained as effective intravascular resuscitation fluid. Use of hypotonic solutions accentuates the patient's natural tendency toward hyponatremia.

Inappropriate use of dextrose solutions in the adult results in a misleading osmotic diuresis. This "pseudodiabetes" leads to an artificially induced urine flow, which negates urine output as a means of assessing kidney perfusion. In addition, osmotic diuresis is associated with hypokalemia, hypophosphatemia, and hypomagnesemia. Equally important, glucose will enter the burn wound, creating an osmotic gradient, attracting more fluid, accentuating wound edema, and complicating resuscitation [26].

In children, however, resuscitation fluid must contain glucose. Small children have neither the equivalent glycogen stores of adults nor the ability to convert fat and proteins into glucose easily. An osmotic diuresis may be encountered in children; therefore, dextrose concentration is decreased if glycosuria occurs. An accurate assessment and an intelligent treatment plan will obviate these problems.

Generally, intravenous fluid resuscitation is required in adults with burns of 15 percent TBSA or greater and in children with burns of 10 percent TBSA or greater. Patients with smaller burns, however, may benefit from resuscitation, for example, a drunk or previously dehydrated patient, or children with facial burns who reject feedings. In small children, the resuscitation volume may calculate to be less than the daily normal maintenance volume of 1500 ml/m^2/day (see Burns in Children). In such a case, one gives the burn formula *plus* daily maintenance for the first 24 hours.

EXAMPLE

In a 10-kg child with a 20 percent TBSA scald burn
Normal maintenance = 750 ml/day
Parkland formula = 10 kg × 4 ml × 20 percent TBSA = 800 ml/day
800 ml/day − 750 ml/day = 50 ml/day allowed for the burn
Therefore, the Parkland formula alone leads to underresuscitation in a child less than 2 years of age.

Colloid in the form of albumen or fresh frozen plasma is added to the intravenous fluid during the second 24 hours or when the primary capillary leakage has stopped. In this way, maximal benefit from an increased colloid oncotic pressure is obtained. A diuretic phase begins on approximately the third to fifth postburn day, during which there is a risk of hypokalemia if potassium is not replaced parenterally.

An intelligent plan for resuscitation requires full evaluation of the burn wound. This cannot be done unless the wound has been mapped. Although the rule of nines is sufficient in an emergency setting, eventual evaluation utilizing a Lund-Browder body surface area chart is essential. Blistered and loose skin must be removed. The extent of an injury can be surprisingly larger or smaller than initially assessed. This is particularly true with heavily pigmented patients and has significant clinical impact on the very young and the elderly.

Tetanus Prophylaxis

Emergency care of the acute injury, either major or minor, dictates adequate tetanus prophylaxis. Clinical tetanus has been described even in superficial second-degree injuries [27]. For patients previously immunized, a booster of tetanus toxoid is given. For those never immunized, active as well as passive immunization is required. For previously immunized patients with large burns or patients with an uncertain immunization history, passive immunization with tetanus immune human globulin (Hyper-Tet) is suggested.

Ocular Injury

Direct ocular injury is uncommon unless chemical agents have come into contact with the orbit [28]. Usually, only the eyelids are injured; the cornea is protected by Bell's phenomenon. Acid or alkaline injury to the eye is a true ophthalmic emergency. The eye should always be inspected early, before facial edema makes evaluation impossible. The eyes should be irrigated with saline to a neutral pH as determined by litmus paper. Smoke and other particulate matter may, however, create a corneal abrasion; therefore, an examination with fluorescein is indicated. There is no indication for early tarsorrhaphy. Superficial corneal injuries reepithelialize within 48 hours, requiring only systemic pain relief and eye patching; local anesthetics are not used. Significant or questionable injuries warrant ophthalmologic consultation.

Post-burn Ileus

During the first 48 hours, patients with burns in excess of 20 percent TBSA have an ileus. The reasons are both pharmacologic and mechanical. The massive catecholamine release associated with the injury shows peristalsis and augments the bowel mesentery edema that occurs during the resuscitation phase. Such an ileus is generally self-limited and resolves during the diuretic phase. Nasogastric suction prevents emesis and pulmonary aspiration. As soon as gastric and intestinal emptying begins at 48 to 72 hours, the rigid nasogastric tube is removed, and nutritional support commences immediately, either orally or through a Silastic feeding tube.

Initial Wound Care

Full assessment of the burn wound is not possible until after thorough debridement. In the emergency department setting, iced saline is not used to debride or cover up the wounds. Although the cold does decrease pain and may decrease edema, it also creates hypothermia, increases metabolic demands, and may injure marginally viable cells; therefore, application of ice or ice water is not advised for burns larger than 10 percent TBSA. All blisters should be debrided except those on the soles of the feet and palms of the hands. In those areas, the skin is relatively thick, and preservation of bullae reduces pain, speeds epithelialization, and allows use of the hands during physiotherapy and early ambulation even with burns of the feet. Elsewhere, the burn wound is debrided, and thick hair in the vicinty of the injury is shaved. Topical therapy can then be instituted (see under Wound Care).

Unless a patient is physically confined to bed by support equipment, a daily tubbing or shower is done in conjunction with one of the dressing changes. Debridement and wound washing are done during this time. Wounds must be inspected daily, since a streptococcal or staphylococcal cellulitis can appear and advance rapidly.

Escharotomy

The major musculoskeletal complication during the early postburn period is a compartment syndrome. Circumferential injuries, because of their effect on the perfusion of an extremity, may create a vascular emergency. The burn need not be full thickness or totally circumferential to produce vascular compromise [29].

The inelastic burned skin acts as a tourniquet; edema from the burn trauma and the subsequent fluid resuscitation lead to increased compartment pressure and resultant venous compression. Compartment pressure continues to build until arterial inflow stops. Thus, the presence of pulses in a circumferentially burned extremity does not preclude against vascular compromise. The pressure within the extremity must exceed arterial pressure before arterial pulsation is no longer felt or heard. Prior to this, venous occlusion results in increased compartment pressure that endangers the viable nerves by compromising small vasa nervorum. Ulnar and peroneal nerve palsies can occur in the absence of classic signs of limb ischemia.

Direct measurement of compartmental pressure is the best way to determine the need for an escharotomy if there is clinical doubt [30]. Commercially made wick catheters are available but not necessary; this procedure can be done with a standard 21-gauge needle connected by high-pressure tubing to a transducer and pressure monitor. Pressure exceeding 30 mm Hg is sufficient to occlude venous outflow and indicates the need for an escharotomy. Individual compartments can be monitored selectively.

Fig. 14-2. Escharotomy of the right arm and hand. Note the separation of the skin edges and the extension of the escharotomy onto the digits.

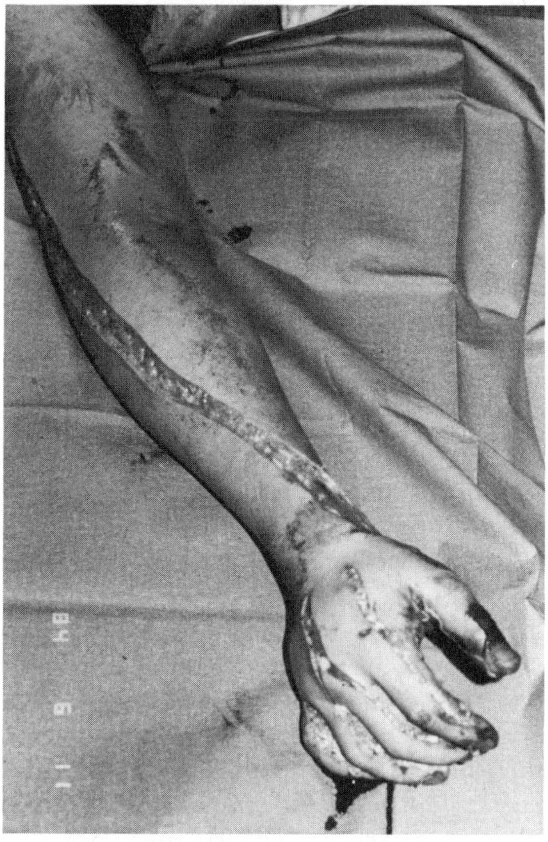

Escharotomy is best done at the time it is considered. It is essentially a bedside procedure, not requiring an operating room. The eschar is incised to the underlying subcutaneous tissue (Fig. 14-2). Fasciotomy is rarely required except in high-voltage electrical injuries. Since the eschar is nonviable, bleeding is minimal. Electrocautery is helpful, however, for small areas of bleeding that occur in the underlying fat. Morphine can often provide adequate pain relief; for larger procedures, ketamine is an excellent short-acting anesthetic.

In distal arm and hand burns, escharotomies must be extended onto the dorsal surface of the hand for maximal benefit. Escharotomy only to the wrist is not sufficient. Severely burned hands may require escharotomies of individual fingers [31]. Occasionally, eschar on the torso creates a restrictive respiratory insufficiency, which is relieved by chest escharotomies. This is most often seen in pediatric patients because of lack of intercostal development, but it may also occur in adults.

WOUND CARE

The mainstay of burn treatment is good wound care. Wounds must be examined and assessed daily, and care plans revised accordingly. Evidence of breakdown in previously closed areas may suggest trauma, poor nutritional support, or infection. Mechanical debridement is necessary; merely submerging the patient in a whirlpool is not by itself sufficient. Topical drug therapy can be used in either an open or closed fashion.

Topical Therapy

Topical drug therapy is now a mainstay of burn care. The goal is control of bacterial colonization of the wound until spontaneous eschar separation or debridement and subsequent wound closure. Teplitz, in pioneering a clinicopathologic model of burn wound sepsis, pointed out that 75 percent of patient deaths were associated with burn wound sepsis, and in 54 percent of these, the infection was limited to the burn wound.

Silver sulfadiazine (Silvadene) is an excellent, all-purpose agent. In the United States, it is the primary topical agent of choice. It is applied at least twice daily, after removing all the old cream and cellular debris before each new application. If left for longer periods or caked up, it will create a neo-eschar. It has a wide antibacterial spectrum but may be less effective against virulent staphylococcus. It has few disadvantages: infrequent hypersensitivity to the sulfa and a transient leukopenia. The leukopenia is both absolute (decrease) and relative (immature forms) [32]. If the white blood cell count falls below 2000, it is best to change to a different topical agent. When the white blood cell count returns to normal, silver sulfadiazine can be restarted, and only rarely will there be a recurrent leukopenia. Silver sulfadiazine is characterized by intermediate penetration into eschar and therefore may not be effective in relatively deeply burned or avascular areas [33].

An alternative topical agent is mafenide acetate (Sulfamylon). Capable of greater penetration into eschar than silver sulfadiazine, it has excellent bacteriostasis. Because mafenide has better eschar penetration than silver sulfadiazine, it is an excellent agent to be used for dressing change on eschar just prior to excision of a burn wound, infected burns, or extremely thick eschar such as seen in electrical injuries. Its disadvantages include pain on application and creating a predisposition to candidal overgrowth in the wound. It must be used with caution in large burns, since it is systemically absorbed and produces a metabolic acidosis secondary to carbonic anhydrase inhibition and bicarbonate excretion in the kidneys. The greater the surface area burn, the greater the absorption. Usually noted after 3 to 5 days of use, this results in hyperventilation [34]. Patients with chronic obstructive pulmonary disease do not compensate well, which can lead to further accentuation of the acidosis.

Povidone-iodine (Betadine) is effective against staphylococcus species; however, it may injure marginally viable cells. Like mafenide, it is painful upon application, and this complaint from patients should be anticipated. When used as a solution or ointment on burns greater than 50-percent TBSA, hypernatremia can be an associated complication. Serum sodium levels of 160 mEq with serum osmolarities of 380 mOsm have been reported [35]. This is reversed when the povidone-iodine is removed and a different topical agent substituted. Povidone-iodine should not be used with silver sulfadiazine, since silver iodine precipitation will inactivate both agents. Hyperiodemia has been described, but the clinical significance has not been determined [36]. Since iodine levels can be increased after prolonged use, povidone-iodine is generally avoided over large surface areas or prolonged periods of use in children.

Silver nitrate is a liquid topical preparation, used as a 0.5% solution and applied as a wet-to-wet dressing saturating the wound. It has excellent antibacterial properties but poor penetration into the eschar. Moreover, it is difficult and messy to use. With its use, both burned and nonburned skin becomes discolored, making serial examination of the wound difficult [33]. Electrolyte imbalances are common; because it is hypotonic, an osmotic gradient may lead to a hyponatremic, volume-depleted state. The required bulky dressings hamper early physical therapy.

Furacin is a nitrofurazone compound that was a mainstay in burn therapy prior to the introduction of silver sulfadiazine. It has a wide batericidal spectrum, especially against *Pseudomonas* and other enteric species. Major drawbacks include hypersensitivity reaction in up to 25 percent of patients and hyperosmolarity secondary to propylene glycol absorption [37].

Moist saline dressings are effective for superficial second-degree wounds. Dakin's solution or another similar sodium hypochlorite solution can also be used on a wet-to-dry or wet-to-wet basis. This type of dressing can be used for preparing a recipient site for grafting or for minor debridement. Wet-to-dry dressings are painful, and increased analgesic medication is needed.

Travase is an enzymatic debriding agent useful in wound care. A proteolytic enzyme derivative of the *Bacillus subtilis,* it has no antibacterial properties itself and must be mixed with another topical agent such as silver sulfadiazine or mafenide acetate. It will not injure viable tissue and can be an effective adjunct to surgical debridement [38]. Disadvantages include pain on application and leeching sodium and water through the wound resulting in hyponatremia and volume depletion. Travase (sutilains) is not compatible with povidone-iodine, which inactivates the enzyme.

To be effective, Travase must have a wetting agent. Saline is applied to the dressings after application of the Travase and topical agent. A dry kerlix is then applied. Some bleeding from the wound may be noted.

Surgical Management

Since the reintroduction of the concept of tangential excision of the burn wound in the 1960s, early operative debridement of the burn wound with wound closure either by autograft or allograft has become a standard of care [39,40]. Improvement in survival correlates with aggressive, prompt excision of burn eschar and immediate physiologic closure of the wound [41]. The presence of the burn wound itself has an impact on the body beyond its potential as a nidus of infection. Once burn wound sepsis is established, debridement can be thought of as analogous to draining an abscess. Debridement and early closure of wounds of indeterminate depth also decrease morbidity over more conservative approaches by speeding closure time, hastening entry into rehabilitation therapy programs, decreasing pain, and retarding formation of hypertrophic scar.

There are two types of burn wound excision: tangential (sequential) and full (fascial) [42]. Dermal injuries can be debrided with a hand-held knife or power-driven dermatome held tangential to the wound, removing eschar serially in layers. Full excision of the eschar is performed with scalpel, electrocautery, or laser and removes the wound and subcutaneous tissue down to the level of the underlying muscle fascia (Fig. 14-3).

Tangential excision is carried down to punctuate bleeding. Unless good bleeding of the wound bed is noted, the excision has not been adequate. Excision over bony prominences can be facilitated by subcutaneous infiltration of saline. Once an adequate excision has taken place, lap pads soaked in epinephrine (1/10,000 solution) are placed on the wound, followed by wrapping with an Ace bandage to stop the bleeding. Although topical epinephrine may be absorbed systemically, it does not result in arrhythmias or hypertension [43]. Occasionally, electrocautery is necessary, especially if the debridement is carried into the underlying subcutaneous tis-

Fig. 14-3. A full excision of the burn eschar to the underlying fascia on the dorsum of the right hand.

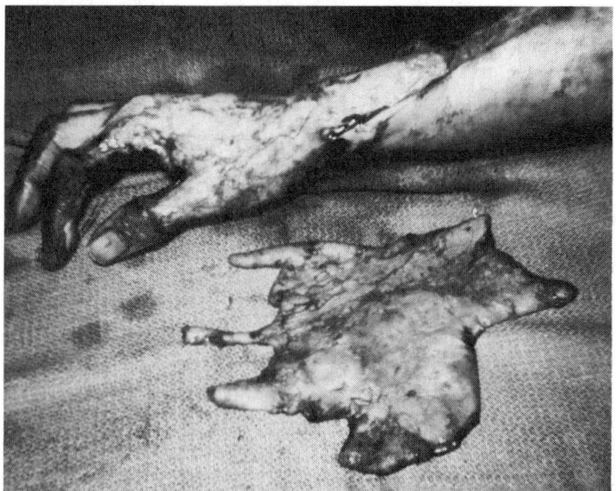

sue. In areas not amenable to Ace wrapping, topical thrombin spray is helpful.

Wounds debrided only superficially into the dermis can be redressed with a topical agent. These are usually left undisturbed until the following day, when a dressing change is done in the tub. Wounds tangentially excised into deeper layers of the dermis require closure to prevent desiccation or formation of a neo-eschar. Wound closure can be achieved utilizing autograft, allograft, other biologic dressings, or synthetic skin substitutes.

For full-thickness injuries, an excision down to the underlying fascia may be indicated. Full (or fascial) excision should also be considered for exposed and desiccated subcutaneous fat and for severe invasive bacterial or fungal wound infection. The advantages of full excision include a more controlled blood loss. The fascial bed may provide a better recipient site for immediate autografting than exposed subcutaneous tissue. Full excision in the face of burn wound sepsis removes the complete eschar and underlying tissue, which is the source of bacterial or fungal invasion of the lymphatics. Disadvantages of full excision are that it results in a poor cosmetic result, commits one to future skin grafts or flaps, may expose underlying tendon, and sacrifices cutaneous sensory nerves.

Operative debridement of the burn wound is not be taken lightly. Each patient undergoing a full-thickness excision or tangential debridement of burn wound greater than 10-percent TBSA should have 4 to 6 units of blood available in the operating room. Prior to the actual excision, the blood is checked and prepared for infusion. All solutions are passed through a warming coil. To prevent hypothermia, the operating room should be preheated. Prolonged exposure is avoided. The key to success is to minimize the operative trauma to the patient; planning and preparation prior to starting debridement is mandatory. Attention to detail is of paramount importance.

The excision is a timed procedure and rarely should exceed more than 20 minutes by the clock. Excision of more than 20-percent TBSA in a single sitting is unusual. A tangential debridement carried out for a longer period of time or over a greater surface area may be more detrimental to the patient than a return to the operating room 1 or 2 days later. Because it is a timed procedure, all potentially necessary equipment should be laid out and available prior to the start of the excision.

The anesthesiologist must be part of the operating team. For example, care must be taken not to inadvertently contaminate the endotracheal tube on the patient's dressing or wounds. A burn patient should never receive succinylcholine [44]. Systemic hyperkalemia is associated with the use of this drug in burn patients, as in all trauma patients. The use of a slower acting, nondepolarizing muscle relaxant such as pancuronium is in order; the use of succinylcholine in a burn patient is absolutely contraindicated until after the wounds heal.

Wound Closure

A number of methods are available to attain wound closure after debridement or excision. Factors such as availability of donor sites, presence or absence of infection, patient stability in the operating room, associated medical factors, and rehabilitation goals will all contribute to the decision. Skin coverage can be thought of as either permanent or temporary. Examples of permanent coverage include autografting or flaps; temporary dressing may be either biologic, such as allograft, or synthetic. Like debridement, wound closure requires advanced planning for optimal results.

There is no substitute for the patient's own skin. Most burn wounds, especially in the acute period, can be adequately managed utilizing split-thickness skin grafts 0.010 to 0.012 inch thick. Local or free flaps are the exception rather than the rule. Thick skin grafts will provide better functional and cosmetic results than thin split-thickness skin grafts, but one must take into account the possible future need for reharvesting donor sites.

Except for the face or other critical cosmetic areas, most skin grafts are meshed, allowing for expansion and larger surface area coverage. In addition, fluids beneath the meshed graft will not collect as a seroma or hematoma, especially on freshly excised areas. Skin meshed at a 1.5 : 1 ratio and minimally expanded will generally give a good cosmetic result everywhere except the face (Fig. 14-4). When donor sites are sparse, a meshing ratio of 3 : 1, or even 6 : 1, may be used. Care should be taken to approximate adjacent pieces of skin graft carefully. This may be done using surgical staples, which are faster to apply than sutures. Steri-strips are also effective.

The most common cause of early graft failure is poor adherence. This is most often the result of motion of the graft on the recipient site. Care must be taken to apply closely con-

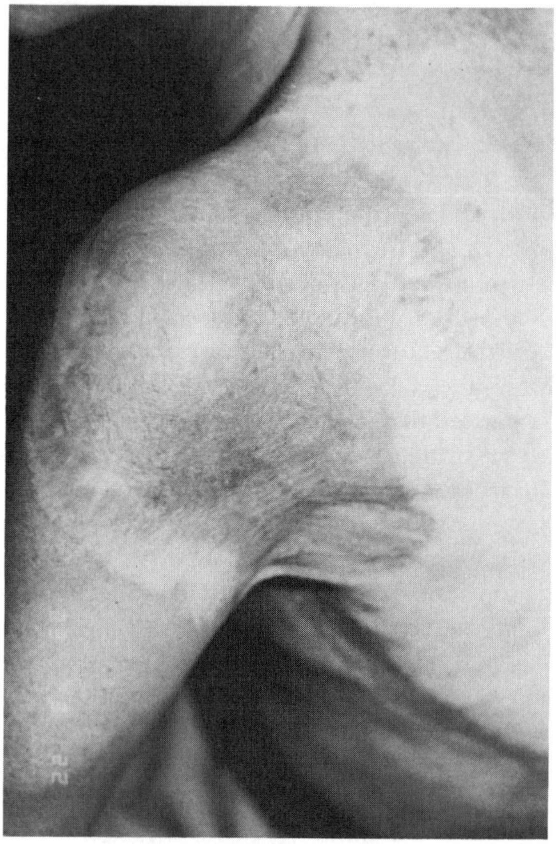

Fig. 14-4. Appearance of a 1.5 : 1 meshed, unexpanded skin graft at maturity.

forming dressings and immobilizing splints. Preoperative consultation with the occupational therapist is invaluable.

If autografting is not feasible, temporary coverage with a biologic dressing such as allograft or xenograft is advisable. Biologic dressings afford the bacteriostasis, pain relief, and diminution of fluid and protein loss seen with autografts [45]. Xenografts, most commonly pigskin, have the disadvantage of increased antigenicity, need for frequent dressing changes, and hyperpyrexia. As such, allograft is the preferred alternative. It has the disadvantage, however, of limited availability, high cost, and the possibility of rejection phenomenon. These disadvantages do not outweigh the benefit, however, and in the absence of the patient's own skin, cadaver allograft is our dressing of choice.

The ideal skin substitute should afford adherence, durability, elasticity, adequate vapor barrier, bacteriostasis, and pain protection [46]. Of these, adherence is the most important factor. Poor wound adherence correlates with increased subgraft suppuration [47]. Skin coverage with biologic dressings will sterilize a contaminated wound, but the bacterial suppression is related more to adherence and subsequent vascular ingrowth than any property inherent to the graft or prosthesis.

Cadaver allograft may be used either fresh or frozen. The results with frozen equal that of fresh allograft and have the advantage of longer shelf life. The slow, controlled-rate freezing coupled with quick thawing results in a product that has oxygen consumption almost equal to live skin [48].

Clinical uses of cadaver allograft are varied (Fig. 14-5). It can provide immediate coverage of fresh second-degree burns or prolonged coverage of debrided wounds. One must take care not to leave allograft that has "taken" on a wound until the point of classic rejection. The resultant inflammation may convert a partial-thickness wound to a full-thickness injury. For similar reasons, allograft cannot be

Fig. 14-5. Sheets of cadaver allograft 12 days after application to the right leg. Note the 3 : 1 mesh autograft on the thigh at 5 days postsurgery.

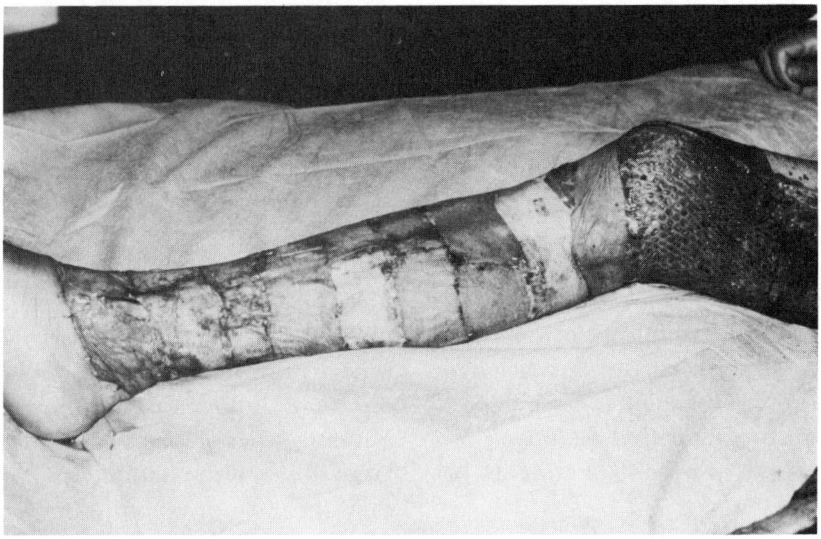

recommended as a dressing for split-thickness skin graft donor site [49]. Allograft may, however, be used to prepare a poor granulating bed for autografting or as a test graft. Finally, it will protect exposed tendon and fat from desiccation until autografting or local flaps can be done.

If allograft is unavailable, a variety of synthetic temporary skin substitutes are available. These dressings are less versatile than biologic dressings. The best of these currently commercially available are Biobrane and Opsite [50,51]. Biobrane is a bilaminar nylon/silicon temporary skin coverage that has semipermeable properties. It can be used as a covering for donor sites, wide-meshed skin grafts, or superficial injuries. Once applied and adherent, it does not need to be covered and can be left open to air, obviating the need for frequent dressing changes. As the new epithelium regenerates from the underlying dermis, the Biobrane will be lifted off the wound, much in the fashion as xeroform gauze is "rejected." Biobrane comes in a variety of thicknesses and with variable pore size. It requires some expertise in application.

Opsite is another semipermeable membrane dressing, an advanced generation of Hydron spray. A polyurethane film, it is more occlusive than Biobrane and therefore less useful over wet, weeping surfaces because of the risk of seroma formation. Like Biobrane, it is transparent, lending itself to observation of the wound through the dressing. Because it is virtually water impermeable, it is a useful dressing for intravenous catheter sites of patients who undergo whirlpool treatments or tubbing.

Pain Control

There is a dichotomy in the treatment of pain in the burn patient. When seen in the emergency room, it is common for the patient to be overmedicated. Once hospitalized, the patient is commonly undermedicated [52]. The individual with a second-degree injury has exposed, functional nerve endings. The changing of a dressing, the debriding of a wound, or a rehabilitation therapy session stimulates these functioning organs.

For dressing changes, an adult will require a minimum of 10 mg of morphine or 100 mg of meperidine (Demerol). This is the recommended starting dosage for an adult. It is improper to consider a lesser dose or the addition of promethazine (Phenergan) as a potentiating agent. For tubbings or large dressing changes, a dose of 20 to 40 mg of morphine may be required. Such a dosage can be titrated. The nursing staff may give increments of 5 to 10 mg until the patient is comfortable but not unconscious. Keep in mind that it is easier to prevent pain than to eradicate pain; adequate analgesia should be given before stimulation [53].

Morphine is a safer drug than diazepam (Valium) because of its easy reversibility with naloxone (Narcan). Naloxone should always be present when large doses of morphine are used. Remember, however, that the half-life of naloxone is less than that of morphine (20–30 minutes), and a second dose may be needed. When morphine is used appropriately (i.e., *only* for painful stimuli), our experience is that patients do not become addicts, even after large doses. If the patient is a known drug addict, he will frequently require additional doses of medication. It is our philosophy to give the drug addict such medication. Attempts at drug withdrawal are only successful within a very controlled environment, where the patient is being mentally and physically supported, not after trauma such as burns where the patient is placed within a strange and often painful environment.

Sharp debridement of eschar done outside the operating room or other procedures such as escharotomies or allograft placement can be facilitated through the judicious use of lidocaine (Xylocaine) field or regional blocks or ketamine anesthesia. Before starting such a procedure, all equipment, drugs, and personnel that might be necessary must be secure. Cardiovascular monitoring is essential; the automated blood pressure cuff is useful. If blood loss is anticipated, blood should be called for and its identification checked prior to starting the procedure.

Ketamine is a dissociative anesthetic that is amenable to short-term use. It is fast acting and associated with a slightly increased skeletal muscle tone, cardiovascular and respiratory stimulation, occasional mild respiratory depression, and normal pharyngeal reflexes. Postanesthetic psychological side effects occur in up to 12 percent of patients. Doses of 2 mg/kg produce anesthesia for 5 to 10 minutes. The adjunct use of atropine decreases salivation. Ketamine should be used with caution in patients in whom increased blood pressure could be dangerous. Mechanical stimulation of the pharynx should be avoided. Intraocular and intracranial pressure may increase; therefore, avoid use in patients with glaucoma or head injury.

Lidocaine is metabolized mainly by the liver and is excreted by the kidneys. Adverse reactions may result from excessive doses, inadvertent intravascular injections, or idiosyncrasy. Central nervous system reactions are excitatory, while cardiovascular effects are depressant. Maximal doses in adults should not exceed 4.5 mg/kg without epinephrine or 7 mg/kg with epinephrine.

NUTRITION

Plans for the nutritional support of the patient are considered at the time of admission to the burn team. The hypercatabolic state in the patient with over 20-percent TBSA burns is characterized by increased oxygen consumption, increased nitrogen excretion, and weight loss [54]. The increased metabolic rate is proportional to the size of the burn up to 50-percent TBSA, where a plateau is reached at near maximal levels of heat production [55]. Metabolic rate may exceed normal levels by 2 to 2½ times. The hypermetabolic state is characterized by the preferential use of lean body mass for gluconeogenesis.

The cause of the extreme hypercatabolism of large burns remains unknown. Conflicting data exist to indicate, as well as refute, the roles of external stimuli and changes in endogenous setpoint as the pathogenesis [56,57]. Since the evaporation of 1 ml of water requires 0.58 kcal, some portion of the hypercatabolism is associated with heat loss due to vaporization of water. Use of occlusive dressings or an increase of ambient temperature, however, does not fully offset the elevated metabolic rate. The increased oxygen consumption is not the result of post-traumatic hyperthyroidism but may be mediated by increased activity of the sympathetic nervous system. Thus, two components may be at work, and the burn patient may be both internally warm and externally cold.

Establishing the minimum daily caloric needs has been difficult, and a number of guidelines and formulas exist. The most commonly used yardstick is the Curreri formula: (25 × kg) + (45 × % burn) [58]. Recent studies employing indirect calorimetry indicate that this formula may best predict the maximal caloric need rather than daily requirements [59]. A more realistic approach is to attempt to achieve this maximal caloric input only during periods of extreme stress such as sepsis and to aim for daily levels of approximately 60 to 70 percent of the Curreri formula. Use of indirect calorimetry is difficult and expensive; daily urine nitrogen levels are unreliable. Modifications of the Harris-Benedict formula to estimate energy requirements have not been validated against measured energy expenditure in burn patients.

The response to a burn injury is one of an ileus that typically resolves in 2 to 3 days. Once the ileus is resolved, the patient is expected to eat. If the patient is unable to do so, tube feedings can be started. There is no reason to institute intravenous hyperalimentation as the primary means for nutritional support when an intact gastrointestinal tract exists. All efforts are made to utilize the gastrointestinal tract before subjecting a patient to the morbidity and mortality associated with intravenous hyperalimentation solutions. There are a number of advantages to enteral feedings. Tube feedings can be tailored to a patient's specific needs while avoiding the risk of line sepsis associated with intravenous hyperalimentation. They protect the gut mucosa lining, neutralize gastric pH, preserve a normal balance of gut flora, and reduce the risk of endotoxemia. Moreover, preliminary data indicate that parenteral nutrition may in fact adversely affect the immunologic host defenses [60]. Tube feedings for the very young and the elderly should be discontinued at night to avoid aspiration. When tube feeding volume exceeds 50 ml/hr, the head of the bed should be elevated. Tube feeding is never begun until radiographic confirmation has been made of placement of the radiopaque tip in the stomach.

Elemental diets such as Vital are begun by infusing one-third strength at a rate of 30 ml/hr. Once begun, there are two options: Increase the infused volume at 15 to 30 ml/hr every 12 to 24 hours, or gradually increase the strength up to double strength. In children, volume is considered first to ensure adequate fluid maintenance and urine output. The concentration is increased after reaching an appropriate volume intake.

If diarrhea occurs because of the high osmolarity of tube feedings, one can decrease the concentration and/or volume. If diarrhea persists, 5 to 10 ml of Lomotil can be added to the tube feeding. If this does not work, a tube feeding with a different osmolarity or use of a bulking agent may give a favorable response.

Burn nutrition should be started as soon as the gastrointestinal tract will tolerate feeding, as early as the third day. Calories equate to survival in severely traumatized patients. Care is taken to provide these calories as fat, proteins, and carbohydrates. To avoid cholestasis, no more than 40 percent of the total caloric load should be in the form of fat. The nonprotein kilocalorie-nitrogen ratio of 100 : 1 will achieve positive nitrogen balance in patients with over 20-percent TBSA wounds more effectively than a 150 : 1 ratio [61]. Trace elements such as copper and zinc are essential. Zinc is lost through the burn wound and is provided orally in the gluconate form to enhance wound healing and augment immunologic defense mechanisms. Vitamin supplementation, especially vitamin C at 1 to 2 gm/day (adult dosage), is used to promote collagen synthesis and wound healing.

Parenteral hyperalimentation is considered only when all other routes of nutrition have failed. Peripheral hyperalimentation using a 7.5% glucose solution in conjunction with a peripheral lipid solution is considered first. The morbidity and mortality associated with centrally infused 20 to 25% glucose solution have to be carefully weighed against the gain.

Fluid taken by mouth must contain calories. Allowing patients to drink large volumes of water is discouraged. Patients may have alcoholic beverages if they wish. This particularly applies to individuals who have been known to be heavy drinkers. Alcohol helps prevent delirium tremens, provides calories, and acts as a mild sedative.

SEPSIS AND INFECTION CONTROL

For victims not killed at the scene, most burn deaths occur during the critical first 2 weeks post injury. The major causes of death are progressive pulmonary insufficiency and sepsis. Uncontrolled infection leading to multisystem failure is a cause of death in over 50 percent of burn patients. For the burn patient, any organism can be a pathogen; it is more a matter of when and where the contamination occurs. Evidence of burn wound infection typically manifests itself first at 5 to 7 days post injury. Usually, the patient is self-contaminated. Common sources are the gastrointestinal tract, upper respiratory tract, nasopharynx, and nonburned skin. In women, vaginal flora secondarily contaminate adjacent wounds, especially with fungal species. The other major source of contamination for the burn wound comes from personnel carrying bacteria from one patient to another. Poor technique by the hospital staff allows bacteria to be passed from patient to patient. In this respect, strict hand washing and other infection control techniques cannot be stressed enough.

The burn team must approach a wound with the intent of not carrying organisms either to or from a patient. Scrub dress rather than street clothes is worn while changing a dressing. A cap is worn whenever a patient's room is entered; masks are necessary only in the presence of open wounds. Gloves are required when handling wounds or dressings. Plastic aprons keep clothing from being contaminated and should be discarded when leaving a patient's room. Shoe covers do not provide additional protection. Strict epidemiologic control avoids introduction of new organisms to a patient. Use of common equipment, such as stethoscopes, blood pressure cuffs, and so on, is avoided. Proper *hand washing* is the foundation on which other infection control measures are built [62].

Certain procedures are unique to the burn

unit with regard to infection. The soil in which plants are kept as well as the water in flower vases are grossly contaminated with bacteria, particularly *Pseudomonas*. Fresh vegetables and fresh fruit are easily contaminated. For these reasons, both plants and fresh fruit are not allowed in the burn unit area. Ice machines and their water are frequently contaminated with *Pseudomonas*; therefore, only sterile ice is allowed in the burn unit.

The burn team should always be aware of the hazards from bacteria. It is never considered an insult when one team member reminds another that an appropriate technique is not being followed. The spirit of such a comment is directed toward better patient care.

Burn Wound Sepsis

After the first postburn week, the major complication facing the burn patient and burn team remains sepsis. Invasive wound infection is a persistent risk until full skin coverage is achieved. The eschar, that is, the coagulated protein exudate and injured skin, provides a growth medium for bacterial and fungal growth. The burn injury leads to an immunosuppressed state, further enhancing the risk of infection [63,64].

Serial observations of the wound are helpful but not definitive. Use of clinical signs and symptoms for the diagnosis of sepsis in the burn patient can be difficult; some of these "classic" signs such as tachycardia, disorientation, and fever are common daily occurrences in the burn patient [65]. Other signs and symptoms are helpful, however: thrombocytopenia, sudden onset of glycosuria, increased fluid requirements, and lethargy [66–68]. Suspect invasive wound infection with the appearance of wound ulcerations surrounded by a dark rim, eschar separation within the first 3 to 5 days, cellulitis in adjacent nonburned skin, or dusky granulation tissue (Fig. 14-6). Definitive bacteriologic surveillance and rational antibiotic therapy depend on the use of quantitative wound biopsy culture.

Invasive wound infection or burn wound sepsis is defined as greater than 100,000 organisms/gm of tissue [68–70]. Quantitative biopsies for wound culture should be obtained after an alcohol preparation of the eschar. The biopsy should include the full thickness of the eschar down to underlying viable tissue. For local anesthesia to obtain the biopsy, use intracardiac lidocaine, since it does not contain preservatives that may interfere

Fig. 14-6. Lesions consistent with burn wound sepsis, in this case due to *Pseudomonas*.

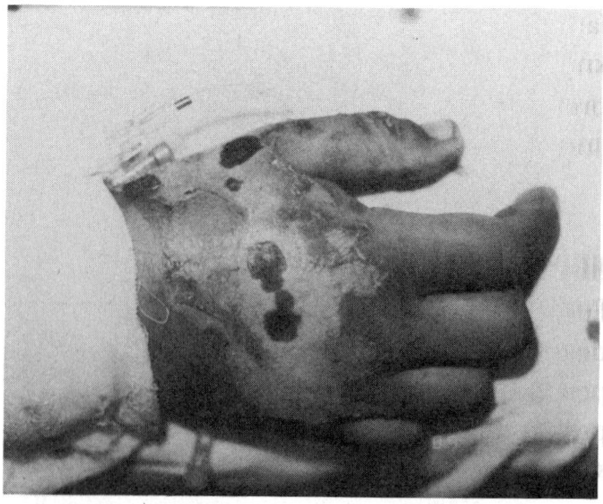

with bacterial growth in the culture. Quantitative wound biopsy cultures are subject to some error, and there is a 60-percent chance that reported values will be plus or minus 1 log unit. They are superior, however, to qualitative (swab) cultures, which reveal only surface colonization, and blood cultures, which have limited yield.

Prophylactic systemic antibiotic therapy is not used, except for diabetics with foot burns or patients with prosthetic devices. Injudicious use of prophylactic antibiotics does not lower the infection rate and will select out more resistant organisms [71,72]. Systemic antibiotic therapy is instituted when a wound biopsy culture identifies an organism growing to the extent of greater than 10^5 colonies. Treatment is also instituted when there is a lower level of bacteriologic growth, but associated clinical signs of sepsis exist.

If systemic administration of aminoglycosides is required, "supernormal" doses may be required to achieve therapeutic serum levels, since there is an increased metabolism and excretion of aminoglycosides in burn patients [73,74]. For this reason, serum aminoglycoside (peak and trough) levels must be drawn to ensure adequate but not toxic drug levels. Peak and trough samples are drawn within 30 minutes of infusion. The patient's doses are then titrated accordingly. Aminoglycoside doses as high as 240 mg may be necessary to obtain adequate serum levels, and "standard" doses will be ineffective. Serum levels should be drawn as early as the third dose to ensure reaching therapeutic levels quickly; increased mortality can be correlated to time delays in reaching therapeutic doses [75].

Non–Burn Wound Sepsis

Burn wound sepsis is not the only cause of sepsis in the burn patient. Other sources of sepsis such as pneumonia and urinary tract infection are common. One insidious and silent source of infection is suppurative (septic) phlebitis. With a reported 4- to 5-percent incidence in major burn centers [76,77], its mortality, untreated, approaches 100 percent. Typically, the complication goes unrecognized as the patient has continued "fevers of unknown origin." Diagnosis is difficult; local signs are uncommon, and attempted aspiration of a suspect vein gives a poor yield. Often, the first sign may be pus draining from an old intravenous site. Diagnosis often rests on clinical suspicion. Treatment requires excision (not stripping or incision and drainage) of the involved vein.

Bacteremias associated with the use of central venous catheters are a risk during nutritional support or cardiovascular monitoring. After 5 days of use, flow-directed pulmonary artery catheters are associated with valvular vegetations [78]. Bacterial endocarditis, with an incidence of 1 to 2 percent, is rarely diagnosed premortem. The associated average time of onset of sepsis is 15 days; previous heart disease is not necessary.

Other sources of sepsis are sinusitis and chondritis. Maxillary sinusitis may result after nasotracheal intubation or extended use of a nasogastric tube [79]. Prolonged nasotracheal intubation causes sinusitis by direct irritation of the nasal mucosa and occlusion of drainage pathways. The diagnosis is made with radiographs (Waters' view) or computed tomography (CT) scans. Occasionally, sinus irrigation and aspiration for culture are necessary. Otitis media may occur in children after intubation through the nose.

Chondritis is reported to occur in 25 percent of burn patients with head involvement [80]. Typically, the patient presents with extremely painful, edematous "Dumbo" ears. Therapy requires bivalving the ear and removal of infected cartilage. Direct instillation of antibiotics with or without iontophoresis has been advocated in the early stages. In our experience, chondritis has been avoided by using the deeply penetrating topical antibacterial mafenide and giving meticulous care to head dressings. Pressure, bending, and kinking of the ear is avoided. Head doughnuts are used in place of pillows.

Over time, progressive decrease in a patient's immunocompetence and previous antibiotic use contribute to the selection of infections by opportunistic organisms. Candidemia is devastating, with a mortality rate as high as 76 percent [81]. Radical debridement or amputation is necessary when fungus is found deep in subcutaneous tissue or muscle. Prophylaxis with oral nystatin (Mycostatin) is used for control of gastrointestinal fungus, which is particularly important in patients with large burns or exposed fat. Nystatin vaginal suppositories are prescribed for women.

Documented disseminated infections and candidemia are treated with amphotericin B. If necessary, amphotericin B can be used every other day in patients with renal compromise. The presence of *Candida* in the sputum, wound, or urine can be treated with a ketoconazole-type drug; the presence of fungus in all three locations, in the blood, or on examination of eye grounds requires the use of amphotericin. Reluctance to use amphotericin pending obtaining a second positive blood culture is usually a fatal error.

Stress Ulceration

The risk of upper gastrointestinal bleeding secondary to gastric mucosal erosions or frank stress ulceration is well documented. The cause of such ulcers is unknown but may be related to increased acid secretions, changes in the stomach mucosal barriers, or alteration in gastric blood flow [82,83]. The presence of sepsis increases the risk of stress bleeding.

Control studies have shown gastric erosions and gastritis to be present in up to 86 percent of burn patients within 72 hours of the injury [84]. The clinical manifestation of these punctate lesions is not always evident. Untreated, however, there is a high incidence of frank gastric or duodenal ulcerations.

The three components of stress ulcerations in trauma patients are ischemia, bile acids, and hydrochloric acid. Though the absolute production of hydrochloric acid may not increase, the sensitivity of the gastric mucosa may become more susceptible to acid destruction. Adequate prophylaxis is maintained by hourly administration of antacids, titrating the therapy to maintain gastric pH above 3.0. Cimetidine is not used routinely and has not been shown to be more effective than appropriate antacid therapy [85,86]. Its use is reserved for patients in whom gastric pH cannot be controlled with antacids or diarrhea results from excessive antacid use. Cimetidine, however, may have untoward side effects, especially in the presence of renal or hepatic insufficiency. Vitamin A is given (10,000 units every other day); it has been described as having a protective effect on the gastric mucosa through its role as a cofactor in the production of mucin [87]. Cholestyramine is given every 6 hours to bind bile acids.

Enteral alimentation by tube feeding serves not only to provide caloric supplementation but also as stress ulcer prophylaxis [88]. Enteral alimentation regimens, such as Vital, have a pH of approximately 5.0. By constant infusion through a feeding tube into the stomach, the effect is similar to that of around-the-clock antacid therapy, and in our experience, stress bleeding has not occurred in any patient successfully tube fed.

SPECIAL PROBLEMS

High-Voltage Electrical Injuries

The high voltage–associated electrical injury presents management problems different from those of thermal injury alone. Major tissue destruction from electricity is usually associated with 500 volts or greater [89]. There are three possible components of such an injury. The first is direct damage from the current, consisting of coagulation and cellular destruction. The major destruction is deep and away from direct observation, and 5 to 10 days may be required to recognize the full extent of the underlying damage. The second type of injury is associated with arcing of the electrical current. The arc has a temperature of up to 2500°C and causes a concentrated, deep injury. The third component is a flame burn resulting from the ignition of clothing by the arc. This aspect of an electrical injury should be treated as any other thermal injury.

During the resuscitation phase, attention should be directed toward maintaining a brisk diuresis to prevent renal tubular damage. Further efforts to prevent deposition of hemochromogens include administration of bicarbonate to alkalinize urine and, rarely, judicious administration of mannitol.

During the first week after a high-voltage electrical injury, the patient is at risk for clostridial infections in necrotic tissue. Injured bone or joint may become exposed. The natural history of this injury is one of progressive tissue necrosis. Like the tip of an iceberg, what one sees on the day of admission is not necessarily the whole extent of the victim's injury (Fig. 14-7). It is not uncommon to have nonadjacent areas of necrotic tissue, creating a challenge in wound care.

Several strategies are possible. Early and radical debridement including amputation will sacrifice viable tissue. Delay in surgical intervention until full wound demarcation takes place risks sepsis. Serial debridement, leaving the wound open, affords the best chance of limb salvage and tissue preservation but requires multiple operations.

Radionuclide scans such as technetium pyrophosphate can augment clinical impressions of muscle viability and aid in establishing areas for surgical debridement or amputation [90]. Technetium scans obtained in the first 48 hours postinjury have up to 95-percent reported accuracy in identifying viable and nonviable muscle bundles (Fig. 14-8). In conjunction with clinical observations, this will help decrease the

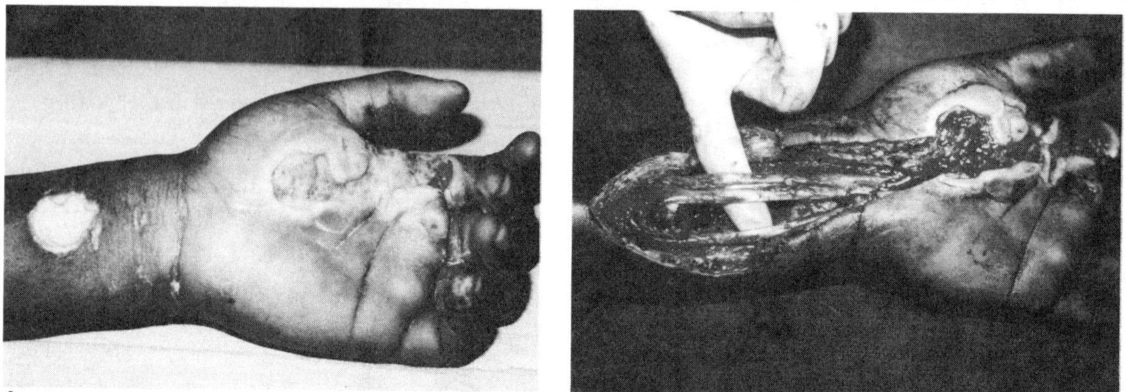

A B

Fig. 14-7. *A.* Entrance wound associated with a high-voltage electrical injury at 3 days postburn. *B.* Same wound 5 days later, showing the extent of progressive necrosis.

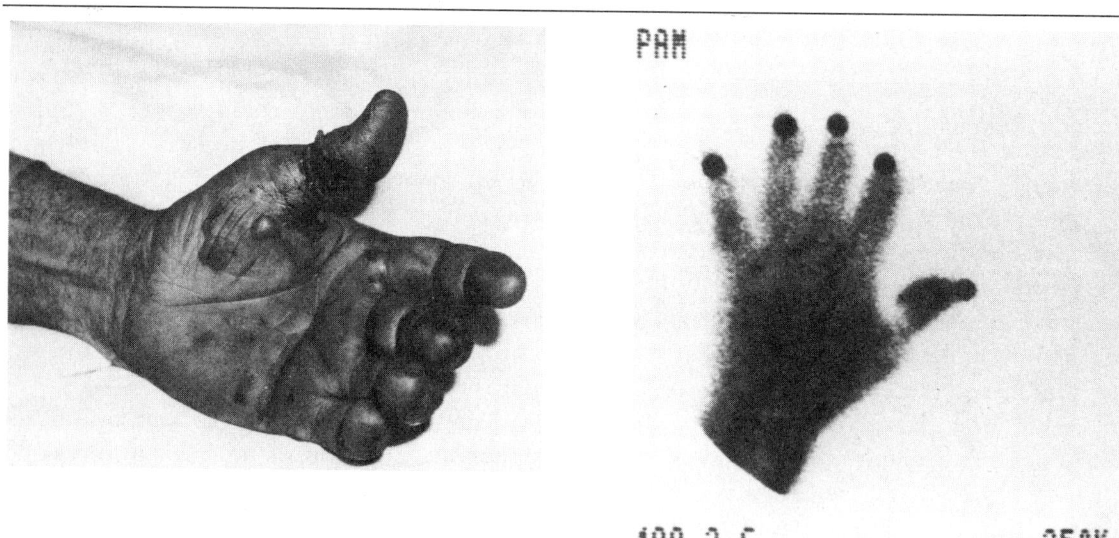

A B

Fig. 14-8. *A.* Entrance wound of high-voltage electrical injury exposes the interphalangeal joint of the left thumb. *B.* Technetium-99m pyrophosphate scan demonstrates blood flow to and viability of the distal thumb.

number of serial debridements necessary and allow a surgeon to pursue early wound closure.

Tar Burns

Tar burns may be deceptively deep. Tar is heated to 500 to 600°F, producing burns that are usually deep second-degree or third-degree. Since the tar has cooled by the time the patient arrives at the hospital, however, there is no emergency in removing it. Although acetone and kerosene are solvents, they should be avoided. Though effective, the treatment is painful, and marginally viable underlying tissue may be injured. Commercial tar removers, such as "Tween 80" or "Goop," or citric acid derivatives such as "Orange-sol" should be used. Silver sulfadiazine or Neosporin ointment will also remove tar over a 24- to 48-hour period because the propylene glycol base acts as a solvent.

Burns in Children

Significant differences exist in the care of pediatric burn patients from that rendered adult victims. Children are not merely "little adults." For example, estimation of burn size in the child requires a different nomogram, since the head comprises a greater surface area and the extremities a lesser surface area in relation to the torso in children than in adults. Size assessment of the child is also important; for example, a 7-kg child has one-tenth the weight of a 70-kg adult but one-fourth of the surface area.

Resuscitation requirements are likewise different in the pediatric burn victim. Resuscitation formulas must account for the higher ratio of total body water to body weight. In infants, resuscitation by the Parkland formula alone is insufficient. Adequate resuscitation requires the Parkland formula plus daily maintenance (see Fluid Resuscitation). In addition, children have limited glycogen stores in the liver. Thus, glucose must be administered as part of the resuscitation regimen, although urine must be monitored closely for glycosuria.

Children have a higher rate of heat exchange than adults and have poorly developed mechanisms of heat conservation. This makes them more susceptible to hypothermia. Infants may have limited renal function with less concentrating ability and higher insensible losses. Limited mechanisms for respiration must be taken into account. These physiologic differences, depending on age, complicate the electrolyte, nutritional, and wound management in burned children.

Hypertension in burned children is a phenomenon first described in 1964 and has been described in up to 24 percent of pediatric burn patients [91]. Correlated with elevated plasma resin, this systolic hypertension is usually paroxysmal and subsides with wound closure [92]. Indications for treatment include persistent hypertension (over 24 hours), diastolic hypertension, or symptomatic hypertension.

Child Abuse

While 2 to 6 percent of burns in children requiring admission to the hospital can be demonstrated to be nonaccidental, as many as one-third of burns in children may be suspicious for child abuse or neglect [93,94]. Examination for additional signs and symptoms of abuse is essential. Historical and social information that may alert the physician or nurse to the possibility of child abuse include differing historical accounts, history of prior accidents, a history attributing the burn to siblings, inappropriate parental affect, treatment delay, or history of the child being brought to the emergency room by nonrelated adults. Physical findings that are cues to child abuse include a passive or introverted child, a burn that is incompatible with the history or the child's developmental age, burns localized to the perineum or buttocks, "mirror image" burns, burns older than the stated age, or unrelated injuries (old or new). A suspicion of a nonaccidental burn warrants admission to the hospital and social service investigation, even if the burn itself is not a medical necessity for hospitalization.

REHABILITATION

Rehabilitation therapy cannot be overemphasized. Therapy strategies are considered at the beginning of the patient's hospitalization. Passive ranging of motion and splinting begin immediately. The only reason not to receive rehabilitation therapy on admission is because of interference with life support systems. Although survival takes precedence in the critically ill patient, physical therapy/occupational therapy objectives are always kept in mind. A coordinated therapy program will increase the chance of maintaining the preoperative level of function, improve protein utilization, speed wound closure, and document the patient's limitations.

An informed rehabilitation therapist can best meet the needs of the patient. The therapist should be notified in advance of the operating room so that range of motion under anesthesia can be planned and prefabricated splints can be constructed. Therapists should be consulted about patients considered to be infection risks so that proper precautions can be taken to protect other patients. Infected patients are seen at the end of the day in their rooms, rather than in the general rehabilitation area.

Physical rehabilitation can be divided into four distinct phases. Preoperative rehabilitation begins at the time of admission. This may involve only assessment but can also include positioning and splinting. Intraoperative rehabilitation includes documentation of the patient's limits, ranging under anesthesia, and splinting following operation. The goal of interoperative rehabilitation is to maintain or restore preoperative function while preparing for the next surgical procedure. Finally, postoperative rehabilitation customarily resumes 3 to 5 days after surgery and aims to maintain or improve the position of the grafted area.

Two important axioms must be remembered. First, the burn wound will shorten by contraction until it meets an opposing force. Across a flexor surface, this results in a contracture. As a corollary, the position of comfort is the position of contracture.

Active and aggressive physical and occupational therapy will prevent or retard the development of contracture. Careful positioning of the patient avoids shortening across flexor angles. Thus, maneuvers such as removing pillows from behind the head, avoiding pillows beneath the knees, nighttime splinting, utilization of the prone position to counteract hip flexion, and proper positioning in bed must be enforced [95]. For bed-bound patients, air-fluidized beds afford some protection against wound breakdown or the formation of decubitus.

All joints should be positioned in an antideformity position [96]. Hands are splinted in an anticlaw position. Efforts to reduce limb edema will facilitate preservation or joint function and may help decrease intradermal scar formation. While lower extremities may be elevated on pillows, adequate venous drainage of the upper extremities necessitates elevation in a stockinette from an IV pole or an over-the-bed trapeze. Since the ultimate goal is independent function, activities of daily living are stressed.

Hypertrophic scar formation results in skin more tender and pruritic than nonhypertrophic reepithelialized areas or skin grafts. Little can be done acutely for pain or itching except supportive care with analgesics and antihistamines. Long-term treatment of scar hypertrophy involves pressure garments, steroid instillation, and scar revision. Although more commonly seen in darker skinned individuals, hypertrophic scar is a potential complication for any wound that requires more than 2 to 3 weeks to reepithelialize [97]. Individuals who are at higher risk because of skin color, length of time with open wounds, location of scar, or prior history of keloid formation are candidates for use of prophylactic pressure garments. For facial burns, use of a transparent face mask (Uvex) has better patient acceptance and provides better pressure to the upper lip and nasolabial folds (Fig. 14-9). Unless functional disability dictates a greater urgency, scar revision is delayed until wound maturity. This typically occurs 6 to 18 months post burn.

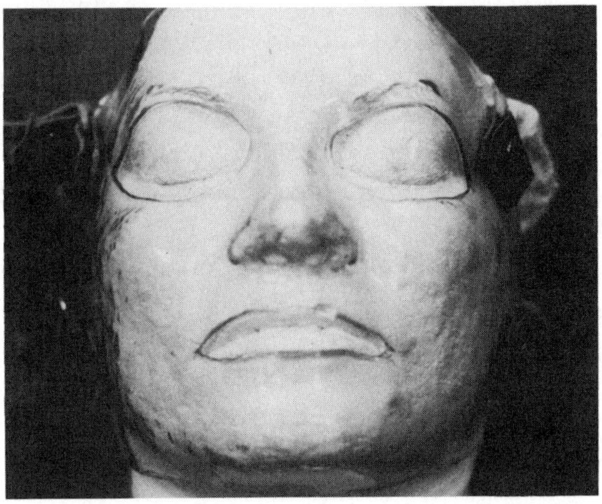

Fig. 14-9. Example of a clear plastic (Uvex) face mask for pressure therapy control of hypertrophic scar. It sits on the life mask bust used for its construction.

Heterotopic ossification occurs with an incidence of 13 to 23 percent [98,99]. Most prominent in the areas of elbows, shoulders, and knees, it has been associated with a delay in skin coverage. Its etiology, however, is controversial, and multiple theories have been advanced. It may occur even though the burn does not involve the bone or the joint.

The onset of heterotopic ossification is 3 to 12 weeks post injury. Signs and symptoms include pain, swelling, and decreased range of motion. Loss of function or pain on movement may occur suddenly. These symptoms precede plain radiographic changes of new bone formation. Although serum alkaline phosphatase levels may be elevated, calcium and phosphorus levels are normal.

Prophylaxis involves an early mobilization program. Once ectopic calcification is documented, forceful stretching and bending of involved muscles and joints is avoided. Range of motion exercises and stretching are only carried to the point of discomfort. Most patients will regain function over time; surgical excision of heterotopic ossification is eventually necessary in only approximately one-third of patients.

Finally, mental rehabilitation is as important as physical rehabilitation [100,101]. The patient's cooperation in his or her own care is essential for a successful outcome. As soon as it is practical, patients enter a teaching program to learn about their burns as they strive to achieve normal function.

REFERENCES

1. Artz, C. P., Moncrief, J. A., and Pruitt, B. A. *Burns: A Team Approach.* Philadelphia: Saunders, 1979.
2. Demling, R. H. Burns. *N. Engl. J. Med.* 313:1389, 1983.
3. Nichter, L. S., Bryant, C. A., and Edlich, R. F. Efficacy of burned surface area estimates calculated from charts: The need for a computer-based model. *J. Trauma* 25:477, 1985.
4. Hammond, J. S., and Ward, C. G. Transfers from emergency room to burn center: Errors in burn size estimate. *J. Trauma,* in press, 1987.
5. Lund, C. C., and Browder, N. C. The estimation of areas of burns. *Surg. Gynecol. Obstet.* 79:352, 1944.
6. Herndon, D. N., Thompson, P. B., and Traber, D. L. Pulmonary injury in burned patients. *Crit. Care Clin.* 1:79, 1985.
7. Trunkey, D. D. Inhalation injury. *Surg. Clin. North Am.* 58:1133, 1978.
8. Achauer, B. M., Allyn, P., Furnas, D. W., et al. Pulmonary complications of burns. *Ann. Surg.* 177:311, 1973.
9. Myers, R. A., Linberg, S. E., Cowley, R. A., et al. Carbon monoxide poisoning: The injury and its treatment. *J.A.C.E.P.* 8:479, 1979.
10. Larkin, J. M., Brahos, G. J., and Moyland, J. A. Treatment of carbon monoxide poisoning: Prognostic factors. *J. Trauma* 16:111, 1976.
11. Divincenti, F. C., Pruitt, B. A., and Reckler, J. M. Inhalation injuries. *J. Trauma* 11:109, 1971.
12. Agee, R. N., Long, J. M., Hunt, J. L., et al. Use of 133 xenon in early diagnosis of inhalation injury. *J. Trauma* 16:218, 1976.
13. Moyland, J. A., Adib, K., and Birnbaum, M. Fiberoptic bronchoscopy following thermal injury. *Surgery Gynecology & Obstetrics* 140:541, 1975.
14. Welch, G. W., Lull, R. J., Petroff, P. A., et al. The use of steroids in inhalation injury. *Surgery Gynecology & Obstetrics* 177:539, 1977.
15. Eckhauser, F. E., Billote, J., Burke, J. F., et al. Tracheostomy complicating massive burn injury: A plea for conservatism. *Am. J. Surg.* 1276:418, 1974.
16. Demling, R. H. Fluid and electrolyte management. *Crit. Care Clin.* 1:27, 1985.
17. Baxter, C. R. Fluid volume and electrolyte changes of the early post-burn period. *Clin. Plast. Surg.* 1:693, 1974.
18. Pruitt, B. A. Fluid and electrolyte replacement in the burned patient. *Surg. Clin. North Am.* 58:1291, 1978.
19. Morton, J. H. Fluid replacement in patients with large area, full- and partial-thickness burns. *Arch. Surg.* 114:247, 1979.
20. Mahler, D., Baruchin, A., Hauben, D., et al. Recent concepts regarding the resuscitation of the burned patient. *Burns* 9:30, 1982.
21. Baxter, C. R. Problems and complications of burn shock resuscitation. *Surg. Clin. North Am.* 58:1313, 1978.
22. Navar, P. D., Saffle, J. R., and Warden, G. D. Effect of inhalation injury on fluid resuscitation requirements after thermal injury. *Am. J. Surg.* 150:716, 1985.
23. Monafo, W. W., Chuntrasakal, C., and Ayvazian, V. H. Hypertonic sodium solutions in the treatment of burn shock. *Am. J. Surg.* 126:778, 1973.
24. Caldwell, F. T., and Bowser, B. H. Critical evaluation of hypertonic and hypotonic solutions to resuscitate severely burned children. *Ann. Surg.* 189:546, 1979.
25. Caldwell, F. T., Casali, R. E., Flannigan, W. J., et al. What constitutes the proper solution for resuscitation of the severely burned patient? *Am. J. Surg.* 12:655, 1971.

26. Baxter, C. R. Burns. In G. T. Shires (ed.), *Care of the Trauma Patient*. New York: McGraw-Hill, 1966. Pp. 201–209.
27. Larkin, J. M., and Moylan, J. A. Tetanus following a minor burn. *J. Trauma* 15:546, 1975.
28. Hammond, J. S., and Ward, C. G. Burns of the head and neck. *Otolaryngol. Clin. North Am.* 16:679, 1983.
29. Kaplan, I., and White, W. L. Incisional decompression of circumferential burns. *Plast. Reconstr. Surg.* 28:609, 1961.
30. Saffle, J. R., Zeliff, G. R., and Warden, G. D. Intramuscular pressure in the burned arm: Measurement and response to escharotomy. *Am. J. Surg.* 140:825, 1980.
31. Salisbury, R. E., Taylor, J., and Levine, N. S. Evaluation of digital escharotomy in burned hands. *Plast. Reconstr. Surg.* 58:440, 1976.
32. Valente, P., and Axelrod, J. L. Acute leukopenia associated with silver sulfadiazine therapy. *J. Trauma* 18:146, 1978.
33. Moncrief, J. A. Topical antibacterial therapy of the burn wound. *Clin. Plast. Surg.* 1:563, 1974.
34. Petroff, P., Hander, E., and Mason, A. D. Ventilatory patterns following burn injury and effect of Sulfamylon. *J. Trauma* 15:650, 1975.
35. Buckner, D. Personal communication, 1981.
36. Hunt, J. L., Sato, R., Heck, E., et al. A critical evaluation of povidone-iodine absorption in thermally injured patients. *J. Trauma* 20:127, 1980.
37. Kulick, M. I., Lewis, N., Bansal, V., et al. Hyperosmolarity in the burn patient: Analysis of an osmolar discrepancy. *J. Trauma* 20:223, 1980.
38. Dimick, A. R. Experience with the use of proteolytic enzyme (Travase®) in burn patients. *J. Trauma* 17:948, 1977.
39. Jackson, D., Topley, E., Cason, J. S., et al. Primary excision and grafting of large burns. *Ann. Surg.* 152:167, 1960.
40. Janzekovic, Z. A new concept in the early excision and immediate grafting of burns. *J. Trauma* 10:1103, 1970.
41. Tompkins, R. G., Schoenfeld, D. A., Behringer, G. C., et al. Prompt eschar excision: A treatment system contributing to reduced burn mortality. *Ann. Surg.* 204:272, 1986.
42. Heimbach, D. M., and Engrav, L. H. (eds.). *Surgical Management of the Burn Wound.* New York: Raven, 1984.
43. Pavlin, E. G. Anesthetic Considerations. In D. M. Heimbach, and L. H. Engrav (eds.), *Surgical Management of the Burn Wound.* New York: Raven, 1984.
44. Belin, R. P., and Karleen, C. I. Cardiac arrest in the burned patient following succinylcholine administration. *Anesthesiology* 27:516, 1966.
45. Zaroff, L. I., Mills, W., Jr., Duckett, J. W., Jr., et al. Multiple uses of viable cutaneous homografts in the burned patient. *Surgery* 59:368, 1966.
46. Atrip, R. G., and Burke, J. F. Skin coverage. *Curr. Prob. Surg.* 20:625, 1983.
47. Robson, M. C., Samburg, J. L., and Krizek, T. J. Quantitative comparison of biological dressings. *J. Surg. Res.* 14:431, 1973.
48. Malinin, T. Personal communication, 1985.
49. Miller, T. A. The deleterious effect of split skin homograft coverage on split skin donor sites. *Plast. Reconstr. Surg.* 53:316, 1974.
50. Tavis, M. J., Thornton, J., Danet, R., et al. Current status of skin substitutes. *Surg. Clin. North Am.* 58:1233, 1978.
51. Frank, D. H., Wachtel, T., Frank, H. A., et al. Comparison of Biobrane, porcine, and human allograft as biologic dressings for burn wounds. *J. Burn Care Rehab.* 4:186, 1983.
52. Perry, S., and Heidrich, G. Management of pain during debridement: A survey of U.S. burn units. *Pain* 13:267, 1982.
53. Foley, K. M. The practical use of narcotic analgesics. *Med. Clin. North Am.* 66:1091, 1982.
54. Wilmore, D. W., and Aulick, L. H. Metabolic changes in burned patients. *Surg. Clin. North Am.* 58:1173, 1978.
55. Wilmore, D. Nutrition and metabolism following thermal injury. *Clin. Plast. Surg.* 1:603, 1974.
56. Aulick, L. H., Handler, E. H., Wilmore, D. W., et al. The relative significance of thermal and metabolic demands on burn hypermetabolism. *J. Trauma* 19:559, 1979.
57. Caldwell, F. T., Bowser, B. H., and Crabtree, J. H. The effect of occlusive dressings on the energy metabolism of severely burned children. *Ann. Surg.* 193:579, 1981.
58. Curreri, P. W., Richmond, D., Marvin, J., et al. Dietary requirements of patients with major burns. *J. Am. Diet. Assoc.* 65:415, 1974.
59. Turner, W. W., Ireton, C. S., Hunt, J. L., et al. Pre-

dicting energy expenditures in burn patients. *J. Trauma* 25:11, 1985.
60. Stein, M. D., Herndon, D. N., Abston, S., et al. Lack of beneficial effects of TPN administration on immunity and mortality in thermal injury patients. Abstract presented at the 18th Annual Meeting of the American Burn Association, Chicago, April 1986.
61. Matsuda, T., Kagan, R. J., Hanumadass, M., et al. The importance of burn wound size in determining the optimal calorie:nitrogen ratio. *Surgery* 94:561, 1983.
62. Gordon, M., Varas, R., Walter, P., et al. Burn care protocols: Infection control in the burn unit. *J. Burn Care Rehab.* 8:61, 1986.
63. Miller, S. E., Miller, C. L., and Trunkey, D. D. The immune consequences of trauma. *Surg. Clin. North Am.* 62:167, 1982.
64. Edelson, R. L., and Funk, J. M. The immunologic function of skin. *Sci. Am.* 252:46, 1985.
65. Parish, R. A., Novack, A. H., Heimbach, D. M., et al. Fever as a predictor of infection in burned children. *J. Trauma* 27:69, 1987.
66. Carvajal, H. F., Feinstein, R., Traber, D. L., et al. An objective method for early diagnosis of gram-negative septicemia in burned children. *J. Trauma* 21:221, 1981.
67. Rowe, M. I., Marchildon, M. B., Arango, A., et al. The mechanisms of thrombocytopenia in experimental gram-negative septicemia. *Surgery* 84:127, 1978.
68. Marvin, J., Heck, E., Loebl, E., et al. Usefulness of blood cultures in confirming septic complications in burn patients: Evaluation of a new culture method. *J. Trauma* 15:657, 1975.
69. Loebl, E., Marvin, J., Heck, E., et al. The method for quantitative burn-wound biopsy cultures and its routine use in the care of the burned patient. *Am. J. Clin. Pathol.* 61:20, 1974.
70. Volenec, F. J., Clark, G., Mani, M. M., et al. Burn wound biopsy bacterial quantitation: A statistical analysis. *Am. J. Surg.* 138:695, 1979.
71. Larkin, J. M., and Moylan, J. A. The role of prophylactic antibiotics in burn care. *Am. Surg.* 42:247, 1976.
72. Boss, W. K., Brand, D. A., Acampora, D., et al. Effectiveness of prophylactic antibiotics in the outpatient treatment of burns. *J. Trauma* 25:224, 1985.
73. Zaske, D. E., Sawchuk, R. J., Gerding, D. N., et al. Increased dosage requirements of gentamicin in burn patients. *J. Trauma* 16:824, 1976.
74. Zaske, D. E., Sawchuk, R. J., and Strate, R. G. The necessity of increased doses of amikacin in burn patients. *Surgery* 84:603, 1978.
75. Jackson, G. G., and Riff, L. J. *Pseudomonas* bacteremia: Pharmacologic and other bases for failure of treatment with gentamicin. *J. Infect. Dis.* 124(suppl.):S185, 1971.
76. Baker, C. C., Peterson, S. R., and Sheldon, G. F. Septic phlebitis: A neglected disease. *Am. J. Surg.* 138:97, 1979.
77. Pruitt, B. A., Jr., McManus, W. F., Kim, S. H., et al. Diagnosis and treatment of cannula-related intravenous sepsis in burn patients. *Ann. Surg.* 191:546, 1980.
78. Ehrie, M., Morgan, A., Moore, F. D., et al. Endocarditis with the indwelling balloon-tipped pulmonary artery catheter in burn patients. *J. Trauma* 18:664, 1978.
79. O'Reilly, M. J., Reddick, E. J., Black, W., et al. Sepsis from sinusitis in nasotracheally intubated patients. *Am. J. Surg.* 147:601, 1984.
80. Hammond, J. S., and Ward, C. G. Burns of the head and neck. *Otolaryngol. Clin. North Am.* 16:679, 1983.
81. Spebar, M. J., and Pruitt, B. A., Jr. Candidiasis in the burned patient. *J. Trauma* 21:237, 1981.
82. Lucas, C. E., Sugawa, C., Riddle, J., et al. Natural history and surgical dilemma of "stress" gastric bleeding. *Arch. Surg.* 102:266, 1971.
83. Rees, M., and Bowen, J. C. Stress ulcers during live *Escherichia coli* sepsis: The role of acid and bile. *Ann. Surg.* 195:646, 1982.
84. Czaja, A. J., McAlhany, J. C., and Pruitt, B. A., Jr. Acute gastrointestinal disease after thermal injury. *N. Engl. J. Med.* 291:926, 1974.
85. Weigelt, J. A., Aurbakken, C. M., Gewertz, B., et al. Cimetidine vs. antacid in prophylaxis for stress ulceration. *Arch. Surg.* 116:597, 1981.
86. Martyn, J. A., Greenblatt, D. J., and Abewathy, D. R. Increased cimetidine clearance in burn patients. *J.A.M.A.* 253:1288, 1985.
87. Chernov, M. S., Hale, H. W., Jr., and Wood, M. Prevention of stress ulcers. *Am. J. Surg.* 122:674, 1971.
88. Choctaw, W. T., Fujita, C., and Zawacki, B. E. Prevention of upper gastrointestinal bleeding in burn patients. *Arch. Surg.* 115:1073, 1980.
89. Sances, A., Jr., Larson, S. J., Mykleburst, J.,

et al. Electrical injuries. *Surg. Gynecol. Obstet.* 149:97, 1979.

90. Hunt, J., Lewis, S., Parkey, R., et al. The use of technetium-99m stannous pyrophosphate scintigraphy to identify muscle damage in acute electric burns. *J. Trauma* 19:409, 1979.
91. Lowrey, G. H. Hypertension in children with burns. *J. Trauma* 7:140, 1967.
92. Popp, M. B., Freidberg, D. L., and MacMillan, B. G. Clinical characteristics of hypertension in burned children. *Ann. Surg.* 191:473, 1980.
93. Stone, H. H., Rinaldo, L., Humprey, C., et al. Child abuse by burning. *Surg. Clin. North Am.* 50:1419, 1970.
94. Watkins, A. H., Gagan, R. J., and Cupoli, J. M. Child abuse by burning. *J. Fla. Med. Assoc.* 72:497, 1985.
95. Helm, P. A., Head, M. J., Pullium, G., et al. Burn rehabilitation: A team approach. *Surg. Clin. North Am.* 58:1263, 1978.
96. Pullium, G. F. Splinting and Positioning. In S. V. Fisher, and P. A. Helm (eds.), *Comprehensive Rehabilitation of Burns.* Baltimore: Williams & Wilkins, 1984. Pp. 64–95.
97. Deitch, E. A., Wheelahan, T. M., Rose, M. P., et al. Hypertrophic burn scars: Analysis of variables. *J. Trauma* 23:895, 1983.
98. Munster, A. M., Bruck, H. M., Johns, L. A., et al. Heterotopic calcification following burns: A prospective study. *J. Trauma* 12:1071, 1972.
99. Edlich, R. F., Horowitz, J. H., Rheuban, K. S., et al. Heterotopic calcification and ossification in the burn patient. *J. Burn Care Rehab.* 6:363, 1985.
100. West, D. A., and Schuck, J. M. Emotional problems of the severely burned patient. *Surg. Clin. North Am.* 58:1189, 1978.
101. Tucker, P. Psychosocial problems among adult burn victims. *Burns* 13:7, 1987.

15

Trauma and the Pediatric Patient

Joseph J. Tepas, III

Trauma continues to be the most common cause of death in children. According to the National Safety Council, 9703 children under age 14 years and 26,206 young people between 15 and 24 years of age died of accidental injury in 1980 [1]. Considered in light of a 24- to 40-percent incidence of preventable death in injured children, this fact becomes tragedy [2]. While the loss of a child is overwhelming to any parent, the wastage of our greatest national resource, compounded by the cost of long-term care for injured children, is a tragedy that encompasses the entire population.

THE CHILD AS A TRAUMA VICTIM

Considering the child as a trauma victim, there are many unique characteristics that must be addressed. The incidence of blunt over penetrating trauma is highest in the pediatric population. Evaluation of the first 3400 patients entered in the National Pediatric Trauma Registry confirms blunt injury to be nine times more common than penetrating lesions in the pediatric population. Multisystem injury is the rule rather than the exception. All organ systems must be assumed to be injured until proved otherwise.

The unique anatomic characteristics of the pediatric population require special considerations in assessing and treating the pediatric trauma victim. The child's smaller size produces a smaller target to which is applied linear forces from fenders, bumpers, and falls. Because of diminished body fat, increased elasticity of connective tissue, and close proximity of multiple organs, these forces are less well dissipated, and a more intense energy is applied to multiple organs. The skeleton of a child is incompletely calcified, contains multiple active growth centers, and is more resilient. It is, therefore, less able to absorb kinetic forces applied during a traumatic event and may produce a situation wherein significant internal derangement has occurred in the face of apparently minimal external damage.

The ratio between a child's body surface area and body volume is highest at birth and diminishes throughout infancy and childhood. As a result, the potentially negative influence of thermal energy loss becomes a significant factor in the smaller child. While this may not be life threatening of and by itself, it frequently provides additional stress to a child who may be hypotensive and in significant pain.

The psychological ramifications of caring for an injured child can also present a significant challenge. As normal human psychological maturation progresses from total dependence to self-sufficiency, a variety of specific phases occur. Unfortunately, in the very young child, emotional lability frequently leads to a regressive psychological behavior when stress, pain, or other perceived threats intervene on the child's environment. The child's ability to interact with unfamiliar individuals in strange environments is usually limited and makes history taking and cooperative manipulation extremely difficult. An understanding of these characteristics and a willingness to cajole and soothe an injured child will frequently be the most effective means of achieving good rapport and a more comprehensive understanding of the child's physiologic state.

A final consideration in dealing with pediatric trauma is the effect that injury may have on subsequent growth and development. Unlike the adult, the child must not only recover from the effects of a traumatic event but must also continue along a normal process of growth and development. The effect of injury on this process, specifically in long-term disability, growth deformity, or abnormal subsequent development, both physiologically and psychologically, cannot be underestimated. Children sustaining even minor injury may have prolonged disability in either cerebral function, psychological adjustment, or organ system disability. The cost of correcting these problems is frequently staggering and lifelong. The effect of inadequate or inappropriate care in the immediate post-traumatic period may have consequences, therefore, not only on the child's survival but perhaps as importantly on the quality of the child's life for years to come [3,4].

INITIAL ASSESSMENT

The small size of the patient, the diminished caliber and size of the vascular system, and the unique anatomic characteristics of the airway frequently cause the standard procedures used in basic life support to be extremely challenging and technically difficult in the pediatric patient. As a result of this, it is far better to "scoop and run" with the patient than it is to waste inordinate time in the field attempting venous access or endotracheal intubation. This does not imply that an attempt at establishment of an adequate airway and adequate venous access should be neglected; rather, it is to be emphasized that untoward amounts of time should not be wasted in the establishment of these modalities. It is far easier to manage an injured child in a better equipped, well-controlled, and well-lighted resuscitation area than it is in the somewhat chaotic, distracting environment of the accident scene.

Essential to the establishment of adequate airway and venous access in the injured child is the availability of appropriate sized equipment. An attempt at placement of an overly large intravenous cannula or inappropriate sized endotracheal tube will more likely increase potential damage and cause greater risk to the patient. It is therefore essential that any pediatric trauma receiving area have immediately available appropriate sized laryngoscope blades, endotracheal tubes, nasogastric tubes, Foley catheters, chest tubes, blood pressure cuffs, oxygen masks, and other associated equipment. Table 15-1 is a graphic illustration of the various sizes of standard rescue equipment required for different size and age groups of children. These charts are available from a variety of sources and should be used as guidelines both for emergency rescue units for field use and for stocking emergency rooms and resuscitation areas.

Airway Control and Ventilation

The primary goal of initial assessment and triage of the injured child is the restoration of adequate tissue oxygenation as effectively and as completely as possible. Oxygenation and circulation are as essential to the injured child as they are to the adult. In this regard, the standard principles of airway control, breathing, and circulation are no differently addressed in the injured child than they are in the injured adult. Accordingly, the first priority of assessment is the child's airway. The smaller the child, the greater the disproportion between the size of the cranium and midface, and the greater the propensity of the posterior pharyngeal areas to "buckle" as the relatively larger occiput forces passive flexion of the cervical spine. As a result, the child's airway is best protected by a slightly superior, anterior position of the midface known as the "sniffing position." Careful attention to maintenance of this position is especially important in the obtunded child whose level of consciousness is waxing and waning.

The larynx of the child is smaller than that of the adult, has a slightly more anterocaudad angle, and is frequently more difficult to visualize for direct cannulation. Despite this, the most reliable means of ventilation in the child with airway compromise remains direct endotracheal intubation. Nasotracheal intubation requires blind passage around the relatively acute posterior nasopharyngeal angle and may cause inadvertent penetration of the cranial vault. In the absence of appropriate intubation equipment, bag-valve-mask ventilation with 100% oxygen is an acceptable alternative. In the child whose craniofacial injuries cause upper airway obstruction, a needle cricothyroidostomy through which high-flow (10 L/min) oxygen can be delivered in 45/15 second on/off cycles may provide enough support until definitive management can be provided.

As in the adult, endotracheal intubation must include careful attention to the cervical spine. The head must be maintained in a neutral position by an assistant while careful laryngoscopy and insertion of an endotracheal tube is performed. In infants and toddlers, an uncuffed endotracheal tube should always be used, the size of which can be readily assessed by evaluating the diameter of the child's fifth finger. A slight amount of cricoid

Table 15-1. Recommended Equipment and Arrangement for Pediatric Trauma Resuscitation Area

Equipment	Premie 3 kg	Newborn 3.5 kg	6 mo 7 kg	1–2 yr 10–12 kg	5 yr 16–18 kg	8–10 yr 24–30 kg
Cervical collars	—	—	Small	Small	Small	Medium
Chest tubes	10–14 Fr	12–18 Fr	14–20 Fr	14–24 Fr	20–32 Fr	28–38 Fr
Nasogastric tubes	5 Fr Feeding	5–8 Fr Feeding	8 Fr	10 Fr	10–12 Fr	14–18 Fr
Foley catheters	5 Fr Feeding	5–8 Fr Feeding	8 Fr	10 Fr	10–12 Fr	12 Fr
IV equipment	22–24 angio 25 scalp	22–24 angio 23–25 scalp	22–24 angio 23–25 scalp	20–22 angio 23 scalp	20–22 angio 19 scalp	20–22 angio 19 scalp
Arm boards	6 in.	6 in.	6–8 in.	8 in.	8–15 in.	15 in.
Blood pressure cuffs	Newborn	Newborn/infant	Infant/child	Child	Child	Child/adult
Laryngoscopes	0 Straight	1 Straight	1 Straight	1 Straight	2 Straight & curved	2–3 Straight & curved
Endotracheal tubes	2.5–3.0 Uncuffed	3.0–3.5 Uncuffed	3.5–4.5 Uncuffed	4.0–4.5 Uncuffed	5.0–5.5 Uncuffed	5.5–6.5 Cuffed
Suction/stylets	6–8 Fr/6 Fr	8 Fr/6 Fr	8–10 Fr/6 Fr	10 Fr/6 Fr	14 Fr/14 Fr	14 Fr/14 Fr
Oral airways	Infant	Infant/small	Small	Small	Medium	Med/large
O_2 masks	Premie/newborn	Newborn	Ped	Ped	Ped	Adult

pressure will frequently bring the anterior structures of the child's larynx into better view and will passively obstruct the esophagus, thereby ensuring accurate cannulation of the trachea. A frequent error that is made in children who are intubated under emergency circumstances is an overly aggressive insertion of the endotracheal tube, causing right main stem bronchial intubation. Accordingly, careful auscultation of the chest must be performed as soon as the endotracheal tube is placed. In addition to confirming the presence of the endotracheal tube above the carina, this will confirm adequate breath sounds bilaterally and rule out the possibility that a tension pneumothorax or other primary pulmonary injury has occurred. A child with a compromised airway and a primary pulmonary parenchymal injury who was successfully intubated may be in greater jeopardy for the development of tension pneumothorax as a result of more efficient delivery of tidal volume to the tracheobronchial tree. It is absolutely essential, therefore, that careful auscultation be a reflex maneuver performed immediately after insertion of the tube to document both the presence of breath sounds and the overall status of ventilatory function.

Fluid Resuscitation

Establishment of intravenous access in a child can be succinctly summarized by the adage that injured children need a good IV, not necessarily a central one. The survival rate from immediate exsanguinating injury is very low in the pediatric population. Fortunately, most injured children usually present with some degree of adequacy to their circulating volume. If initial assessment suggests severe hypotension or shock, the most likely reason for this is blood loss either through a major external wound (readily observable), an intrathoracic wound (identifiable by diminished ventilatory mechanics and auscultatory findings), or a major abdominal visceral injury. Since blood is a nondistensible medium, the last will frequently produce abdominal distention and increasing abdominal girth. Consequently, any attempt at repletion of a child with severe hypotension or frank shock must deliver adequate fluid volume to the right atrium. The most appropriate site for initial venous access is above the diaphragm and should address first the antecubital fossa. If the antecubital veins cannot be cannulated, either percutaneous cannulation or direct cannulation of the external or internal jugular veins should be considered. Placement of a subclavian catheter in an injured child should be performed only under the most controlled of circumstances. The area beneath the clavicle is extremely small and has in close proximity most of the major neurovascular components of the upper extremity. A misguided catheter not only may be unsuccessful in attaining venous access but actually may worsen the child's overall status by causing either a pneumothorax or brachial injury.

There are multiple sites beneath the level of the diaphragm that are much more easily approachable for direct surgical cannulation. A saphenous venous cutdown at the level of the ankle and direct cannulation of the femoral vein at the groin are both appropriate and adequate resuscitative measures, and they should be considered after an attempt is made above the diaphragm. Obviously, in the severely hypovolemic child, multiple IV sites are required, and use of the subdiaphragmatic areas are to be encouraged as secondary sites.

As in the adult, lactated Ringer's or other balanced electrolyte solutions are considered to be the best initial resuscitating fluid for the hypovolemic child. Since the intravascular phase of crystalloid is so short, a 3 : 1 ratio for crystalloid resuscitation must be followed. As in the adult, signs of significant hypotension develop with the loss of approximately 25 percent of the circulating volume. Thus, an initial resuscitative bolus should reflect approximately 25 percent of the standard circulating volume in the pediatric patient, which calculates to be approximately 20 ml/kg. Considering the 3 : 1 ratio, it becomes obvious that a bolus of 40 to 60 ml/kg is actually what is required to achieve adequate and rapid initial repletion of significant volume loss.

Injured children usually present in one of three ways. The greater majority demonstrate very little evidence of blood loss and hypotension. With the high incidence of head injury, it becomes obvious that volume repletion of these children must consider not only the restoration of adequate circulating volumes but also the possibility of overresuscitation with potentially detrimental effect on evolving cerebral edema. Children who present in hypovolemic shock must receive both large bolus (50–60 ml/kg) crystalloid resuscitation as well as fresh red cells as soon as possible. This group, fortunately very small, are the children in whom a high potential for preventable deaths occur. These patients frequently regain adequate cardiac output of a circulating volume with minimal oxygen-carrying capacity. Tissue oxygenation plummets because of the diminished circulating red cell mass as well as the diminished oxygen-carrying capacity of senescent red cells usually transfused during initial resuscitation. The child who presents in shock, therefore, must be aggressively resuscitated with at least 60 ml/kg as an initial fluid bolus and must be transfused with red cells that are as fresh and as warm as possible as soon as possible. Only under these circumstances will these unfortunate children have even a slight chance of successful correction of their hemorrhagic injury and hopefully complete recovery.

A major consideration in the assessment of the pediatric trauma victim is the concept of "evolving shock." By nature of their increased physiologic reserve, children frequently will sustain hemorrhagic injury and present to the emergency room with only slightly abnormal vital signs. Initial tachycardia may be the result not only of hypovolemia, but also of the effect of psychological stress, pain, and fear. Moreover, a very small child may have a systolic blood pressure that, while considered alarmingly low for an adult, may reflect normal homeostasis for a young, healthy child. Accordingly, all injured children must be monitored continuously with close observation of blood pressure, heart rate, respiratory rate, and overall central nervous system (CNS) status. The child with a hemorrhagic injury can maintain adequate circulating volume by increasing peripheral vascular resistance to maintain mean arterial pressure. If initial resuscitation is inadequate, circulating volume will eventually diminish to a point below which increased peripheral resistance can maintain arterial pressure. Tragically, this may occur hours after the injury when the child is either being inadequately observed or undergoing secondary assessment at a location remote from adequate resuscitative facilities. The concept of "silent shock" must therefore constantly be considered, and the ability to monitor injured children closely and resuscitate them appropriately must be provided until it is absolutely confirmed that no evidence of significant hemorrhagic injury exists.

Physical Examination

Once initial assessment, airway control, and fluid resuscitation have been accomplished, attention can be addressed to a thorough examination of the entire child. The overall guidelines for this assessment must be a high index of suspicion that every major organ system is injured until proved otherwise. Examination must first assess neurologic status. While the child's level of consciousness remains a reliable prognostic indicator of severity of CNS injury, this assessment must be expanded to include pupillary and ocular muscle function, midbrain function, motor function, orientation, and sensory perception. The Glasgow Coma Scale (see Table 6-1) is an excellent guideline for assessment of neurologic status and should be repeated frequently throughout the evaluation process of the child to determine progression or regression of any central nervous system findings.

Completion of the child's physical examination follows a standard head-to-toe protocol. Intrathoracic organs must be evaluated with special consideration of potential cardiac or pulmonary contusions, both of which may be worsened by overly aggressive fluid resuscitation. Since the increased resiliency of the child's ribs may have allowed transmission of significantly greater energy to underlying thoracic organs, there may be an extensive direct pulmonary contusion that could be worsened by aspiration should the child's level of consciousness diminish. Examination of the abdomen must focus on distention, tenderness, discoloration, or presence of an abdominal mass. A careful rectal examination must be performed, addressing the status of the rectal sphincter, the presence of blood in the rectal ampulla, and the overall status of the intrapelvic structures. Careful palpation of the ileac crests will provide evidence of an unstable pelvic fracture and increase suspicion for possible retroperitoneal injury. A nasogastric tube should be passed and the contents aspirated carefully assessed for the presence of blood. In the unstable child, a Foley catheter should be passed into the bladder after exclusion of a pelvic, perineal, or direct urethral injury. When auscultating the injured child's abdomen, the presence of bowel sounds is highly suggestive of normal peristalsis with lessened potential for significant injury. The absence of bowel sounds may be the effect of aerophagia, ileus, stress, or a primary intraperitoneal process. Bowel sounds thus play an extremely minor role in the overall assessment of the child's abdomen, although their status should be assessed and documented for future comparison.

Each extremity must be palpated to rule out deformity, diminished vascular supply, or neurologic deficit. The child's incompletely calcified skeleton with its multiple growth centers increases the possibility of epiphyseal disruption. Accordingly, any area of edema, pain, tenderness, or diminished range of motion should be carefully evaluated and radiographed. A missed orthopedic injury may have little effect on mortality and a major long-term effect on deformity and disability.

Once anoxia and hypoprofusion have been excluded or treated, the next major threat to the injured child is sepsis secondary to disruption of a hollow viscus. Because of this, the most efficacious means of assessing the injured child is the combination of repeated thorough physical examinations and appropriate imaging techniques determined on the basis of initial findings.

As the number of reports documenting the successful healing of splenic, hepatic, and renal injuries without operative intervention have increased, a consensus has developed among pediatric surgeons that the presence of blood within the abdominal cavity does not necessarily mandate operative intervention [5–7]. Because of this, peritoneal lavage by itself is not a particularly specific tool for the assessment of an injured child's abdomen. While analysis of lavage return for increased leukocyte count or the presence of bile, amylase, or feces may be helpful, in reality most types of injuries suggested by these findings can be easily diagnosed by thorough physical examination complemented by computed tomography (CT) when indicated. Because head trauma is frequently the most severe and life-threatening injury, the probability of an injured child requiring immediate CT scan for assessment of the central nervous system is quite high. Accordingly, in children with abdominal trauma who are hemodynamically stable, it is appropriate to complement the CT scan of the head with a scan of the abdomen and pelvis. The instillation of contrast intravenously will identify both renal units as well as provide an indication of their functional capacity. The instillation of contrast into the stomach by swallowing or direct nasogastric tube will also highlight the status of the upper gastrointestinal tract and further emphasize any abnormalities in architecture of the spleen, liver, or retroperitoneum.

In the absence of positive findings on initial physical examination and CT scan, the most effective means of further evaluation of the child is continued careful abdominal physical examination. The development of increasing tenderness, abdominal guarding, or distention is a sign suggestive of evolving peritonitis, which mandates further evaluation and, if necessary, prompt operative intervention.

Laboratory Studies

Upon arrival in the emergency department, all pediatric trauma patients must have blood drawn for complete blood count and transfusion cross match. Other than the hematocrit, there is very little laboratory support required for the accurate initial assessment and triage of an injured child. Serum electrolytes, coagulation profile, platelet count, arterial blood gases, and all of the other myriad laboratory tests that attend routine medical care are frequently noncontributory in the first phase of assessment of the injured child. For all children, it is essential that a white blood count, hematocrit, and urinalysis be obtained so that subsequent assessments can assist documentation of either evolving inflammatory process (i.e., peritonitis) or primary urologic dysfunction (i.e., renal contusion). The remainder of the "standard laboratory battery" including serum electrolytes, amylase, coagulation parameters, and platelet count are frequently superfluous studies in all but the most seriously injured child. When we recently reviewed the contribution of emergency room laboratory studies to the initial assessment and triage of the injured child, we identified one out of every three dollars spent for laboratory assessment were wasted on laboratory tests that frequently returned too late to be considered in initial assessment of the child or with results that were completely within normal limits and noncontributory to clinical decision making [8]. It is obvious that in all but the most seriously injured child, most of these laboratory values reflect the normal baseline homeostasis that existed at the time of injury. Accordingly, they should be considered in the very severely injured child as baseline laboratory function; however, in the mildly or moderately injured child, most of these laboratory tests will usually be unrewarding and unnecessarily costly.

PEDIATRIC TRAUMA TRIAGE

The tragedy of preventable traumatic death has been well documented in multiple studies reported over the past three decades. In regard to the pediatric population, Ramenofsky and coworkers [9] identified an incidence of 53 out of 100 pediatric trauma deaths that could be classified as preventable. These statistics have been one of the prime motivations for development of regional trauma referral systems intended to provide continuous high-quality, sophisticated care in a few centers specifically designated for this function.

Since the level of care and commitment is extremely expensive, the functional efficiency of such systems depends on accurate and judicious triage of appropriately injured patients to appropriately designated centers. This problem becomes even more acute for pediatric trauma patients, since the few hospitals that are designed as pediatric trauma centers frequently serve relatively larger population areas. Intelligent triage of an injured child thus becomes a major factor not only in the determination of initial care, but also in the overall function and impact of the regional trauma system as a whole.

The Pediatric Trauma Score (PTS) was developed specifically as a triage tool for pediatric trauma victims. It consists of a grading system wherein six components of pediatric injury are each graded and added to produce a score that is predictive of injury severity and mortality potential (Table 15-2). Size is considered first because it is readily obvious and is a major consideration in the infant-toddler group in whom mortality from injury is highest. Airway is assessed not just as a functional status but as a descriptor of what care is required to provide adequate management. Systolic blood pressure assessment is arranged primarily to identify those children in whom evolving, preventable shock may occur (50–90 mm Hg systolic pressure [+1]). Regardless of size, a child whose systolic pressure is below 50 mm Hg (−1) is in obvious jeopardy. On the other hand, a child whose systolic pressure exceeds 90 mm Hg (+2) probably falls into a

Table 15-2. Pediatric Trauma Score (PTS)

	Category		
Component	+2	+1	−1
Size	⩾20 kg	10–20 kg	<10 kg
Airway	Normal	Maintainable	Unmaintainable
Systolic BP	⩽90 mm Hg	90–50 mm Hg	<50 mm Hg
Central nervous system	Awake	Obtunded/loss of consciousness	Coma/decerebrate
Open wound	None	Minor	Major/penetrating
Skeletal	None	Closed fracture	Open/multiple fractures
			Sum________(PTS)

If proper sized BP cuff not available: BP can be assessed by assigning
+2 pulse palpable at wrist
+1 pulse palpable at groin
−1 no pulse palpable

Source: Adapted from J. J. Tepas et al.: The pediatric trauma score as a predictor of injury severity. *J. Trauma* 28:425, 1988.

better outcome category than a child with even a slight degree of hypotension.

The most important factor in initial assessment of the central nervous system is level of consciousness. Because children frequently sustain very transient loss of consciousness during injury, the "obtunded" (+1) grade is applied to any child with loss of consciousness, no matter how fleeting [10]. This thereby identifies this patient as able to develop potentially fatal and frequently treatable intracranial sequellae secondary to head injury. Because of the high incidence of skeletal injury in the pediatric population and its potential contribution to mortality, it is also a consideration in determining PTS [11]. Finally, cutaneous injury both as an adjunct to common pediatric injury patterns and as an injury category that includes penetrating wounds is considered in computing the PTS.

By nature of its simple design, the PTS serves as a simple checklist ensuring that all components critical to initial assessment of the injured child have been considered. It is utilizable by paramedics in the field as well as by physicians in facilities other than pediatric trauma units. As a predictor of injury, the PTS has a statistically significant inverse linear relationship with both the Injury Severity Score (ISS) and mortality (Fig. 15-1). Analysis of this relationship has identified a threshold PTS of eight, below which all injured children should be triaged to an appropriate pediatric trauma center.

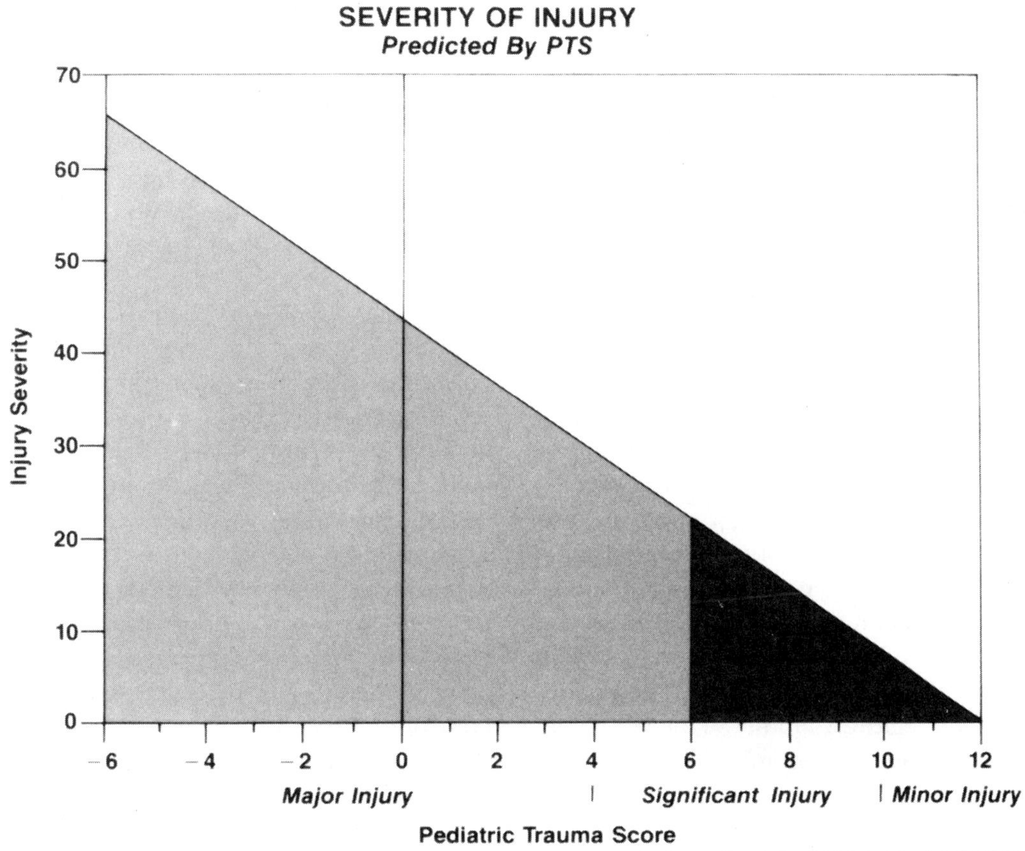

Fig. 15-1. Relationship between PTS and severity of injury. (Adapted from J. J. Tepas et al., The pediatric trauma score as a predictor of injury severity. *J. Trauma* 28:425, 1988.)

SPECIFIC ORGAN SYSTEM CONSIDERATIONS

Head Injury

Head injury continues to be the most common cause of death in the pediatric trauma patient [12]. While many of the most severe injuries are treatable only by prevention, there are many initial resuscitative measures that may at least ameliorate the initial effect of the child's CNS injury. Again the premise of adequate oxygenation, ventilation, and circulation must be addressed, and in the head-injured child, hyperventilation with adequate oxygenation should be considered. From the moment of injury, the reflex responses occurring within the closed cranial vault are partially related to perfusion pressure, tissue oxygenation, and evolving edema. Thus, any child who sustains head trauma in which there has been any prolonged diminution in level of consciousness should be considered for hyperventilation as soon as initial therapy is begun. Tissue perfusion can be improved considerably by simply hyperventilating the patient to a PCO_2 level of 25 mm Hg. This is easily achieved in the obtunded or comatose child by initial airway control and ventilation with either mask or endotracheal tube with 100% oxygen given at 35 to 40 breaths/min.

Initial assessment of the level of consciousness is a rapid and reliably prognostic exercise. It must be considered that any child, regardless of the adequacy of neurologic status on initial assessment, may be susceptible to the secondary changes post CNS injury as the result of even the most minor trauma. Loss of consciousness is an excellent criterion indicating which children should be more aggressively monitored and carefully observed. Any child who sustains even a transient loss of consciousness must be assumed to have sustained adequate degree of mechanical trauma to the brain stem and reticular activating system to allow at least transient depolarization and dysfunction. If the level of consciousness returns to normal, careful observation should be considered to rule out the possibility of evolving secondary dysfunction as a result of cerebral edema or a space-occupying lesion in the form of subdural or epidural hematoma. A careful Glasgow Coma Scale assessment and follow-up examination are therefore paramount to successful monitoring and management of these children.

Children whose Glasgow Coma Score is seven or below or who have sustained severe intracerebral injury require direct monitoring of the intracerebral pressure. While this modality is somewhat imperfect in its reflection of the status of the neuronal metabolism, it is still a relatively good predictor of the overall status of the circulation and perfusion pressures within the cranial vault. Other nonsurgical methods of coma management include initiation of hypothermia, barbiturate coma, and chronic mannitol or glycerol drip therapy. All of these modalities require extremely aggressive and careful monitoring and must be performed under the direct observation and control of a physician in a pediatric critical care unit. The child who presents to a hospital incapable of this level of care should be stabilized, hyperventilated, and transported to an appropriate center. Obviously, the modality of transport must be secure enough to allow careful monitoring and control of the child's airway during transit so that adequate oxygenation, ventilation, and tissue perfusion can be maintained.

Recent work by Andrassy and Dubois [13] has identified the rapid development of catabolism in children sustaining head injury. Their study compared nitrogen balance in children who had sustained primary head injury with children who had sustained orthopedic injury requiring prolonged immobilization. They demonstrated that children with head injury had a severe shift into a negative nitrogen balance and, as a result of this, demonstrated significant catabolism. It stands to reason then that individuals providing comprehensive care to children with multiple injuries, especially those with head injuries, may well improve the overall rehabilitative function of the child as well as rapidity of recovery by the provision of adequate nutrition as soon after stabilization as possible. Multiple studies are presently underway to identify further some of the characteristics of the postinjury catabolism syndrome as well as means of effectively controlling and reversing it. There is no question, however, that rapid institution of adequate nutritional support, by either enteric or intravenous means, is a very significantly positive factor in promoting rapid and complete recovery in brain-injured children.

Finally, the initiation of physical therapy in the form of passive range of motion and active rehabilitation is essential to an improved outcome in pediatric CNS injury. Here again, as soon as adequate stabilization is achieved, input from the rehabilitative and physical therapy service should be provided so that recovery can proceed as expeditiously as possible.

Thoracic Injuries

As has been mentioned, the extremely resilient rib cage of the child with its incomplete calcification provides a means wherein energy transferred through the thoracic cage to intrathoracic organs is frequently more devastating than in the adult population. As a result, the child may have sustained a significant parenchymal injury, disruption of vascular anatomy, or simple contusion without manifestation of even the slightest degree of abnormality on external examination. A high index of suspicion is key to diagnosis of these injuries. Every child sustaining injury to the chest and torso should be carefully monitored, should have anteroposterior lateral chest x-rays in an upright position, and should be carefully assessed as to normal cardiopulmonary and ventilatory function. Finally, the possibility of cardiac contusion in children sustaining blunt thoracic trauma must be considered. Accordingly, any child who has sustained a high-impact blunt thoracic injury should at least have a comprehensive 12-lead electrocardiogram to rule out the possibility of a subtle cardiac contusion.

Abdominal Injuries

Because of the increased size of the torso relative to the extremities in children, abdominal injuries continue to be an extremely common problem. As has been discussed, the presence of blood within the peritoneal cavity does not necessarily mandate immediate laparotomy.

Since the initial description of overwhelming postsplenectomy sepsis in asplenic individuals by King and Schumaker [14] in 1952, there has been a gradually increasing ground swell among the pediatric surgical community to minimize splenectomy whenever possible. Multiple studies have confirmed successful nonoperative management of splenic injuries and have most recently documented similar success with hepatic and renal injuries. Obviously, common sense and good clinical judgment must be applied in management of children with blunt abdominal trauma. A child who is unstable on presentation and remains so or a child who requires large volumes of blood transfusion to maintain adequate cardiovascular stability must be explored. Figure 15-2 demonstrates a commonly used protocol initially developed at the Hospital for Sick Children in Toronto that mandates transfusion of somewhere on the order of 50 to 70 percent normal circulating

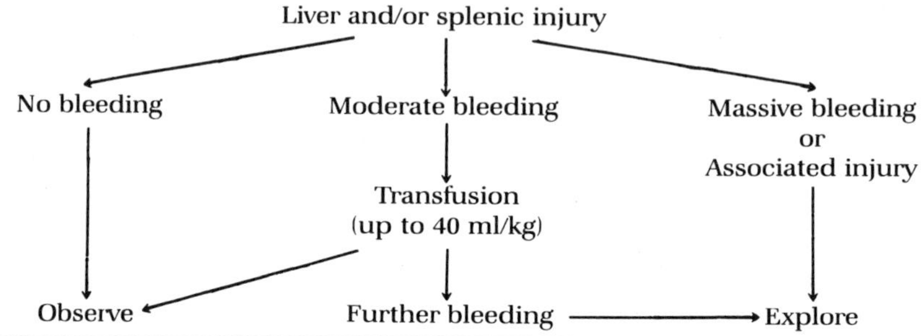

Fig. 15-2. Protocol for management of hepatic or splenic trauma. (From D. E. Wesson et al., Ruptured spleen: When to operate. *J. Pediatr. Surg.* 16:324, 1981.)

volume prior to the consideration for operative intervention [5]. Repeat careful clinical examination of the abdomen is absolutely mandatory. Abdominal distention, tenderness to palpation, evolving rebound, and guarding are all signs suggestive that either a hemoperitonium or rupture of a hollow viscus may be present.

When operative intervention must be considered, splenorrhaphy should be attempted whenever possible. The amount of time required to complete splenorrhaphy must be titrated against potential threat to the patient by prolonged operative intervention and evolving or poorly controlled hypovolemic shock. Hepatic injuries are best treated by simple debridement and, whenever possible, direct vascular ligation [15]. The main premise of management is elimination of devitalized tissue, which may provide substrate for ongoing sepsis or abscess formation.

Although complex pancreatic or duodenal injuries seem to be somewhat infrequent in the pediatric age group, duodenal perforation can and does occur. A simple x-ray of the abdominal cavity with careful attention to the presence of gas in the retroduodenal area on lateral projection may indicate the possibility of a subtle duodenal injury. The incidence of isolated midbody pancreatic injuries secondary to falls and blunt trauma is quite significant. It cannot be overemphasized that the actual traumatic incident causing these types of injuries may actually be very minor and that a high index of suspicion is essential to successful identification and treatment of these injuries. Abdominal CT scan is an extremely sensitive tool for assessment of the status of the pancreas and can be very effective in identifying these injuries. Adequate therapy of these lesions requires operative intervention and, in most cases, resection of the segment of pancreas distal to the area of disruption. Since this is usually the midportion of the body of the pancreas as it overlies the vertebral column, a distal subtotal pancreatectomy without splenectomy is frequently the procedure of choice in treatment of this injury.

The development of peritonitis secondary to perforation of a hollow viscus is both an immediate and long-term possibility. Children who are injured wearing seat belts in an incorrect manner frequently sustain an avulsion injury in which part of the distal small bowel is torn from its underlying mesentery. This in combination with a direct contusive injury to the abdomen may cause immediate blowout of the involved segment of gut, with purulent fecal peritonitis developing shortly thereafter. It may, however, cause a simple area of devascularization and ischemia that will progress to necrosis and perforation within 48 to 72 hours post injury. Therefore, any child sustaining significant blunt abdominal trauma must be carefully observed for this possibility and explored immediately should signs or symptoms of acute abdominal distress suddenly develop.

Extremity Trauma

In comparison to the adult, the child's skeleton is incompletely calcified and consists of a high degree of cartilagenous tissue and metabolically active growth plates. The collateral ligamentous structure binding this skeleton is frequently stronger and better able to withstand mechanical disruption than the boney elements to which it is attached. As a result, children sustaining skeletal trauma frequently sustain major deforming forces prior to development of fractures or disruptions of their boney skeleton. Primary joint disruption from other than penetrating injury is uncommon in comparison to disruption of the diaphyseal or epiphyseal segments of bone. Fractures involving the growth plate must be carefully identified and treated in a manner that will ensure not only adequate healing but also prevention of subsequent displacement or deformity.

The association of vascular injuries with orthopedic injuries must always be excluded in the pediatric population. Besides the obvious injury to the brachial artery secondary to suprachondylar fracture of the humerus, the possibility of minor vascular disruptions causing growth plate ischemia or major vascular disruption causing low-flow or hypoprofusion states must be considered. Since the pediatric population does not usually suffer from advanced atherosclerosis, mechanical forces will temporarily deform rather than disrupt major vessels. The adventitia and media of the child's arterial system can well tolerate this transient deformity and immediately return to a normal anatomic state. The intima of these vessels, however, will frequently fracture as a result of this stretching deformity and, upon return to the normal anatomic position, develop an intimal flap that will impede vascular flow. Rather than gross disruption of the vessel with hypovolemia and hemorrhagic shock, a child sustaining blunt vascular injury either primarily or in association with an orthopedic injury may sustain diminution of flow as a result of a silent intimal flap. Here again, a high index of suspicion and careful assessment of the distal vascular runoff of the injured child must be routinely considered. When there is the slightest suggestion of decrease in perfusion, arteriography should be considered. While the natural history of these lesions remains unclear, there is no question that a major disruption of blood flow as the result of an intimal flap within the aorta may well warrant at least careful observation if not immediate operative correction.

LONG-TERM FOLLOW-UP

According to Gallagher and associates [16], for every child that dies of traumatic injury, 45 others require admission and intensive hospital care, and 1300 additional children require at least emergency room assessment and therapy. It becomes obvious, therefore, that the effect of traumatic injury on our pediatric population is extensive. Unfortunately, long-term follow-up of injured children has focused primarily on that very small segment with severe injury who have identifiable CNS dysfunction requiring prolonged rehabilitation. In reality, a variety of other injuries, some of which are "survivable," are being poorly followed and yet are providing ongoing morbidity and health care problems for these children. Careful follow-up must be provided for all injured children, specifically in regard to developmental anomalies and propensity for repeat injuries. Centers providing care for the injured child and individuals committed to this end should ensure that all children to whom care is provided are given careful long-term scrutiny so that the effects of injury can be analyzed and hopefully their detrimental results minimized. This type of program should focus on subtle residual deficits in CNS function as well as psychological effects and the identification of "accident-prone" children.

In conclusion, initial and definitive care of the injured child requires careful application of the standard trauma life support principles to the unique characteristics of this patient population. An individual who understands the types of injuries that frequently affect children, the mechanical forces at play when children are injured, and the unique characteristics of the child as a patient will be most likely to provide a level of care that will be expeditious, effective, comprehensive, and successful. Achievement of this goal not only will provide a tremendous sense of personal satisfaction, but also will be a major step forward in diminishing the most common cause of death and disability in our pediatric population.

REFERENCES

1. National Safety Council. Chicago *Accident Facts—1984 Edition.* National Safety Council, 1984.
2. Cales, R. H., and Trunky, D. D. Preventable trauma deaths. *J.A.M.A.* 245:1059, 1985.
3. Rimel, R., Geordani, B., Barth, J., et al. Disability caused by minor head injury. *J. Neurosurg.* 9:221, 1981.
4. Plant, M., and Gifford, R. Trivial head trauma and its consequences in a perspective of regional health care. *Milit. Med.* 141:244, 1976.
5. Wesson, D. E., Filler, R. M., Ein, S. H., et al. Ruptured spleen: When to operate. *J. Pediatr. Surg.* 16:324, 1981.
6. Karp, M. P., Cooney, D. R., Pros, G. A., et al. The nonoperative management of pediatric hepatic trauma. *J. Pediatr. Surg.* 18:512, 1983.
7. Polley, T. Z., and Coran, A. C. Special problems in management of pediatric trauma. *Crit. Care Clin.* 2(4):775, 1986.
8. Bryant, M. S., Tepas, J. J., Mollitt, D. L., and Talbert, J. L. Impact of emergency room laboratory studies on the ultimate triage and disposition of the injured child. *Am. Surg.* 54:209, 1988.
9. Ramenofsky, M. D., Luterman, A., Quindlen, E., et al. Maximum survival in pediatric trauma: The ideal system. *J. Trauma* 24:818, 1984.
10. Stablein, D. M., Miller, J. D., Choi, S. C., et al. Sta-

tistical methods for determining prognosis in severe head injury. *Neurosurgery* 6(3):243, 1980.
11. Champion, H. R., and Sacco, W. J. Measurement of injury severity and its practical application. *Trauma Q.* 1:25, 1984.
12. Kraus, J. F., Fife, D., Cox, P., et al. Incidence, severity and external causes of pediatric brain injury. *Am. J. Dis. Child.* 140:687, 1986.
13. Andrassy, R. J., and Dubois, T. Modified injury severity scale and concurrent steroid therapy: Independent correlates of negative nitrogen balance in pediatric trauma. *J. Pediatr. Surg.* 20(6):799, 1985.
14. King, H., and Schumacker, H. B. Susceptibility to infection after splenectomy performed in injury. *Ann. Surg.* 136(2):239, 1952.
15. Feleciano, D. V., Mattox, K. L., Jordan, G. L., et al. Management of 1000 consecutive cases of hepatic trauma (1979–1984). *Ann. Surg.* 204(4):438, 1986.
16. Gallagher, S. S., Finison, K., Guyer, B., and Goodenough, S. Incidence of injuries among 87,000 Massachusetts children and adolescents. *Am. J. Public Health* 74(12):1340, 1984.

16

Trauma and the Geriatric Patient

George M. Watkins

It is evident from this study that the aged person who survives can often expect longevity. This is satisfactory from a surgeon's point of view. . . .
Born Bjorn Anderson [1]

It is unknown whether the humor of redundancy was intended or whether the author was coping with an unfamiliar subtlety of a foreign language. The fact remains that the elderly surgical patient who survives hospitalization and attendant surgeries after trauma will usually return to a state that is similar to what he had before injury or is altered only by the specific injury [2]. If the quality of life as measured by the elderly person himself is taken into account, then individuals who underwent a variety of surgical procedures generally were satisfied with the outcome [3]. One study of patients over 70 years of age, however, concluded that 92 percent of a group of elderly traumatized patients either were in nursing homes (72 percent) or needed medical assistance (20 percent) after trauma, while 96 percent of the same patients were independent prior to injury [4]. In this study, the mortality rate was only 15 percent. Most of the mortality was due to burn injuries, whereby the patients were moribund on arrival at the hospital, or was secondary to trauma received after falls. The latter were not broken down as to mechanism of injury. In addition, the number of patients who had fractures was not specified. Fractures of the hip have a very detrimental outcome [5]. Up to 50 percent die within 6 months. Part of the mortality rate is in-hospital and may be due to associated diseases. The most prevalent of the risk factors for death is thromboembolism in some series [6].

Falls are often the result of permanently disabling diseases being present. At times, they are part of the first expression of such chronic disabling diseases. In studies where falls were documented as being a result of an individual's having a multitude of diseases, the falls themselves were not a major component causing posthospital long-term care. When the elderly received specific geriatric therapy with a goal toward rehabilitation, "... a cardinal geriatric principle: impaired elderly patients can respond dramatically to treatment" [7] was the conclusion reached.

In many areas of trauma statistics, the elderly and young children have similarities. The four leading causes of death in these extremes of age are the same. For severe injuries such as burns, the mortality is much higher at the start and the end of the life cycle. Also the mortality for the same injury may be higher than in the general population. Falls and auto-pedestrian–related injuries are two of the first four causes of death resulting from trauma. In both groups, the incidence of injury is lower than in the general population, while the mortality from similar injuries is higher than the norm.

Major differences between the injured young and old lie not only in associated disease but also in youth's ability to recuperate and adapt to any limitations in a short period of time. The most obvious case is the head injury, wherein a child may recover from amazing damage, while a head-injured elder may never survive any prolonged derangement of consciousness. The elderly, on the other hand, not only adapt poorly to new limitations but also take a long time to recover even if there are no permanent changes. Of course, there remains the true old adage that "one can not keep a youngster in bed while one may not be able to get an elder out of bed." Still, with perseverance, most elderly can recover to near their preinjury state if some mechanical or chronic nervous system factor does not prevent such.

Life expectancy is continuing to climb in the United States and presently is about 75 years [8]. The U.S. population between the ages of 65 and 74 is increasing at the rate of 2 percent per year. The increase in the over 74 age group is 3 percent per year. These changes are in contrast to the population increase of 1 percent per year in the United States as a whole [9]. The outcome is that the United States has significantly more individuals living to an older age every year. Traumatic injuries in the elderly will inevitably be consuming a greater part of our resources.

For a variety of reasons, we see these older individuals living independently while having a series of discovered [10] and undiscovered illnesses [11]. Modern control of such illness may allow afflicted individuals to exist in the routines of modern living while being at risk for dangers such as automobile accidents or the increasing violence of our society. On the other hand, as exemplified by Malcolm Forbes, a person who is old in years may be physiologically quite healthy and lead the lifestyles of the middle-aged but with higher risks [12]. In either situation, an injury that would have resulted in short-term disability for a young person may lead to marked morbidity or death in an elder.

Numerous articles have been written concerning outcomes of surgery in the aged. Many are a hodgepodge of elective and emergency cases with and without trauma being included. These series usually include fractures with emergency surgery but do not distinguish between these and other emergencies. Other series are specific to organ systems but do not either include trauma or identify trauma cases [13–18]. The unexpected nature of trauma in the elderly, the mixing of trauma cases with total operations or total emergency operations, and the use of retrospective trauma analysis make definitive treatment protocols more subjective than usual. Surgical judgment increases in importance.

Also, the term *elderly* has different meanings in various series. The age defining the biologic time that marks the start of elderly years varies from a high of 70 to a low of 50 years. Many series use 65 years either because it is the age of usual retirement or because of governmental decree making that age "elderly" for Medicare purposes. Interestingly, the Trauma Score was originally supposed to predict outcomes in injured individuals under the age of 60 years [19]. Later the decision was made to use 55 years of age to "consider taking to trauma hospital for moderately severe injury" [20]. No scientific reason was given for changing the age recommendation, but one author stated that the change was because of increased risk above that age [21]. The trauma algorithm still does not make any allowance for age in altering scoring, but a recent simple modification is a crude start [22]. No series has been able to sort trauma to include risk factors of co-morbidity. Yet co-morbidity is known to affect outcome adversely [23].

Few absolutes are present to define *elderly*. Different systems of the body deteriorate at different rates. It is safe to say that the human is not a "one-horse shay." While multiorgan failure is often the cascade of events that occur in elderly who are ill, systems deteriorate at different aging rates. Different reserves are present that are more dependent on heredity and environmental factors than on any biologic age. Many of these factors can be manipulated by influences such as exercise. The outcomes, however, may be in a positive or negative manner. As an example, the lifetime athlete may alter the normal progressive decreases in cardiac output from birth to death for a while. But the wear and tear on his musculoskeletal system can make him a nonathlete or even a cripple in later life, negating the effects of earlier conditioning.

The skin is one system that has been immune to positive manipulation. While the declination of skin function and structure goes on through adult life, significant clinical skin changes almost inevitably take place by the time an individual is 60 years old. Even though Retin-A has some effects on slowing the aging process and continued contact with the elements may have some negative changes, both effects are limited to exposed parts of the body, usually the face, neck, and hands [24].

Whether this change is the reason that 60 years has been used so often as the start of the elderly years is uncertain. Part of the usage may be historical, because 60 years is the start of the seventh decade, because of tradition, or because of unknown reasons. The author has found no reason why 60 is the year used for "aged." He uses such age in part because of historical precedent [25,26] and in part because many body functions begin to have important or rapid declinations about the sixtieth year when the average of a broad population is examined.

EPIDEMIOLOGY OF TRAUMA IN THE ELDERLY

The leading causes of death in the United States are the same as they were prior to

World War II. Cardiovascular diseases were far and away the leading killer. Next was cancer. Third was trauma. Arteriosclerosis and cancer tend to strike at the end of an individual's life [27]. Moreover, the toll of coronary artery deaths has dramatically decreased over the last 25 years [28]. Generally, trauma is thought to be a disease of younger age groups. Injury rate, however, changes little with age after the forty-fifth year. Mortality rate due to trauma of both vehicular and nonvehicular origins increases exponentially with advancing age [29].

Automobile-induced pedestrian injuries, burns, and when adjusted for age, automobile crashes are more frequent in the elderly. Traffic-light timing, habits, and "senility" are all thought to contribute [30]. Until recently, little attention has been paid to suicide, the rate of which climbs steadily with age greater than 40. Abuse of the elderly and hidden alcoholism are cofactors in injuries of the elderly.

Ironically, old chronologic age may mean bias against aggressive treatment of the elderly ill. Such a bias in health care personnel often means the prophecy of poor outcome is fulfilled [31].

SPECIFIC OPERATION AND TECHNICAL MANEUVERS IN THE ELDERLY

There are no specific operations for the elderly who are injured, and the technical aspects are covered elsewhere in this book or in standard texts and atlases. Certain operations may be modified. For example, the author is much more likely to perform a splenectomy in an elderly person with a possibly salvagable spleen that is damaged even if there are no other injuries. He certainly will remove the spleen if there are multiple injuries besides. The risk-benefit ratio is too high because of the time constraints and possible continued bleeding requiring reoperation. Such problems must be compared to the lower protection splenic salvage offers in the elderly. The length of time an operation takes may or may not be a factor by itself in increasing morbidity and mortality of the injured elderly. Certainly, the length of anesthesia time causes much greater heat loss in the elderly individual than in a younger cohort. It is reasonable to perform an ileostomy rather than carry out an anastomosis or do other more conservative treatments than subject an older injured person to a prolonged hypothermia. Delayed primary closure probably should be undertaken more frequently as age increases. In some individuals who are already bedridden, have bowel control problems, and/or have decubitus ulcers, a colostomy may be a better definitive procedure than a colonic anastomosis.

ASSESSMENT AND TREATMENT OF THE INJURED ELDER

An elderly person who is injured is initially assessed as any trauma victim: *a*irway with cervical spine control, *b*reathing, *c*irculation with control of hemorrhage, *d*isability, and *e*xposure. As previously noted, the older individual often has severe hidden or overt preexisting diseases. These diseases have an effect on the survival after severe injury, such as burns, if two or more factors are preexistent [2], but the true effect of co-morbidity on the outcome of injury remains to be defined. Probably the preexisting disease will be scored as if it were an anatomic area injured. The square of the severity would be added to be a part of the injury severity score or other indicator of relative injury severity. To an extent, age itself is already factored into need to triage to trauma centers. Still, it is the co-morbidity that exists in an older person, not age itself, that increases mortality and morbidity.

When taking the history of an injured older person, there may be little objective evidence of preexisting illness or the treatment of that illness may alter the body composition. Unlike in the young, electrocardiogram monitoring, blood gases, and full chemistries can alter the course of treatment. Also transfusion should be considered earlier in the elderly for at least two reasons: Arteriosclerotic cardiovascular heart disease may inhibit increased flow through the coronary vessels, and the older individuals usually will not be able to offset loss in oxygen- and carbon dioxide–carrying capacity and/or increase needs by a major increase in cardiac output and/or ventilation.

If the person taking an injured elder's history is not able to get an adequate history from the patient, an omission may be ominous. Serious illnesses may be totally hidden until the stress of operation or the postoperative period occurs. The illnesses may be exhibited as immediately occurring abnormalities such as heart attack, or they may be expressed over time, as when a patient with heart failure does not have digitalis continued after admission. They may be physically apparent, such as the residua of an old stroke, or they may be picked up from laboratory data such as severe chronic anemia. While not all of the preexisting illnesses may be controllable, many are amenable to therapy. It is incumbent on treating physicians to get a history as soon as possible, even if extraordinary measures are required.

OPERATIVE MEASURES

When the elderly individual is transferred to the operating room for treatment of acute trauma, the surgery itself is similar to that of other injured individuals. The way in which surgery is carried out is the important feature. The operating room temperature usually is set for the comfort of the operating room team. Like children, older individuals rapidly lose heat while in operating room and recovery room environments. The heat loss is more difficult to reverse than in younger adults. The author's personal opinion from treating a large volume of elderly injured, including for burns [2,23], is that a drop in rectal or esophageal temperature to less than 96.5°F is associated with a rapidly accelerating and continuing drop in temperature. Such declines lead to coagulopathies, prolonged stuporous states, and prolonged discomfort. In turn, usually there is increased catabolic hormone and interleukin release plus shivering. The results are a series of adverse effects including rapid protein breakdown. Since most elders start with a diminished muscle mass, any proteolytic effects should be magnified. How much such problems affect the outcome overall in the traumatized elderly is not certain, but morbidity and mortality dropped when hypothermia was minimized in the burned elderly [2].

Heating pads, coverage of unused body parts with "space blankets," warm fluids, room temperature of 85°F, and incandescent heating lamps are important. If possible, any nonoperated area of the body should be kept dry to avoid insensible heat loss. The risk-benefit of raising humidity in the room is an unsettled issue.

While the same aids should be used in the recovery room, it is usually impractical to control temperature as effectively. The recovery room is a shared facility. The patient can be encased front and back with heating pads, and the aluminum-mylar film "space blanket" can be placed over the patient with or without or blankets beneath.

POSTOPERATIVE AND POST-TRAUMA CARE

Pneumonia is the friend of the elderly.
Sir William Osler.

This statement must be borne in mind in the care of older traumatized patients. The axiom that an older person who is not totally mobilized within a week after being placed at bed rest will not get out of bed is not always true. Still, it is a good rule to remember when planning the postoperative care of such patients.

The role of early enteral feeding in the elderly has not been studied prospectively. It appears to be at least as important, if not more so, than in younger individuals. The liberal use of intraoperative needle feeding jejunostomies is strongly encouraged. When the abdomen is not opened or the jejunostomy was not performed at operation, radiographically placed transoral, transgastroduodenal jejunostomy should be carried out as an urgent procedure when the patient has any risk of not eating immediately. If full diet needs are met within 48 to 72 hours after injury, a whole series of unwanted morbidities may be avoided [32–35].

Severely injured elderly or those who are less injured but have significant underlying disease tend to die of two causes: respiratory failure/pneumonia or arteriosclerotic cardiovascular occlusive disease. Early extubation, transfusion, mobilization, and early enteral feeding all play vital roles in lessening the severity of these diseases. Particularly because of underlying disease and diminished reserves, fluid and electrolyte balance should be rigorously maintained. Excess sodium and water, which may be easily handled in others, will often be very injurious to the older person who is postinjury.

Renal failure is usually the result of the above or because of therapy or lack thereof. Intravascular hypovolemia is the norm post-trauma, even though the patient usually has an increased extracellular, extravascular space. Aminoglycosides and/or diuretics should be avoided if such body composition changes are suspected. Restricting total salt intake including calculation of "piggyback" medication sodium may be preferable. Antibiotics of low nephrotoxicity should be used.

While the specifics of decision making are on an individual basis, one caveat of trauma care in the elderly is that the patient, family, and surgeon often must accept less than optimum results as far as an organ to avoid morbidity or mortality of the entire body. Two examples are accepting the deformity of a Colles' fractures by early mobilization to keep wrist and hand function and leaving a colostomy in place in a high-risk elder who is bedridden rather than have the risks of reoperative bowel surgery.

REHABILITATION

Rehabilitation should start at the time of first treatment. Rehabilitation of the elderly is often long and even tedious. Whatever is done to shorten the lag interval until rehabilitation is started will usually lessen the rehabilitation time.

Only 20 percent of the injured population of the United States has adequate rehabilitation. Facilities, trained personnel, costs, and availability all hinder the process. Presently there are bills before the Senate and House of Representatives that will in some part help rectify the problem.

REFERENCES

1. Anderson, B., and Ostberg, J. Long-term prognosis in geriatric surgery: 2–17 year follow-up of 7922 patients. *J. Am. Geriatr. Soc.* 20:255, 1972.
2. Watkins, G. M. Burns in the Elderly. In Meakins and Maclarin, (eds.), *Surgical Care of the Elderly.* Chicago: Year Book, 1988.
3. Midgett, M. C. Social and emotional need for geriatric patients. *Soc. Work Health Care* 6:69, 1981.
4. Oreskovich, M. R., Howard, J. D., Copass, M. K., et al. Geriatric trauma: Injury patterns and outcome. *J. Trauma* 24:565, 1984.
5. Smith, C. Trauma in the elderly. *Nurs. Mirror* 17:36, 1985.
6. Palmberg, S., and Hirsjarvi, E. Mortality in geriatric surgery. *Gerontology* 25:103, 1979.
7. Rubinstein, R. Z. Geriatric evaluation units. *N. Engl. J. Med.* 311:664, 1981.
8. Life expectancy in the United States. *Stat. Bull. Metrop. Life Found.* 64:12, 1983.
9. U.S. Department of Commerce. *Statistical Abstract of the United States.* Washington, D.C.: Government Printing Office, 1984.
10. Moore, A. R. Surgery and the aged. *Aust. Fam. Physician* 1:1045, 1978.
11. Del Guercio, L. R. Monitoring operative risk in the elderly. *J.A.M.A.* 243:1350, 1980.
12. Brady, J. In step with Malcolm Forbes. *Parade,* vol. 22, April 10, 1988.
13. Ziffren, S. E. Comparison of mortality rates for various surgical operations according to age groups, 1951–1977. *J. Am. Geriatr. Soc.* 27:4337, 1979.
14. Greenburg, A. G. Mortality and gastrointestinal surgery in the aged. *Arch. Surg.* 116:788, 1981.
15. Linn, S. L., Linn, M. W., and Wallen, N. Evaluation of results of surgical procedures in the elderly. *Ann. Surg.* 195:90, 1982.
16. Devine, R. M., Farnell, B. F., and Mucha, P. Acute cholecystitis as a complication in surgical patients. *Arch. Surg.* 119:389, 1984.
17. Warner, M. A. Hosking, M. D., Lobdell, C. M., et al. Surgical procedures among ≥ 90 years of age: A population-based in Olmstead, Minnesota; 1975–1985. *Ann. Surg.* 4:380, 1988.
18. Schwab, C. W. Trauma and the elderly. Presented at the 15th Annual Meeting of the American Trauma Society, Washington, D.C., May 1988.
19. Sacco, W. J., Champion, H. R., and Carnazzo, A. J., et al. Trauma score. *Crit. Care Med.* 9:672, 1981.
20. Committee on Trauma of the American College of Surgeons. Appendix F to the hospital resources: Field categorization of trauma patients (field triage). *A.C.S. Bull.* 71:17, 1986.
21. Aprahamian, C. Personal communication, 1988.
22. Boyd, C. R., Tolson, M. A., and Capes, W. S. Evaluating trauma care: The TRISS method. *J. Trauma* 27:370, 1987.
23. Watkins, G. M., and Cruse, W. C. Burns in the elderly. Presented at the 40th Annual Meeting of The American Association for the Surgery of Trauma, Phoenix, Arizona, 1980.
24. Gilchrest, B. A. Age-associated changes in the skin. *J. Am. Geriatr. Soc.* 30:139, 1982.

25. Bull, J. P. Current trends in research on burns. *Proc. R. Soc. Med.* 65:27, 1972.
26. Feller, I., Tholen, D., and Cornell, R. G. Improvements in burn care, 1965 to 1979. *J.A.M.A.* 244:2074, 1980.
27. National Center for Health Statistics. *Health in the U.S. Chart Book.* DHEW Pub. No. (PHS) 80:1233, 1980.
28. Goldman, L. Analyzing the decline in the CAD death rate. *Hosp. Pract.* 109-17, 1988.
29. Fife, D. D., Barancik, J. I., and Chatterjee, M. S. Northeastern Ohio trauma study: II. Injury rates by age, sex, and cause. *Am. J. Public Health* 74:473, 1984.
30. Haddon, W., and Baker, S. J. in Disease Etiology and Prevention, 8. Injury Control; 109-38, 1981. As cited by S. J. Baker, B. O'Neill, and R. S. Karpf, *The Injury Fact Book.* Lexington, Mass.: D.C. Heath, 1984.
31. Wetle, T. Age as a risk factor for inadequate treatment. *J.A.M.A.* 258:516, 1987.
32. Deitch, E. A., Winterton, J., and Berg, R. The gut as a portal of entry for bacteremia: The role of protein malnutrition. *Ann. Surg.* 205:681, 1987.
33. Alexander, J. W., MacMillan, B. G., Stinnet, J. D., et al. Beneficial effects of aggressive protein feeding in severely burned children. *Ann. Surg.* 192:505, 1980.
34. Moore, E. E., and Jones, T. N. Benefits of immediate jejunostomy feeding after major abdominal trauma: A prospective randomized approach. *J. Trauma* 26:874, 1986.
35. Alverdy, J., Chi, H. S., and Sheldon, G. F. The effect of parenteral nutrition on gastro-intestinal immunity. *Ann. Surg.* 24:681, 1985.

17

Trauma During Pregnancy

Jeffrey S. Augenstein

There is possibly no problem in trauma care that is as worrisome as the care of a woman injured during pregnancy. The clinical and medicolegal considerations weigh heavily. The social stature and the accepted excellent prognosis of mother and unborn child in American society enhance the pressure to achieve a good outcome from post-trauma clinical interventions. Yet, the outcome is a function of the same factors as with any injured patient: magnitude of injury, organ systems involved directly and indirectly, success and rapidity of the resuscitation, adequacy of repairs and other interventions, and the ability of physiologic responses to respond to the various perturbations and reach the presumably normal preinjury state.

There is no difference in the approach to the diagnosis or treatment of most injuries in the pregnant or nonpregnant patient. The cardinal rule is that the mother must have the anatomic and physiologic competence required for pregnancy to achieve normal delivery. The embarrassments of the injury must quickly be overcome to reach this end. Errors in management arise from two directions: (1) not recognizing the "normal" anatomy and physiology of pregnancy, thereby over- or underreacting clinically; and (2) attending too much to theoretical injuries to the fetus from diagnostic and therapeutic interventions and, as a consequence, not providing the full measure of clinical care required by the mother to define and treat.the problems. Simply stated, the standards of trauma care are not different for the pregnant trauma patient than for any other patient.

A subset of issues relate to the unique decision making that is appropriate for this group of patients:

1. The approach to positioning the patient for diagnostic and therapeutic interventions.
2. Strategies for repairing the injured uterus and considerations for hysterectomy.
3. Choices in pharmacologic interventions that minimize insult to the fetus.
4. Choices in radiologic diagnostics that minimize fetal radiation exposure.

The strategy of this chapter will be to define a structure to help emergency room physicians and the general surgeon in their approach to the injured pregnant patient. It is assumed that an obstetric surgeon and a pediatric surgeon will address specific issues of delivery and direct care of the fetus or neonate. First, the "normal" physiology of pregnancy will be described. Second, generally accepted techniques in diagnosis and therapy of injury will be described. Third, the approach to injuries specific to pregnancy will be addressed. There will also be discussion of the approach to the fetus when the mother's life cannot be saved. There will be no attempt to review injury management that does not differ in the pregnant and nonpregnant patient, which is the case for most extra-abdominal injuries. The scope of pharmacologic therapeutics in pregnancy is too great and of too critical a nature to hope to address more than the most general concepts in this chapter. The goal is to provide the emergency room physician and the general surgeon responsible as the "captain" of the trauma team a framework with which to approach diagnosis, initial therapy of these patients, and evaluation of the recommendations of the consulting services.

PHYSIOLOGIC CHANGES OF PREGNANCY

Cardiovascular System

The physical examination and electrocardiogram (ECG) are changed from normal during pregnancy. It is imperative that these normal-for-pregnancy findings be understood so that overtreatment does not occur. The heart rate increases by about 15 beats/min by the third trimester; the resting pulse remains less than 100 beats/min. Systolic flow murmurs of grade 1 to 2 as well as a third heart sound are often auscultated. The ECG can show progressive left-axis deviation as a function of the elevation of the heart causing counterclockwise rotation. The T waves become flattened or inverted in leads III, V_1, and V_2 [1].

During the first trimester, the maternal blood volume increases until it plateaus at about 50 percent above prepregnancy levels. This occurs at 30 weeks' gestation. The clinical significance is that the patient has a better than normal response to hemorrhage. However, the severity of the blood loss may be masked. The pregnant patient can maintain stable vital signs and adequate perfusion of most vital organs with a 30- to 35-percent gradual blood loss and a 10- to 20-percent acute loss. Unfortunately, the fetus may not survive the marked decrease in uterine blood flow from uterine artery vasoconstriction.

The cardiac output increases by 40 percent early in the pregnancy. Toward the end of the gestation, the output is extremely sensitive to position. At this point, the inferior vena cava can be nearly occluded by the uterus when the patient is supine. Normally, the pregnant patient is able to compensate for this decrease in blood flow with an increase in peripheral resistance. The injured patient is often maximally vasoconstricted, and this supine positioning may produce catastrophic hypotension.

Systemic vascular resistance decreases during pregnancy. The maximum effect occurs during the second trimester with a fall of 5 to 15 mm Hg in the mean pressure. Peripheral venous pressure may significantly increase in the lower extremities. The clinical consequence is that there may be increased bleeding from the legs after injury. The peripheral blood flow may increase significantly. The augmentation of pelvic vascularity may enhance the risk of hemorrhage and hematoma with injury [2].

Pulmonary System

During pregnancy, hypoxia and hypocarbia occur more often than in nonpregnant women, as hypoventilation is produced by a reduced functional residual capacity. The increased levels of progesterone stimulate hyperventilation. An increased tidal volume causes the arterial PCO_2 to be about 30 mm Hg and the PO_2 to rise to between 100 and 108 mm Hg. The PO_2 decreases in the supine position as pregnancy advances. The pH remains normal by a compensation of increased renal excretion of bicarbonate. During the latter stages of pregnancy, the enlarged uterus elevates the diaphragm, making the pregnant patient more susceptible to postoperative atelectasis and pneumonia [3].

Hematopoietic System

Plasma volume increases by 50 percent, while red cell volume increases by 25 percent. This hemodilution produces the so-called physiologic anemia of pregnancy and should not be assumed to represent loss of blood. It is not uncommon to see a hemoglobin of 10 gm/dl in normal, pregnant patients not receiving iron supplements. During the second and third trimesters, a white blood cell count up to 18,000/μl can be expected normally [3]. During labor, this can increase to 25,000 without pathology. The increase is attributable to enhancement of the neutrophils; occasionally immature forms may be seen on the peripheral smear. Thus, in the normal pregnant patient, the differential may be shifted to the left, although a true left shift with toxic granulations is rarely seen. Platelet counts may be depressed, but significant decreases indicate a consumption coagulopathy. Circulating plasminogen activator and increases in fibrinogen and some of the other clotting factors are normal physiologic responses that seemingly prepare the gravid female for delivery. Unfortunately, these responses predispose the patient to thromboembolic complications following trauma, prolonged bed rest, or surgery. When anticoagulation is deemed necessary, the drug of choice is heparin, as it does not cross the placenta. The placenta contains large amounts of thromboplastin, and the uterus is a major source of plasminogen activator. Injury to either of these structures may precipitate disseminated intravascular coagulation. Elevated levels of fibrin degradation products are normal in pregnancy, as intravascular coagulation occurs routinely; it is abnormal when these levels are not increased.

Central Nervous System

There is little known about the effects of pregnancy on the central nervous system. Some neurologic abnormalities are seen reasonably frequently during pregnancy. This may affect the postinjury physical examination in looking for trauma-induced neuropathology. Vascular headaches, which can be accompanied by parasthesias and visual changes, are seen more frequently than in nongravid females, particularly during the first half of gestation. Eclampsia, which occurs during the third trimester, may be mistaken for post-traumatic seizures. An injured patient in the third trimester who presents with seizures should have as part of the therapeutic considerations the treatment of eclampsia. Eclampsia-related seizures require a different approach than typical post-traumatic seizures; the former require infusion of magnesium sulfate and delivery of the fetus [3]. Treatment of seizures not caused by eclampsia would include investigation for the presence of head injuries and neurosurgery and/or standard anticonvulsants. It is thus critical that the right strategies be initiated.

Gastrointestinal System

The pregnant patient is at greater risk for regurgitating gastric contents and aspiration because of a reduction in lower esophageal sphincter function [1]. Gastric emptying and intestinal motility are slowed. If emergency surgery is considered, it should be assumed that the gravida has a full stomach; thus placement of a nasogastric tube and decompression should be done prior to induction of anesthesia. However, this is not documented in the trauma literature. The liver is relatively unchanged with pregnancy; the blood flow and size are unaltered. However, some confusion can occur because a common liver enzyme, alkaline phosphatase, is two to four times increased over normal values by the third trimester due to increased placental production. Since this enzyme is often used as a marker for intrahepatic masses and biliary obstruction, awareness of normalcy for pregnancy is important to reduce overtreatment. It should be noted that the aspartate aminotransferase and alamine aminotransferase remain within normal values. Total serum protein levels decline, mainly due to a reduction in the albumin levels of 1.0 gm/dl.

The pregnancy, particularly in the latter stages, affects the anatomic relation of organs. This along with the flaccid, stretched abdomen may affect the ability to assess for injury. Pain may radiate to uncharacteristic locations or may even be masked. Because of the concentration of the small bowel in the upper abdomen in the latter stages of the pregnancy, injuries may involve a number of loops. On the other hand, the important physical findings of nausea and vomiting, which increase the index of suspicion of intra-abdominal pathology after trauma, are normal findings in pregnancy.

Urogenital System

From the time of early pregnancy, the renal collecting system is dilated [1]. This physiologic hydronephrosis is more pronounced on the right than on the left. The bladder is elevated out of the pelvis and is compressed by the uterus, thus making it more prone to rupture. The creatinine clearance increases beyond 150 ml/min, and the blood area nitrogen falls, mostly due to increased renal plasma flow. The finding of a serum creatinine level of more than 0.8 mg/dl or a blood urea nitrogen level of greater than 10 mg/dl is abnormal [3].

CLINICAL EVALUATION

Overall Concerns

Before addressing the general considerations, it is important to note a very real difference in the approach to a very small group of severely injured pregnant patients. One of the major differences in the resuscitation of the pregnant versus nonpregnant patient is in the approach to the patient presenting without vital signs. The strategy would be to pursue resuscitation aggressively in the pregnant patient. Even if the mother has a fatal injury, the possibility remains for a postmortem cesarean section to provide a perfectly viable neonate. This area is one of the most complex in all of trauma care, however. The ethical, social, and medical considerations are tremendous. It remains that a newborn capable of a totally normal life can be delivered after as much as 15 minutes of maternal loss of vital signs. By maintaining life support in the brain-dead mother, perfectly viable newborns have been delivered weeks after the initial trauma [4]. The scope of this chapter does not allow further discussion of this topic. The clinician must individualize each case.

The approach to the patient maintains the well-documented prioritization of *a*irway, *b*reathing, *c*irculation, and so on. There is no difference in the first two in the gravid trauma patient. The resuscitation should emphasize maintaining the maternal PO_2 minimally at 80 mm Hg at all times. Confirmation of this requires arterial blood gas monitoring. Liberal use of supplemental oxygen is indicated at any point there is question of the maintenance of this level of PO_2.

The patient is maintained in the left lateral tilt position whenever possible. This limits the reduction in cardiac output from the enlarged uterus compressing the inferior vena cava and impeding venous return to the heart. The resuscitative fluid requirements may be much greater than in the nonpregnant patient, as the pregnant patient is normally hypervolemic with respect to the nonpregnant stage. Vasopressors for the most part will reduce fetal blood flow and increase fetal hypoxia. As with all trauma patients, resumption of normal blood pressure and flow is a function of replenishment of intravascular volume with fluid, correction of any cardiovascular mechanical embarrassments (e.g. tension pneumothorax), and control of any ongoing bleeding. If, after the initiation of these efforts, it is deemed that a cardiotonic drug is needed or a pressor is required for an immediate response, dopamine or ephedrine is the drug of choice. They seem to have the least deleterious effects on uterine blood flow.

Diagnosing Intra-abdominal Hemorrhage

The standard of diagnostic tests for intra-abdominal injury after blunt trauma is the peritoneal lavage. It can be performed at any time during pregnancy. The supraumbilical open approach is probably the safest and should be considered in the latter stages of gestation. In all cases, 1 liter of lactated Ringer's solution should be instilled, and at least 700 ml returned. The criteria for a positive test are identical in the pregnant and nonpregnant state [5]:

1. More than 100,000 red blood cells/μl of blood
2. More than 500 white blood cells/μl of blood
3. Amylase concentration higher than serum
4. Any bile
5. Any bacteria or food particles on Gram stain

In the pregnant patient, the presence of amniotic fluid in the effluent is also considered a positive sign of intra-abdominal injury.

A significant area for concern is the retroperitoneum. Injury to the duodenum or pancreas can escape the lavage detection if the peritoneum has not been violated. Signs of injury include persistent pain in the epigastrium, elevated serum amylase, retroperitoneal air, and persistent vomiting. If the patient is hemodynamically stable, a "noninvasive" workup can be performed. The accepted workup has two parts: that for the pancreas and that for the duodenum. The strategy in the pancreatic evaluation is to use a computed tomography (CT) scan to look for retroperitoneal hemorrhage about the pancreas. If that is found, then an endoscopic retrograde pancreaticoduodenography should be performed to visualize the pancreatic duct. If the major duct shows any leakage, then immediate surgery should be performed. The duodenum is evaluated by an upper gastrointestinal series, carefully visualizing all portions. An intraluminal hematoma can be treated nonoperatively with nasogastric suction. Any perforation demands immediate surgical intervention.

As described previously, CT scanning is being given an increasingly important role in the diagnosis of intra-abdominal injury after blunt trauma [5]. Some feel that a well-performed study including intravenous and gastrointestinal contrast can provide complete evaluation of the peritoneum and retroperitoneum. The data are not yet complete enough to substantiate that claim, in the opinion of this author.

The diagnosis of injury to the abdomen after penetrating trauma has no generally accepted test. The controversy centers on the cardiovascularly stable patient with no obvious signs of intraperitoneal injury [5]. All other patients demand immediate surgery. Most would agree that bullet injuries in the confines of the abdomen should be evaluated by an exploratory laparotomy. They have about an 80-percent incidence of significant intra-abdominal injury. Stab wounds receive the spectrum of opinion on evaluation including observation; local exploration and, if peritoneal penetration is discovered, peritoneal lavage (with a red blood cell count of 25,000–50,000 cells/μl considered grounds for exploration); and mandatory exploratory laparotomy. Stab wounds of the abdomen have an approximately 20-percent incidence of significant injury. On one hand, exploratory laparotomy has a very high accuracy and very low morbidity, even in the pregnant woman. However, the low yield has influenced some to take a less invasive approach, particularly with stab wounds. There is no controlled study that systematically evaluates the approach to the evaluation of these injuries in the gravid patient. The literature is replete with anecdotal reports. A general theme is that the mother, particularly at the latter stage of pregnancy, is well protected from significant injury by the uterus. It is the most common organ to be injured. Fetal viability is often compromised; the mothers typically have a good outcome, even from gunshot wounds. In most of the reported literature, exploratory laparotomy is the diagnostic procedure employed.

Obstetric Evaluation

After initial resuscitation, if the patient is stable, an obstetric examination should be performed. The strategy is to obtain information in four areas: the gestational age, the status of uterine pain, the integrity of the cervix, and the status of the fetus according to heart rate.

Abdominal palpation of the uterus provides information on the gestational age in addition to detecting uterine trauma. The fundus cannot be palpated until the fetus is 12 weeks of age. By 20 weeks' gestation, the fundus is at the level of the umbilicus. Until 32 weeks, fetal age is approximately equal to the distance in centimeters between the top of the symphysis pubis and the top of the fundus. The finding of a localized area of uterine tenderness is suggestive of injury or abruption. The other entities that produce uterine tenderness can typically be differentiated from injury. Labor produces pains that are mostly bilateral, involve the major portion of the organ, and resolve at the termination of the contraction. The other common uterine pain is a benign condition, round ligament stretching. This occurs most often between 16 and 18 weeks of gestation and is localized to the upper lateral portion of the fundus unilaterally or bilaterally.

Whenever the patient is stable enough to assume the lithotomy position, a sterile speculum examination should be performed. The examiner can then determine if there is cervical bleeding and possibly its source, the degree of cervical dilation, and if there is leakage of amniotic fluid. The diagnosis of leakage of amniotic fluid can be suspected if blood is detected at the os. This impression can be confirmed if pH-sensitive nitrazine paper is turned blue by the fluid drained from the posterior vaginal fornix. A bimanual examination is usually avoided to reduce the incidence of infection. Moreover, if the membranes are no longer intact, cultures should be obtained for *Neisseria gonorrhoeae*, group B streptococcus, and *Chlamydia trachomatis*.

By 12 weeks' gestation, a Doppler sonographic device will permit auscultation of the fetal heart tones [3]. By 20 weeks' gestation, fetal heart tones should be heard with a fetoscope. If no heart tones can be detected, a complete ultrasonographic examination should be performed to evaluate the status of heart activity in the fetal chest. The maternal heart tones should be obtained simultaneously to make sure that the supposed fetal tones are not maternal. Normal fetal heart rate is 120 to 160 beats/min. The major concern is fetal bradycardia, which is defined as rates below 100 beats/min. The causes include separation of the placenta and more commonly inadequacy of maternal circulation and/or oxygenation. Immediate augmentation of oxygen availability by mask or tracheal intubation should be performed. Fetal perfusion should be maximized by placing the mother in a Trendelenburg position and avoiding the dorsal supine position. Crystalloid fluid and blood should be given as necessary.

X-ray Considerations

Radiologic studies that clearly help define therapy are indicated and should be performed at any point during the pregnancy. There is a very small risk to the developing fetus, particularly in the earliest stages of gestation. However, the overriding principle is that fetal viability is directly related to maternal physiologic integrity. Any chest, abdominal, and skeletal films that are essential to decision making should not be deleted. Reasonable safeguards should be employed, however. Shielding the uterus from x-rays when this will not obscure the image is indicated. If two studies will provide the same information within the same time frame and with similar manipulation of the patient, obviously the one that requires the least radiation is the study of choice. The refinement of CT scanning techniques has allowed a single examination with relatively low radiation to provide information similar to that of a combination of relatively high-exposure studies [6]. In abdominal evaluation for example, a CT scan taken after infusion of gastrointestinal and intravenous contrast media can, in some cases, provide comparable information to an intravenous pyelogram, an upper gastrointestinal series looking at the duodenum for contusion or perforation, and detailed skeletal views of the lumbar spine and pelvis. If the patient is deemed stable enough to allow a radiographic workup, the decision to use the CT scan has to be based on its availability and the capability of the various physicians to diagnose injury versus more traditional techniques.

Patient Monitoring

So-called noninvasive procedures are often time-consuming, involving patient transport as well as execution of the studies. The greatest importance must be placed on monitoring the patient at all times during workup and therapy. Frequent direct observations of the patient for cardiovascular, respiratory, neurologic, and bleeding status; uterine contraction state; and fetal heart tones are mandatory. In addition, invasive and noninvasive monitoring provides continuous indices of important functions. The ability to use alarms and to place the electronic displays in positions that allow continuous surveillance, even during a long radiologic study, is a great advantage in patient monitoring. Current, well-accepted, readily available portable monitors are

1. Multilead ECG.
2. Arterial pressure recorders through invasive intra-arterial catheters and noninvasive, intermittently inflated sphygmomanometers.
3. Intracranial pressure monitors through invasive bolts or catheters.
4. Noninvasive transcutaneous oxygen saturation monitors, which provide reasonably accurate indications of arterial PO_2.
5. Invasive, multifunctional Swan-Ganz catheters, which provide continuous monitoring of mixed venous oxygen saturation. This is an excellent integrative measurement that can be an early indicator of decreases in oxygen delivery.
6. Noninvasive and intrauterine fetal heart rate monitors.

At the very least, maternal ECG should be continuously monitored with frequent physical examinations and manual measurements of the various cardiovascular, respiratory, bleeding, and neurologic functions of the mother and heart rate of the fetus.

SURGICAL INTERVENTION

Overall Considerations

One of the concerns often voiced with respect to the care of the pregnant patient is that exploratory surgery is very dangerous to the fetus. There are ample data that the fetus is reasonably tolerant of the stresses of surgery and anesthesia. Even premature labor is of minimal risk after laparotomy. On the other hand, the fetus is not very tolerant of maternal hypoxia or hypovolemia. Thus, if surgery is indicated by standard trauma criteria, it should be performed without delay.

During laparotomy, the uterus may be packed or retracted out of the field if the blood flow through the uterine vessels is not compromised. If uterine contraction begins, a tocolytic agent like ritodrine may be used. However, stabilization of the maternal vital signs should be accomplished prior to its use.

Cesarean section is only rarely indicated [3]. Direct injury to the uterus is the major indication, particularly if there are signs of fetal compromise. Need for exposure, onset of labor during laparotomy, or the presence of a pelvic fracture is by no means an absolute reason for a surgical delivery. The goal is to allow the pregnancy to reach reasonable maturity and not to "anticipate" problems with a cesarean section.

In general, there is no difference in the antibiotic approach to pregnant versus nonpregnant patients. Various regimens of antibiotics that cover the full spectrum of enteric flora, including colonic anaerobes, are described in the trauma literature. The dosing includes preoperative, intraoperative, and postoperative coverage, with limited postoperative coverage if no significant distal small bowel or colonic spillage is found. If an aminoglycoside is used, peak and trough blood levels should be obtained; pregnancy may increase the dosage required to achieve therapeutic levels. Tetracycline and chloramphenicol should be avoided, as they can produce fetal damage.

Premature Labor

The presence and frequency of uterine contractions are best documented by monitoring the patient with a tocodynamometer. In the absence of this instrument, manual evaluation can be accomplished by placing a hand on the uterine fundus and palpating for episodic increases in uterine tone. Contractions last at least 40 seconds and generally must occur at regular intervals of less than 8 minutes to cause cervical effacement and dilation. The diagnosis of premature labor is made when the gestational age is less than 36 weeks and contractions occur that are sufficiently intense and frequent to produce cervical change. Pathologic causes should be evaluated and, if possible, treated. Hypoxia and hypovolemia are two etiologies of premature labor that must be addressed if the mother is to survive. Uterine injury, intra-abdominal bleeding, and placental abruption are other causes that should be investigated.

If the cervix continues to ripen, in association with contractions that persist despite maternal cardiorespiratory resuscitation and bed rest, then tocolytic therapy should be instituted. If no cervical dilation occurs, nothing need be done. On the other hand, if the cervix is dilated more than 4 cm, no tocolytic drug is likely to be effective. The most popular tocolytic drug is ritodrine. However, its side effects of tachycardia, hypokalemia, widened pulse pressure, and hemodilution may be life-threatening in the cardiovascular-unstable pregnant trauma patient. Strict contraindications to the use of ritodrine in the pregnant patient include maternal heart rate of more than 120 beats/min, hypotension, significant bleeding, and fetal distress [3]. Magnesium sulfate is less effective as a tocolytic agent but is safer from a cardiovascular perspective and can be considered in the injured gravida in premature labor.

Uterine Rupture

Traumatic rupture of the uterus is uncommon because the myometrium is very elastic. The incidence reported in the literature is that 1 percent of pregnant victims of severe automobile trauma will sustain this injury. The point of rupture is frequently at the placental implantation site, where increased vascularity weakens this portion of the uterine wall. The etiology of the injury often is that the abdomen of the gravida is run over by a car tire. It appears from the literature that the use of seat belts reduces maternal injury. However, improved fetal as well as maternal survival occurs when the pregnant victim wears a shoulder harness as well as a lap belt.

Major uterine rupture is often connected with findings associated with intra-abdominal bleeding and shock. If the fetus is separated from the uterus, it can often be palpated as a separate abdominal mass with distinct fetal anatomy identified; the uterus in this situation is a separate mass in the normal location. Vaginal bleeding occurs typically if the laceration involves the lower uterine segment and cervix. Peritoneal lavage is almost always positive and may contain a liter of amniotic fluid. Minor uterine injuries may reveal only localized uterine tenderness.

This injury is always a surgical emergency. There are some reported cases of repairing minor uterine injuries and achieving viable deliveries. However, in the majority of reported cases, the fetus is not viable, and all attention is directed to maternal survival. The uterus should be repaired if at all possible. Hysterectomy is required in the rare patient and only if bleeding cannot be controlled with less ablative techniques.

Uterine Penetration

Penetrating abdominal injuries may involve the uterus and the fetus. In gunshot wounds to the abdomen, the uterus is the most commonly injured organ. It acts as a shield apparently, as less than 20 percent of women injured by gunshots have other associated visceral injuries. There is a frequent reference in the literature to there having been no maternal deaths from gunshot wounds to the uterus since 1912. This should not encourage a cavalier attitude to these injuries, as most still are very serious. However, the perinatal mortality reported ranges from 41 to 71 percent [7].

As with the general trauma literature, there is a spectrum of opinion on how to approach penetrating abdominal injuries in the pregnant woman who is stable. Most agree that bullet wounds should all be explored. The greatest controversy surrounds knife injuries. The recommendations range from mandatory exploration to continued observation in the patient without obvious signs of intra-abdominal injury. A position that seems to be gaining favor is the use of local exploration combined with peritoneal lavage for injuries anterior to the anterior axillary line. The index of positivity on lavage is generally based on a red blood cell count of from 25,000 to 50,000 red cells/μl of returned effluent. In addition, the finding of amniotic fluid is considered grounds for exploration. Flank and back injuries in the region of the abdomen are even more controversial. Local exploration is less useful, but techniques include lavage, contrast enema of the colon, and intravenous pyelogram.

Unfortunately, the direction to follow for the evaluation of intra-abdominal injury in the stable gravid patient with penetrating trauma, but without obvious peritoneal irritation signs, is not clear. It is important to remember that the stresses of anesthesia and surgery, even a negative exploratory laparotomy, are much better tolerated by the mother and fetus than untreated injuries that include significant intraperitoneal bleeding and/or soilage.

If at laparotomy the uterus is found to be injured, it usually can be repaired by debridement and multilayer closure [7]. The only indication for hysterectomy is uncontrollable bleeding or such major devitalization that a repair could not safely be performed. If bleeding cannot be managed by direct control, ligation sequentially of the internal iliac and ovarian arteries can be done. Apparently this can be accomplished without impairing future reproductive capacity. There is no clear recommendation from the literature on what to do when a uterine injury occurs in association with other injuries. It seems that the presence of other injuries, including colonic, do not necessarily change the recommendation that repair rather than resection of the uterus be performed if possible.

Some controversy seems to surround the question of what to do about the fetus if the uterus is injured. In most cases, the fetus is injured if the uterus is involved. If the gestational age is more than 34 weeks, the incidence of mortality caused by complications of prematurity is less than 3 percent. Therefore, delivery by cesarean section is indicated. When the fetus is less than 34 weeks of gestational age, decisions must be individualized. There are reports in the literature of cases wherein the injured fetus underwent surgery and was replaced in the uterus, as well as reports of potentially injured fetuses not being examined and allowed to complete gestation in utero. In these limited reports, there have been some normal, full-term deliveries. Yet, no clear direction to follow emerges from these experiences, and thus each case below 34 weeks' gestation must be individualized. If the fetus is clearly dead by auscultation, but the uterus is not injured requiring hysterotomy, there is no absolute indication to perform a cesarean section. A spontaneous per vaginal abortion can be allowed to occur.

Placental Abruption

After the twentieth week of pregnancy, premature separation of the normally implanted placenta with resultant retroplacental bleeding is defined as abruptio placentae. It occurs in less than 1 percent of all deliveries. However, it is much more common in trauma victims. Shock, inertial forces, and uterine penetration have all been implicated as causes. One study shows a 3.4-percent incidence of abruption in severely injured gravidas [8]. It is much more common than uterine rupture. It occurs most commonly in association with severe pelvic fractures. It is the most common cause of fetal death after maternal death.

The findings with abruptio placentae are vaginal bleeding, uterine tenderness, increased uterine tone or hypercontractility, increased uterine size, and signs of fetal distress. In milder cases, the only finding may be vaginal bleeding as blood insinuates its way between the membranes and the uterus and escapes through the cervix. Sterile speculum examination is the best way to make the diagnosis. Ultrasound is very good at localizing the placenta, but the relatively small size of most clots makes this technique not very useful in diagnosing abruption. In some patients, the bleeding is concealed, and no vaginal bleeding is noted. In this situation, often there are uterine tetany and tenderness, fetal distress, and possibly maternal shock.

The severity of illness is a function of the sequelae of fetal materials entering the maternal bloodstream. The problems stem from two areas: (1) the triggering of intravascular coagulation by thromboplastin from the decidua and placenta entering the maternal circulation and (2) the entry of amniotic fluid into the maternal circulation through subplacental sinusoids. The latter, which is described as amniotic fluid embolus, occurs less frequently than the former. It can also be caused by an interruption of the amniotic membrane. The particulate matter is filtered out in the distal pulmonary circulation, producing mechanical obstruction. There is a decrease in cardiac output and a reflex bronchospasm; severe hypoxia often results. The overall syndrome is characterized by a rapid onset and includes dyspnea, cyanosis, cardiovascular collapse, hemorrhage, coma, and seizures. The bleeding diathesis results from a consumptive and fibrinolytic coagulopathy. Rarely is there time for a confirmation of the diagnosis by blood tests. However, the finding of amniotic debris floating over the buffy coat of white cells is confirmatory. Treatment is supportive, directed toward cardiopulmonary stabilization with fluids and inotropic agents, intubation, ventilation, and blood and clotting factor replacement. The mortality for amniotic fluid embolus is about 75 percent; 50 percent die at the time of the embolus, and the additional 25 percent die subsequently.

The more common complication from abruptio placentae is the coagulopathy from the release of thromboplastin. Most of the blood loss is maternal. However, there can be a loss of fetal blood into the maternal circulation as well. A Kleihauer-Betke stain of maternal blood can be used to reveal fetomaternal hemorrhage. The important point about this is that $Rh_0(D)$ immunoglobin may be required by the mother, if she is Rh-negative, to prevent maternal Rh sensitization.

Minor degrees of abruptio placentae require only careful monitoring of fetal and maternal vital signs, blood loss, and uterine and labor status. A fetal heart rate monitor and a tocodynamometer are very useful to this end. Obviously, cardiopulmonary integrity must be maintained with fluids, including blood, and support of oxygenation and ventilation.

The component of this problem that is unique to this injury is the possibility of disseminated intravascular coagulopathy (DIC). This entity occurs in about 30 percent of abruptions where fetal death occurs but is rare when the fetus survives. If unusual clinical bleeding occurs, the diagnosis must be entertained. The confirmation can be made grossly when a sample of blood drawn from a peripheral site shows no clotting after more than 5 minutes. The differential always includes consumptive coagulopathy from untreated bleeding. The combination of a markedly increased prothrombin time and partial thromboplastin time; increased fibrin split products; fibrinogen level below 40 mg/dl; platelet count below 50,000/hpf power field confirms the diagnosis. The treatment includes the maintenance of adequate hematocrit, platelets, and clotting factors. Most of the last can be provided by fresh frozen plasma. However, cryoprecipitate must be used to correct significant hypofibrinogemia.

The definitive therapy for DIC associated with abruptio placentae is delivery [3]. There is little controversy that in the third-trimester fetus in distress, immediate delivery is indicated if the maternal status permits. The other cases must be individualized.

REFERENCES

1. Chatterjee, M. S. Physiology of Pregnancy. In C. E. Haycock (ed.), *Trauma and Pregnancy.* PSG, Littleton, Massachusetts 1985. Pp. 1–7.
2. Baker, D. P. Trauma in the pregnant patient. *Surg. Clin. North Am.* 62:275, 1982.
3. Alger, L. S., and Crenshaw, M. C., Jr. Management of the Obstetric Patient After Trauma. In J. G. Siegel (ed.), *Trauma Emergency Surgery and Critical Care.* London: Churchill Livingstone, 1987. Pp. 1075–1098.
4. Aderet, N. B., Cohen, I., and Abramowicz, J. S. Traumatic coma during pregnancy with persistent vegetative state: Case report. *Br. J. Obstet. Gynaecol.* 91:939, 1984.
5. Flint, L. M., and Malangoni, M. A. Abdominal Injuries. In J. D. Richardson, H. C. Polk, and L. M. Flint (eds.), *Trauma: Clinical Care and Pathophysiology.* Chicago: Year Book, Publishers, 1987. Pp. 353–395.
6. Eliot, G., and Rao, D. Pregnancy and Radiographic Examination. In C. E. Haycock (ed.), *Trauma and Pregnancy.* Littleton, Ma.: PSG, 1985. Pp. 69–79.
7. Buchsbaum, H. J., and Staples, P. P., Jr. Self-inflicted gunshot wound to the pregnant uterus: Report of two cases. *Obstet. Gynecol.* 65:32, 1985.
8. Crosbym, W. M., and Costiloe, J. P. Safety of lap-belt restraint for pregnant victims of automobile collisions. *N. Engl. J. Med.* 284:632, 1971.

18

ICU Management of the Trauma Patient

Scott H. Norwood and
Joseph M. Civetta

Trauma has been described as the last great plague of modern society [1]. Intensive care units (ICUs), which began in the 1960s, now provide laboratory and monitoring capabilities for the physiologic evaluation of life-threatening problems in these trauma patients. Systematic, coordinated, and coherent therapeutic plans, if utilized properly, are invaluable in addressing life-threatening factors by priority to improve outcome similar to the approach used in emergency assessment and resuscitations. Although there is a perception that many surgeons are abandoning their patients to nonsurgical specialists in the postoperative period [2], we believe that the roles of the surgical intensivist and the ICU team are to provide critical care postoperatively and provide early recognition of life-threatening complications. While it is the surgeon who best knows when a patient is too ill to have an operation and when a patient is too ill not to have an operation [3], lifesaving decisions and therapy must be rapidly employed in the ICU, and postoperative management can be significantly improved by a well-trained individual who can act appropriately in the absence of the trauma surgeon. Communication between the traumatologist and the intensivist is extremely important, and clear lines of authority and responsibility should be developed and enforced [3].

PHILOSOPHY OF CARE

A fundamental early goal of critical care is to maintain adequate oxygen delivery to vital tissues. Therapeutic interventions often precede or occur simultaneously with diagnostic testing to achieve this end. Next, potential complications of surgically repaired injuries must

All opinions stated are those of the authors and not necessarily those of the United States Air Force.

be known and evaluated in the postoperative period. Further, the physiologic effects of trauma on each organ system must be understood, adverse phylogenetic mechanisms appropriately controlled, and anticipatory monitoring/evaluation and treatment initiated. Sepsis is the leading cause of death in surgical patients [4], and an evaluation for sepsis should be developed.

The second major goal of postoperative critical care is to provide secondary triage. Specific admission and discharge criteria along with criteria for withdrawing support must be developed to prevent overutilization of critical care resources in patients with little hope for survival. Such practice may deny lifesaving care to patients who have a much better prognosis.

Given the general goals for the evaluation and treatment of the trauma patient who needs intensive care, an approach to the common problems can be formulated.

EVALUATING SUDDEN HYPOTENSION IN THE ICU TRAUMA PATIENT

Crucial steps in the initial management of a catastrophic and immediately life-threatening complication consist of immediate resuscitative efforts, rapid evaluation, especially exclusion of "mechanical" etiologies, and immediate notification of the surgical team. Table 18-1 lists the most common causes of sudden hypotension in the postoperative trauma patient. Any evidence of inadequate tissue oxygenation, such as low venous oxygen saturation ($\bar{V}sat$) and venous oxygen tension ($P\bar{v}O_2$), acidemia, arterial hypotension suggests that oxygen delivery is inadequate and death may be imminent unless corrective measures are taken.

Table 18-1. Common Causes of Sudden Hypotension in Critically Ill Trauma Patients

Loss of airway
Tension pneumothorax
Cardiac tamponade
Hemothorax
Intra-abdominal hemorrhage
Acute myocardial infarction
Septicemia
Reaction to medication

Hypotension associated with bradycardia indicates severe hypoxemia and, if an acute event, is usually due to a mechanical complication such as loss of airway, tension pneumothorax, or cardiac tamponade. A rapid evaluation to search for these possibilities must be done.

Loss of a patent airway can lead quickly to cardiac arrest secondary to hypoxemia, especially in patients being treated for acute respiratory failure. Direct laryngoscopy should be done if there is any suspicion or evidence that the airway has become displaced. Decreased breath sounds, tracheal deviation, a sharp rise in peak inspiratory pressure during mechanical ventilation, increased $PaCO_2$, and hypoxemia are all signs of tension pneumothorax. A chest roentgenogram should be obtained if time permits. However, if systolic pressure falls below 90 mm Hg or the patient develops severe bradycardia, aspiration of the chest with a small-gauge needle should be performed, and if air is withdrawn, surgical decompression should be performed immediately. If high positive end-expiratory pressure (PEEP) levels are needed to maintain oxygenation, removal from the ventilator may only worsen the clinical situation. A previously placed chest tube *does not* eliminate the possibility of ipsilateral tension pneumothorax. The tube may be plugged, the lung may be adherent to the tube, or in the case of adhesions, a loculated pneumothorax may still develop. The clinical diagnosis is often difficult to make in the ICU.

Hemothorax may occur after the initial evaluation, or the rate of intrathoracic bleeding may be so slow that a significant deficit in blood volume first occurs in the ICU. This may be diagnosed and treated in a manner similar for pneumothorax.

Muffled heart sounds, jugular venous distention, and equalization of left and right atrial chamber pressures implicate cardiac tamponade as the etiology for hypotension. These signs may also follow tension pneumothorax, and if bilateral chest decompression does not result in clinical improvement, pericardiocentesis or pericardiotomy should be performed.

While the diagnostic possibilities are being considered, it is generally good practice to begin volume resuscitation unless hypovolemia can definitely be eliminated. Rapid crystalloid infusion and Trendelenburg positioning will improve cerebral perfusion and usually increase blood pressure while the rapid evaluation is being performed. A dopamine infusion should be available if the patient does not respond to vigorous volume replacement. A bolus of 0.2 to 1.0 mg of epinephrine may be required to maintain perfusion to vital organs. The patient should temporarily be placed on 100% oxygen until the situation is corrected.

Once extra-abdominal sources have been ruled out, intra-abdominal bleeding should be considered in patients who have suffered blunt trauma or previous abdominal exploration. The abdomen should be rapidly assessed for any obvious signs such as abdominal distention or increased bloody discharge through an incision or abdominal drain. Other catastrophic abdominal problems include ischemic bowel from embolization or volvulus, missed or later perforation of the alimentary tract, hemorrhagic pancreatitis, and streptococcal or clostridial wound infections. All of these complications require immediate surgical intervention for survival.

Hypotension secondary to the administration of medications may represent unmasking of previously compensated hypovolemia or the first presentation of progressive hypovolemia due to ongoing fluid losses, bleeding, or the development of sepsis.

SUPPORTIVE MEASURES PRIOR TO ABDOMINAL REEXPLORATION

Volume resuscitation is the most important therapy prior to abdominal reexploration. Crystalloid solution should be rapidly administered in lieu of type-specific blood until stabilization occurs. Four to six units of blood should also be made available for surgery. Fluid resuscitation is continued until mean arterial pressure is stabilized above 80 mm Hg. Rapid access to the venous system may be crucial. It is often quicker and easier to provide access centrally through the subclavian, internal jugular, or femoral veins in the ICU patient who has peripheral edema or previously used peripheral sites. Large venous access catheters, such as the 8.5 Fr introducers used for inserting pulmonary artery (PA) catheters, work very well for rapid access and volume resuscitation. The side port can be removed, with the IV tubing placed directly into the end of the introducer to provide a faster flow rate. In cases of extreme emergency, one should not hesitate to utilize previously placed hyperalimentation catheters for resuscitation. A new catheter for hyperalimentation can be inserted later.

PA catheters are not usually needed for treatment of hypovolemia from intra-abdominal bleeding in young, previously healthy patients. Many critically ill patients may already have a PA catheter in place, which will aid in directing volume resuscitation, evaluation of pulmonary and cardiac function, and oxygen delivery to the tissues. Elderly patients, especially those with cardiac dysfunction, may be more easily managed both preoperatively and intraoperatively if time permits placement of a PA catheter. However, definitive correction of the abdominal problem in the operating room should not be delayed.

The pneumatic antishock garment (PASG) may be useful as a temporary measure to increase blood pressure in patients with obvious intra-abdominal or retroperitoneal hemorrhage. The PASG may slow the rate of pelvic or abdominal bleeding and allow for more rapid stabilization of vital signs prior to reexploration. ICU personnel should be familiar with the proper positioning and inflation of the PASG prior to use, since improper application may be inefficient or cause serious complications.

Other Intra-abdominal Emergencies

The majority of complications involving perforation, obstruction, or ischemia of abdominal organs present with severe abdominal pain. Many ICU patients are not capable of communicating their discomfort, and restlessness, hypertension, and tachycardia may be the only manifestations unless physical examination reveals increased abdominal distention. Gastric or colonic perforation will lead to peritonitis and hypovolemic or septic shock. Resuscitative efforts are similar to those described for intra-abdominal bleeding with the addition of broad-spectrum antibiotics preoperatively. Since the actual site of perforation cannot usually be determined preoperatively, a combination of antibiotics that will cover hospital-acquired aerobes and anaerobes as well as normal gut flora is indicated. A plain film of the abdomen and a semi-upright chest roentgenogram may identify dilated loops of large or small bowel or free intraperitoneal air under the diaphragm. Early surgical intervention is crucial to survival regardless of the specific diagnosis in most patients.

Intra-abdominal Sepsis

Sepsis remains the most common cause of death in critically ill surgical patients [4,5]. The onset is usually progressive and indolent, often with extra-abdominal signs such as persistent respiratory failure and hyperglycemia. Hypotension, especially associated with gram-negative bacteremia, can also develop. The evaluation of intra-abdominal sepsis in the postoperative period is discussed in detail later in the chapter.

Trauma patients with massively contaminated wounds may develop profound septic shock within 24 to 36 hours of injury due to clostridial or streptococcal abdominal wound infections. This may occasionally occur following colon or biliary tract injuries. Early diagnosis and radical debridement are crucial to survival.

Table 18-2. Risk Factors for Development of ARDS in Trauma Patients

Sepsis
Aspiration
Pulmonary contusion
Fat embolism
Acute pancreatitis
Multiple blood transfusions

MANAGING PATHOPHYSIOLOGIC EFFECTS OF TRAUMA

Respiratory System

Acute respiratory failure following trauma was reported as early as World War I [6]. The spectrum of pathophysiologic abnormalities can range from mild pulmonary edema from fluid overload to severe noncardiogenic pulmonary edema and profound hypoxemia. The latter abnormality, often called the adult respiratory distress syndrome (ARDS), generally results from multiple etiologies due to direct or indirect damage to the alveolar capillary interface [7]. The mortality rate from ARDS is still reported to be approximately 50 to 60 percent [8,9]. The exact incidence in trauma patients is not known, although it has been estimated that approximately 150,000 people a year in the United States are afflicted with ARDS [10].

Long lists of causes and associated syndromes have been previously reported as possible etiologies for ARDS [11,12]. Potential risk factors specific to the trauma patient are listed in Table 18-2. Many associated etiologies, such as disseminated intravascular coagulopathy (DIC), multiple blood transfusions, and various forms of nonseptic shock, may represent a constellation of related phenomena that result from the severity of illness rather than true etiologic risk factors.

Several studies identify sepsis as one of the most common factors leading to ARDS [6,13–15]. This risk factor also appears to be the most serious because the pulmonary abnormalities usually cannot be corrected unless the underlying source for sepsis can be identified and eliminated. One study [16] prospectively evaluated 136 patients who were placed on mechanical ventilation and had at least one of eight preselected conditions historically considered to be risk factors for development of ARDS. These risk factors were sepsis, aspiration, pulmonary contusion, multiple emergency blood transfusions, multiple major fractures, near drowning, pancreatitis, and prolonged hypotension. ARDS developed in 25 percent of patients with only one condition, 42 percent with two conditions, and 85 percent with three conditions. Thirty-eight percent of patients with the single condition of sepsis, 30 percent with aspiration, and 17 percent with pulmonary contusion as their only risk factor developed ARDS. The number of emergency blood transfusions received in a 12-hour period also correlated with increased risk. Twenty-four percent of patients who had no other predisposing factors and who received at least 22 units of blood in 12 hours or less developed ARDS in this study [16].

In summary, trauma patients who develop systemic sepsis or who have direct pulmonary injury from aspiration or pulmonary contusion are generally believed to be at increased risk for developing pulmonary complications that may lead to ARDS. In addition, patients with severe pancreatitis and those patients who have required multiple rapid emergency blood transfusions may also be at increased risk.

Pathophysiology

Under normal conditions, many forces are related to and responsible for a constant egress of water from the pulmonary capillaries to the interstitium [17,18]. The hydrostatic pressure gradient to the pulmonary interstitium is partially balanced by the oncotic pressure gradient between capillary and interstitial fluid. The positive capillary hydrostatic pressure tends to drive water out of the capillary and into the interstitium, which has a slight negative pressure under normal conditions. Since the hydrostatic gradient exceeds the oncotic gradient, the net effect is a slight flux of water from the capillaries to the interstitial space. Normally, lymphatic flow removes this filtered fluid from the pulmonary interstitium.

Three physiologic safety features tend to prevent pulmonary edema under normal conditions [19]: (1) interstitial protein washout, which lowers interstitial oncotic pressure and increases the oncotic pressure gradient; (2) the elevation of interstitial pressure toward atmospheric pressure, which occurs without a significant increase in interstitial volume; this decreases the capillary interstitial pressure gradient; and (3) increased lymphatic flow from the interstitial space to evacuate the increased volume of fluid. These safety factors can prevent pulmonary edema until the pulmonary microvascular pressure exceeds about 20 mm Hg [20]. In most patients with respiratory failure associated with trauma, increased lung water develops because of disruption of the alveolar capillary membrane, which increases capillary permeability. Interstitial edema can form even with a normal hydrostatic pressure gradient.

Neutrophils as mediators of tissue injury provide the most plausible concept for the cause of the alveolar-capillary damage and increased capillary permeability in ARDS [21]. Superoxide radicals, hydroxyl ions, lysosomal enzymes, and hydrogen peroxide are all released from activated neutrophils, which are sequestered in pulmonary capillaries and are probably involved in mediating the cellular pulmonary injury [22]. Various other metabolites and cellular particles have also been implicated and are listed in Table 18-3.

Treatment

Positive end-expiratory pressure (PEEP) is still considered the most effective therapy for ARDS. PEEP improves functional residual capacity and usually reverses the hypoxemia associated with acute respiratory failure so that nontoxic levels of inspired oxygen may be used to provide adequate arterial oxygenation. The goals of ventilatory support should be adequate oxygenation [23,24], a safe fraction of inspired oxygen (FIO_2), adequate oxy-

Table 18-3. Metabolites, Cells, and Cellular Particles Implicated in the Development of ARDS

Neutrophil products	
	Proteases
	Elastases
	Lysozyme
Oxygen products	
	Hydrogen peroxide
	Hydroxyl ions
	Superoxide radicals
Arachidonic acid metabolites	
	Prostacyclin
	Thromboxane A_2
	Leukotrienes
Other humoral factors	
	Histamine
	Serotonin
	Kinins
	Bacterial endotoxins
	Complement products
	Fibrin degradation products (fragment D)
	Fatty acids
	Factor VII
	Factor XIII
	Platelets

gen delivery, and judicious use of ancillary testing only as needed [25].

Empiric treatment of advanced ARDS (because there is no specific therapy to correct the pathophysiology) usually will result in an unsuccessful outcome. A more appealing approach is close early monitoring and simple interventions to restore pulmonary function to near normal levels as soon as signs of acute respiratory failure develop in patients with one or more risk factors for ARDS. An appropriate regimen may include sequential blood gas measurements, airway control, low levels (5 cm H_2O) of PEEP to maintain oxygenation, and sufficient mechanical ventilation to ensure elimination of carbon dioxide. Quantitation of PaO_2 is very important after each major therapeutic intervention because both mechanical ventilation and PEEP may compromise myocardial function, which could then reduce oxygen delivery [25].

In the setting of acute respiratory failure following trauma, increased airway pressure is the preferred treatment, since it directly counteracts the pulmonary changes causing hypoxemia (a reduced functional residual capacity and expiratory reserve volume). This may be measured at the end of expiration (PEEP) or maintained during the entire spontaneous breathing cycle (continuous positive airway pressure [CPAP]). Mechanical ventilation alone has little applicability in treating this problem because it affects only inspiratory lung volumes. Since most trauma patients with acute respiratory failure demonstrate hypocapnea, reflecting an increased minute ventilation, therapy designed solely to increase ventilation, such as controlled mechanical ventilation (CMV) or assist control ventilation (AMV), is almost never needed or efficacious. Furthermore, there are specific detrimental effects that may be caused by these therapeutic modalities [26].

In treating acute respiratory failure, the first priority must always be reversal of life-threatening hypoxemia. We generally begin PEEP or CPAP therapy if PaO_2 falls to 55 mm Hg or less ($FIO_2 = 0.21$) and the patient experiences the clinical signs of tachypnea or labored breathing. If the disease process is not discovered until late in its course, then high inspired oxygen concentrations may be necessary as a temporary measure to maintain PaO_2 greater than 70 mm Hg. As soon as possible, however, FIO_2 should be reduced to less than 50 percent. If acute respiratory failure is recognized early, most patients can maintain a PaO_2 of at least 70 mm Hg with an FIO_2 equal to 0.45, although higher levels of PEEP may be required to achieve this goal.

Generally, PEEP should be increased in increments of 2 to 3 cm H_2O until a PaO_2/FIO_2 of approximately 250 to 300 : 1 is reached. This ratio corresponds to an intrapulmonary shunt fraction of approximately 15 to 25 percent if the arteriovenous oxygen content difference ($Ca - C\bar{v}$) is normal [27]. A PA catheter should be used if compromise of cardiac function is suspected, or if PaO_2/FIO_2 has not been corrected after the application of PEEP at 15 cm H_2O. Younger patients without cardiac disease can often be treated safely with even higher PEEP levels, since the PA catheter does not add a significant amount of important information regarding therapy. However, when significant doubt remains, measurement of cardiovascular parameters and calculations of $\dot{Q}S/\dot{Q}T$ are necessary.

We prefer intermittent mandatory ventilation (IMV) to CMV or AMV in conjunction with PEEP because most trauma patients can ventilate spontaneously and the detrimental effects of controlled mechanical ventilation can be avoided. IMV is increased in increments of 1 to 2 breath/min to maintain pH at 7.35 to 7.45 and $PaCO_2$ at 35 to 45 mm Hg (in previously eucapneic patients). The ventilator is usually set to deliver a tidal volume of 12 to 15 ml/kg of body weight. Most trauma patients will receive adequate ventilatory assistance with only 2 to 4 breaths/min. In general, work of breathing is not significantly increased once optimal levels of PEEP are reached because compliance is usually improved [26]. However, it is important to ensure that proper ventilatory IMV circuits are being utilized. Blood gases should be measured and IMV rates should be evaluated if the spontaneous rate is greater than 30 breaths/min, labored breathing is noted, or the patient becomes anxious or subjectively uncomfortable.

An assessment of the patient's total clinical condition in terms of diagnoses and complications since the initiation of ventilatory support is the most important step in selecting an appropriate point to attempt weaning. If the underlying cause for acute respiratory failure, such as sepsis or pulmonary contusion, has not significantly resolved, weaning is certain to fail. We have found that if the pulmonary disease process is mild, of rapid onset, and has been swiftly treated, it may be necessary only to maintain PEEP at the highest level for 6 to 12 hours before attempting to wean the patient. If the underlying disease process has been difficult to control, however, or if support was begun late in the course of the disease, it is often necessary to continue treatment for at least 24 hours before attempting to wean.

Priorities for weaning are based on consideration of the detrimental effects of therapy. The first priority should be to decrease the FIO_2 to less than 0.5. Higher levels of oxygen may cause lung units with low $\dot{V}/\dot{Q}$ to collapse when oxygen is absorbed from the alveoli at a rate exceeding its replacement [28]. An even more important consideration concerns the relationship between oxygen toxicity and high inspired oxygen tensions. No cases of oxygen toxicity have been reported in humans after prolonged administration of oxygen in less than 50-percent concentrations. Some authors have suggested that FIO_2 values of 0.4 or lower should be attained [26,29]. However, it is probably safe to assume that no significant difference in outcome will be related to these differing end points of FIO_2 below 0.5 in critically ill patients.

The second priority is reduction of the percentage of minute ventilation provided by the ventilator by lowering the number of IMV breaths to a level that permits a normal pH (7.35–7.45) and a normal $PaCO_2$ (35–45 mm Hg) at a satisfactory spontaneous respiratory rate (< 30 breaths/min). This process should be continued until the rate has been reduced to 2 mechanical breaths/min. We usually maintain patients at 2 breaths/min until just before extubation, although lower levels are certainly acceptable.

Finally, PEEP is lowered in increments of 2 to 3 cm H_2O as long as oxygenation remains satisfactory, that is, there is no major diminution in PaO_2. PEEP should not be decreased at a rate greater than 10 cm H_2O during a 24-hour period. This empiric plateau avoids the setbacks of sudden hypoxemia, which is then often followed by a period of augmented therapy. Weaning from PEEP therapy should be continued until the pressure has been lowered to 5 cm H_2O.

Therefore, minimal ventilatory support is defined as an IMV rate of 2 breaths/min, a PEEP level of 5 cm H_2O, and an FIO_2 value of less than 0.5. Patients who tolerate minimal ventilatory support are considered for extubation if protection of the upper airway is no longer necessary and the disease process has resolved. IMV is decreased to 0 breath/min while maintaining CPAP of 5 cm H_2O. If extubation criteria are met—pH 7.35 or more, $PaCO_2$ 45 mm Hg or less, spontaneous ventilatory rate 30 breaths/min or less, and PaO_2 55 mm Hg or more while breathing room air—the patient can be extubated. Our choice of these values as extubation criteria is based on our clinical experiences. Blood gas values taken when the patient inspires room air at a CPAP of 5 cm H_2O are the closest approximation of those gases obtained after the patient has been extubated. Since the purpose of weaning is to determine whether the patient will be capable of maintaining adequate unassisted ventilation (and oxygenation), we have found that the CPAP of 5 cm H_2O while breathing room air is our best predictor of a successful extubation [30,31].

Measurement of negative inspiratory force and vital capacity is usually not necessary if the previously described approach to weaning and blood gas criteria has been used. Such mechanical criteria may be useful in the weaning of patients who have received ventilatory support for longer periods (>4 weeks) or in patients with neuromuscular disorders.

Cardiovascular Support

Supporting the cardiac function of patients following trauma often requires manipulation of physiologic determinants of cardiac output to ensure adequate oxygen delivery. This is especially important if the patient also has coexistent acute respiratory failure. Since the pulmonary and cardiovascular systems are integrally related in determining oxygen delivery, both must be very carefully monitored, especially if mechanical ventilation and PEEP are required to maintain arterial oxygenation [32].

Cardiovascular Physiology

The Fick equation describes the relationship among cardiac output, oxygen consumption, and arterial (Ca) and mixed venous oxygen content ($C_{\bar{v}}$) as follows [33]:

$$\text{Cardiac output} = \frac{\text{oxygen consumption}}{(C_a - C_{\bar{v}})O_2}$$

For the short period required to measure cardiac output and obtain arterial and mixed venous blood samples, oxygen consumption remains relatively constant. An increased arteriovenous content difference [$(C_a - C_{\bar{v}})O_2$] usually results in a decrease in $C_{\bar{v}}$, oxygen tension ($P_{\bar{v}}O_2$), and venous saturation ($\bar{V}_{sat}$) because arterial content does not spontaneously increase. If oxygen consumption remains constant, an increase in $(C_a - C_{\bar{v}})O_2$, or more specifically a decreased $P_{\bar{v}}O_2$ and $\bar{V}_{sat}$, suggests that cardiac output is inadequate for the existing level of oxygen consumption [32]. A decrease in $P_{\bar{v}}O_2$ and $\bar{V}_{sat}$ often occurs before other clinical signs of cardiovascular dysfunction, such as decreasing urine output and metabolic acidosis, develop, and monitoring of $\bar{V}_{sat}$ may be useful as an "early warning system" [34].

Cardiac output is the product of stroke volume and heart rate. There are three major factors that influence stroke volume: preload, afterload, and contractility. The interaction of these factors and their effects on "muscle work" were first described in 1898 [35] and later emphasized in 1914 [36].

Preload defines the relationship between end-diastolic fiber length and work performed by the contracting cardiac muscle [37]. Clinically, ventricular muscle fiber length is considered proportional to end-diastolic volume, which in turn is proportional to end-diastolic pressure. Measurement of wedge pressure (otherwise called pulmonary artery occlusion pressure [PAOP]) provides a reasonable approximation of left ventricular end-diastolic and left atrial pressures. Likewise, right ventricular preload can be assessed by right atrial or central venous pressure measurements, which approximate right ventricular end-diastolic pressures. Although clinically very useful, these measurements do not always reflect volume status accurately, especially in elderly patients whose ventricular compliance may be poor.

Afterload is defined as the "load" the cardiac muscle must move when it contracts [37] or, more specifically, the ventricular wall tension that is required to eject a given stroke volume [38]. Systemic vascular resistance (SVR) and left ventricular radius are the two primary factors influencing afterload [38].

The formula for calculating SVR is as follows:

$$\text{SVR} = \frac{\text{MAP} - \text{CVP}}{\text{C.O.}} \times 79.9$$

where MAP = mean arterial pressure
CVP = central venous pressure
C.O. = cardiac output
Normal SVR = 900–1200 dynes cm^{-5}

Ventricular radius and ventricular wall tension are also related:

$$\text{Wall tension} = \frac{\text{distending pressure} \times \text{radius}}{\text{wall thickness}}$$

As ventricular radius increases, wall tension increases exponentially to produce the same amount of work at a constant pressure (preload) and wall thickness [38]. Increasing afterload when preload and contractility remain constant results in decreased muscle shortening with contraction, that is, a less efficient ventricle [39]. Increasing afterload prolongs the presystolic ejection time. Increasing this period of isovolemic contraction markedly increases myocardial oxygen consumption, which can be detrimental to trauma patients with coronary artery disease and limited myocardial blood flow.

The rate of generation of cross linkings between actin and myosin determines the state of myocardial contractility [40]. The state of contractility controls stroke volume when preload and afterload are constant. This process is intimately related to the quantity of available ionized calcium and the level of norepinephrine, the intrinsic cardiac adrenergic transmitter [38]. There are no readily available studies that are helpful in the ICU trauma patient to allow for quantitation of contractility. Therapeutically induced augmentation of contractility is thus usually empiric, and improved cardiac output and oxygen delivery at a constant preload and afterload are used to gauge the appropriate end point [32].

If stroke volume remains constant, cardiac output increases linearly up to a heart rate of approximately 150 beats/min. Rate is determined primarily by a balance between the parasympathetic nervous system's cholinergic receptors in the sinoatrial node (for a decreased rate) and the sympathetic nervous system's release of catecholamines peripherally and within the myocardium, causing stimulation of beta-adrenergic receptors (for an increased rate) [41,42]. Cardiac output in younger individuals with normal cardiac function generally is rate-dependent. The benefits of improving cardiac output by increasing heart rate must be weighed against the detrimental increases in myocardial oxygen consumption, especially in patients with coronary artery disease [38,41].

Therapeutic Approach to Cardiovascular Support

The usual first step to improving cardiac output in trauma patients is augmentation of preload. Volume expansion has little detrimental effect on myocardial oxygen consumption [41]. However, the principal reason for using preload augmentation as the first intervention is that many trauma patients are relatively hypovolemic, especially if there is any element of sepsis, and the detrimental effects of ventilatory support can almost always be overcome by volume infusion [42].

The type of fluid (crystalloid or colloid) remains controversial. Clinically, there is no advantage in using colloids over crystalloids [43–46]. Today, in the intense scrutiny related to cost containment, if there are clearly no significant differences between therapies, one should choose the least expensive solution [21].

Afterload reduction may be necessary to improve oxygen delivery if cardiac output is diminished as a result of elevated SVR. Preload must always be optimized before using afterload reducing agents such as sodium nitroprusside. Hypertension can occur with hypovolemic states, especially in younger patients, when high catecholamine levels cause intense peripheral vasoconstriction. If afterload reducing agents are given in the presence of hypovolemia, severe hypotension can develop. Sodium nitroprusside should be administered slowly through a central venous catheter, beginning at a rate of 0.1 to 0.3 μg/kg/min and increased until mean arterial pressure is reduced to near normal levels. The effects on oxygen delivery should be confirmed by direct measurements.

If preload and afterload are optimized and oxygen delivery remains inadequate, agents affecting contractility, such as dopamine or dobutamine, should be considered to increase cardiac output. The inotropic dose for both drugs is in the range of 5 to 15 μg/kg/min. These agents significantly increase myocardial oxygen consumption and must be used judiciously, especially in patients with a previous history of coronary artery disease [38]. Increased systemic blood pressure does not necessarily reflect improvement in oxygen delivery and myocardial efficiency. These measures must be evaluated more directly through measurement of $\bar{V}_{sat}$ and cardiac output.

Dopamine is generally our drug of choice to augment contractility. Its wide range of clinically useful effects at various dosage levels makes it valuable in a number of clinical settings in trauma patients [41]. Dobutamine is reported to be more specific in cardiac beta-receptor stimulation (less chronotrophy) [47,48], but we have found the chronotropic effects to be variable. Significant tachycardia can be induced by either drug in certain individuals.

An increased heart rate not only increases myocardial oxygen consumption but may also decrease presystolic ejection time to the point that stroke volume may be reduced. Therefore, heart rate should be maintained at 100 to 120 beats/min to reduce these detrimental side effects. Intermittent doses of intravenous propranolol (1–2 mg) are very useful in counteracting the adverse effects of tachycardia and generally do not significantly reduce cardiac output or mean arterial pressure if preload is optimized.

Renal Support

The most common cause of acute renal failure following trauma is acute tubular necrosis from diminished renal blood flow, which develops from systemic hypotension, sepsis, or a combination of both. Factors predisposing to acute renal failure are listed in Table 18-4. Oliguric renal failure is one of the most serious complications affecting ICU trauma patients. Although acute renal failure as an isolated abnormality in nonsurgical patients is associated with only an 8-percent mortality [49], acute renal failure in combination with other organ system dysfunction increases mortality up to 60 to 100 percent [49–52].

Acute renal failure is defined as an abrupt decline in renal function sufficient to cause retention of nitrogenous waste [53]. Oliguric

Table 18-4. Factors Predisposing to Acute Renal Failure in Trauma Patients

Renal hypoperfusion (hypovolemia, sepsis)
Nephrotoxic drugs and anesthetics
Iodinated contrast dyes
Aminoglycosides
Amphotericin B
Aspirin
Nonsteroidal anti-inflammatory agents
Hemoglobinuria
Myoglobinuria
Preexisting renal or cardiac disease

renal failure is defined as less than 400 ml of urine produced in 24 hours [53]. It appears that with advances in ICU support, hemodynamic monitoring, and increased use of nephrotoxic drugs, nonoliguric renal failure is becoming more common [54]. It also seems that nonoliguric forms of acute renal failure are associated with less morbidity and mortality, and diuretic therapy may successfully convert oliguric renal failure to the nonoliguric form [54].

Acute renal failure is most commonly recognized following a period of critical underperfusion of the kidney (mean arterial pressure < 80 mm Hg), which consequently causes vasoconstriction of the renal afferent arterioles by norepinephrine and angiotensin [55,56], resulting in tubular cellular hypoxia. If not corrected, renal dysfunction persists secondary to intraluminal tubular obstruction by cellular debris, proteins, and cellular edema [57]. Persistent vasoconstriction by overactivity of the renin-angiotensin system may also be an important factor in sustaining acute renal failure [56]. Resulting metabolic abnormalities include metabolic acidosis, hyperkalemia, hyponatremia, hypermagnesemia, hyperphosphatemia, and hypocalcemia [53].

Oliguria in the postoperative period should create a sense of urgency to diagnose and correct the problem. If urine output falls below 30 ml/hr for 2 consecutive hours (< 0.5 ml/kg/hr), prerenal and postrenal causes must be rapidly ruled out and corrected to prevent renal parenchymal deterioration. An approach to evaluating and treating oliguria is summarized in Figure 18-1.

Various laboratory tests that can be helpful in determining prerenal from intrinsic renal failure are listed in Table 18-5. If prerenal and postrenal causes are eliminated, every effort should be made to convert oliguric intrinsic renal failure to the nonoliguric state, since prognosis may be improved [58]. In fact, the major goal in critically injured trauma patients is prevention of renal failure, which is much more effective than any treatment presently available [53].

Neurologic Support

Intracranial injury combined with other organ system dysfunction creates a very difficult clinical setting for optimal management, since modalities used to improve cardiorespiratory function and oxygen delivery may have detrimental effects on factors determining optimal intracranial hemodynamics and cerebral oxygen delivery. A satisfactory outcome requires recognition and successful treatment of the alterations in intracranial hemodynamics, brain metabolism, and brain water compartmentation, since the magnitude of the insult to brain parenchyma is ultimately dependent

Urine output <0.5 ml/kg/hr for two consecutive hours
↓
Irrigate/replace Foley catheter
↓
Consider undiagnosed urological injury
↓
Give 500 ml rapid bolus of crystalloid
↓
Consider repeating 500 ml fluid bolus
↓
Place pulmonary artery catheter if hypovolemia no longer likely
↓
Continue fluid administration until PAOP = 15–18 torr
↓
Send 5 ml urine and blood for diagnostic tests (Table 5) (do not wait for tests to return)
↓
Infuse dopamine 3 to 5 micrograms/kg/min
↓
Mannitol 25 gm I.V. bolus
↓
Furosemide 40 mg I.V. bolus
↓
Furosemide 200 mg I.V. bolus
↓
Assume acute renal failure
↓
Consider hemodialysis as indicated

Fig. 18-1. An approach to evaluating and treating oliguria in the postoperative trauma patient.

Table 18-5. Tests for Determining Prerenal Versus Renal Oliguric Dysfunction

Test	Prerenal	Renal
U/P osmolality	>1.25	<1.1
Urine sodium	<20	>40
Fractional excretion (FE) of sodium*	<0.01	>0.03

U = urine; P = plasma; Na = sodium; creat = creatinine.

$$*FE_{Na} = \frac{U_{Na} \times P_{creat}}{P_{Na} \times U_{creat}}$$

on the degree of ischemia sustained by the neurons [59].

As with any organ system, the final common pathway of brain injury is impairment of oxygen delivery and metabolic nutrients to the cells. Thus, cardiorespiratory function must be adequately maintained in the multiply injured patient to protect from further brain injury. There are many systemic manifestations of head injury that also may complicate not only the prognosis for the brain injury per se, but also other organ systems. Hypertension and tachycardia from elevated catecholamine levels may adversely affect cardiac output, as previously described, and also cause significant negative nitrogen balance [60]. Neurogenic pulmonary edema, although uncommon, may further complicate acute lung injury from direct trauma or sepsis. Coagulopathies may develop from liberated stores of brain tissue thromboplastin following severe head injury [59].

There is little doubt that intracranial pressure (ICP) monitoring is helpful in managing the multiply injured patient with head injury, although it is controversial whether monitoring has improved outcome in these critically ill patients [61]. Although it is recognized that ICP control does not necessarily correlate with optimal cerebral blood flow, cerebral perfusion pressure, or oxygen delivery to the brain, maintenance of ICP below 20 mm Hg remains the standard clinical end point of

Table 18-6. Therapeutic Interventions for Reducing ICP and Potential Side Effects

Therapy	Side effects
Hyperventilation ($PaCO_2$ = 25–30 mm Hg)	Reduced O_2 utilization from respiratory alkalosis
Mannitol (0.5–1.5 gm/kg q4h)	Serum hyperosmolarity
	Renal dysfunction
	Hypotension
	Hyponatremia, hypokalemia
	Cardiac dysrhythmias
Ventricular CSF drain	Nosocomial infection
Dexamethasone[a] (10 mg loading, 4 mg q6h)	Nosocomial infection
	Increased caloric expenditure
Induced barbiturate coma[b] (pentobarbital sodium, 3–5 mg/kg loading, 1–2 mg/kg q1–2h)	Hypotension
	Cardiac failure

[a]Steroids have not been shown to reduce ICP consistently in head injury patients.
[b]From M. A. Rockoff, L. F. Marshall, and H. M. Shapiro. High-dose barbiturate therapy in humans: A clinical review of 60 patients. *Ann. Neurol.* 6:194, 1979.

therapy [62]. ICP monitoring offers the ability to recognize and correct changes in ICP that may develop from therapeutic interventions on other organ systems, such as PEEP for hypoxemic respiratory failure and inotropic support for cardiac dysfunction.

Various therapeutic modalities for achieving ICP less than 20 mm Hg along with potential systemic side effects of these therapies are listed in Table 18-6. The treatment for intracranial trauma is discussed in greater detail in Chapter 6.

EVALUATING THE SEPSIS SYNDROME

The evaluation of sepsis should include a knowledge of the trauma patient's history, especially intraoperative technical details, a thorough physical examination with the high-risk areas highlighted, and specified tests to delineate or confirm the source. Rote ordering of tests (e.g., the "fever workup") that is not directed by clinical findings may only confuse the issue and increase patient charges [63,64]. Although ICU patients have three times the risk of developing a nosocomial infection when compared to ward patients [65], a sense of urgency often leads to reflex fever workups that are difficult to justify, interrupt, or curtail.

The importance of a directed evaluation was highlighted in a study of postoperative fever in 15 percent of 464 patients during the first 6 days following abdominal operation [64]. Upon analysis, infection was found in 19 patients (27 percent of the febrile group). A correct diagnosis could have been made on clinical findings and confirmed by a single appropriate test in 14 (74 percent) of the patients with infection. Frequently used tests ordered in combination, the habitual "battery," had very low positive yields in this study. Urine culture was obtained in 86 percent of patients but was positive in only 10 percent. Chest x-rays were performed in 75 percent of patients, with one positive result. Blood cultures were obtained in 60 percent of patients with only two (5 percent) positive results [64].

Similar reasoning can be applied to the evaluation of sepsis in critically ill trauma patients. Minor elevations of temperature on the day of surgery are usually insignificant, and generally even a 2°F elevation should not require investigation beyond physical examination and careful inspection of the patient's wounds unless fever recurs.

The initial septic evaluation should include urinalysis only if urosepsis is suspected (generally only when the urinary tract has been instrumented). A urine culture should be obtained *only* if pyuria is present. The absence of white blood cells in the urine makes the diagnosis of urinary tract infection very unlikely [66]. If anaerobic urinary infection is suspected, a suprapubic urine specimen should be obtained [67]. Urinary tract infections causing systemic sepsis are more likely in elderly men and in patients catheterized longer than 7 days [68].

Pulmonary sources are commonly suspected. Physical examination and review of recent chest x-rays should precede routine cultures as the sole diagnostic step. Further, a sputum Gram stain, containing numerous white cells and a predominant organism, is more likely to provide immediate information concerning the likelihood of true pulmonary infection than the sputum culture. Gram stain provides more rapid information as well because the culture result will not be available for 2 or 3 days. Routine cultures obtained through the endotracheal tube or with bronchial washings are reportedly very unreliable [69–76]. Since gram-negative organisms are the predominant cause of nosocomial pneumonias [71,72], antibiotic therapy can initially be based on Gram stain, since *some type* of gram-negative organism will most likely grow in the culture (due to colonization). If cultures are crucial to rule out other pathogens or direct therapy, then brush cultures by bronchoscopy may be more reliable [75,77,78], although the cost-effectiveness and superiority of this technique has recently been questioned [79].

Most wound infections are diagnosed by physical examination and Gram stain. Patients with contaminated wounds who develop severe pain, agitation, and high fevers within the first 48 to 72 hours postoperatively must be closely examined for streptococcal or clostridial wound infections [80–87]. Large open wounds that are healing secondarily should not be routinely cultured. Quantitative bacterial cultures should be performed to confirm the wound as the septic source if suspected [88–94].

We believe that intravascular devices placed during emergency resuscitation should routinely be removed after stabilization and admission to the ICU. Thereafter, peripheral intravenous cannulas should be routinely replaced every 72 hours. The percutaneous entry site should be inspected daily for signs of erythema or purulent drainage. Similar recommendations are made for arterial lines, although the duration of catheterization is more dependent on preservation of a clean entry site [95]. No specific duration for arterial catheterization is proposed because it is a very uncommon cause of systemic sepsis [95].

Central catheters are often implicated if an otherwise unexplained fever spike occurs. The first priority, however, is to perform a directed physical examination and specific laboratory tests because half of the cases of suspected catheter sepsis may be eliminated by this process. Of those patients remaining, only 20 percent will have line sepsis confirmed.

Populations can be considered in terms of the likelihood of line sepsis [96]:

1. Septic patients: The longer the duration of the illness, the more likely the possibility that line sepsis will occur.
2. Clean patients: Fever is less frequent; there are fewer sources of bacteria, shorter duration of monitoring, and better host resistance.
3. Patients in whom fever develops soon after line placement: It is rare to find a catheter-related infection in less than 48 hours.

Catheters placed under controlled circumstances are less likely causes for line sepsis than catheters placed under unknown circumstances, in emergency situations, or after repeated attempts.

Our suggested PA catheter protocol consists of the following: If there is no evidence of infection at the percutaneous site, patients having had contaminated surgical procedures ("dirty" cases) should have the catheter and introducer guidewire exchanged at 72 hours following a 2-minute scrub of the entry site with povidone-iodine and alcohol. At 6 days, the catheter/introducer is removed and replaced to a different site. In patients having had clean or clean-contaminated surgery, the catheter/introducer is guidewire exchanged on the fourth day if further hemodynamic monitoring is required.

The tip and intracutaneous segment of the catheter (or introducer if used) are semiquantitatively cultured following every replacement over a guidewire. If either culture returns positive for catheter infection (defined as $\geqslant$ 15 colonies), the new catheter and introducer (which had been placed over the guidewire) are removed, and a new line, if necessary, is started at a different site.

Blood cultures drawn through PA catheters, central catheters, or arterial lines are not beneficial in diagnosing bacteremia or catheter-related infection. Routine peripheral cultures are not indicated, even in the febrile patient [97]. Although the number and timing of peripheral blood cultures remain controversial [97], blood cultures at or just before the highest fever are often helpful.

In a confirmed central catheter–related bacteremia, the catheter should be removed. Antibiotics are not usually necessary. When the bacteremia can conceivably be related to another site or source, or if the problem was not promptly discovered, antibiotic therapy can be considered.

Hyperalimentation lines are not subjected to the frequent breaks in sterility for medications and blood sampling and are an unlikely source for sepsis in critically ill patients unless the catheter has been in place for several weeks. If the hyperalimentation catheter is suspected, it should be replaced over a guidewire and cultured semiquantitatively [96,98].

Meningitis in trauma patients is rare and almost never occurs until after the seventh hospital day [99]. Spinal fluid cultures are probably indicated if a significant change in mental status develops with no clinical cause *and* a positive culture would alter antibiotic therapy. A fever workup in the trauma patient should not routinely include lumbar puncture.

Abdominal computed tomography (CT) scanning to rule out abscess should not be performed within the first week postoperatively and should only be done if the information obtained would be used to direct therapy [100]. Patients with multisystem organ failure generally do not benefit from abdominal CT [100], and perhaps early reexploration should be the only diagnostic test [101–104], especially in patients with unexplained single-system organ failure. Portable ultrasonography is a safe and relatively inexpensive method for diagnosing acute cholecystitis in the postoperative trauma patient if the clinical examination suggests this diagnosis [105,106].

REFERENCES

1. Maull, K. I. *Advances in Trauma* (Vol. 1). Chicago: Year Book, 1986.
2. Maloney, J. V. Intinerant surgery: At home and on the road. *Ann. Surg.* 200:115, 1984.
3. Walt, A. J. The training and role of the surgeon in the intensive care unit. *Surg. Clin. North Am.* 65:753, 1985.
4. Meakins, J. L., Wickland, B., Forse, R. A., et al. The surgical intensive care unit: Current concepts in infection. *Surg. Clin. North Am.* 60:117, 1980.
5. Shires, G. T., and Dineen, P. Sepsis following burns, trauma, and intra-abdominal infections. *Arch. Intern. Med.* 142:2012, 1982.
6. Petty, T. L. Adult respiratory distress syndrome: Definition and historical perspective. *Clin. Chest Med.* 3:3, 1982.
7. Fein, A. M., Goldberg, S. K., Lippman, M. L., et al. Adult respiratory distress syndrome. *Br. J. Anaesth.* 54:723, 1982.
8. Balk, R., and Bone, R. L. The adult respiratory distress syndrome. *Med. Clin. North Am.* 67:685, 1983.
9. Bell, R. C., Coalson, J. J., Smith, J. D., et al. Multiple organ system failure and infection in adult respiratory distress syndrome. *Ann. Intern. Med.* 99:293, 1983.
10. Rinaldo, J. E., and Rogers, R. M. Adult respiratory distress syndrome: Changing concepts of lung injury and repair. *N. Engl. J. Med.* 306:900, 1982.
11. Myers, T. J., Cole, S. R., Klatsky, A. U., et al. Respiratory failure due to pulmonary leukostasis following chemotherapy of acute nonlymphocytic leukemia. *Cancer* 51:1808, 1983.
12. Zimmerman, G. A. Adult respiratory distress syndrome secondary to high altitude pulmonary edema. *West. J. Med.* 133:335, 1980.
13. Fulton, R. L., and Jones, C. E. The cause of posttraumatic pulmonary insufficiency in man. *Surg. Gynecol. Obstet.* 140:179, 1975.
14. Kaplan, R. L., Sahns, S. A., and Petty, T. L. Incidence and outcome of adult respiratory distress syndrome in gram-negative sepsis. *Arch. Intern. Med.* 139:867, 1979.
15. Taylor, R. W. The Adult Respiratory Distress Syndrome. In R. R. Kirby and R. W. Taylor (eds.), *Respiratory Failure* (1st ed.). Chicago: Year Book, 1986.
16. Pepe, P. E., Potkin, R. T., Reus, D. H., et al. Clinical predictors of the adult respiratory distress syndrome. *Am. J. Surg.* 144:124, 1982.
17. Robin, E. D., Cross, C. E., and Aelis, R. Pulmonary edema. *N. Engl. J. Med.* 288:239, 1973.
18. Staub, N. C. Pulmonary edema. *Physiol. Rev.* 54:678, 1974.
19. Taylor, A. E. Capillary fluid filtration: Starling forces and lymph flow. *Circ. Res.* 49:557, 1981.
20. Borzotta, A. P., and Polk, H. C. Multiple system organ failure. *Surg. Clin. North Am.* 63:315, 1983.
21. Norwood, S. H., and Civetta, J. M. The adult respiratory distress syndrome. *Surg. Gynecol. Obstet.* 161:497, 1985.

22. Taylor, A. E., Martin, D., and Parker, J. C. The effects of oxygen radicals on pulmonary edema formation. *Surgery* 94:433, 1983.
23. Rose, D. M., Downs, J. B., and Heenan, T. J. Temporal responses of functional residual capacity and oxygen tension to changes in positive end-expiratory pressure. *Crit. Care Med.* 9:79, 1981.
24. Shapiro, B. A., Cane, R. D., and Harrison, R. A. Positive end-expiratory pressure in acute lung injury. *Chest* 3:558, 1983.
25. Norwood, S. H., and Civetta, J. M. Ventilatory support in patients with ARDS. *Surg. Clin. North Am.* 65:895, 1985.
26. Downs, J. B., and Douglas, M. E. Applied Physiology and Respiratory Care. In W. C. Shoemaker (ed.), *Critical Care State of the Art* (Vol. 3). Anaheim: Society of Critical Care Medicine, 1982.
27. Keighley, G. R. The arterial/alveolar oxygen tension ratio: An index of gas exchange applicable to varying inspired oxygen concentrations. *Am. Rev. Respir. Dis.* 109:142, 1974.
28. Dantzker, D. R., Wagner, P. D., and West, J. B. Instability of lung units with low V/Q ratio during O_2 breathing. *J. Appl. Physiol.* 35:886, 1975.
29. West, J. B. *Respiratory Physiology.* Baltimore: Williams & Wilkins, 1974.
30. Norwood, S. H., Silva, J. S., Civetta, J. M., et al. The value of room air blood gases to predict successful tracheal extubation (Abstract). *Crit. Care Med.* 14:376, 1986.
31. Norwood, S. H., and Silva, J. S. Room air blood gases versus traditional criteria for predicting successful tracheal extubation. In press.
32. Norwood, S. H., and Duncan, C. A. Cardiac Function During Respiratory Failure. In R. R. Kirby and R. W. Taylor (eds.), *Respiratory Failure* (1st ed.). Chicago: Year Book, 1986.
33. Giovannini, I., Boldrini, G., Sgonga, G., et al. Quantification of the determinants of arterial hypoxemia in critically ill patients. *Crit. Care Med.* 11:644, 1983.
34. Nelson, L. D. Continuous venous oximetry in surgical patients. *Ann. Surg.* 203:329, 1986.
35. Frank, O. Die Grundform des arteriellen pulses. *Z. Biol.* 37:483, 1898.
36. Patterson, S. W., Piper, H., and Starling, E. H. The regulation of the heart beat. *J. Physiol.* 48:465, 1914.
37. Ayres, S. M. Ventricular Function. In W. C. Shoemaker (ed.), *Critical Care State of the Art* (Vol. 1). Fullerton: Society of Critical Care Medicine, 1980.
38. Glass, D. D. Cardiovascular Drugs. In J. M. Civetta (ed.), *Intensive Care Therapeutics.* New York: Appleton-Century-Crofts, 1980.
39. Sonnenblick, E. H., Ross, J., and Braunwald, E. Oxygen consumption of the heart: Newer concepts of its multifactorial determination. *Am. J. Cardiol.* 22:238, 1968.
40. Sonnenblick, E. H. Determinants of active state in heart muscle: Force, velocity, instantaneous muscle length, time. *Fed. Proc.* 24:1396, 1965.
41. Sibbald, W. J., Calvin, J. E., Holliday, R. L., et al. Concepts in the pharmacologic support of cardiovascular function in critically ill surgical patients. *Surg. Clin. North Am.* 63:445, 1983.
42. Smith, P. K., Tyson, G. S., Hammon, J. W., et al. Cardiovascular effects of ventilation with positive end-expiratory airway pressure. *Ann. Surg.* 195:121, 1982.
43. Civetta, J. M. Crystalloids and Colloids: Is There a Clinical Controversy? Part II. *Weekly Anesthesiology Update* (Vol. 1, Lesson 39). Princeton: Biomedia, 1978.
44. Poole, G. V., Meredith, J. W., Pennell, T., et al. Comparison of colloids and crystalloids in resuscitation from hemorrhagic shock. *Surg. Gynecol. Obstet.* 154:577, 1982.
45. Virgilio, R. W., Matildi, L. A., Shackford, S. R., et al. Crystalloids vs. colloids in fluid resuscitation in patients with severe pulmonary insufficiency. *Surg. Gynecol. Obstet.* 158:207, 1984.
46. Virgilio, R. W., Rice, C. L., Smith, D. E., et al. Crystalloid versus colloid resuscitation: Is one better? *Surgery* 85:129, 1979.
47. Loeb, H. S., Khan, I. M., Saudye, A., et al. Acute hemodynamic effects of dobutamine and isoproteronol in patients with low output cardiac failure. *Circ. Shock* 3:55, 1976.
48. Robie, N. W., Nutter, D. O., and Moody, C. In vivo analysis of adrenergic receptor activity of dobutamine. *Circ. Res.* 34:663, 1974.
49. Cameron, J. S. Acute renal failure in the ICU today. *Intensive Care Med.* 12:64, 1986.
50. Conger, J. D. A controlled evaluation of prophylactic dialysis in post-traumatic acute renal failure. *J. Trauma* 15:1056, 1975.
51. Cox, S. C., Norwood, S. H., and Duncan, C. A.

Acute respiratory failure: Mortality associated with underlying disease. *Crit. Care Med.* 13:1005, 1985.
52. Fischer, R. P. High mortality of post-traumatic renal insufficiency in Vietnam: A review of 96 cases. *Am. Surg.* 40:172, 1974.
53. Bollinger, R. R., and Mahnensmith, R. L. Acute Renal Failure in Surgical Patients: Prevention and Treatment. In D. C. Sabiston (ed.), *Textbook of Surgery* (13th ed.). Philadelphia: Saunders, 1986.
54. Dixon, B. S., and Anderson, R. J. Nonoliguric acute renal failure. *Am. J. Kidney Dis.* 6:71, 1985.
55. Daughtry, T. M., Ueki, I. F., Mercer, P. F., et al. Dynamics of glomerular ultrafiltration in the rat: V. Response to ischemic injury. *J. Clin. Invest.* 53:105, 1974.
56. Hofstetter, T. H., Wilkes, B. M., and Brenner, B. M. Renal Circulatory and Nephron Function in Experimental Acute Renal Failure. In B. M. Brenner and J. M. Lazarus (eds.), *Acute Renal Failure.* Philadelphia: Saunders, 1983.
57. Stein, J. H., Lifschitz, M. D., and Barnes, L. D. Current concepts on the pathophysiology of acute renal failure. *Am. J. Physiol.* 234:F171, 1978.
58. Anderson, R. J., Linas, S. L., Berns, A. S., et al. Non-oliguric acute renal failure. *N. Engl. J. Med.* 296:1134, 1977.
59. Popp, J. A., and Bourke, R. S. Pathophysiology of Head Injury. In R. H. Wilkins and S. S. Rengachary (eds.), *Neurosurgery.* New York: McGraw-Hill, 1985.
60. Clifton, G. L., Ziegler, M. G., and Grossman, R. G. Circulating catecholamines and sympathetic activity after head injury. *Neurosurgery* 8:10, 1981.
61. Silverberg, G. D. Intracranial Pressure Monitoring. In R. H. Wilkins and S. S. Rengachary (eds.), *Neurosurgery.* New York: McGraw-Hill, 1985.
62. Quest, D. O. Increased Intracranial Pressure, Brain Herniation, and Their Control. In R. H. Wilkins and S. S. Rengachary (eds.), *Neurosurgery.* New York: McGraw-Hill, 1985.
63. Civetta, J. M., and Hudson-Civetta, J. A. Maintaining quality of care while reducing changes in the ICU. *Ann. Surg.* 202:524, 1985.
64. Freischlag, J., and Busuttil, R. W. The value of postoperative fever evaluation. *Surgery* 94:358, 1983.
65. Donowitz, L. G., Wenzel, R. P., and Hoyt, J. W. High risk of hospital-acquired infection in the ICU patient. *Crit. Care Med.* 10:355, 1982.
66. Martinez, O. V., Civetta, J. M., Anderson, K., et al. Bacteriura in the catheterized surgical intensive care patient: A prospective survey of 100 patients. *Crit. Care Med.* 14:188, 1986.
67. Bromberg, K., Gleich, S., and Ginsberg, M. B. *Clostridia* in urinary tract infections. *South. Med. J.* 75:1298, 1982.
68. Shapiro, M., Simchen, E., Izraeli, S., et al. A multivariate analysis of risk factors for acquiring bacteriuria in patients with indwelling urinary catheters for longer than 24 hours. *Infect. Control* 5:525, 1984.
69. Bartlett, J. G., Alexander, J., Mayhew, J., et al. Should fiberoptic bronchoscopy aspirates be cultured? *Am. Rev. Respir. Dis.* 114:73, 1976.
70. Benner, E. J., Munzinger, J. P., and Chan, R. Superinfections of the lung: An evaluation by serial transtracheal aspirations. *West. J. Med.* 121:173, 1974.
71. Greenfield, S., Teres, D., Bushnell, L. S., et al. Prevention of gram-negative bacillary pneumonia using aerosol polymixin as prophylaxis. *J. Clin. Invest.* 52:2935, 1973.
72. Johanson, W. G., Pierce, A. K., Sanford, J. P., et al. Nosocomial respiratory infections with gram-negative bacilli. *Ann. Intern. Med.* 77:701, 1972.
73. Laurenzi, G. A., Potter, R. T., and Kass, E. H. Bacteriologic flora of the lower respiratory tract. *N. Engl. J. Med.* 265:1273, 1961.
74. Murray, P. R., and Washington, J. A. Microscopic and bacteriologic analysis of expectorated sputum. *Mayo Clin. Proc.* 50:339, 1975.
75. Tobin, M. J., and Grenvik, A. Nosocomial lung infection and its diagnosis. *Crit. Care Med.* 12:191, 1984.
76. Wanner, A., Amikam, B., Robinson, M. J., et al. Comparison between the bacteriologic flora of different segments of the airways. *Respiration* 30:561, 1973.
77. Wimberly, N. W., Bass, J. B., Boyd, B. W., et al. Use of a bronchoscopic protected catheter brush for the diagnosis of pulmonary infections. *Chest* 81:556, 1982.
78. Wimberly, N., Faling, J. C., and Bartlett, J. G. A fiberoptic bronchoscopy technique to obtain uncontaminated lower airway secretions for

bacterial culture. *Am. Rev. Respir. Dis.* 119:337, 1979.
79. Baigelman, W., Bellin, S., Cupples, L. A., et al. Bacteriologic assessment of the lower respiratory tract in intubated patients. *Crit. Care Med.* 14:864, 1986.
80. Giuliano, A., Lewis, F., Hadley, K., et al. Bacteriology of necrotizing fasciitis. *Am. J. Surg.* 134:52, 1977.
81. Hart, G. B., Lamb, R. C., and Strauss, M. B. Gas gangrene. *J. Trauma* 23:991, 1983.
82. Janevicius, R. V., and Martin, J. D. Necrotizing fasciitis. *Surg. Gynecol. Obstet.* 154:97, 1982.
83. Majeski, J. A., and Alexander, J. W. Early diagnosis, nutritional support, and immediate extensive debridement improve survival in necrotizing fasciitis. *Am. J. Surg.* 145:784, 1983.
84. Majeski, J. A. Necrotizing fasciitis of the extremities. *Prob. Gen. Surg.* 1:500, 1984.
85. Simmons, R. L. Wound infections: A review of diagnosis and treatment. *Infect. Control* 3:44, 1982.
86. Stone, H. H. Gas gangrene of the abdominal wall. *Prob. Gen. Surg.* 1:659, 1984.
87. Stone, H. H., and Martin, J. D. Synergistic necrotizing cellulitis. *Ann. Surg.* 175:702, 1972.
88. Heggers, J. P., Robson, M. C., and Doran, E. T. Quantitative assessment of bacterial contamination of open wounds by a slide technique. *Trans. R. Soc. Trop. Med. Hyg.* 63:532, 1969.
89. Krizek, T. J., and Cossman, D. V. Experimental burn wound sepsis: Variations in response to topical agents. *J. Trauma* 12:553, 1972.
90. Krizek, T. J., and Robson, M. C. Evolution of quantitative bacteriology in wound management. *Am. J. Surg.* 130:579, 1975.
91. Loebl, E. C., Marvin, J. A., Heck, E. L., et al. The method of quantitative burn-wound biopsy cultures and its use in the care of the burned patient. *Am. J. Clin. Pathol.* 61:20, 1974.
92. Nagee, C., Harry, B., Rodeheaver, G., et al. A rapid technique for quantitating wound bacterial counts. *Am. J. Surg.* 133:760, 1977.
93. Robson, M. C., Duke, W. F., and Krizek, T. J. Rapid bacterial screening in the treatment of civilian wounds. *J. Surg. Res.* 14:426, 1973.
94. Robson, M. D., and Heggers, J. P. Bacterial quantification of open wounds. *Milit. Med.* 134:19, 1969.
95. Norwood, S. H., Cormier, B. A., Moss, A. M., et al. A prospective evaluation of catheter-related infection during prolonged arterial catheterization. *Crit. Care Med.* 16:836, 1988.
96. Maki, D. Infections Associated with Intravascular Lines. In J. S. Remington and M. N. Swartz (eds.), *Current Clinical Topics in Infectious Diseases.* New York: McGraw-Hill, 1982.
97. Neu, H. C. Cost-effective blood cultures: Is it possible or impossible to modify behavior? *Infect. Control* 7:32, 1986.
98. Sitzman, J. V., Townsend, T. R., Siler, M. C., et al. Septic and technical complications of central venous catheterization. *Ann. Surg.* 202:766, 1985.
99. Mombelli, G., Klastersky, J., Coppens, L., et al. Gram-negative bacillary meningitis in neurosurgical patients. *J. Neurosurg.* 59:634, 1983.
100. Norwood, S. H., and Civetta, J. M. Abdominal CT scanning in critically ill surgical patients. *Ann. Surg.* 202:166, 1985.
101. Driver, T., Kelly, G. L., and Eiseman, B. Reoperation after abdominal trauma. *Am. J. Surg.* 135:747, 1978.
102. Feraris, V. A. Exploratory laparotomy for potential abdominal sepsis in patients with multiple-organ failure. *Arch. Surg.* 118:1130, 1983.
103. Hinsdale, J. G., and Jaffe, B. M. Re-operation for intra-abdominal sepsis. *Ann. Surg.* 199:31, 1984.
104. Machiedo, G. W., Tikellis, J., Suval, W., et al. Reoperation for sepsis. *Am. Surg.* 51:149, 1985.
105. Clark, R. A., and Tobin, R. Abscess drainage with CT and ultrasound guidance. *Radiol. Clin. North Am.* 21:445, 1983.
106. Mueller, P. R., and Simeone, J. F. Intra-abdominal abscesses: Diagnosis by sonography and computed tomography. *Radiol. Clin. North Am.* 21:425, 1983.

19

Comprehensive Monitoring of the Critically Injured Patient

Loren D. Nelson

APPROACH TO COMPREHENSIVE MONITORING

Continuous physiologic evaluation of the critically injured patient begins at the scene of the injury and continues throughout the hospitalization of the patient. Comprehensive monitoring is a goal-directed method of evaluation intended to detect all the changes in a patient's status. Properly applied monitoring will warn the clinical team of a status change when appropriate intervention may affect the outcome of the patient.

This chapter will describe a comprehensive method of patient evaluation. While the concepts may be applied to any critically ill patient, they are intended specifically for the acutely injured patient who may be in or on the verge of shock.

Monitoring should be goal-directed toward specific end points and tailored to the needs of the patient. Since the needs of the patient vary over time, it is convenient to divide monitoring into preoperative, perioperative, and postoperative phases.

Preoperative Monitoring

The preoperative monitoring requirements of the patient have been stressed in Chapters 3, 4, and 5. The emphasis in this phase of trauma care is on rapid evaluation, stabilization of vital signs, and rapid movement to definitive operative therapy. Frequent assessment of heart rate, blood pressure, ventilatory rate, mental status, skin perfusion, and perhaps urine output will usually meet the monitoring needs of the critically injured patient in the preoperative period. These factors plus careful assessment of the injuries sustained serve as a guide for blood and fluid resuscitation preoperatively. Inspection of the patient's neck veins may also provide important information regarding the differential diagnosis between hypovolemic shock related to acute blood loss and obstructive forms of shock such as pericardial tamponade or tension pneumothorax [1,2].

Intraoperative Monitoring

The second phase of monitoring begins when the patient arrives in the operating room. Induction of anesthesia obscures monitoring of the patient's neurologic status and the signs of adequate cerebral perfusion. It is common in this phase of monitoring that more invasive and continuous monitoring be instituted. Electrocardiographic monitoring, arterial catheterization, and continuous assessment of urine output provide the minimal monitoring required in the critically injured patient.

An indwelling arterial catheter not only provides heart rate and blood pressure information but also allows observation of the waveform, which may give the anesthesiologist information regarding cardiac contractility and peripheral perfusion. Equally important to pressure monitoring is the ability to obtain arterial blood samples for assessment of oxygenation, ventilation, and acid-base balance of the patient. Determination of acid-base data is particularly important, as the finding of a metabolic acidosis is highly suggestive of inadequate tissue perfusion—that is, shock.

One of the most important monitors of volume resuscitation and peripheral perfusion in the operating room is urinary output. While an adequate urine output does not universally ensure normal peripheral perfusion, a low urine output (< 0.5 ml/kg/hr) in the absence of underlying renal disease or acute injury to the urinary tract suggests inadequate volume resuscitation.

In patients without massive blood loss or severe underlying systemic illness, additional monitoring in the operating room is needed very infrequently. Measurement of central venous pressure (CVP) has been advocated as a monitor in more complex patients. While the placement of a central venous catheter is associated with some risk to the patient, it may provide some useful intraoperative information. The details of central venous catheterization will be discussed in the section on cardiovascular monitoring. Suffice to say here that, when properly measured, a low CVP usually indicates that the right ventricle is capable of accepting a larger volume load; little other information is gained from this finding. However, the finding of a high CVP dictates that more information regarding the patient's cardiovascular system is necessary. An abrupt increase in CVP may be associated with the onset of tension pneumothorax, pericardial tamponade, fluid overload, and right-sided heart failure, as well as a variety of other disorders of the cardiovascular or pulmonary systems. A high CVP detected intraoperatively means that further assessment is necessary.

Central venous catheterization may also provide a useful means by which to assess central venous oxygenation. Sampling of central venous blood for oxygen saturation measurements may indicate severe imbalances of oxygen supply and demand [3]. While central venous oxygenation cannot be equated to mixed venous oxygenation [3,4], the finding of significant desaturation should alert the clinician that adequate resuscitation has not been achieved. Details of the interpretation of mixed venous oxygen saturation will be discussed later in this chapter.

Postoperative Monitoring

The final and most complex phase of comprehensive monitoring of the injured patient occurs in the intensive care unit. As stated earlier, comprehensive monitoring of the critically injured patient must be tailored to the magnitude of injury and the underlying disease status of the patient. To avoid errors of omission, a systematic approach is suggested. Since nearly all organ systems can be affected by prolonged shock following injury, the monitoring survey must include all systems (Table 19-1). A systematic survey should include medical history, physical examination, vital signs, laboratory data, radiologic and imaging data, and physiologic data where appropriate for each system. The frequency with which each system should be monitored and the extent of monitoring for each system is determined by the severity of injury, underlying medical problems, baseline information gathered previously on each system, and the current condition of the patient.

Table 19-1. Systematic Monitoring

Cardiac
Pulmonary
Gastrointestinal
Pancreatic
Coagulative
Psychiatric
Nutrition
Infection
Vascular
Renal
Hepatobiliary
Hematologic
Neurologic
Integument
Medications
Tubes, lines, drains

CARDIOVASCULAR MONITORING

Monitoring of the cardiovascular system is designed to detect arrhythmias, cardiac conduction disturbances, myocardial ischemia, and malperfusion of vital organs and the periphery. Historical information of importance includes underlying coronary artery; myocardial, valvular, or peripheral vascular disease; prior medications; and the likelihood of thoracic injuries. The physical examination of the cardiovascular system should include serial auscultation of the heart and palpation of the major peripheral pulses (radial, brachial, carotid, femoral, popliteal, dorsal pedal, and posterior tibial). Careful documentation of the physical findings will be important for other examiners to detect changes in any of the physical findings.

Traditional vital signs of pulse rate and blood pressure are routinely recorded in nearly all patients. The monitoring of fluid intake and output is one of the most important indicators of vital organ perfusion. While continuous cardiac rhythm monitoring has not been shown to alter mortality or morbidity in surgical patients without a history of myocardial ischemia [5], electrocardiogram (ECG) equipment has become standard in all intensive care units and is a convenient way to observe heart rate and allow early diagnosis of cardiac rhythm disorders. However, if myocardial ischemia is suspected, unipolar ECG monitoring is of only limited value, and a traditional 12-lead ECG should be obtained.

Evaluation for potential myocardial contusion should be included as part of the assessment of any patient sustaining thoracic trauma. While controversial, the measurement of CK-MB fraction will give an indication of significant myocardial necrosis [6]. While necrosis is not universally present in myocardial contusion nor is the finding of myocardial necrosis always indicative of myocardial contusion [7], the measurement of CK-MB fractions is common in the first 24 hours following thoracic injury.

Serial chest radiographs, while of limited value as a cardiovascular monitor, are an important adjunct to intensive care monitoring. Chest x-rays may allow early detection of pleural or pericardial fluid accumulations. More importantly, serial chest x-rays allow repeated evaluation of the position of invasive lines, tubes, and drains, which may be crucial to the safe use of these monitoring and support devices [8].

Invasive cardiovascular monitoring may be required postoperatively in critically ill patients. The multiple components of invasive cardiovascular monitoring will be considered individually.

Arterial Catheterization

Percutaneous arterial catheterization is fundamental to cardiovascular monitoring in critically injured patients. Arterial catheterization allows both continuous assessment of systolic, diastolic, and mean arterial pressures and access for frequent arterial blood sampling [9]. There are no specific contraindications to arterial catheterization, but bleeding diatheses increase the risk of hemorrhagic complications. Arterial occlusive disease, the presence of vascular prosthesis, and local infections are contraindications to specific sites for arterial catheterization. Several peripheral vessels have been advocated as sites of choice for indwelling arterial catheters. Advantages and disadvantages of each site must be weighed according to the individual patient. The collateral blood supply and the superficial location of the radial artery make it a common site for arterial catheterization. Adequate collateral blood flow to the hand through the ulnar artery should be confirmed by a modified Allen test prior to cannulation of the radial artery. If collateral flow is insufficient, alternative sites should be considered. The dorsal pedal, axillary, and femoral arteries are also commonly used for indwelling catheters. The brachial artery, because of the potential limb loss resulting from thrombotic complications, should rarely be used as a site for an indwelling arterial catheter in critically ill patients.

The two most common procedural problems related to arterial catheterization are failure to cannulate the vessel and localized bleeding with hematoma. Following successful cannulation, dislodgement of the catheter, or disconnection of the monitoring system with resultant bleeding, thrombosis, localized infection, and catheter-related infection are the most common complications [10]. Severe complications such as digital ischemia following radial artery catheterization occur in less than 1 percent of patients. The catheter site should be carefully evaluated, and any sign of inflammation, infection, or distal ischemia should be considered an indication to remove the catheter promptly. If ischemia occurs, sympathetic blockade with long-acting local anesthetics may relieve the symptoms and minimize the chance for tissue loss.

Central Venous Catheterization

Central venous catheterization has become one of the most frequently performed procedures in critically ill patients. Central lines are useful when secure access to the circulation is required for fluid therapy, drug infusion, frequent blood sampling, parenteral nutrition, and measurement of CVP. There are no absolute contraindications to central venous catheterization, although bleeding diatheses increase the risk of hemorrhagic complications. The most commonly used sites for central venous catheterization are the internal and external jugular veins and the subclavian vein. Long catheters passed by peripheral veins or the femoral vein are associated with a high incidence of thrombotic and infective complications. While the risk of central venous catheterization is significant, it may be minimized by meticulous attention to proper technique [10].

Many new types of central venous catheters are available for use in critically ill patients. Multiple-lumen catheters allow simultaneous administration of central venous nutrition, other intravenous fluids and medications, and CVP measurement (Fig. 19-1). These multiple-lumen catheters are likely to be cost-effective in that they lessen the risk of complications from multiple central venous catheterizations and reduce the need for

Fig. 19-1. Triple-lumen catheter. The multiple-lumen central venous catheter may be used for simultaneous administration of parenteral nutrition, medications and intravenous fluid, and measurement of central venous pressure. (Courtesy Arrow International, Inc., Reading, Penn.)

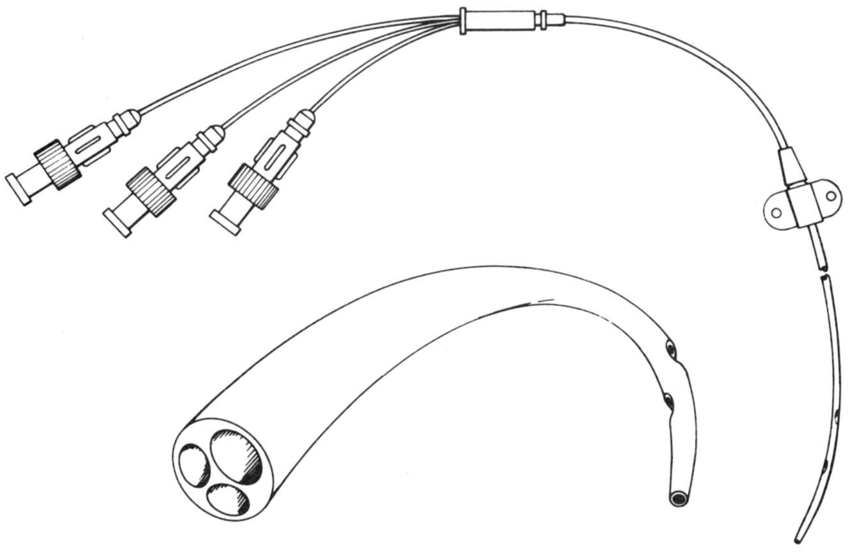

chest radiographs following each line insertion.

When central venous lines are used to measure CVP, they should be connected to an electromechanical transducer so that the waveform can be displayed on the bedside monitor. Water column manometers have a frequency response that is too low to respond to the pressure changes in the central circulation. Since the waveform cannot be displayed using water manometers, the catheter tip may inadvertently enter the right ventricle and erroneous mean pressure values, which are significantly higher than CVP, may be recorded [11]. A properly placed central venous line is capable of accurately measuring right atrial pressure, which, in the absence of tricuspid valve disease, will reflect right ventricular end-diastolic pressure. The right ventricular end-diastolic pressure indicates the *relationship* between intravascular volume and right ventricular function. Therefore, CVP cannot be used to assess either of these factors independent from the other [12]. Furthermore, CVP cannot be used to assess left ventricular pressures or left ventricular function. Disparate ventricular function has been documented in surgical patients since the availability of pulmonary artery (PA) catheters [13]. Significant differences in left and right ventricular function are documented in critically ill surgical patients [14], in patients with shock, or following trauma [15,16]. CVP is an unreliable monitor of intravascular volume and resuscitation in shock [17], complex surgical patients [18], and burn patients [19]. CVP does not reliably predict left-sided filling pressures in any identifiable population of critically ill patients.

Central venous catheters may also be used for repeated blood sampling and for measuring of central venous oxygen saturation. Low values of central venous oxygen saturation require further assessment because these values imply imbalance between oxygen delivery and tissue oxygen consumption. Normal values of central venous oxygen saturation are unreliable because they may reflect more localized changes in the distribution of peripheral blood flow. When there is a serious question as to the adequacy of oxygen transport, true mixed venous samples should be obtained by PA catheterization [3].

Pulmonary Artery Catheterization

Pulmonary artery (PA) catheterization has provided a "quantum leap" in the ability to assess cardiopulmonary function accurately in critically ill patients [11]. While the ability to measure left-sided filling pressures (PA occlusion pressure [PAOP], or "wedge") rather than right ventricular filling pressures (CVP) is an advantage of PA catheterization, the real utility is the measurement of blood flow (cardiac output) and true mixed venous oxygen saturation ($S\bar{v}O_2$) so that all of the derived parameters describing oxygen transport can be assessed. Since the major risk of PA catheterization is that of the central venous puncture, PA rather than central venous cannulation alone should be performed when hemodynamic information is necessary to assess cardiopulmonary function.

PA catheterization allows the clinician to answer two very important questions regarding the critically ill patient: (1) Is oxygen delivery to the tissue adequate to meet the body's need? and (2) What options are available to improve oxygen delivery? The adequacy of tissue oxygen delivery may be assessed clinically in some patients by observing pulse rate, blood pressure, cutaneous perfusion, mentation, and urine output. Unfortunately, in critically ill patients, none of these parameters can be used to estimate either cardiac output or blood volume deficits [20]. The important issue is whether the delivery of oxygen to the tissue satisfies the tissue oxygen requirement for efficient aerobic metabolism.

Monitoring Oxygen Transport

Oxygen delivery (DO_2) is calculated as the product of cardiac output (C.O.) and arterial oxygen content (CaO_2):

$$DO_2 = C.O. \times 10 \times CaO_2$$

The CaO_2 determinant of DO_2 may be accessed by measuring hemoglobin concentration (Hgb), arterial oxygen saturation (SaO_2), and arterial oxygen tension (PaO_2):

$$CaO_2 = (Hgb \times 1.38 \times SaO_2) + (PaO_2 \times 0.0031)$$

A complete assessment of CaO_2 may be made by arterial blood gas analysis. However, since estimates of cardiac output are not clinically accurate, cardiac output must be measured to access oxygen delivery adequately. This is done using the thermodilution technique through the PA catheter.

Thermodilution is used to determine cardiac output by injecting a known volume of fluid at a known temperature into the central circulation. After adequate mixing in the right atrium and right ventricle, the change in blood temperature in the proximal PA is measured by a thermistor imbedded in the wall of the PA catheter. The temperature change produced in the blood is inversely proportional to cardiac output. This technique for the measurement of cardiac output is accurate, reproducible, and simply performed using available instrumentation [12].

The measurement of cardiac output and the calculation of DO_2, however, do not indicate the adequacy of either of these parameters. The adequacy of DO_2 can only be assessed in terms of the amount of oxygen being consumed at the time of measurement (Table 19-2). Oxygen consumption or uptake (VO_2) can be measured by analyzing inspired and expired oxygen concentrations and expired minute volume, or it can be calculated using the Fick equation:

$$VO_2 = C.O.. \times C(a\text{-}v)O_2$$

Utilizing the Fick equation, the clinician can estimate the adequacy of DO_2 in terms of the amount of oxygen being consumed by the patient. The oxygen utilization coefficient (OUC) is equal to VO_2 divided by DO_2.

$$OUC = VO_2 / DO_2$$

When arterial oxygenation is maintained at a high level, SvO_2 can be used to estimate oxygen transport balance (OUC). Since SvO_2 can be monitored continuously using fiberoptic technology, it is a clinically useful on-line technique (Fig. 19-2). If SaO_2 is greater than 0.90, the SvO_2 is equal to 1 − OUC. So, in many patients, SvO_2 can be used to assess the balance between DO_2 and the body's oxygen re-

Table 19-2. Normal Ranges and Units for Oxygen Transport Variables

Term	Units	Normal range
Arterial oxygen tension (PaO_2)	mm Hg	70–100
Arterial oxygen saturation (SaO_2)	(fraction)	0.93–0.98
Arterial oxygen content (CaO_2)	ml/dl	16–22
Mixed venous oxygen tension ($P\bar{v}O_2$)	mm Hg	36–42
Mixed venous oxygen saturation ($5\bar{v}O_2$)	(fraction)	0.68–0.77
Mixed venous oxygen content ($C\bar{v}O_2$)	ml/dl	12–17
Arterio venous content difference ($C[a\text{-}v]O_2$)	ml/dl	3.5–5.5
Oxygen delivery (DO_2)	ml/min	640–1400
Oxygen consumption (VO_2)	ml/min	180–280
Oxygen utilization coefficient (OUC)	(fraction)	0.23–0.32
Intrapulmonary shunt ($\dot{Q}S/\dot{Q}T$)	(fraction)	0.03–0.08

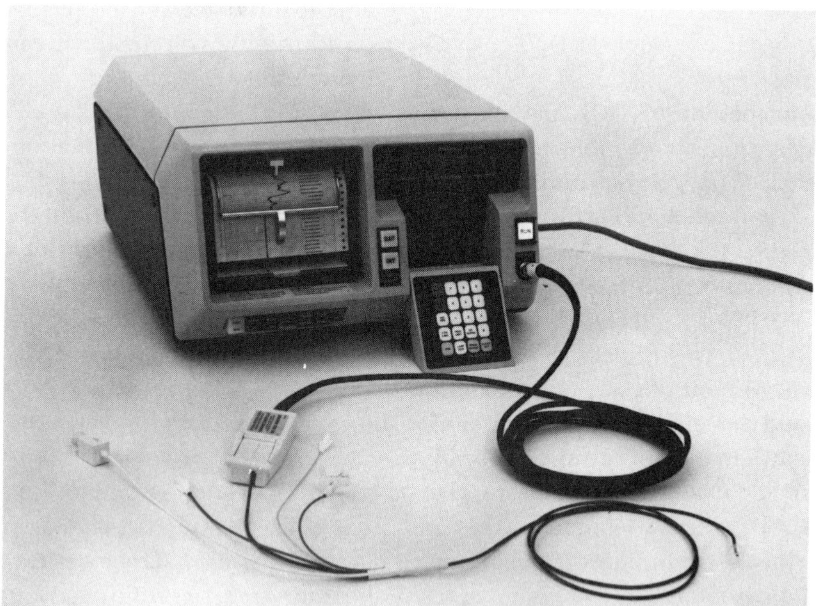

Fig. 19-2. Continuous oximetry pulmonary artery catheter and oximeter. (Courtesy Oximetrix, Inc., Moutain View, Calif.)

quirement. It must be recognized, however, that there are four determinants of SvO_2: hemoglobin concentration, SaO_2, cardiac output, and VO_2 [21]. Alteration in any of these four parameters can upset the oxygen supply-demand balance.

The adequacy of cardiac output (and therefore oxygen transport) can also be assessed by looking at the arteriovenous oxygen content difference [$C(a-v)O_2$]. Increases in $C(a-v)O_2$ of greater than 5.5 ml/dl indicate increased oxygen extraction. This may be associated with either increased consumption or decreased cardiac output.

Finally, the adequacy of oxygen delivery to meet the demand of the tissue can be assessed by looking at the metabolic acid-base status of the patient. Progressive metabolic acidosis is associated with inadequate tissue perfusion and lactate accumulation caused by anaerobic metabolism. Unfortunately, lactic acidosis occurs late in the shock state (after compensatory mechanisms have failed) and is associated with a poor prognosis [22].

When oxygen delivery has been determined to be inadequate to meet the body's needs, what can be done to improve the patient's status? Therapeutic efforts must be directed toward correcting the major cause of the deficiency of oxygen transport. If CaO_2 is inadequate, the most efficient means to improve DO_2 will be either to increase hemoglobin concentration (carrying capacity) or to increase SaO_2. When SaO_2 is greater than 0.90 to 0.95, the efficacy of raising saturation further is quite low. Furthermore, increasing hemoglobin concentration to levels greater than approximately 12 to 14 gm/dl has little benefit and may actually interfere with microvascular blood flow and tissue oxygen delivery. Therefore, once CaO_2 has been increased by improving oxygenation and optimizing hemoglobin concentration, the only means to improve DO_2 further is to increase cardiac output.

Utilizing Pulmonary Artery Catheter Measurements

The determinants of cardiac output are heart rate and stroke volume. Gross alterations in heart rate occur in children and younger patients to maintain or increase cardiac output in times of stress. However, tachycardia is inefficient in that it causes a great increase in myocardial oxygen consumption. In older patients, especially those with coronary artery disease, tachycardia may be extremely detrimental to the myocardial oxygen supply-demand balance. Heart rates greater than 100 to 110 probably should be avoided in patients with suspected coronary artery disease. In these patients, cardiac output may be increased by raising stroke volume. Stroke volume is determined by preload (the volume of blood presented to the ventricle for ejection), afterload (the impedance to blood flow from the left ventricle), and contractility. The PA catheter can be used to assess each of these determinants of stroke volume (Table 19-3).

Starling's law of the heart says that work performed will be proportional to the resting length of the myocardial fibers. In a given geometric shape, the fiber length will be proportional to the end-diastolic volume of the ventricle. When ventricular compliance does not change, the left ventricular end-diastolic pres-

Table 19-3. Normal Ranges and Units for Hemodynamic Variables

Term	Units	Normal ranges
Mean arterial pressure	mm Hg	70–105
Mean pulmonary arterial pressure	mm Hg	10–20
Pulmonary artery occlusion pressure	mm Hg	2–12
Central venous pressure	mm Hg	0–8
Cardiac index	$L/min/m^2$	2.8–4.2
Systemic vascular resistance	dyne s cm^{-5}	900–1400
Pulmonary vascular resistance	dyne s cm^{-5}	150–250
Left ventricular stroke work index	$gm \cdot m/m^2$	43–61
Right ventricular stroke work index	$gm \cdot m/m^2$	7–12

sure is proportional to the left ventricular end-diastolic volume. In the absence of mitral valve disease, the left atrial pressure is equal to the left ventricular end-diastolic pressure. Finally, in the vast majority of clinical situations, a properly measured PAOP ("wedge") will be equal to left atrial pressure. Using these assumptions, changes in PAOP may be used to estimate the magnitude and direction of change of left ventricular preload. There are many pitfalls in making these assumptions, but they are valid in many clinical circumstances [12]. Volume loading can be used to increase stroke volume while the PAOP is less than 18 mm Hg. Above this level, PAOP must be carefully assessed to determine if further volume loading is indicated.

Afterload of the left ventricle is the impedance to flow created by the mass and viscosity of blood, the compliance of the great vessels, and the systemic vascular resistance (SVR). For practical purposes, the only parameter over which we have major control is the SVR. SVR can be calculated from mean arterial pressure (MAP), CVP, and cardiac output (C.O.) using a modification of Ohms law:

$$\text{SVR} = \frac{(\text{MAP} - \text{CVP})}{\text{C.O.}} \times 80$$

When there are extreme increases in SVR (usually > 2000 dyne s cm^{-5}), afterload reduction using an arterial vasodilator may be effective to increase forward blood flow and stroke volume. It is important to note that preload (adequate ventricular filling as assessed by PAOP) must be maintained when using vasodilator therapy to augment stroke volume.

Contractility is the third determinant of stroke volume. While contractility is difficult to quantitate serially in the ICU, ventricular function can be assessed by relating ventricular work to preload. Calculation of left ventricular stroke work index (LVSWI) accounts for the work performed by the ventricle while controlling for changes in heart rate (HR) and the size of the patient (BSA):

$$\text{LVSWI} = \frac{(\text{MAP} - \text{PAOP}) \times \text{C.O.}}{\text{HR} \times \text{BSA}} \times 0.0136$$

Changes in LVSWI occur with changes in preload, afterload, and contractility, but when PAOP and SVR are unchanged, changes in LVSWI correlate with changes in contractility [12]. Contractility may be affected by using inotropic agents. These agents should be reserved for volume-resuscitated patients following injury but at times may be indicated for short periods to "catch up" with volume losses.

CASE 1. POST-TRAUMATIC SHOCK

A 45-year-old man was involved in a high-speed motor vehicle accident, pinning him behind the steering wheel for 30 minutes. Following extrication, he was transported to a level I trauma center by helicopter. He received 1.8 liters of Ringer's lactate during extrication and transport. During transport, his pulse was 120 and blood pressure (BP) 100/50. On arrival in the emergency department, pulse was 128 and BP palpable at 80 systolic. He was intubated transnasally, ventilated, and two additional large-bore IVs were established. He was given 2 liters of Ringer's lactate rapidly, and blood was sent for type and cross match and laboratory analysis for hematocrit, electrolytes, creatinine, glucose, blood urea nitrogen (BUN), and amylase. An arterial blood gas was sent during manual ventilation with 40% oxygen. Initial assessment showed a lethargic and confused man with facial lacerations, contusions of the anterior chest and decreased breath sounds on the left, a distended abdomen, and cool, clammy, mottled skin. BP was palpable at 90, and pulse was 130. Neck veins were now distended. [Fifteen minutes have now elapsed since arrival in the emergency department, and it is clear that the patient has sustained severe trauma with multiple injuries. He is in shock, at least a component of which is hypovolemic. The distended neck veins and decreased breath sounds strongly suggest a left tension pneumothorax.] A left tube thoracostomy was performed, and 100 ml of blood and a large gush of air were obtained. Two units of O-negative blood were started, and x-rays of the chest and lateral cervical spine were obtained. BP was then 100/70 and pulse 120; neck veins were flat. Blood gas results showed PO_2 = 100, PCO_2 = 29, pH = 7.25, and base deficit = −18 mEq/L. [The obstructive component of shock has apparently been resolved by tube thoracostomy, but the patient remains in shock.] The abdomen was found to be more distended, and the patient was rushed to the operating room (OR) for immediate laparotomy. Exploration revealed a shattered spleen, a grade IV liver laceration, and transected body of the pancreas. Splenectomy, distal pancreatectomy, debridement, oversewing of bleeding points, and drainage of the liver were performed. The patient received 12 liters of Ringer's lactate and 6 units of blood during the 3½ hours in the OR. The estimated blood loss was 3500 ml (including initial 2500-ml hemoperitoneum); the patient put out 400 ml of urine. [Preoperative monitoring was sufficient with pulse, BP, and rapid physical examination. Intraoperative monitoring added a radial arterial line placed during (not before) the procedure and measurement of urine output. Had significant complications occurred in the OR, further monitoring may have been necessary. Postoperative monitoring needs will be determined by the patients immediate ICU course.]

PULMONARY MONITORING

The pulmonary system is vulnerable to both direct and indirect injury following trauma. As with all aspects of comprehensive monitoring, an appropriate medical history should be obtained regarding the mechanism of injury, likelihood of thoracic trauma, prior pulmonary disease and medications, and other information that may affect patient management. The physical examination of the pulmonary system is useful to detect mechanical problems regarding endotracheal tube placement, pneumothorax, hemothorax, and bronchospasm. However, the presence of nonspecific signs, including rales and rhonchi, are of limited value in intubated patients receiving mechanical ventilatory support. Vital signs of the pulmonary system include respiratory rate but also include monitored data available from the ventilator. Tidal volume and peak airway pressure may be useful in determining the presence of pulmonary complications.

By far the most common laboratory test used to assess pulmonary function is arterial blood gas analysis. This has rapidly become the most frequently utilized test in the surgical intensive care unit. Arterial blood gases indicate the adequacy of arterial oxygenation, ventilation (carbon dioxide excretion), and acid-base status of the patient.

The portable chest x-ray has greatly supplemented physical examination in critically ill patients receiving mechanical ventilatory support [23]. Chest x-rays following invasive vascular or airway procedures should always be performed to rule out complications and to ensure the proper positioning of catheters [8]. Serial chest x-rays are also of value in detecting subclinical changes in effusions and lung parenchyma.

The physiologic monitoring of the pulmonary system can be divided into three discrete parts: pulmonary mechanics, oxygenation, and ventilation.

Pulmonary Mechanics

Pulmonary mechanics in intubated patients may be monitored by observing ventilatory rate, tidal volume (spontaneous and mechanical), peak inspiratory airway pressure, and expiratory airway pressure [24]. Pulmonary compliance describes the distensibility of the lungs by relating the pressure change required to produce a volume change. The effective dynamic compliance (EDC) of the pulmonary system can be calculated as the exhaled tidal volume (TV) divided by the difference between peak inspiratory (PIP) and end-expiratory (EEP) airway pressures:

$$\text{EDC} = \frac{\text{TV}}{\text{PIP} - \text{EEP}}$$

The EDC is affected by both the total thoracic compliance and flow-resistive properties of the airways. Increases in airway resistance secondary to secretions, partial obstruction, malpositioning of the tracheal tube, or bronchospasm will affect peak inspiratory airway pressure [24,25]. If, however, the exhalation valve of the ventilator is maintained in the closed position following inspiration, air flow ceases so that resistive effects on airway pressure are negated. This so-called plateau or pause pressure is always lower than peak inspiratory pressure, and when it is substituted in the compliance calculation, a quasi-static compliance is obtained.

The quasi-static compliance reflects the compliance of the lung and chest wall but is not affected by changes in airway resistance. Factors that affect chest wall compliance include edema, muscle tone, splinting secondary to pain, abdominal distention, pneumothorax, hemothorax, abdominal incisional pain, and respiratory efforts on the part of the patient. When changes in these factors are minimized, changes in plateau airway pressure will reflect changes in lung compliance. Decreases in lung compliance are associated with acute restrictive diseases such as the adult respiratory distress syndrome [26]. Therefore, continuous monitoring of airway pressure may be a useful on-line monitor of pulmonary injury (Table 19-4).

Table 19-4. Factors Affecting Peak Inspiratory Airway Pressure

Peak inspiratory gas flow
Airway resistance
End-expiratory airway pressure
Chest wall compliance
Musculature—pain or paralysis
Chest wall edema
Rib fractures, incisions, tubes
Pneumothorax, hemothorax, effusions
Pleural thickening, inflammation
Diaphragm elevation—ascites, distention
Abdominal pain—incisions, inflammation
Abdominal musculature—paralysis
Lung compliance
Pulmonary edema
Atelectasis
Resting lung volume

Oxygenation Monitoring

The measurement of arterial blood gases and analysis of oxygen tension and saturation have been the key to monitoring the oxygenation function of the lung. When patients require supplemental oxygen, changes in PaO_2 become difficult to associate with changes in lung function. For this reason, many indices have been developed to interpret lung function while the patient receives supplemental oxygen [24]. Of these, the PaO_2/FIO_2 ratio is simple to calculate and has clinical utility [27]. A PaO_2/FIO_2 of less than 300 mm Hg indicates significant oxygenation dysfunction.

The problem with all of the derived oxygenation indices is that they are all partially dependent on mixed venous oxygen saturation [$S\bar{v}O_2$). As pulmonary function worsens, as in adult respiratory distress syndrome, increasing intrapulmonary shunting makes the PaO_2 and indices derived from PaO_2 even more dependent on $S\bar{v}O_2$. The calculation of intrapulmonary shunt fraction ($\dot{Q}S/\dot{Q}T$) accounts for changes in $S\bar{v}O_2$ and therefore is a more valid parameter for assessing oxygenation function. The calculation of $\dot{Q}S/\dot{Q}T$ requires near complete saturation of pulmonary capillary blood ($FIO_2 > 0.30$) and the measurement of hemoglobin, SaO_2, and $S\bar{v}O_2$ and the calculation of pulmonary capillary oxygen content (CcO_2), arterial content (CaO_2), and mixed venous content ($C\bar{v}O_2$):

$$CcO_2 = (Hgb \times 1.38) + (P_AO_2 \times 0.0031)$$

Where $P_AO_2 = F_IO_2 \times$ (barometric pressure $- 47) - PaCO_2/RQ$
And intrapulmonary physiologic shunt fraction is as follows:

$$\dot{Q}S/\dot{Q}T = \frac{CcO_2 - CaO_2}{CcO_2 - CvO_2}$$

This requires PA catheterization and is usually reserved for patients with severe cardiovascular or pulmonary impairment.

All of these measurements are intermittent and are often measured either too frequently or not frequently enough. Continuous noninvasive arterial saturation indicators such as pulse oximetry (Fig. 19-3) allows a continuous assessment of arterial oxygenation, provided that perfusion to the sensor is maintained [28]. This monitoring technique is likely to be both cost-effective and efficacious in improving patient care in critically injured patients.

Ventilation Monitoring

The adequacy of ventilation is assessed by the measurement of arterial carbon dioxide tension ($PaCO_2$). $PaCO_2$ is determined by carbon dioxide production (VCO_2) and alveolar minute ventilation. VCO_2 is determined by oxygen consumption (VO_2) and substrate utilization (respiratory quotient). Alveolar ventilation is determined by total exhaled ventilation (tidal volume $\times$ ventilatory rate) and the fraction of tidal volume that is dead-space ventilation (V_D/V_T). When the ventilatory needs of the patient are not met ($PaCO_2$ is high), supplemental mechanical ventilation may be required.

Fig. 19-3. Pulse oximeter. (Courtesy Nellcor, Inc., Hayward, Calif.)

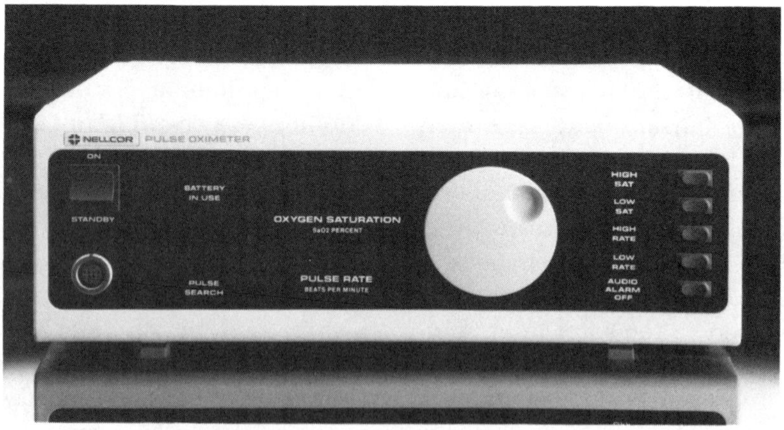

CASE 1 (CONTINUED). ACUTE RESPIRATORY FAILURE

The patient was admitted to the surgical ICU postoperatively. Initial BP was 140/90 and pulse 110. The patient's muscle relaxants had not been reversed, and he was placed on controlled mechanical ventilation with a volume cycled ventilator at a rate of 8 breaths/min, a tidal volume of 1000 ml (15 ml/kg), 45% oxygen, and positive end-expiratory pressure (PEEP) of 5 cm H_2O. Peak inspiratory airway pressure (PIP) was 30 cm H_2O. Breath sounds were clear and equal bilaterally; there were occasional rhonchi and some scattered rales. The trachea was midline, and the chest wall rose symmetrically during inspiration. There was no significant chest tube drainage, no air leak, and the water column fluctuated with each mechanical breath. Initial chest x-ray showed the nasotracheal, left thoracostomy, and nasogastric tubes to be in proper position. There was a small residual left pleural effusion, multiple anterior and lateral left rib fractures, and a large parenchymal infiltrate in the midportion of the left lung. Initial blood gases drawn from the radial arterial line were $PaO_2 = 78$, $PaCO_2 = 32$, ph = 7.32, and base deficit = −9. [Interpretation at this time is that effective dynamic compliance is satisfactory (40 ml/cm H_2O), there is moderate oxygenation dysfunction ($PaO_2/FIO_2 = 173$), induced hyperventilation ($PaCO_2 = 32$), and continued moderate to severe metabolic acidosis. The level of cardiopulmonary monitoring seems adequate.] Over the next 2 hours, the patient began breathing spontaneously and became more alert. His ventilatory mode was changed to intermittent mandatory ventilation (IMV) at a rate of 4. Spontaneous ventilatory rate was 24 with a tidal volume of 500 ml. PIP was 42 cm H_2O. Arterial blood gases showed $PaO_2 = 65$, $PCO_2 = 34$, pH = 7.35, and base deficit = −6. Physical examination was unchanged. [The metabolic acidosis is improving, but the hypoxemia has worsened ($PaO_2/FIO_2 = 144$), and hyperventilation persists in spite of a reduction in mechanical ventilatory support. PIP has also increased somewhat, suggesting either increased airway resistance or decreased total thoracic compliance.] During the next 2 hours, the IMV rate was reduced to 2 breaths/min. The patient's spontaneous breathing rate remained at 24, and there was no significant change in physical examination. The PIP was 45 cm H_2O and arterial blood gases were $PaO_2 = 55$, $PCO_2 = 34$, pH = 7.40, and base deficit = −4. (Hypoxemia is clearly present with continued hyperventilation and resolving metabolic acidosis. There is no clinical evidence of bronchospasm, yet PIP is increasing suggesting a further decrease in compliance [EDC = 27 ml/cm H_2O].) Chest x-ray now showed an extensive left pulmonary contusion and early parenchymal infiltrates on the right. Pulse oximetry monitoring was instituted, showing an SaO_2 of 0.88. The PEEP was incremented in 2 to 3 cm H_2O steps to 12 cm H_2O, and SaO_2 was noted to increase to 0.95. Repeat arterial blood gases were $PaO_2 = 80$, $PCO_2 = 35$, pH = 7.42, and base deficit = −1. The PIP remained at 42 cm H_2O on the same tidal volume. [The acute loss of lung functional residual capacity due to the pulmonary contusion, prolonged shock, and thoracic and abdominal injuries has responded to therapy. Oxygenation has improved somewhat ($PaO_2/FIO_2 = 178$), as has EDC (33 ml/cm H_2O), and further increases in pulmonary monitoring are not indicated at this time. However, if there is further progression of pulmonary dysfunction, PA catheterization for mixed venous blood gas analysis and hemodynamic monitoring would be indicated.]

RENAL MONITORING

The two purposes of monitoring the renal system are to assess the adequacy of cardiac output and to prevent acute renal failure. Historical information of importance regarding the renal system includes the history of underlying renal disease, nephrotoxic medications, exposure to nephrotoxic radiographic contrast media, hypotension or other hypoperfused states, severe crush injury, hemolysis, or direct injury to the urinary tract. Physical findings associated with postoperative renal complications are few, except for the external evidence of trauma to the urinary tract.

Measurement of urine output is essential in all aspects of the monitoring of the injured patient. It may often give an indication of inadequate renal perfusion due to decreased intravascular volume or low cardiac output. Unfortunately, diuresis may be induced by an osmotic load (from radiographic contrast agents or hyperglycemia), diabetes insipidus, administration of diuretics, or the presence of nonoliguric renal failure.

Biochemical tests performed on blood and urine are the most sensitive indicators of abnormalities in renal function. Since critical illness is associated with factors causing great variability in urea synthesis, blood urea nitrogen is of little value as a reliable monitor of renal function. Serum creatinine is a better indicator of overall renal function but also is affected by muscle mass, catabolic stress, rhabdomyolysis, and glomerular filtration. Calculation of creatinine clearance (in the presence of a stable serum creatinine) will give an indication of the approximate glomerular filtration rate.

Alterations in renal function may be divided into prerenal, renal intrinsic, or postrenal causes. More than 80 percent of patients with postoperative oliguria have a prerenal etiology. Two to fifteen percent of patients with oliguria have a postrenal obstructive cause. Appropriate urethral catheterization can eliminate bladder outlet obstruction as a cause and is an essential diagnostic tool to rule out postrenal causes for oliguria.

The most difficult and common differential diagnosis is between prerenal and renal intrinsic causes for azotemia. Assessment of renal tubular function by measuring urine sodium and osmolality is the key to differentiate between renal intrinsic and prerenal causes of oliguria. Calculation of free water clearance and the fraction of excreted sodium may provide additional information for the interpretation of these numbers [29,30]. The interpretation of tests of tubular function is predicated on two conditions. First, the patient must be oliguric (i.e., urine output < 0.5 ml/kg/hr). Second, the patient must not have had loop diuretics in the 6 to 12 hours preceding the test. The administration of loop diuretics interferes with tubular function in a manner that will bias the test in the direction of favoring a diagnosis of renal intrinsic disorders (Table 19-5). While these tests are often useful to distinguish prerenal from intrinsic failure, the complex interplay of many factors makes the absolute value of these tests less significant [31].

Table 19-5. Differential Diagnosis of Azotemia

Parameter	Prerenal	Renal
Specific gravity	1.015–1.030	1.010 (fixed)
Urine osmolality	>500	<350
Urine-plasma osmolality ratio	>1.3:1	<1.1:1
Urine sodium	<20	>40
Fraction excreted sodium	<1%	>2%
Free water clearance	Negative	Zero

CASE 1 (CONTINUED). ACUTE RENAL FAILURE

Eighteen hours postoperatively, the patient's blood pressure was 110/80 and pulse 120. There was cyclic variation in systolic blood pressure during mechanical ventilations. Urine output had been 40 ml/hr for the last 6 hours but then dropped to 20 ml/hr. Since surgery, the patient had received 3 liters of crystalloid solution and passed 1200 ml of urine. Physical examination was unchanged. Urinalysis showed 3+ glycosuria since surgery; specific gravity was 1.028. Blood glucose was 450. A fluid challenge of 1000 ml IV over 20 minutes was given; 30 ml of urine was passed in the following hour. [There is evidence of hypovolemia secondary to inadequate fluid administration and an osmotic diuresis postoperatively caused by hyperglycemia. The low BP, tachycardia, cyclic variation with ventilation, and oliguria suggest hypovolemia may be present. The poor response to a fluid challenge is concerning but may indicate that the problem was more severe than anticipated or that the fluid challenge was too little.] Two more liters of crystalloid were given over the next hour, but urine output remained at 20 to 30 ml/hr. Urine sodium was 25 mEq/L, osmolality was 500 mOsm/kg, and free water clearance was negative. [The laboratory data suggest a prerenal cause for the oliguria in spite of the fluid boluses.] A PA catheter was placed to assess cardiovascular function. Initial values were PAOP = 8 mm Hg, CVP = 10 mm Hg, cardiac output = 6.0 L/min, LVSWI = 56 gm·m/m^2, and SVR = 1400 dyne s cm^{-5}. [The data are compatible with mild vasoconstriction and low left ventricular filling pressures.] Hematocrit at this time was 24 ml/dl. The diagnosis of postoperative bleeding was made, and 3 units of packed RBCs were given. Urine output increased to 50 ml/hr, heart rate decreased to 90, and blood pressure increased to 130/80. [The PA catheter was used to aid in the diagnosis and therapy of postoperative oliguria in a patient who has sustained prolonged shock and had acute respiratory failure. The utility of PA catheterization increases with the complexity of the clinical situation.]

MONITORING OF OTHER SYSTEMS

The monitoring and fine tuning of other systems (see Table 19-1) is what distinguishes mediocre intensive care from comprehensive intensive care. While it is beyond the scope of this chapter to discuss monitoring of these other systems in great detail, the approach should be a systematic review of each of the systems in a degree sufficient to detect compromise of any of the systems and a time in which organ system failure may be prevented. The monitoring of these systems is dictated by the severity of the illness of the patient and the underlying medical illnesses.

REFERENCES

1. Blaisdell, F. W. General Assessment, Resuscitation and Exploration of Penetrating and Blunt Abdominal Trauma. In F. W. Blaisdell and D. D. Trunkey (eds.), *Trauma Management*. Vol. 1, Abdominal Trauma. New York: Thieme-Stratton, 1982.
2. Nelson, L. D. Management of shock. *Acute Care Therap.* 2:1, 1986.
3. Nelson, L. D. Mixed Venous Oximetry. In J. V. Snyder and M. R. Pinsky (eds.), *Oxygen Transport in the Critically Ill.* Chicago: Year Book, 1987.
4. Lee, J., Wright, F., Barber, R., et al. Central venous oxygen saturation in shock: A study in man. *Anesthesiology* 36:472, 1972.
5. Lewis, F. J., and Quinn, M. L. Continuous electrocardiogram monitoring in a surgical intensive care unit. *Crit. Care Med.* 5:73, 1977.
6. Tenzer, M. L. The spectrum of myocardial contusion: A review. *J. Trauma* 25:620, 1985.
7. Frazee, R. C., Mucha, P., Farnell, M. B., et al. Objective evaluation of blunt cardiac trauma. *J. Trauma* 26:510, 1986.
8. Henschke, C. I., Pasternack, G. S., Schroeder, S., et al. Bedside chest radiography: Diagnostic efficacy. *Radiology* 149:23, 1983.
9. Nelson, L. D. Monitoring and Measurement in Shock. In J. Barret and L. M. Nyhus (eds.), *Treatment of Shock: Principles and Practice.* Philadelphia: Lea & Febiger, 1986.
10. Nelson, L. D., and Civetta, J. M. Surgical Intensive Care and Perioperative Monitoring. In A. P. Monaco, R. S. Jones, P. Elbert, et al. (eds.), *Textbook of Surgery.* New York: Macmillan, in press, 1988.
11. Civetta, J. M. Invasive Catheterization. In W. C. Shoemaker and W. L. Thompson (eds.), *Critical Care: State of the Art* (Vol. 1). Fullerton: Society of Critical Care California Medicine, 1980.
12. Nelson, L. D., and Snyder, J. V. Technical Problems with Data Acquisition. In J. V. Snyder and M. R. Pinsky (eds.), *Oxygen Transport in the Critically Ill.* Chicago: Year Book, 1987.
13. Civetta, J. M., Gabel, J. C., and Laver, M. B. Disparate ventricular function in surgical patients. *Surg. Forum* 22:136, 1971.
14. Toussaint, G. P., Burgess, J. H., and Hampson, L. G. Central venous pressure and pulmonary wedge pressure in critical surgical illness. *Arch. Surg.* 109:265, 1974.
15. DeLaurentis, D. A., Hayes, M., Matsumoto, T., et al. Does central venous pressure accurately reflect hemodynamic and fluid volume patterns in the critically ill surgical patient? *Am. J. Surg.* 126:414, 1973.
16. Hartong, J. M., and Dixon, R. S. Monitoring resuscitation in the injured patient. *J.A.M.A.* 237:242, 1977.
17. Wilson, R. F., Sarver, E., and Birks, R. Central venous pressure and blood volume determinations in clinical shock. *Surg. Gynecol. Obstet.* 132:631, 1971.
18. Brisman, R., Parks, L. C., and Benson, D. W. Pitfalls in the use of central venous pressure. *Arch. Surg.* 95:902, 1967.
19. Rubin, L. R., and Bongiovi, J. Central venous pressure: An unreliable guide to fluid therapy in burns. *Arch. Surg.* 100:269, 1970.
20. Connors, A. F., McCaffree, D. R., and Gray, B. A. Evaluation of right heart catheterization in the critically ill patient without myocardial infarction. *N. Engl. J. Med.* 308:263, 1983.
21. Nelson, L. D. Continuous venous oximetry in critically ill surgical patients. *Ann. Surg.* 203:329, 1986.
22. Kasnitz, P., Druger, G. L., Yorra, F., et al. Mixed venous oxygen tension and hyperlactatemia: Survival in severe cardiopulmonary disease. *J.A.M.A.* 236:570, 1976.
23. Bekemeyer, W. B., Crapo, R. O., Calhoon, S., et al. Efficacy of chest radiography in a respiratory intensive care unit. *Chest* 88:691, 1985.
24. Nelson, L. D. Monitoring Lung Injury. In B. Chernow and W. C. Shoemaker (eds.), *Critical*

Care: State of the Art (Vol. 8). Fullerton: The Society of Critical Care Medicine, 1987.
25. Bone, R. C. Compliance and dynamic characteristics curves in acute respiratory failure. *Crit. Care Med.* 4:173, 1976.
26. Milic-Emili, J., and Ploysongsang, Y. Respiratory mechanics in the adult respiratory distress syndrome. *Crit. Care Clin.* 2:573, 1986.
27. Horowitz, H. H., Carrico, C. J., and Shires, G. T. Pulmonary response to major injury. *Arch. Surg.* 108:349, 1974.
28. New, W. Pulse oximetry. *J. Clin. Monit.* 1:126, 1985.
29. Brown, R., Babcock, R., Talbert, J., et al. Renal function in critically ill postoperative patients: Sequential assessment of creatinine, osmolat, and free water clearance. *Crit. Care Med.* 8:68, 1980.
30. Schrier, R. W., Acute renal failure. *J.A.M.A.* 247:2518, 1982.
31. Zarich, S., Fang, L. S. T., and Diamond, J. R. Fractional excretion of sodium: Exceptions to its diagnostic value. *Arch. Intern. Med.* 145:108, 1985.

SUGGESTED READINGS

Barrett, J., and Nyhus, L. M. (eds.). *Treatment of Shock: Principles and Practice* (2nd ed.). Philadelphia: Lea & Febiger, 1986.
Nelson, L. D. Monitoring Lung Injury. In B. Chernow and W. C. Shoemaker (eds.), *Critical Care: State of the Art* (Vol. 8). Fullerton: The Society of Critical Care Medicine, 1987.
Snyder, J. V., and Pinsky, M. R. (eds.). *Oxygen Transport in the Critically Ill.* Chicago: Year Book, 1987.
Sprung, C. L. (ed.). *The Pulmonary Artery Catheter: Methodology and Clinical Applications.* Baltimore: University Park Press, 1983.

20

Trauma and Multiple Organ Failure: The Clinical Challenge

Christopher C. Baker
Linda C. Degutis

Trauma, with its unpredictable and devastating impact on individuals and society, continues to provide clinical challenges to surgeons. Initial experience with large numbers of trauma cases in this century occurred in World Wars I and II, in which hemorrhagic shock was the major cause of battlefield fatalities [1,2]. As a result, the importance of volume resuscitation in hemorrhagic shock became established, initially by Blalock [3] and later by Shires [4]. During the Korean War [5] and early in the Vietnam War [6], as better resuscitation of hemorrhagic shock occurred, larger numbers of soldiers developed acute renal failure, with a mortality of 50 percent [5]. In the 1970s, the late causes of death in both civilian and military trauma patients shifted to pulmonary failure [6,7] and adult respiratory distress syndrome (ARDS). More recently, multiple organ failure (MOF) and sepsis [8,9] have developed as major problems. Recent data suggest that late deaths following trauma constitute roughly 20 percent of trauma deaths [10] and that 75 to 80 percent of these late deaths are due to sepsis and/or MOF [8].

The area of MOF and sepsis is extremely complex, multifactorial, and still incompletely understood despite multiple clinical and basic laboratory studies. An exhaustive review of MOF and sepsis following trauma is beyond the scope of a single chapter, and the interested reader is referred to Suggested Readings for more detail. The goals of this chapter are as follows:

1. To characterize the MOF syndrome.
2. To present illustrative cases of patients with MOF with comments on their management.
3. To describe strategies to prevent MOF and/or to treat it when it arises.
4. To make some suggestions for future clinical and research efforts in this area.

CHARACTERIZATION OF MULTIPLE ORGAN FAILURE

Multiple organ failure is really a by-product of improvements in the management of critically ill and injured patients. Prior to 1970, these patients generally died early of hemorrhagic shock or single organ failure (SOF)—most commonly of the lung or kidney. Nonetheless, improvements in surgery, anesthesia, resuscitation techniques, ventilatory management, pharmacologic support, nutritional support, dialysis techniques, and intensive care management have led to the salvage of patients who then are at risk for developing MOF. Baue [11] was one of the first authors to describe the sequential nature of various organ systems failing in patients with MOF. Somewhat earlier, Tilney and coworkers [12] had identified this pattern in patients undergoing surgery for ruptured abdominal aortic aneurysms; Eisman and colleagues [13] later analyzed MOF in a diverse group of 42 patients. In the early writings on this subject, several key concepts emerged: (1) patients often had shock or major injury occur shortly before MOF (early), or they developed MOF later, often in association with sepsis; (2) previous medical diseases (especially chronic obstructive pulmonary disease [COPD], atherosclerotic cardiovascular disease, diabetes mellitus, or cirrhosis) placed patients at higher risk for developing MOF or hastened its progression; (3) organs tended to fail in a sequential or cascade fashion; (4) the etiology of MOF was (and still is) multifactorial and poorly understood; and (5) the mortality rate was high for MOF and rose exponentially toward 100 percent when four or more organs had failed. A partial list of risk factors for MOF is shown in Table 20-1.

As the pattern of MOF has been observed, it is clear that patients with MOF have a severe metabolic insult, often have been subjected to a clinical error of omission (e.g., missed esophageal injury) or commission (24 of 42

Table 20-1. Risk Factors for MOF

Premorbid diseases
Chronic obstructive pulmonary disease
Adult onset diabetes mellitus
Cirrhosis
Cancer
Peripheral vascular disease/coronary artery disease
Injury-related factors
Major trauma
Major thermal injury
Soft-tissue crush injury
Major surgery
Drug overdose
Physiologic states
Prolonged shock
Hypotension
Hypothermia
Treatment factors
Massive blood transfusions
Prolonged immobilization
Nosocomial devices
Antibiotic abuse
Inadequate nutritional support
Steroids
Immunosuppressive drugs
Complications
Untreated sepsis
Coagulopathies
Necrotic tissue
Nosocomial infection

patients in the series by Eiseman and colleagues [13]), and have sepsis as a concomitant problem 50 [9] to 75 percent [8,13] of the time. Intra-abdominal sepsis was identified in 22 of the 29 patients with sepsis and MOF in the series by Eiseman and colleagues [13], and this point has been emphasized more recently by Fry and associates [14]. As more data have accumulated, investigators have examined the prognosis of MOF. Recently, Knaus and coworkers [15], in a large, multicenter study of 5677 intensive care unit (ICU) patients, correlated mortality with the number of organs failing and the number of days in MOF. In this study, when organ failure had persisted for more than 4 days, the mortality was 40 percent for SOF, 56 percent when two organs failed, and 100 percent for MOF [15].

Characterization of MOF has been very difficult and has been attempted by a number of authors [8,9,13–15]. Clinically, this process has been largely phenomenologic. In terms of basic research, most of the studies have examined various mediators of inflammation [16] and coagulation [17] as they relate to MOF. These issues will be discussed later in this section.

An outline for characterization of MOF is presented in Table 20-2. As can be seen, clinical, radiographic, laboratory, and pathologic findings are listed for the various organs involved in MOF. In addition, an attempt has been made to list the organs in the order in which they fail, although this sequence may often vary in specific patients. It should be noted that the diagnosis of MOF is usually suspected on clinical grounds and confirmed by radiographic and laboratory studies. For organs such as the lung and kidney, the diagnosis of organ failure can often be made quite specifically; in other cases (e.g., immune and gastrointestinal systems), the abnormalities are often clinical or inferential. Nonetheless, this characterization is offered as a framework to aid clinicians in thinking about patients with suspected MOF.

Efforts to describe and delineate the basic pathophysiologic alterations and mechanisms underlying MOF have been complex and confusing. Much of the difficulty in this area arises from the multifactorial nature of MOF and the complex interactions of the immune and coagulation systems. A stylized diagram of the sequence of events in MOF is represented in Figure 20-1. Injury places metabolic demands on the individual that set the stage for upsetting the balance of homeostasis. Sepsis is often the underlying factor that tips the scale in favor of organ failure. Several candidates exist as mediators of MOF. One of the early manifestations of MOF is a defect in oxygen utilization with an elevation of the lactate-pyruvate ratio [18]. It is probable that the pathogenesis of MOF is "the biologic summation of numerous humoral mediators," as stated by Fry [19]. Two of the more prominent mediators studied have been interleukin-1 and prostaglandins. It is clear from studies by Clowes and colleagues [20] that interleukin-1 can cause fever, proteolysis, and an acute phase response as is often seen in sepsis. Other authors have demonstrated elevated levels of thromboxane B_2 [21] and 6-ketoprostaglandin F_{1a} [22] in patients dying of sepsis. Some preliminary data exist that indomethacin treatment, which suppresses production

Table 20-2. Characterization of Multiple Organ Failure

Organ system	Clinical findings	Radiographic findings	Laboratory findings	Pathologic findings
Respiratory	Tachypnea Dyspnea Cyanosis	Interstitial edema (early) Diffuse alveolar infiltrates/ consolidation (late)	$PaO_2 \leq 50$ ($FIO_2 > 0.6$) $PaCO_2 \geq 55$ Compliance 50 cc/cm $QS/QT \geq 0.3$ $VD/VT \geq 0.6$	↑ Lung weight (≥ 1000 gm) Congestive atelectasis Hyaline membranes Fibrosis (late)
Renal	Oliguria or polyuria Hypervolemia Peripheral edema	Renal scan (↓ blood flow and/or excretion) IVP (↓ excretion) Ultrasound (occasionally hydronephrosis)	Urine S.G. ≤ 1.010 Urinary casts BUN ≥ 100 mg/dl U_{Na} ≥ 20 mEq/L Cr ≥ 3.5 mg/dl $K^+ \geq 5.0$ mEq/L	Acute tubular necrosis (early) ↑ Kidney weight Tubular casts Cortical necrosis (late)
Immune	Disorientation Temperature ≥ 101°F ≤ 97°F DIC	Pneumonia Intra-abdominal abscess Occult abscess (bone, brain)	WBC ≥ 13,000 ≤ 3000 Glucose ≥ 250 Platelet count ≤ 50,000 Abnormal immunologic studies	Septic emboli Peritonitis Pulmonary infiltrates Endocardial vegetations Brain abscesses
Hepatic	Jaundice Encephalopathy Coagulopathy	Liver-spleen scan (↓ uptake) HIDA scan (↓ excretion)	Bilirubin ≥ 3 mg/dl AST ≥ 500 U/ml PT ≥ 15 sec Alk phos ≥ 200 U/ml	Bile stasis (early) Centrilobular inflammation and/ or necrosis Periportal fibrosis (late)

Gastrointestinal (GI)	GI bleeding Ileus	Ileus pattern Intramural air (late)	N/A	Loss of villi (early) Submucosal hemorrhage (late)
Coagulation	DIC	N/A	Platelet count $\leqslant$ 40,000/mm PT $\geqslant$ 15 sec PTT $\geqslant$ 55 sec Fibrinogen $\leqslant$ FSP	Intravascular and intrapulmonary microaggregates (early) Intersitial hemorrhage—various organs (late)
Cardiovascular	Hypotension Congestive failure Dysrhythmias	Cardiomegaly Pulmonary edema	PCW $\geqslant$ 25 mm Hg CI $\leqslant$ 1.5 L/min/m^2 $\dot{Q}S/\dot{Q}T \geqslant 0.3$	Cardiac contusion (early) Myofibrillar disruption Subendocardial infarction (late)
Neurologic	Decreased mental status Obtundation GCS $\leqslant$ 6	Variable and nonspecific	ICP $\geqslant$ 30 cm H_2O	Nonspecific Interstitial edema (early) Hemorrhage/infarction (late)

PaO_2 = arterial oxygen tension; $PaCO_2$ = arterial carbon dioxide tension; QS/QT = shunt fraction; VD/VT = dead space to tidal volume ratio; IVP = intravenous pyelogram; S.G. = specific gravity; BUN = blood urea nitrogen; Cr = serum creatinine; K^+ = serum potassium; FSP = fibrin split products; CT = computed tomography; ICP = intracranial pressure; U_{Na} = urinary sodium; HIDA = ^{99m}Tc–dimethyl iminodiacetic acid; AST = aspartate aminotransferase; PT = prothrombin time; Alk phos = alkaline phosphate; N/A = not applicable; PCW = pulmonary capillary wedge pressure; CI = cardiac index; DIC = disseminated intravascular coagulation; PTT = Partial thromboplastin time; GCS = Glasgow Coma Scale.

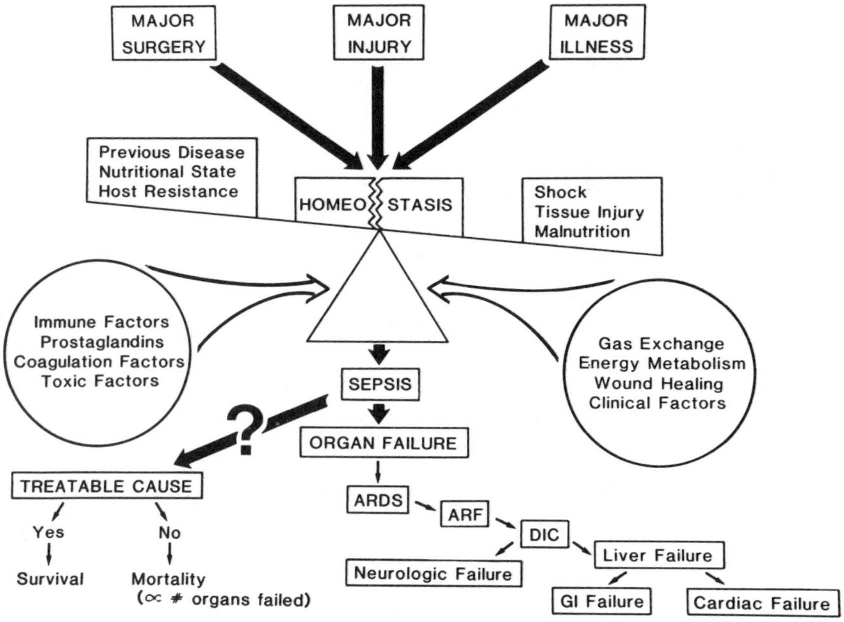

Fig. 20-1. This schematic depicts the major factors leading to disruption of homeostasis, setting the stage for sepsis and MOF. ARDS = adult respiratory disease syndrome; ARF = acute renal failure; DIC = disseminated intravascular coagulation; GI = gastrointestinal.

of thromboxane and 6-ketoprostaglandin F_{1a}, may be protective in a rat fecal peritonitis model [23].

A number of other possible etiologies of MOF have been suggested. Complement activation, leading to leukocyte aggregation and release of vasoactive amines, may be the initial event leading to defects in oxygen delivery and MOF [24]. The coagulation cascade, interacting with plasminogen activator from macrophage, may also be an inciting event for MOF in the microcirculation [25]. Meakins and Marshall [26] have suggested that the gastrointestinal tract following critical illness may cease to be an effective barrier to microorganisms and endotoxin. Unfortunately, it is hard to tell whether this breakdown is occurring as a primary cause of MOF or occurs as a result of MOF. It may be that bacterial translocation across the gut leads to Kupffer cell dysfunction [27]. Finally, activation of polymorphonuclear leukocytes, with generation of oxygen radicals and proteases, has clearly been shown to be related to organ failure in ARDS [28]. As pointed out by Maier [29], the macrophage may also be a central effector cell in the genesis of MOF, by virtue of its production of vasoactive mediators (e.g., thromboxane A_2, prostaglandin E_2, leukotrienes C_4 and D_4), chemotactic agents (e.g., LTB_4 and C_5a), proteases, oxygen intermediates, and procoagulant factors. The macrophage, when stimulated with endotoxin, can be a particularly potent stimulus to microvascular thrombosis [30], thereby leading to oxygen deficits and MOF. Finally, more recent studies have suggested that the endothelial cell, by producing vasoactive amines and oxygen radicals, may actually play a more active role in MOF than was previously realized [31]. Although newer studies are coming to light each day, it is clear that our understanding of the basic pathophysiology of MOF is still rather rudimentary. Significant breakthroughs will be required before we can hope to prevent MOF by therapeutic alterations in host response.

CLINICAL CASES OF MULTIPLE ORGAN FAILURE

As will be discussed later, we seem to be seeing fewer patients dying of MOF as prehospital and early hospital care of trauma patients improves [32]. The most important factors accounting for this apparent decline include endotracheal intubation and ventilation in the prehospital phase, early and rapid resuscitation from shock, and aggressive ICU care. Nonetheless, selected patients still do develop MOF, and undoubtedly small numbers will continue to do so. This section is devoted to a discussion of two such patients, with comments addressing illustrative points of MOF as a clinical challenge.

CASE 1

A 34-year-old white man was admitted to the ICU at 5:30 A.M. following a motor vehicle crash. He was thrown 25 feet from the vehicle he was driving and landed flat on his back. He was hypotensive with a systolic blood pressure (BP) of 70 mm Hg and was paraplegic at the scene. On arrival in the emergency room with the MAST inflated and an IV of Ringer's lactate infusing, initial BP was 90 mm Hg systolic. Physical examination revealed good breath sounds bilaterally, a distended abdomen, paraplegia with a T3 sensory level, multiple abrasions, and soft tissue contusions. Chest x-ray demonstrated haziness in both lung fields, multiple bilateral rib fractures, and a vertebral fracture with subluxation at T3. Initial arterial blood gases (ABGs) on room air were pH 7.23, $PaCO_2$ 38, and PaO_2 57. ABGs on 100% oxygen were pH 7.22, $PaCO_2$ 31, and PaO_2 82. Urinalysis was positive for blood, but intravenous pyelogram was normal. A computed tomography (CT) scan of the chest showed the T3 fracture and pulmonary contusions (Fig. 20-2A). The patient was intubated and transferred to the ICU.

A Neo-Synephrine drip was initiated to maintain the patient's BP above 100 Mm Hg systolic. During the night, he spiked a temperature to 101.4°F, and breath sounds were absent almost three-fourths of the way up the thorax bilaterally with coarse ronchi centrally. His urine output remained stable at 40 to 50 ml/hr (specific gravity 1.030–1.035). The patient extubated himself in the morning of the second hospital day (HD 2) and was reintubated. On HD 3, he developed a brief episode of hypotension (systolic BP 30) and bradycardia. His PaO_2 was 30. Chest x-ray revealed a large left pneumothorax. After placement of a chest tube, which immediately drained 300 ml of serosanguinous fluid, his ABGs were pH 7.47, $PaCO_2$ 32, and PaO_2 420. Over the next several days, he continued to have ventilatory problems despite increasing amounts of pos-

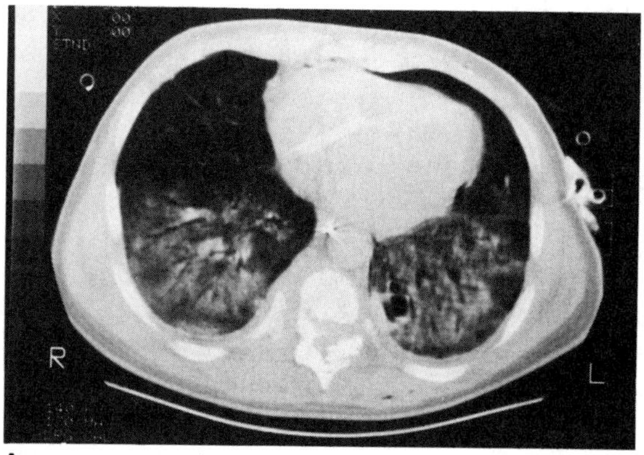

A

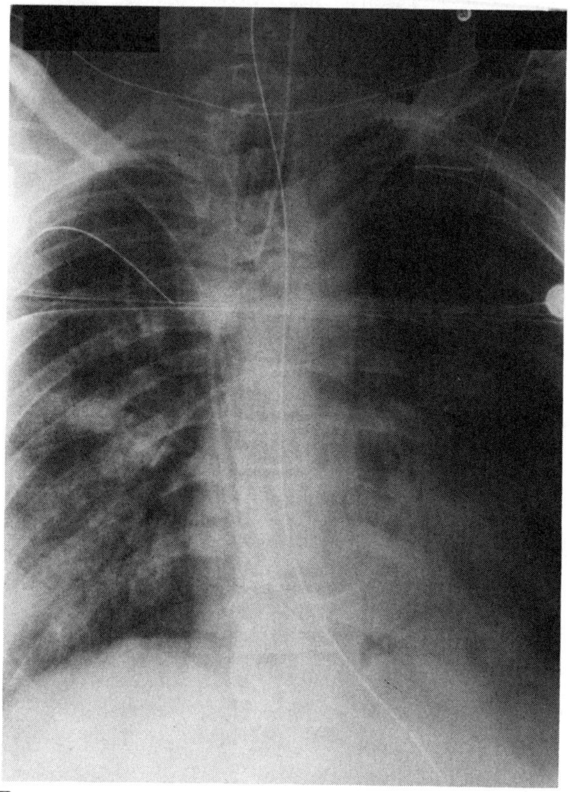

B

Fig. 20-2. Case 1. *A.* This CT scan of the chest demonstrates the major disruption of the third thoracic vertebra with bony fragments in the spinal canal. In addition, severe bilateral pulmonary contusions are seen. *B.* A portable chest film taken 5 days postinjury shows bilateral fluffy infiltrates characteristic of ARDS.

itive end-expiratory pressure (PEEP). An example of a chest film taken on HD 5 is shown in Figure 20-2B. On HD 5, a sputum culture grew 4+ *Staphylococcus aureus,* and 4+ streptococci. His urine output decreased, and urine studies showed osmolarity 736, potassium 92, sodium less than 10, and creatinine 110. Serum creatinine was 2.1, and blood urea nitrogen (BUN) was 40. A renal angiogram demonstrated very slow renal flow with persistence of contrast in renal vessels. The creatinine and BUN continued to rise, and ventilatory problems persisted. By HD 7, MOF was full-blown, with sepsis, disseminated intravascular coagulation (DIC), renal failure, and respiratory compromise. Dialysis was performed and antibiotic therapy initiated. Nonetheless, the patient began to develop hypotension and bradycardia whenever he was disconnected from the ventilator for suctioning. On HD 9, ventilatory function and gas exchange had deteriorated, with continued renal impairment and sepsis. The patient was placed on high-frequency jet ventilation (rate = 150, FIO_2 = 65, PEEP = 20, I/E = 0.45:0.55, driving pressure = 35). On HD 11, he sustained a cardiac arrest shortly after a necessary endotracheal tube change. Maximum resuscitation with closed chest cardiac massage resulted in electromechanical dissociation. The left chest was opened, and cardiac activity returned with internal massage. The patient was epinephrine dependent with a tenuous rhythm and BP for 2 to 3 hours. At this point, he became hypotensive, bradycardic, and then asystolic despite epinephrine and a pacing wire. The family was aware of the situation and requested that no further heroic measures be taken, and he expired on HD 12.

An autopsy was performed by the medical examiner that revealed the lungs to weigh 1600 g (right) and 1610 g (left) with uniform consolidation throughout. Copious quantities of cloudy edema fluid flowed from the cut sections. There was an area of advanced change in the posteromedial left lung field with a 4 × 2 × 2 cm pocket of completely necrotic, red, softened, semiliquid lung tissue. The liver weighed 2230 g, with no focal lesions or evidence of fibrosis. The spleen weighed 230 g, with an extremely soft and near-liquified parenchyma. The gastric mucosa was partially autolyzed. The kidneys weighed 270 g (right) and 280 g (left) and exhibited mottled cortical surfaces. On cut section, 90 to 95 percent of the cortex was yellow with a hemorrhagic border between the cortex and the medulla. The brain weighed 1400 g and was mildly swollen, with closure of the sulci and ventricles. The cause of death was determined to be MOF secondary to trauma (fractures of the thoracic spine and severe pulmonary contusions).

This patient represented the first death from MOF secondary to trauma in 11 months during a recent academic year. Although he would have had a high-level paraplegia, his death left his wife a widow and was frustrating to us all. His ARDS was clearly related to his severe bilateral pulmonary contusions, but it is unclear what therapeutic changes might have reversed the situation. Should he have had earlier institution of jet ventilation? Should negative pressure ventilation (e.g., "iron lung") have been tried? These are the imponderable questions. The etiology of his renal failure is also quite unclear. There may have been some nephrotoxicity from contrast studies, but he was well hydrated. The severe postmortem changes in the kidneys are hard to explain. It may be that this patient had a sudden massive increase in microvascular pressures in multiple organs due to the high kinetic energy transferred at the time of injury. The authors feel that this hypothesis may have some validity in selected patients and may shed some light on the clinical course of this patient and the next patient to be described.

CASE 2

A 37-year-old white man crashed into a tidal river while flying his stunt plane. He was found partially submerged. There was a 1-hour delay in transport to the hospital due to difficulties in access to the patient and extrication. He was brought to the emergency room unconscious with his third liter of Ringer's lactate infusing, MAST on and inflated, and a systolic BP of 70 mm Hg. Physical examination revealed multiple soft tissue injuries, including a partial avulsion of his right ear. He had decreased breath sounds on the right but was moving air bilaterally. Abdominal examination was normal. Chest x-ray revealed diffuse pulmonary contusions bilaterally. He also had a left compound tibial fracture. The patient was taken to CT scan and was alert and responsive with a BP of 120/60 mm Hg at that time. After moving to the CT table, he became unresponsive to deep pain, with a systolic BP of 70 mm Hg. He was intubated and placed on the ventilator at this time. CT of the head showed mild to moderate diffuse hypodensity with small ventricles. The initial hematocrit was 31.8, a second hematocrit was 25.5, and a third hematocrit was 12.

The patient was taken to the operating room for an exploratory laparotomy and placement of feeding gastrostomy. A large retroperitoneal hematoma was found, but he had no intra-abdominal injuries. His soft tissue wounds were repaired, and a Hoffman apparatus was placed on his left leg.

On postoperative day 1 (POD 1), the patient experienced a rapid deterioration of ABGs, requiring an FIO_2 of 100% and PEEP of 18. Despite this, his ABGs remained poor (pH 7.22, $PaCO_2$ 43, PaO_2 53). A bronchoscopy was done and showed a small amount of bloody fluid in the right upper lobe. Chest x-ray showed a patchy infiltrate on the left with total opacification of the right lung field. He was placed on ampicillin, gentamicin, and cefamandole, and fluid resuscitation continued. Systolic BP was 80 to 100 mm Hg and responded to dopamine and fluid. He developed increased hematuria and an elevated serum creatinine. Urine output improved with mannitol. On POD 4, his clinical status deteriorated, with a BP drop to 70 mm Hg. BP continued to drop despite adequate filling pressures and pressors. He had decreased white blood cell and platelet counts, with a fever and further deterioration of renal function. Dopamine was given without response, epinephrine and Neo-Synephrine drips were started, and his BP remained in the 60s. Chest x-ray showed aeration bilaterally without pneumothorax. Treatment with epinephrine, Neo-Synephrine, sodium bicarbonate, naloxone, increased FIO_2, and increased ventilatory support was unsuccessful. The patient experienced a cardiac arrest, resuscitative measures were unsuccessful, and he expired late on POD 4.

An autopsy was performed by the medical examiner. Lungs weighed 1600 g (right) and 1440 g (left) and were firm and rubbery throughout. There was no evidence of pulmonary embolus. The liver weighed 1960 g and exhibited a nutmeg pattern on cut section. The spleen weighed 220 g. The kidneys weighed 210 g (right) and 200 g (left), with swollen and pale renal cortices. The brain weighed 1560 g and was moderately swollen, with closure of sulci and slight closure of the ventricles. The cause of death was determined to be multiple fractures and soft tissue injuries with accompanying sepsis.

This patient had a delay in transport and a delay in performance of laparotomy that may have set the stage for his subsequent deterioration. On the other hand, his initial salvage was a major triumph given his multiple injuries superimposed on aspiration and significant saltwater drowning. In addition, the laparotomy did not show an ongoing bleeding source that might have mandated an earlier laparotomy. This rapid, fulminant pattern of organ failure and death (within 4 days of injury) is less common than the more slowly progressive type of MOF exemplified by patient 1. It is unclear why patients follow one pattern or the other. Obviously more rapid transport should have occurred in patient 2, but the authors are not sure that this would have changed the ultimate outcome. Some of the issues raised by these two patients constitute the challenges facing clinicians who care for patients with MOF.

STRATEGIES FOR PREVENTING AND TREATING MOF

Clearly, clinicians must continue to grapple with the challenge of caring for patients with MOF. Since care of specific SOF has been outlined elsewhere, and since the mortality of treated MOF is so high, most of this section will be devoted to discussing strategies for preventing MOF.

The major goal in preventing MOF must be to block or avoid factors that stimulate the generation of the multiple mediators that lead to MOF. Although it sounds rather simplistic, the two most important early aspects in prevention of MOF are airway control (oxygenation, intubation, and ventilation) and prompt resuscitation of patients from hypovolemic shock. Although many clinicians have noted that prolonged shock is a major risk factor for the subsequent development of sepsis and MOF, few basic scientific studies have addressed this issue. Several years ago, Baker and Miller [33] correlated a depression in immunocompetence following shock with later sepsis, but a causal relationship remains to be established. The care of critically ill surgical patients is complex, expensive, and labor-intensive and requires a major institutional commitment of resources and personnel. Since numerous books have been written on this subject (see Suggested Readings), only salient issues will be emphasized here.

First and foremost, it must be emphasized that ICU care of these patients requires a systems approach directed at maintaining or restoring physiologic organ function. To achieve this goal, a team composed of physicians, nurses, respiratory therapists, pharmacists, and consultants must work together cooperatively and must pay compulsive attention to detail.

An outline of strategies for meeting the clinical challenge of MOF is presented in Table 20-3. The lung is listed first, since it is often the first organ to fail. Recent evidence suggests that although the lung may initially be *affected* by organ failure, it may subsequently become an *effector* organ—leading to MOF through the elaboration of various vasoactive, inflammatory, and immunologic mediators [29,34]. Therefore, restoration and preservation of normal pulmonary homeostasis must assume a very high priority in the clinical management of ICU patients at risk of developing MOF. Aggressive chest physiotherapy, early mechanical ventilation (often with PEEP), and early patient mobilization (often with internal fixation of fractures) are some of the key ingredients for success in averting ARDS.

A number of "do's and don'ts" are listed for other organ systems in Table 20-3. Several areas deserve special emphasis. Because of the immunosuppressive effects of major injury [35–37], strict asepsis must be practiced

Table 20-3. Strategies for Clinical Care of MOF

Organ system	Problem	Prevention/treatment
Lung	Atelectasis/edema/fibrosis	1. Chest PT 2. PEEP 3. Early mobilization 4. ?PGE_1/?NSAID
Kidney	Acute tubular necrosis	1. Optimal resuscitation 2. Avoid nephrotic agents 3. Avoid diuretics 4. ?ATP-$MgCl_2$
Immune system	Sepsis/immunosuppression	1. Asepsis 2. Remove contaminated liver 3. Maximize nutritional support 4. Minimize instrumentation 5. Avoid steroids 6. Avoid antibiotic abuse 7. ?NSAID/?fibronectin
Liver	Hepatocellular dysfunction	1. Avoid hepatotoxic drugs 2. Treat intra-abdominal sepsis 3. ?ATP-$MgCl_2$/?fibronectin
Gastrointestinal	Breakdown of mucosal barriers	1. Antacids 2. Promote enteral feeding 3. Oral nystatin
Coagulation	Disseminated intravascular coagulation	1. Prompt resuscitation of shock 2. Debridement of necrotic tissue 3. Reversal of hypothermia 4. ?NSAID/?heparin
Cardiovascular	Progressive pump failure	1. Prompt resuscitation of shock 2. Treatment of dysrhythmias 3. Optimize hemodynamics 4. Avoid vasopressors and diuretics
Neurologic	Progressive brain swelling	1. Evacuate hematomas 2. Treat elevated ICP 3. Optimize gas exchange 4. Minimize fluid overload 5. ?Oxygen radical scavengers
Metabolic	Progressive oxygen deficit	1. Optimize gas exchange and hemodynamics 2. Maximize nutritional support 3. ?Thyroid hormone 4. ?glutamine

PT = physiotherapy; PEEP = positive end-expiratory pressure; PGE_1 = prostaglandin E_1; NSAID = nonsteroidal anti-inflammatory drugs; ICP = intracranial pressure.

and steroids should be avoided. Optimization of early resuscitation and hemodynamic status later in the course of therapy are critical and cannot be overemphasized. Since metabolic failure is the hallmark of MOF, adequate support of caloric and energy needs assumes a very high priority. The early metabolic response to trauma precludes nutritional support in the first 48 hours, but careful metabolic planning and therapy should begin in a *prospective* fashion shortly thereafter. The metabolic changes following injury have been studied extensively [18,20,38,39], but it is still unclear what is the optimal nutritional source and route in these patients. Cerra and associates [39,40] have advocated the use of branched-chain amino acids. Although total parenteral nutrition has been the preferred technique for refeeding many trauma patients, there are some recent studies suggesting that enteral feeding may be superior [41]. If this is so, it may be due to a restoration of immunity and prevention of bacterial translocation by maintaining the mucosal barrier of the gut.

Clearly, prevention of complications is tantamount to avoiding the ravages of MOF. Aggressive surveillance for sepsis and septic foci must assume a high priority in the harsh nosocomial environment of the ICU. Numerous studies have demonstrated the fact that a disproportionate share of expense generated and resources utilized occurs in patients who subsequently die. At the Massachusetts General Hospital, Cullen and associates [42] reported that 70 percent of their most seriously ill ICU patients were dead at 1 year (57 percent in the first month), having consumed $22,000 per patient in 1978 dollars. In our experience, the mortality of ICU patients was 83 percent when ICU stay exceeded 21 days [43]. The ethical implications of these data are beyond the scope of this chapter, but these considerations face all of us involved in the care of these patients.

Is it possible to make an impact on MOF, and if so, how? Our experience at Yale suggests that it *is* possible for us to make an impact—primarily through an organized and systematic team approach to the care of the trauma patient. Prior to July 1983 at Yale–New Haven Hospital (YNHH), multiple trauma patients were shared between two general surgery services that also performed elective cases daily. Thereafter, elective patients were all placed on one service, and a dedicated trauma service was created to handle trauma patients, emergency general surgical patients, and consultations. Simultaneously, trauma protocols were implemented in the emergency service, an ICU team was created, a weekly trauma conference was begun, and all attendings and upper level residents completed the Advanced Trauma Life Support course sponsored by the American College of Surgeons. Our initial experience following this reorganization has been reported previously [32] and will be updated here. Data for trauma patients admitted to the ICU are presented in Table 20-4. For the first year, mortality of trauma patients admitted specifically to the surgical ICU fell from 21 to 6.1 percent ($p < 0.05$ by chi-square). As can be seen from Table 20-4, overall mortality for ICU patients has fallen progressively during the time of this *prospective* study. Far more importantly for

Table 20-4. Outcome Data for ICU Trauma Admissions

Group/year	Admissions (% of total)	Deaths (%)
Group I (pre–trauma service)		
7/82–6/83	193 (17.4)	31 (16.1)
Group II (trauma service)		
7/83–6/84	170 (16.6)	20 (11.8)
7/84–6/85	259 (20.6)	11 (4.2)*
7/85–6/86	175 (12.9)	7 (4.0)*

*Significantly lower than group I mortality by chi-square ($p < 0.001$).

purposes of the present discussion, both the incidence and mortality rates (decreased from 70 to 25 percent) of MOF have fallen since the creation of a dedicated trauma service. Prior to the trauma service, five of nine patients dying of MOF and sepsis were on the general surgery services, whereas none of the three patients dying of MOF in the second year of the study were on the trauma service. The number of patients dying of MOF has been maintained at this level; in fact, in the last year for which complete data are available, only *one* patient died of MOF and sepsis. It appears that this organized team approach, based on some of the sound physiologic principles previously outlined, can not only decrease the number of trauma patients who develop MOF, but also improve salvage in those who do develop MOF. Although this study is hampered somewhat by the use of historical controls, all data were gathered on a prospective basis, and clinical decisions about outcome were made independently by the authors. The two groups of trauma patients being compared in this study were similar with regard to age, sex, race, and mechanism of injury. Injury severity scores were comparable during both study periods; in fact, the mean injury severity score was higher in the trauma service group. Therefore, one can say that the two groups are comparable. Interestingly, the overall outcome data for all trauma admissions (approximately 1100 patients/year) changed very little from the first year of the study (3.4 percent) to the last (2.9 percent). Therefore, it appears that the major impact on mortality in the seriously injured patient can be made in the ICU—the battleground where the war against MOF is fought.

FUTURE CLINICAL AND RESEARCH EFFORTS

Major advances have been made in the care of trauma patients over the last four decades [3,5–6]. To some extent, MOF and sepsis are the by-products of our successes. To make strides in our battle against these formidable challenges, we must continue to work hard in the clinical arena while undertaking and cooperating with basic research in this area. This section will highlight some future directions for clinical and research efforts related to MOF.

Obviously, prevention and injury control will be key factors in decreasing the incidence of MOF [8,10]. Organization of prehospital care, emergency services, trauma services, intensive care units, and trauma systems to meet the highest standards is paramount. Clinical efforts to define and identify the patients at risk for MOF should continue.

With respect to specific organ system management, a few comments can be made. A great deal of experimental work has accumulated on the problem of ARDS. Sugerman and colleagues have demonstrated improvement of pulmonary function, but not capillary leak, with ibuprofen in the pig *Pseudomonas* ARDS model [44] and with methylprednisolone, ibuprofen, and prostacyclin following acid aspiration in dogs [45]. Recently in humans, Holcroft and coworkers [46] noted that survival following ARDS improved from 35 to 71 percent with prostaglandin E_1. It appears that therapy of established ARDS may eventually require a polypharmaceutical approach. Meanwhile, ventilatory techniques will continue to improve (witness jet ventilation). It is our bias that pulmonary contusion, as seen in both our patients presented earlier, constitutes a particularly significant risk factor. Prevention of ARDS must be our goal. This will require a better understanding of clinical risk factors and basic pathophysiologic mechanisms than is currently available.

Acute renal failure, the second great nemesis to the trauma patient, has decreased substantially as a clinical problem. Further areas for research include studies to develop a better understanding of myonecrosis, hypovolemic shock, and nephrotoxic drugs as they affect renal function. Preliminary evidence suggests that there is a protective effect of ATP-$MgCl_2$ [47], and we have had success in a couple of selected patients with this agent. It should be noted that this agent may also have a positive effect on the metabolic imbalances and Kupffer cell dysfunction seen in the liver following shock [36].

The remaining problems appear to be largely related to the activation of the various mediators. Coagulopathies must continue to be treated by removing the inciting cause. Inasmuch as the macrophage has a role to play in the clotting system through its generation of plasminogen activator, the use of nonsteroidal anti-inflammatory drugs (NSAIDs) may merit study. Clearly, in the area of immunology and sepsis, NSAIDs may have a role [36]. It may be that neurologic and other organ dysfunction may be prevented or improved with the use of free radical scavengers such as catalase and superoxide dismutase. Finally, the whole area of metabolism and nutritional support will continue to provide a fruitful area for research. In addition to branched-chain amino acids [37,40], studies of specific amino acids such as glutamine and arginine need to be done. The role of enteral versus parenteral therapy in nutritional support should be explored.

The future, as always, is hard to predict. Several things are clear, however. Human beings will continue to traumatize themselves and each other. Organ failure will continue to pose a challenge to clinicians. The answer to these problems lies both at the macrocosmic level—a systems approach to the organization of trauma care—and at the microcosmic level—cellular and subcellular mechanisms of function and dysfunction. The authors feel that the future holds exciting discoveries and advances on all these fronts in the battle against MOF and sepsis.

REFERENCES

1. Cannon, W. B. *Traumatic Shock*. New York: Appleton, 1923.
2. Cournand, A., Riley, R. L., Bradley, S. F., et al. Studies of the circulation in clinical shock. *Surgery* 13:964, 1943.

3. Brooks, B., and Blalock, A. Shock with particular reference to that due to haemorphagic and trauma to muscles. *Ann. Surg.* 100:728, 1934.
4. Shires, G. T., Carrico, C. J., and Canizaro, P. C. *Shock.* Philadelphia: Saunders, 1973.
5. Howard, J. M. (ed.). *Battle Casualties in Korea: Studies of the Surgical Research Team.* IV. Post-traumatic Renal Insufficiency. Washington, D.C.: Government Printing Office, 1955.
6. Iaian, J., Reisin, E., and Eliahou, H. Acute renal failure in combat injuries. *J. Trauma* 15:281, 1975.
7. Hardaway, R. M., III. Vietnam wound analysis. *J. Trauma* 18:635, 1978.
8. Baker, C. C., Oppenheimer, L., Stephens, B., et al. Epidemiology of trauma deaths. *Am. J. Surg.* 140:144, 1980.
9. Faist, E., Baue, A. E., Dittmer, H., et al. Multiple organ failure in polytrauma patients. *J. Trauma* 23:775, 1983.
10. Trunkey, D. D. Trauma. *Sci. Am.* 249:28, 1983.
11. Baue, A. E. Multiple, progressive, or sequential systems failure: A syndrome of the 1970's. *Arch. Surg.* 110:779, 1975.
12. Clemens, M. G., McDonough, P. F., Chaudry, I. H., et al. Hepatic microcirculatory failure following ischemia and reperfusion: Improvement with ATP-$MgCl_2$ treatment. *Am. J. Physiol.* 248:H 804, 1985.
13. Eiseman, B., Beart, R., and Norton, L. Multiple organ failure. *Surg. Gynecol. Obstet.* 144:323, 1977.
14. Fry, D. E., Pearlstein, L., Fulton, R. L., et al. Multiple system organ failure. *Arch. Surg.* 115:1316, 1980.
15. Knaus, W. A., Draper, E. A., Wagner, D. P., et al. Prognosis in acute organ-system failure. *Ann. Surg.* 202:685, 1985.
16. Pierce, C. W. Macrophages: Modulators of immunity. *Am. J. Pathol.* 98:10, 1980.
17. Graziano, C., Miller, C. L., and Lim, R. C. Role of the monocyte function in alteration of the thrombofibrinolytic system after shock. *Surg. Forum* 31:25, 1980.
18. Cerra, F. B., Siegel, J. H., Borden, J. R., et al. The hepatitic failure of sepsis: Cellular versus substrate. *Surgery* 86:409, 1979.
19. Fry, D. E. Humeral mediators of MOF. *Arch Surg.* 121:201, 1986.
20. Clowes, G. H. A., Jr., Hirsch, E., George, B. C., et al. Survival from sepsis: The significance of altered protein metabolism regulated by proteolysis including factor, the circulating cleavage product of interleukin 1. *Ann. Surg.* 202:446, 1985.
21. Reines, H. D., Haluska, P. V., Cook, J. A., et al. Plasma thromboxane levels are elevated in patients dying with septic shock. *Lancet* 2:174, 1982.
22. Haluska, P. V., Reines, H. D., Barrow, S. E., et al. Elevated plasma 6-keto-prostaglandin F-1-alpha in patients with septic shock. *Crit. Care Med.* 13:451, 1985.
23. Wise, W. C., Cook, J. A., Haluska, P. V., et al. Protective effects of thromboxane synthetase inhibitors in rats in endotoxic shock. *Circ. Res.* 46:854, 1980.
24. Craddock, P. R., Fehr, J., Brigham, K. L., et al. Complement and leukocyte-mediated pulmonary dysfunction in hemodialysis. *N. Engl. J. Med.* 296:769, 1977.
25. Takemura, R., and Werb, A. Secretory products of macrophages and their physiological functions. *Am. J. Physiol.* 256:C1, 1984.
26. Meakins, J. L., and Marshall, J. C. The gastrointestinal tract: The "motor" of MOF. *Arch. Surg.* 121:197, 1986.
27. Rogoff, T. M., and Lipsky, P. E. Role of the Kupffer cells in local and systemic immune responses. *Gastroenterology* 80:854, 1981.
28. Fantone, J. C., and Ward, P. A. Role of oxygen-derived free radicals and metabolytes in leukocyte-dependent inflammatory reactions. *Am. J. Pathol.* 107:397, 1982.
29. Maier, R. V. Multisystem organ failure. *Arch. Surg.* 121:204, 1986.
30. Maier, R. V., and Hahnel, G. B. Microthrombosis during endotoxemia: Potential role of hepatic vs. alveolar macrophages. *J. Surg. Res.* 36:362, 1984.
31. Colucci, M., Balconi, G., Lorenzet, R., et al. Cultured human endothelial cells generate tissue factor in response to endotoxin. *J. Clin. Invest.* 71:1893, 1983.
32. Baker, C. C., Degutis, L. C., DeSantis, J. S., et al. The impact of a trauma service on trauma care in a university hospital. *Am. J. Surg.* 149:453, 1985.

33. Baker, C. C., and Miller, C. L. Correlation of traumatic shock with immunocompetence and sepsis. *Surg. Forum* XXX:20, 1979.
34. R. Demling. Personal communication, 1987.
35. Baker, C. C., Miller, C. L., and Trunkey, D. D. Identity of leukocytes which compromise trauma patients' resistance. *J. Surg. Res.* 26:478, 1979.
36. Faist, E., Kupper, T. S., Baker, C. C., et al. Depression of cellular immunity after major injury: Its association with post-traumatic complications and its restoration with immunomodulating agents. *Arch. Surg.* 121:1000, 1986.
37. Miller, C. L., and Baker, C. C. Changes in lymphocyte activity after thermal injury: The role of suppressor cells. *J. Clin. Invest.* 63:202, 1979.
38. Duke, J. H., Jr., Jorgensen, S. B., Broell, J. R., et al. Contribution of protein to calorie expenditure following injury. *Surgery* 68:168, 1970.
39. McMenamy, R. H., Birkhahn, R., Oswald, G., et al. Multiple organ systems failure: I. The basal state. *J. Trauma* 21:99, 1981.
40. Cerra, F. B., Jazuski, J., Teasley, K., et al. Nitrogen retention in critically ill patients is proportional to branched chain amino acid load. *Crit. Care Med.* 11:775, 1983.
41. McMenamy, R. H., Birkhahn, R., Oswald, M. S., et al. Multiple organ systems failure: II. The effect of infusion of amino acids and glucose. *J. Trauma* 21:228, 1981.
42. Cullen, D. J., Keene, R., Waternaux, C., et al. Results, charges, and benefits of intensive care for critically injured patients: Update 1983. *Crit. Care Med.* 12:102, 1984.
43. DeSantis, J. G. The Value of Admission Parameters in Predicting Mortality and Complications in the Surgical Intensive Care Unit. M.D. thesis, Yale University, 1984.
44. Lee, C. C., Sugerman, H. J., Tatum, J. L., et al. Effects of ibuprofen in a pig *Pseudomonas* ARDS model. *J. Surg. Res.* 40:438, 1986.
45. Buchanan, S. R., Sugerman, H. J., Tatum, J. L., et al. Failure of methylprednisolone, ibuprofen, of prostacyclin to reduce HCl-induced pulmonary albumin leak in dogs. *Surgery* 96:163, 1984.
46. Holcroft, J. W., Vassar, M. J., and Webber, C. J. Prostaglandin E_1 and survival in patients with the adult respiratory distress syndrome. *Ann. Surg.* 203:371, 1986.
47. Sumpio, B. E., Hull, M. J., Baue, A. E., et al. Comparison of effects of ATP-$MgCl_2$ and adenosine-$MgCl_2$ on renal function following ischemia. *Circ. Shock* 18:375, 1986.

SUGGESTED READINGS

Blaisdell, F. W., and Lewis, F. R. *Respiratory Distress Syndrome of Shock and Trauma.* Philadelphia: Saunders, 1977.

Cerra, F. B. *Manual of Critical Care.* St. Louis: Mosby, 1987.

Kreis, D. J., Jr., and Baue, A. E. *Clinical Management of Shock.* Baltimore: University Park Press, 1984.

Moore, F. D., Lyons, J. H., Jr., Pierce, E. C., Jr., et al. *Post-Traumatic Pulmonary Insufficiency.* Philadelphia: Saunders, 1969.

Ninnemann, J. L. (ed.). *The Immune Consequences of Thermal Injury.* Baltimore: Williams & Wilkins, 1981.

Ninnemann, J. L. (ed.). *Traumatic Injury: Infection and Other Immunologic Sequelae.* Baltimore: University Park Press, 1983.

Suskind, R. M. (ed.). *Malnutrition and the Immune Response.* New York: Raven, 1977.

Unanue, E. R., and Benacenaf, B. *Textbook of Immunology* (2nd ed.). Baltimore: Williams & Wilkins, 1984.

Wilmore, D. W. *The Metabolic Management of the Critically Ill.* New York: Plenum, 1977.

21

Trauma and Nutritional Support

Patricia M. Byers

There has been a great deal of progress in the field of nutritional support since 1843 when Claude Bernard infused intravenous sugar, egg white, and milk into animals [1]. One of the major forefronts remaining involves the support of traumatized and septic patients. Whereas the work of Cuthbertson [2] established the groundwork, it was not until the last 10 to 20 years that an understanding of the altered pathways of metabolism and the development of more efficacious regimens of nutritional support for the traumatized and septic patient have evolved.

This chapter will develop some of the basic concepts of nutritional pathways and demonstrate how they differ in the injured patient. In addition, nutritional assessment and monitoring will be reviewed with emphasis on those measurements that are most important in the traumatized patient. A description of currently available therapy will be described, reviewing both parenteral and enteral formulas. Finally, the special problems involved in organ system failure will be discussed.

NUTRITIONAL PATHWAYS

Fuel Sources

There are three different organic fuel sources available to the human body. The stable, nonfasting individual utilizes carbohydrates and fats as primary fuel sources and proteins for structural and functional roles. During periods of fasting, however, tissue reserves must be mobilized. Table 21-1 demonstrates that fat in the form of triglyceride is available in the largest quantity, muscle protein is next, while limited supplies of glycogen are stored in muscle and liver [3]. The oxidation of different substrates produces varying amounts of energy per gram (Table 21-2).

Table 21-1. Fuel Composition of Normal Man

Fuel	Kg	Kilocalories
Tissues		
Fat (adipose triglyceride)	15	141,000
Protein (mainly muscle)	6	24,000
Glycogen (muscle)	0.150	600
Glycogen (liver)	0.075	300
Total		165,900
Circulating fuels		
Glucose (extracellular fluid)	0.020	80
Free fatty acids (plasma)	0.0003	3
Triglycerides (plasma)	0.003	30
Total		113

Source: Reprinted by permission from G. F. Cahill, Starvation in man. *N. Engl. J. Med.* 282:668, 1970.

Table 21-2. Caloric Energy Available from Major Substrates

Substrate	Kcal/gm
Carbohydrate	4*
Fats	9
Protein	4

*Note that the parenteral form of carbohydrate has only 3.4 kcal/gm.

Carbohydrate Metabolism

The major energy source for human tissues in the fed state is glucose; however, certain tissues such as brain, adrenal medulla, and erythrocytes utilize glucose almost exclusively [4]. Glucose may be supplied exogenously in the diet, derived from the breakdown of the stored carbohydrate through glycogenolysis, or synthesized directly from amino acids, pyruvate, glycogen, or lactate. The major metabolic pathways utilizing glucose oxidation to generate adenosine triphosphate (ATP) are glycolysis and the tricarboxylic acid cycle [5] (Fig. 21-1).

Fat Metabolism

Lipids are important to the human body primarily as a source of stored energy; however, they also play a role in structure and function [6]. Simple lipids, such as the triglycerides, are an important fuel source and are the major storage form of lipid and fatty acids (see Table 21-1).

Triglycerides are composed of three fatty acid chains that are esterified to a glycerol molecule. Fatty acids are classified into medium-chain (6–10 carbons) and long-chain (12–26 carbons) fatty acids. They may be saturated and contain no double bonds or unsaturated and contain one or more double bonds. Linoleic and linolenic are unsaturated fatty acids that are considered essential be-

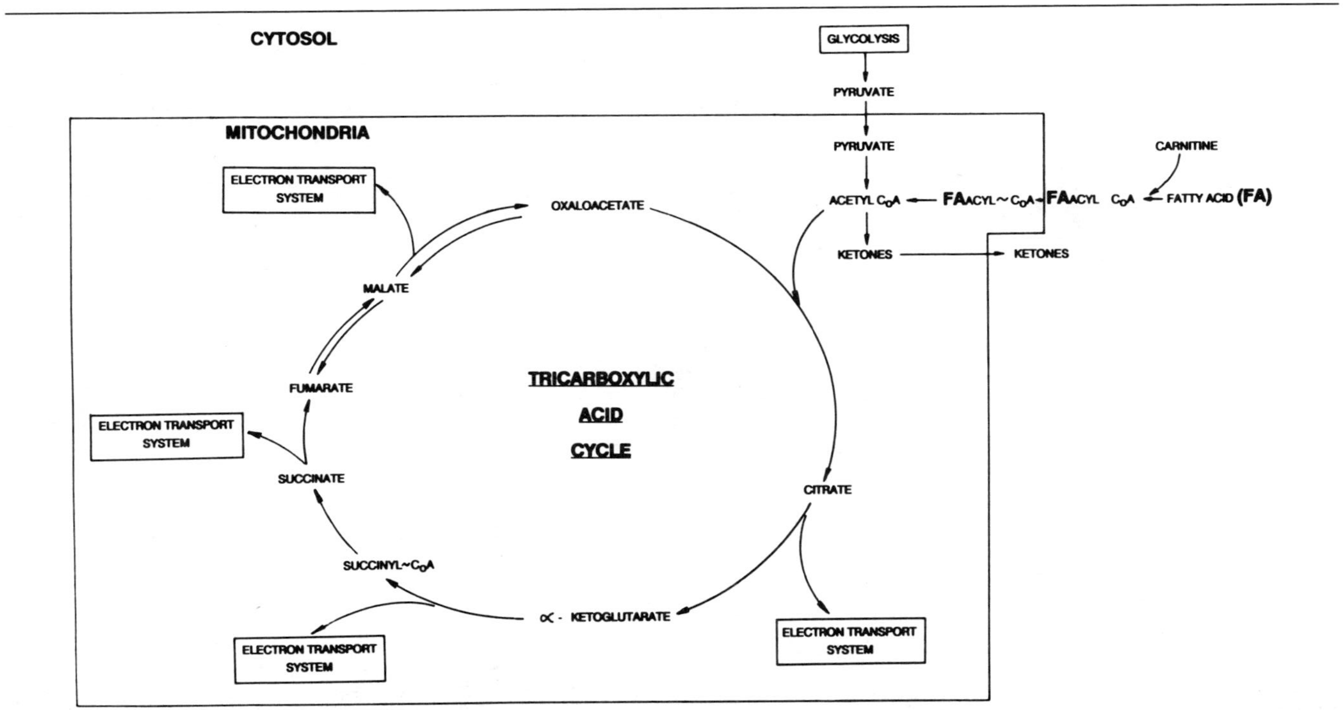

Fig. 21-1. The oxidation of carbohydrate and fat. Note that when oxaloacetate is not available to condense with acetyl CoA because of its shift to gluconeogenic pathways, ketone bodies are produced.

cause they cannot be synthesized and must be ingested [4,7,8].

Beta oxidation of fatty acids occurs within mitochondria, by the cleavage of two carbon fragments that can enter the tricarboxylic acid cycle or undergo ketogenesis (Fig. 21-1). These ketones can be either a fuel source following transport to the periphery or can be excreted intact through the urine.

Protein Metabolism

Protein composes approximately 20 percent of lean body mass or 15 percent of total body weight, which equals approximately 13 kg in a well-nourished, 70-kg adult [9,10] (Fig. 21-2). Unlike carbohydrates and fats, protein is not stored, so that any decrease in the body's protein supply results in decreased functional capacity or diminished structural integrity. The dynamic protein mass, which has also been referred to as the body cell mass, is in a continual state of flux [9,11]. Although the dietary protein requirement necessary to maintain nitrogen balance is only 0.8 gm/kg, over 300 gm of protein is degraded and synthesized each day [12] (Fig. 21-3). Teleologically speaking, this rapid protein turnover allows for metabolic control by regulatory enzymes while at the same time enabling priority utilization of a limited amino acid pool [13].

Protein synthesis from amino acids requires energy from nonprotein substrates. It has been reported that, up to a point, an increase in caloric intake increases nitrogen retention [10,12,14]. The ratio of 150 calories to support the retention of 1 gm of nitrogen was noted by Francis Moore in 1959 to be optimal in stable patients, but since that time this ratio has been noted to vary in different metabolic states [11,14–16]. Insulin must be present in sufficient quantity to promote protein synthesis over degradation, but there are also many cofactors, vitamins, minerals, and electrolytes that are necessary [12,14].

Zero nitrogen balance exists when nitrogen intake is equal to nitrogen losses. Negative nitrogen balance occurs when nitrogen losses exceed nitrogen retention. This involves an increase in protein catabolism over synthesis, as occurs with injury and infection, malnutrition, and immobilization. A net positive balance is present when protein synthesis exceeds protein breakdown. This is the case in growth, in increases in muscle mass, or in the correction of protein malnutrition [17]. Excess protein is metabolized into urea and excreted

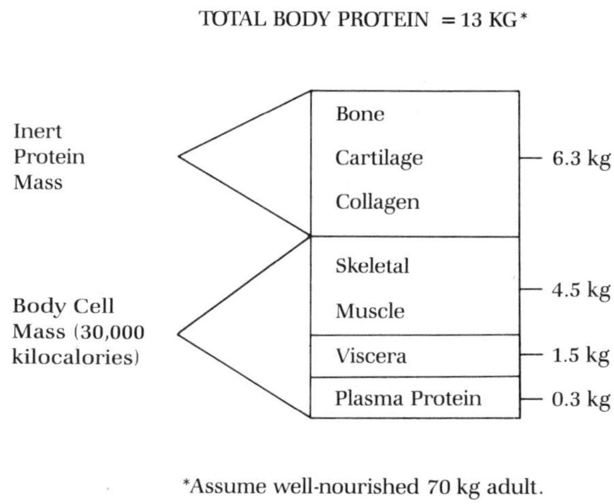

Fig. 21-2. The body protein compartment. (Adapted from G. L. Blackburn et al. Protein Metabolism in the Surgical Patient. In J. R. Kirkpatrick, *Nutrition and Metabolism in the Surgical Patient*. Mt. Kisco, N.Y.: Futura, 1983. With permission.)

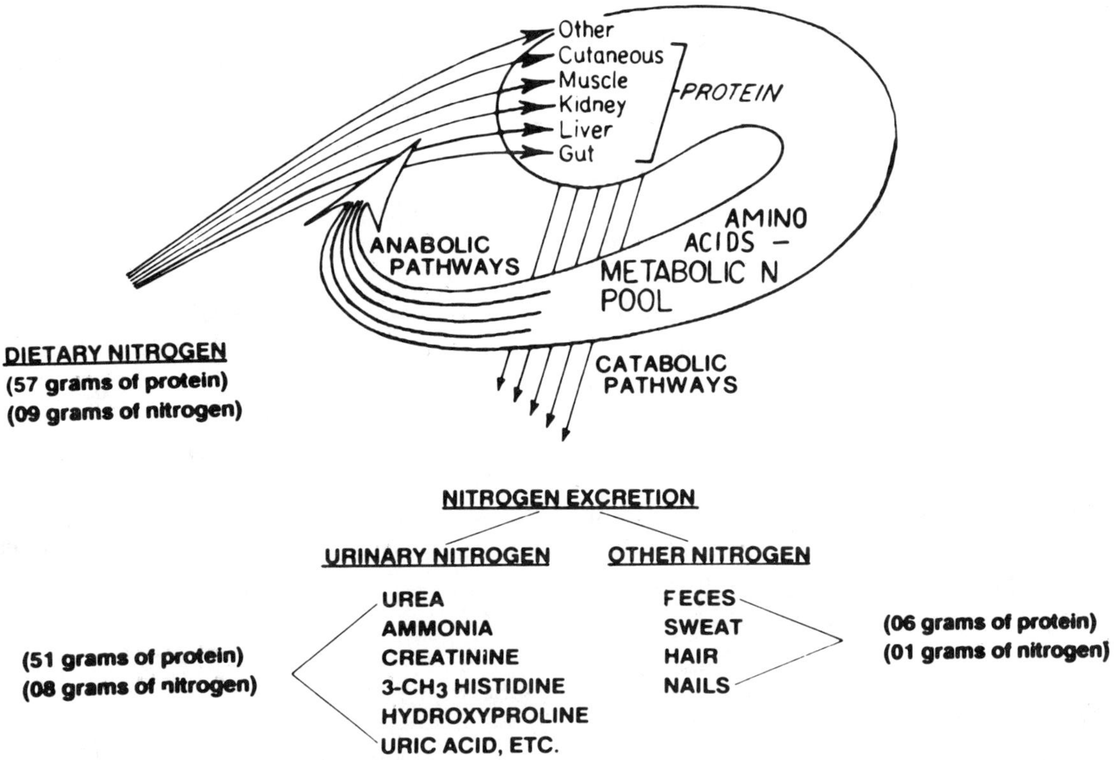

Fig. 21-3. Nitrogen flux through the key body compartments. (Adapted from G. L. Blackburn et al. Protein Metabolism in the Surgical Patient. In J. R. Kirkpatrick, *Nutrition and Metabolism in the Surgical Patient.* Mt. Kisco, N.Y.: Futura, 1983; and T. P. Stein, Protein Metabolism and Parenteral Nutrition. In J. L. Rombeau, and M. D. Caldwell, *Clinical Nutrition. Vol. 2: Parenteral Nutrition.* Philadelphia: Saunders, 1986. With permission.)

into the urine so that in certain circumstances toxicity may result [18].

Amino acids are the building blocks of protein synthesis, and there are 20 naturally occurring amino acids [9]. All amino acids have a carbon backbone structure with an amino group attached [19]. Some undergo oxidative deamination with the carbon skeleton entering the tricarboxylic acid cycle and the nitrogen being excreted as ammonia or urea [13]. Amino acids can be classified according to their utilization. For example, there are essential, semi-essential, and nonessential amino acids [12,20]. Amino acids are also classified according to structure. Two important structural groups of amino acids are the branched-chain amino acids and the aromatic amino acids. Branched-chain amino acids have a role in the metabolism of the injured patient and perhaps in their therapy, while aromatic amino acids are useful in the therapy of patients with hepatic failure.

Starvation

Understanding the metabolic alterations that occur in the stressed patient is facilitated by a knowledge of the physiologic and biochemical changes that characterize starvation. The adaptations discussed in the text occur in the stable, uninjured, and nonstressed patient who is deprived of exogenous substrate.

Circulating levels of glucose and insulin fall in the postabsorptive state. As the primary anabolic hormone, insulin has a significant inhibitory effect on the release of free fatty acids from adipose tissue and or amino acids from skeletal muscle [21]. Declining insulin levels promote amino and fatty acid release from these sources to contribute to gluconeogenesis. In addition, glucagon stimulates glycogenolysis, which provides another source of glucose [10]. However, glycogen supplies are exhausted within 24 hours, since man partially preserves his liver glycogen when fasting for acute emergency utilization in the "fight or flight" response [3]. Thus gluconeogenesis is the major source of body glucose in the absence of exogenous substrate.

Despite the utilization of fatty acids for fuel in most tissues, a large amount of muscle protein must be catabolized on a daily basis in early fasting to support the glucose-dependent tissues [4]. Gamble demonstrated that the administration of only 100 gm/day of glucose significantly decreased the rate of muscle catabolism [22]. Presumably this is sufficient to stimulate insulin release, therefore inhibiting the mobilization of amino acids from muscle. This therapy effectively spares protein only in the stable, noninjured patient without stress.

Clearly, in the absence of further adaptation, humans could never survive weeks and months of starvation. The major adaptation that occurs in humans is the ability of the brain to substitute ketones for approximately 50 percent of its fuel requirements. This allows protein conservation, with the majority of the body utilizing fat-derived fuel sources. The finding of ketones in the urine is evidence of this level of adaptation [10].

The Metabolic Responses to Injury and Infection

The metabolic response to injury was initially described by Cuthbertson in the 1930s in a study of muscle catabolism following fracture injuries and in a subsequent report that delineated the metabolic response to shock [2,23]. Since that time, investigators have attempted to describe these metabolic responses further with multiple schemata [11,23–25] (Fig. 21-4). In general, injured and septic patients are hypermetabolic with an increased energy expenditure and hypercatabolic with an increased rate of nitrogen excretion. These responses serve to maintain function, preserve vital organs and initiate recovery [26]. The degree of hypermetabolism and hypercatabolism that develops is almost always proportional to the magnitude of injury [26,27].

Immediately following a severe injury, pa-

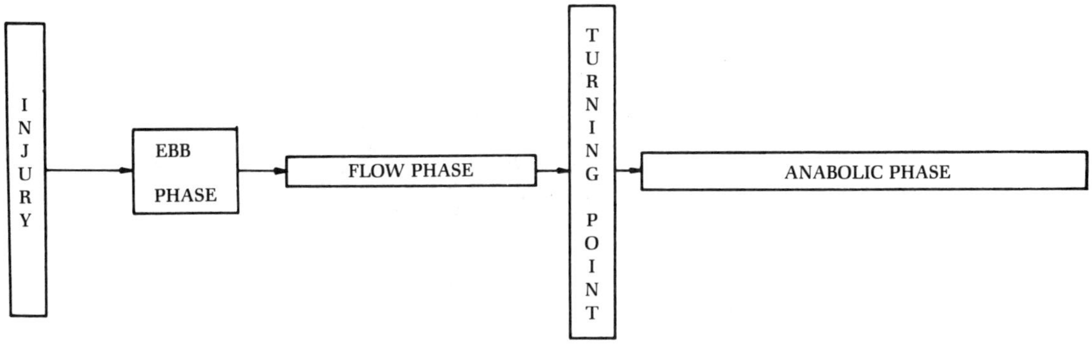

Fig. 21-4. The metabolic phases of injury.

tients enter into an "ebb" or "shock phase" for a period of 1 or 2 days [11,23,25,27–29]. In severely burned patients, however, this phase can last as long as 6 days [29,30]. The body responds with an "alarm signal," which involves rapid hemodynamic and metabolic changes [26,31] (Fig. 21-5). The subsequent increase in circulating catecholamines induces capillary vasoconstriction, tachycardia, and dilatation of coronary blood vessels. In this environment of relative hypofusion, there is decreased oxidative metabolism and increased glycolysis with a diminished capacity for heat production [29]. Simultaneously, there is an outpouring of substrate secondary to increased rates of gluconeogenesis, lipolysis, and glycogenolysis, which may be so dramatic as to deplete hepatic glycogen stores within 6 hours [25,26,29]. Hyperglycemia is common during this phase of injury due to an impaired insulin response and a decrease in the peripheral utilization of substrate [10,14,27,29].

The "flow phase" begins approximately 2 or 3 days following a severe injury at which time the patient would have been stabilized and completely resuscitated [11,27–29]. This phase lasts approximately 5 to 10 days, at which point the patient either reaches the "turning point" and begins to recover or develops septic complications [11]. The flow phase is characterized by an increase in metabolic rate, body temperature, oxygen consumption, and protein turnover [11,27–29]. Although, there is a relative decrease in circulating catecholamines, there still may be marked hyperglycemia as the increases in glucagon and cortisol stimulate the hepatic production of glucose from gluconeogenic precursors [10,25]. End-organ resistance to the action of insulin in muscle and fat is common in this setting and is referred to as "traumatic diabetes" [10,27,29,32–36].

Studies involving burn patients have demonstrated that the wound is central to the metabolic alterations that follow [27,37]. Hyperglycemia and increased blood flow to the wound and splanchnic bed ensure the delivery of required glucose substrate to the regenerating wound tissue [27,37]. Importantly, it has been noted that the hypermetabolic re-

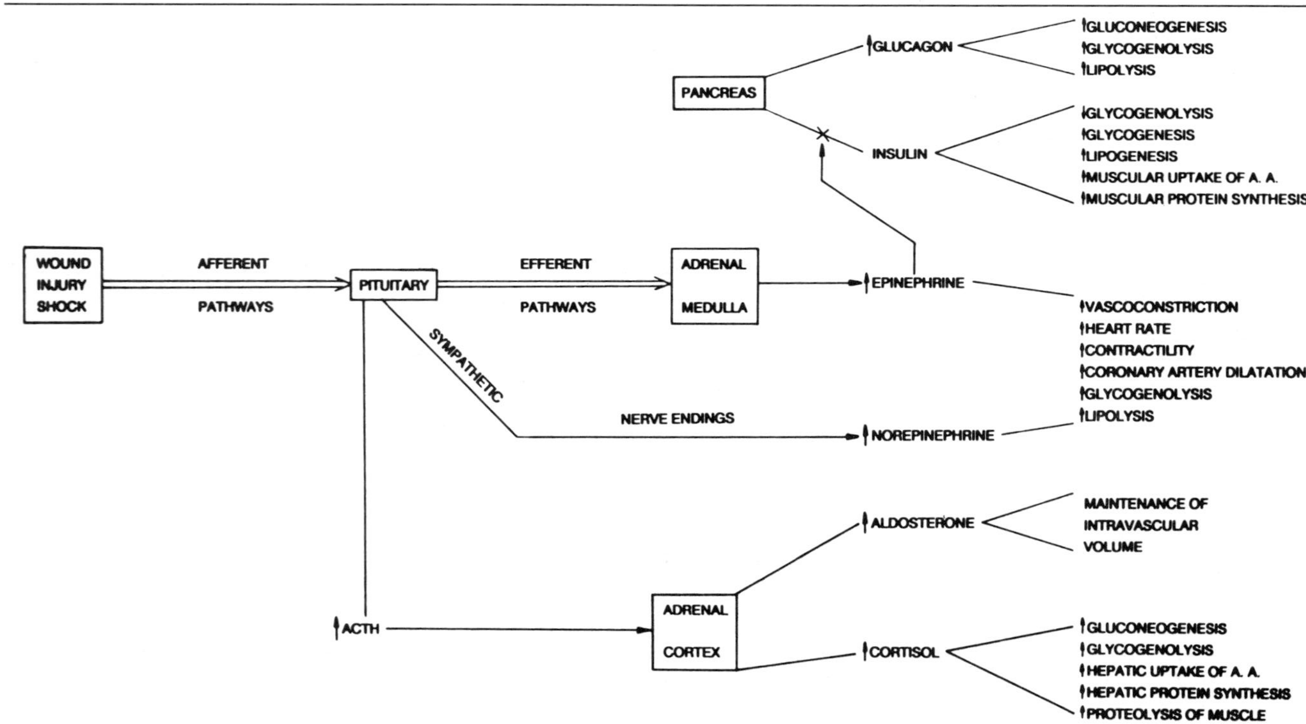

Fig. 21-5. The hormonal response to stress. The metabolic and vasoactive actions of the various hormones involved in the stress response are outlined. Note that the response of insulin is blocked by epinephrine.

sponse is blunted in malnourished patients [35].

Epinephrine, glucagon, and cortisol also serve to increase the rate of fatty and keto acid metabolism seen after trauma [25,26]. In fact, muscle and adipose tissue tend to exclude glucose as a fuel while maintaining a preference for fatty and keto acids [26,32] (Fig. 21-6). A supply of fatty acids is ensured by the fact that lipolysis in liver, muscle, and adipose tissue is not suppressed by elevated levels of glucose and that there is a resistance to lipogenesis even in the face of excess glucose administration [14,29].

In addition to this state of heightened metabolism, there is also a state of heightened catabolism with increased protein turnover and nitrogen excretion [13]. The magnitude of this response is also dependent on the sever-

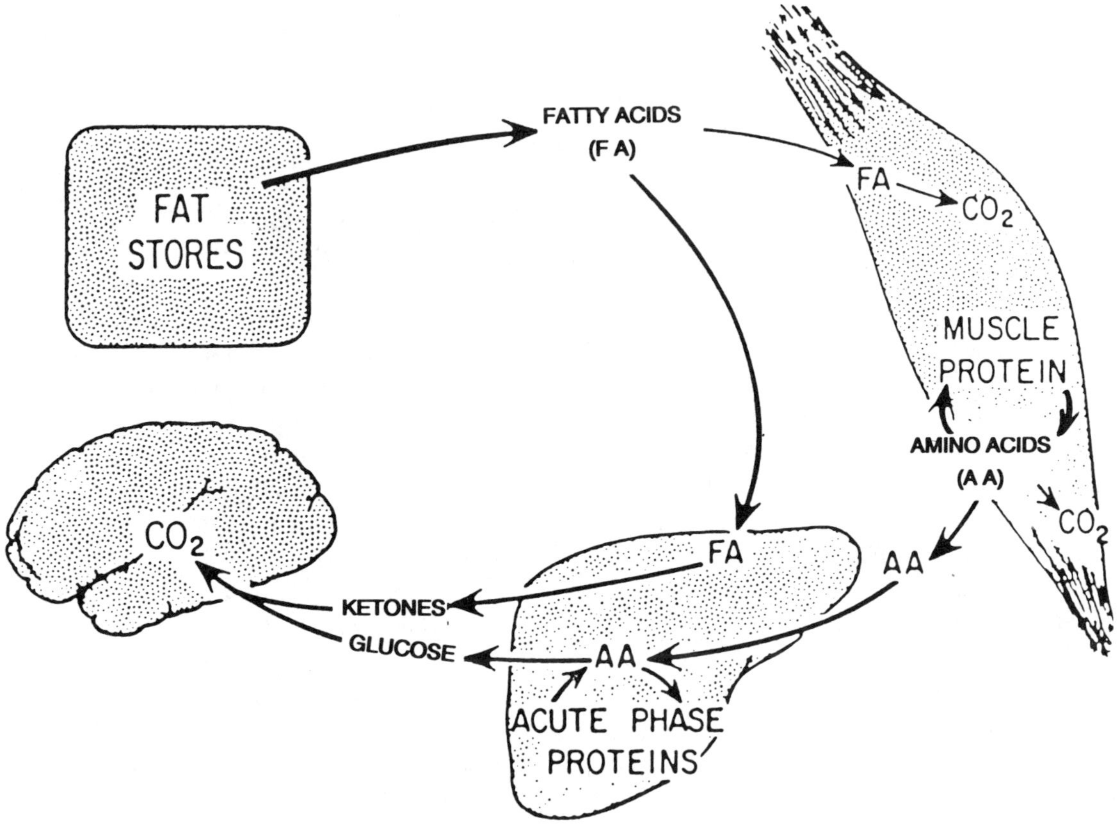

Fig. 21-6. The metabolic response to injury in muscle and liver tissue. (From G. L. Blackburn et al. Protein Metabolism in the Surgical Patient. In J. R. Kirkpatrick, *Nutrition and Metabolism in the Surgical Patient.* Mt. Kisco, N.Y.: Futura, 1983. With permission.

ity of the injury as well as the prior nutritional status of the patient [12,13,23,26]. Although, it was previously felt that the stress response was characterized primarily by an increase in muscle breakdown, it has recently been demonstrated that there is a concomitant increase in protein synthesis. This is an adaptive maneuver by which the body degrades nonpriority peripheral muscle to expand the amino acid pool to provide available substrate for the synthesis of high-priority proteins [26] (Fig. 21-6). By so doing, the amino acids of skeletal muscle are diverted to healing wounds, the immune system, and acute phase proteins [12,13]. The blunted mobilization of the body cell mass seen in malnourished patients may result in delayed wound healing and increased septic morbidity [9,12,13,26].

Despite the increased rate of protein synthesis that follows injury, there is negative nitrogen balance because of the additional sacrifice of muscle protein for use as energy substrate [9,10] (Fig. 21-6). Branched-chain amino acids share fatty acid metabolic pathways in muscle and may thus provide substrate that is needed to support gluconeogenesis [15,26,38–40]. Since the branched-chain amino acids released by muscle proteolysis are preferentially utilized as fuel for the production of high-energy phosphate bonds in muscle, it has been hypothesized that a deficiency of these amino acids may ensue [9,12,26,38]. Therefore, increased muscle catabolism would be required to replete the amino acid profile. This would lead to increased nitrogen excretion and urea production as the excess amino acids that were not utilized for synthesis were deaminated and oxidized [12,15].

Survival of the initial injury with continued improvement enables the patient to approach the "turning point" [11,41] (Fig. 21-4). Circulating catecholamine, glucagon, and glucocorticoid levels all normalize, with subsequent improvement in the serum glucose [9]. Insulin levels also normalize but maintain an influence as the patient enters into a period of anabolism during which time there is a repletion of the body cell mass with a resulting positive nitrogen balance [9]. Eventually, lipolysis gives way to lipogenesis as the body lipid stores are replaced. This process usually takes several months and becomes more obvious after discharge.

METABOLIC SUPPORT

The Basis for Therapy

The initial metabolic therapy of the trauma patient during the "ebb phase" of injury must include a rapid and definitive resuscitation [27]. After airway protection is achieved, adequate volumes of crystalloid and blood products must be administered to avoid prolonged hypoxemia and anaerobic metabolism [42]. Expeditious surgical intervention is beneficial to control hemorrhage, stabilize fractures, and repair any injuries. Rapid closure of all open wounds will help to decrease the catecholamine-dependent metabolic rate. Whenever possible, the patient should be kept warm and free of pain [27].

With entry into the flow phase of injury, the goal of nutritional therapy is primarily to support the patient [42]. Early intervention with nutritional support impacts on protein synthesis, involving the wound, blood cells, immune globulins, and acute-phase hepatic proteins [10,15,43]. Given the difficulty in repairing protein deficits in the critically ill patient, early nutritional intervention is advised, usually between days 2 and 4 [27,44].

Although there is little definitive data in the literature demonstrating that nutritional support improves the outcome of trauma victims, several facts seem to suggest a beneficial role [41]. Firstly, a 40-percent loss of pre-injury body weight in burn victims has been demonstrated to be uniformly fatal, while a loss of less than 10 percent is associated with little disability [45]. Because a critically ill patient can lose 10 percent of body weight in 10 days, early and aggressive nutritional support is necessary to limit these losses [27]. Recent improvements in the salvage rates of massively burned victims have been attributed in part to aggressive parenteral feedings [26,46,47].

Numerous studies have demonstrated that when protein-calorie malnutrition is present, there is an increase in morbidity and mortality above and beyond that which would be expected from the primary disease process [48–51]. Mullen and coworkers [50] were able to show a reduction in postoperative morbidity and mortality by instituting preoperative nutritional support in patients identified as high risk by the prognostic nutritional index [52].

The major cause of late death in trauma patients continues to be sepsis. Important parameters of immune function including the humoral response, T-cell activities, and opsonization are adversely affected by malnutrition [48]. Clinically, the rate of wound infections and other septic complications is greater in the malnourished patient [42,47,52].

As the patient reaches the "turning point" and enters the recuperative phase, the goal is to repair preexisting or hospital-acquired nutritional deficits. Since protein catabolism is diminished while protein synthesis continues, a positive nitrogen balance can be expected. Hopefully, nutritional therapy at this point can be achieved with a house diet. Otherwise, other forms of nutritional support must be continued.

Nutritional Assessment

Malnutrition has been formally defined as a state of calorie, protein, or micronutrient deficiency that is acute or chronic and adversely affects prognosis [49]. Proper nutritional assessment of the trauma patient requires a method to diagnose, characterize, and quantitate malnutrition. Moreover, it is important that patients who are at nutritional risk secondary to their injuries are readily identified [43,48]. Although many trauma patients are young and nutritionally sound, there are patients who present malnourished and will need early institution of nutritional support [47]. Considerable controversy exists regarding the identifcation of clinically significant malnutrition [10]. However, there is a consensus of opinion that all patients with major trauma should have a nutritional assessment performed within 3 days of injury [42]. If an adequate diet is not projected within 5 to 7 days, aggressive nutritional support should be instituted [41,42,53].

Although there are numerous sophisticated methods available to evaluate nutritional status, the information gained from a careful history and physical can be invaluable [49,54,55]. The interview should elicit social and dietary information, any history of recent weight loss, and anything to suggest chronic disease or absorptive abnormalities [48,55,56]. A weight loss of greater than 10 percent of previous body weight is considered to be a risk factor for malnutrition, while a weight loss exceeding 35 percent may contribute to mortality [55–57]. Examination of the patient should include a measurement of current body weight, which can be compared with standard weight tables [49,56]. Body weights less than 80 percent of ideal are considered to be a risk factor for malnutrition [14,48].

Measurements that assess static caloric and skeletal muscle protein reserves, such as anthropometrics and the creatinine height index, may be difficult to obtain in the trauma patient due to soft tissue injury and edema and generally are not useful [9,42,43,47–49,55,58]. Although the assessment of the visceral protein compartment can be performed by most chemistry laboratories, these values have not been found to be useful when applied to trauma patients in the acute phase of injury [9,25,26,44,47–49,59] (Table 21-3). An assessment of the patient's immunologic status can be obtained from the total lymphocyte count and delayed hypersensitivity testing [48,49]. It is important to realize that the effects of severe trauma, infection, and steroid therapy may render these tests to be unreliable in the diagnosis of malnutrition [43,47,49,54,55,59]. They do, however, continue to be reliable indicators of increased morbidity and mortality [42,49,60].

The Prognostic Nutritional Index (PNI) was developed to identify more accurately the patient at increased risk for complications secondary to malnutrition [49,61].

$$\text{PNI}(\%) = 158 - 16.6\,(\text{ALB}) - 0.78\,(\text{TSF}) - 0.20\,(\text{TFN}) - 5.8\,(\text{DH})$$

where ALB = serum albumin (mg/dl)
TSF = triceps skinfold (mm)
TFN = serum transferrin (mg/dl)
DH = delayed hypersensitivity wheal (mm)

Although initially designed to predict morbidity and mortality in patients undergoing gastrointestinal surgery, the PNI has been applied to trauma patients with good success [26,62] (Fig. 21-7). A PNI of greater than 50 percent was associated with a 30-percent risk of complications, while a PNI less than 50 percent was only associated with a 6-percent risk of complications.

Moore and Jones [47] found that the sever-

Table 21-3. Measurement of the Visceral Protein Compartment

Protein marker	Normal values	Half-life (days)
Albumin	>3.5 gm/dl	20
Transferrin	>200 mg/dl	8.5
Prealbumin	200–300 μg/ml	1.3
Retinol-binding protein	40–50 μg/ml	0.4

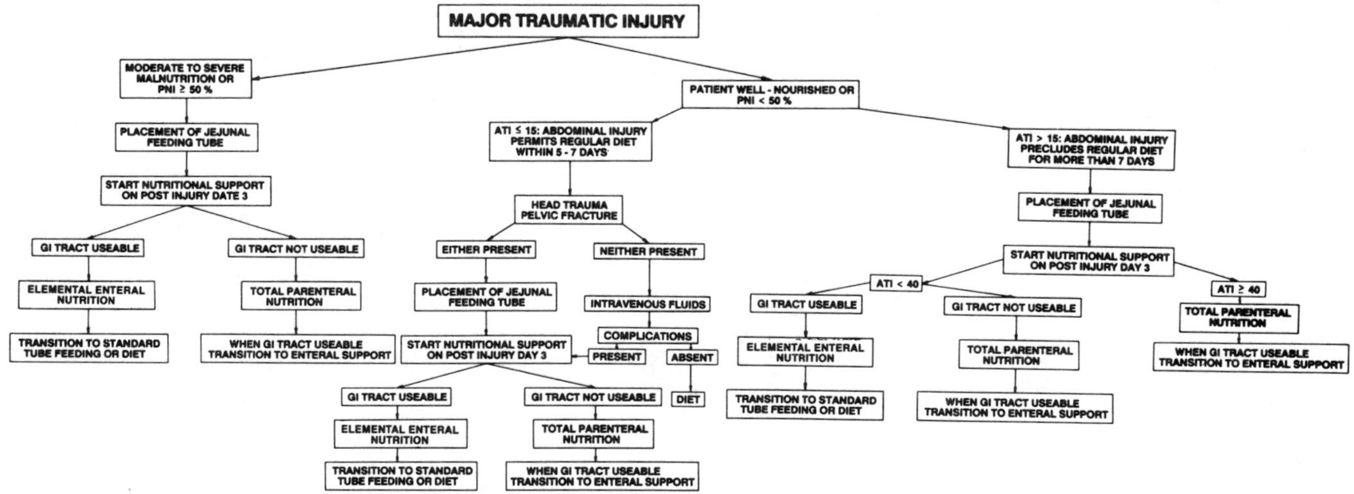

Fig. 21-7. **An approach to nutritional support in major traumatic injury. Risk factor scoring techniques or clinical criteria can be utilized to determine the need for early nutritional support. Note that it should be possible to support most patients with enteral feedings when jejunal tubes are utilized. PNI = Prognostic Nutritional Index, ATI = Abdominal Trauma Index. (Taken in part from E. E. Moore, Enteral elemental nutrition in major trauma. *Contemp. Surg.* 28:18, 1986. With permission.)**

ity of injury was a superior predictor of septic morbidity than standard nutritional markers (Table 21-4). Moore modified the Penetrating Abdominal Trauma Index (ATI) that he had reported in 1981, applied it to all abdominal trauma, and was able to select out which patients needed early nutritional intervention [47,59,62]. Although an ATI greater than 25 percent was associated with an increased rate of complications, Moore suggests early support in all patients with an ATI greater than 15 percent [47,62]. In our institution, we assess the patient clinically on postinjury day 3. If the patient has moderate to severe malnutrition or if the injury is severe enough that we feel that the patient will not be on a regular diet by day 5, we institute nutritional support (Fig. 21-7).

Following a decision to institute nutritional support, a determination of the caloric requirement is needed [14,42,43,63]. The resting energy expenditure (REE) can either be estimated or measured [43]. The metabolic cart provides a way in which the REE can be "measured." Indirect calorimetry is performed, and the metabolic rate is calculated from measurements of oxygen consumption and carbon dioxide production [27,49]:

$$\text{REE (kcal/m}_2\text{/hr)} = \frac{[3.9 \times \text{VO}_2\text{ (L/min)} + 1.1 \times \text{VCO}_2\text{(L/min)}] \times 60\text{ min/hr}}{\text{body surface area (m}^2\text{)}}$$

The basal energy expenditure (BEE) can be calculated either by using conventional metabolic rate tables or from the Harris-Benedict equations:

Table 21-4. The Abdominal Trauma Index (ATI)

Organ injured	Complication risk factor	Injury severity score
Duodenum	5	1. Single wall 2. <25% wall 3. >25% wall 4. Duodenal wall and blood supply 5. Pancreaticoduodenectomy
Liver	4	1. Nonbleeding peripheral 2. Bleeding, central or minor debridement 3. Major debridement or hepatic artery ligation 4. Lobectomy 5. Lobectomy with caval repair or extensive bilobar debridement

A sample of the ATI is provided to demonstrate its calculation. For example an isolated duodenal injury that involves the blood supply would have an ATI = 5 × 4 = 20.
Source: from E. E. Moore, et al., Penetrating abdominal trauma index. *J. Trauma* 21:439, 1981. © by Williams & Wilkins. With permission.

$$
\begin{aligned}
0\ \text{BEE} &= 66 + (13.7 \times \text{wt in kg}) \\
&\quad + (5 \times \text{ht in cm}) \\
&\quad - (6.8 \times \text{age in yr}) \\
0^{+}\ \text{BEE} &= 655 + (9.6 \times \text{wt in kg}) \\
&\quad + (1.7 \times \text{ht in cm}) \\
&\quad - (4.7 \times \text{age in yr})
\end{aligned}
$$

When the BEE is used, proper estimation of energy needs requires the use of a stress factor to adjust for hypermetabolism [14,27,43] (Fig. 21-8). Usually a factor between 1.5 and 1.7 applies to most traumatic injuries [43]. The upper limit of this increased metabolic rate occurs in burn patients at a rate of twice the BEE [27,64]. To simplify matters, the caloric re-

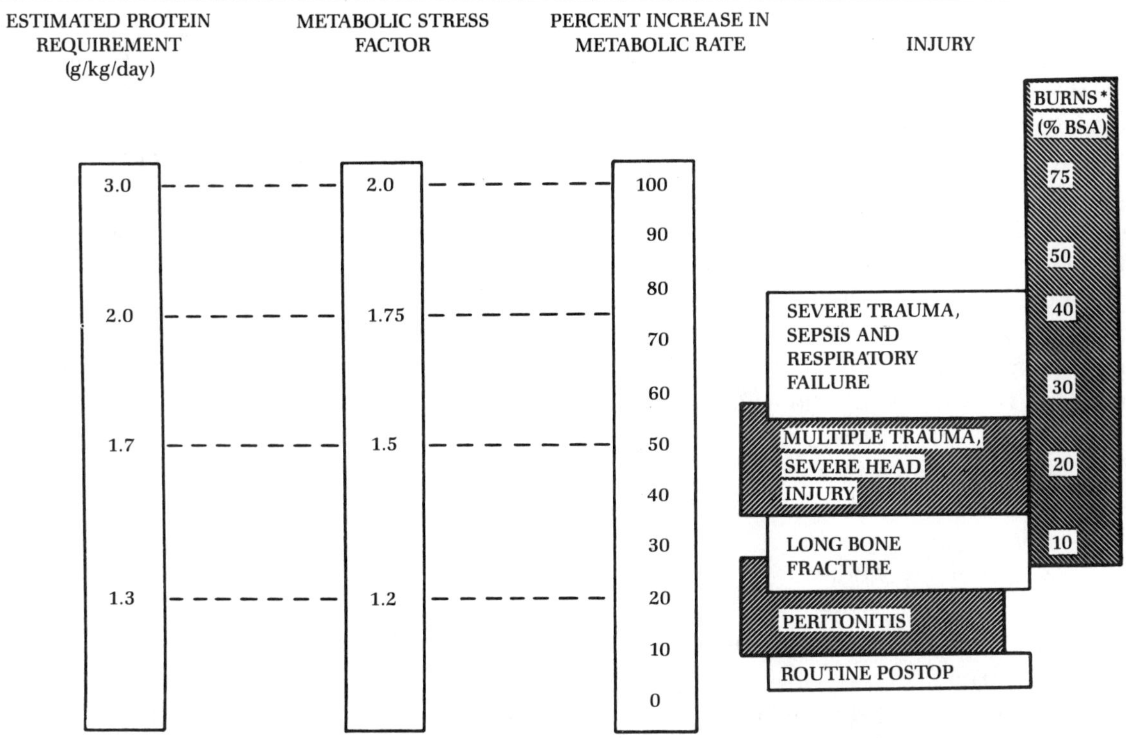

Fig. 21-8. The effect of injury and infection on calorie and protein requirements. Note that as the severity of injury increases there are increased protein and calorie requirements. For example, an estimate of the daily calorie requirements of a patient with a 50% body surface area (BSA) burn would be 2 times the calculated basal energy expenditure. Protein requirements should be met by giving amino acids at a dose of 3 gm/kg. (Adapted from D. H. Elwyn, Nutritional requirements for adult surgical patients. *Crit. Care Med.* 8:15, 1980 © by Williams & Wilkins; and F. B. Cerra, Sepsis and Trauma. Kirkpatrick, J.R. *Nutrition and Metabolism in the Surgical Patient.* Mt. Kisco, N.Y.: Futura, 1983. With permission.)

quirements can be grossly estimated by using 35 kcal/kg/day for stable patients and 45 kcal/kg/day for stressed patients [55].

After the patient reaches the turning point in the illness, in some instances it will be necessary to give extra calories for weight gain, since from this point onward repletion can be accomplished. Patients on an enteral regimen will require 1.5 times the BEE for anabolism, while patients on a parenteral regimen will require 1.75 times the BEE [56].

After the appropriate caloric requirements have been established, the patient's protein requirement must be determined. The degree of stress that has been assigned can also be used to estimate protein needs [56] (Fig. 21-8). A nonstressed individual without excessive losses will require 0.8 gm/kg/day of protein (see Fig. 21-3). As the stress level increases, the protein requirement increases to as high as 3 gm/kg/day [42,55] (Fig. 21-8).

There are techniques that can be utilized to quantitate the daily protein requirement. The simplest is to measure the 24-hour urinary urea nitrogen (UUN) value. The amount of urea produced will depend on the severity of injury, the amount of protein intake, and the previous nutritional status [13,28]. After a major injury, the UUN would be expected to be as high as 18 to 25 gm/day.

Although UUN is easily measured in most hospital laboratories and has been advocated as a readily available index of total nitrogen excretion, many studies have been done that demonstrate that the measurement of total urinary nitrogen (TUN) is most accurate [27,42,56,65]. The UUN may compose less than 50 percent of the TUN in patients with previous starvation and may be falsely low in severely catabolic patients [27]. For this reason, we recommend basing protein therapy on TUN values whenever they are available.

A nitrogen balance study is necessary to determine accurately whether the proper amount of protein therapy is being administered. Nitrogen balance is the difference between the amount of nitrogen administered and the amount of nitrogen lost [9,27,56,57]:

$$\text{Nitrogen balance} = \text{N (in)} - \text{N (out)}$$
$$= \frac{\text{protein (gm/day)}}{6.25} - \text{N (out)}$$

with 1 gm of nitrogen corresponding to 6.25 gm of protein [42]. Losses of nitrogen other than those secondary to muscle catabolism include loss of tissue secondary to injury, loss of blood and exudate in the wound, loss of muscle protein due to disuse atrophy, and cutaneous and fecal losses [27,57]. Urinary losses are most accurately represented by the TUN. If UUN is used, either the addition of 2 gm or an additional 20 percent of the UUN will most closely approximate the losses, which may be equal to an additional 2 gm of nitrogen in patients who are not stressed and as high as 4 gm in patients who are stressed and have increased losses [16,27]. Cutaneous losses are negligible except in patients with large body surface wounds, in whom they may equal up to 4 gm/day of nitrogen [27]. A special problem exists in patients who have a rising blood urea nitrogen (BUN). In this case, not all of the urea that is produced will be present in the urine. The amount of nitrogen sequestered in the extracellular space must be added to the TUN. This is calculated by multiplying the change in BUN by the total body urea space, which is equal to approximately 55 percent of the total body weight in kilograms [16].

There will be occasions when there will be difficulty in providing all of the calorie and nitrogen requirements to a particular patient. Because fat stores are usually plentiful, the provision of adequate protein should take precedence over providing energy needs [14,43,66]. After the amount of calorie and nitrogen support has been calculated, the calorie-to-nitrogen ratio should equal from 150 : 1 to 100 : 1 in the trauma patient and from 100 : 1 to 80 : 1 in the septic patient [15,27,55,67].

In addition to macronutrient requirements of calories and protein, there are micronutrient requirements that must be met with nutritional therapy [14]. These include the major electrolytes sodium, potassium, phosphate, chloride, calcium, magnesium, and iron, which are required for tissue maintenance and repletion [14,66,68]. Vitamins are also required and are usually given prophylactically in commercial preparations [66,69]. Zinc requirements are increased in catabolic states [14,69]. Other trace elements such as copper, chromium, and manganese become essential when parenteral nutrition is required for more than 2 weeks [14].

Because the metabolic response to injury is a dynamic process, nutritional requirements are subject to change. For this reason, we need a mechanism to monitor the results of nutritional therapy [48]. In the critically ill patient, weights, electrolytes, and BUN should be followed at least on a daily basis [48,49]. Urine sugar and acetone as well as serum glucose should be checked by fingerstick at least 2 to 4 times a day. Methods to assess protein and immunologic status can be repeated at weekly intervals, but we have found nitrogen balance studies to be most useful in the acute phase of injury [48,49]. Visceral protein levels will slowly increase as the patient recovers [48]. Liver function tests, prothrombin time, and platelet counts should be checked at least every 7 to 10 days. Zinc and copper levels need to be checked if the acute illness persists for more than 2 weeks and more often in patients with signs of organ system failure or increased losses [14]. Sepsis requires that triglyceride levels be monitored frequently to ensure tolerance to fat administration [14]. Finally, a reassessment of caloric needs should be performed with any change in clinical status, preferably by indirect calorimetry or by using the Harris-Benedict equations with appropriate stress factors.

Enteral Therapy

Enteral therapy offers several advantages when providing nutritional support for the trauma victim. These include safety, lower cost, and a more physiologic route of administration [42,43,47]. Whenever the gastrointestinal tract is functional and accessible, it should be used for feeding [27,41]. Gastric feedings neutralize the luminal pH and thereby decrease the incidence of gastric hemorrhage, while also stimulating the biliary tract and lessening the incidence of acalculous cholecystitis [42,70]. Recently, it has been suggested that the incidence of septic complications following trauma is decreased by early enteral feedings [47].

The recent trend has been to initiate enteral feedings in the immediate postinjury period, in lieu of parental support in the patient with major trauma. Moore and Jones [47] have demonstrated the feasibility of this approach in the trauma victim requiring exploratory laparotomy (see Fig. 21-7). In their study [47], all patients with an ATI greater than 15 had operative jejunostomy catheters placed [71]. All patients with an ATI less than 40 tolerated immediate postoperative feedings with an elemental formula. If an operative jejunostomy catheter cannot be placed, a weighted feeding tube can be placed transnasally distal to the pylorus and allowed to migrate further distally. In many patients, this will require fluoroscopy [42,43,72]. In this way, patients with head injuries, thoracic injuries, or multiple fractures can be managed with nasoenteral tubes.

Other situations arise in the care of the trauma patient where enteral nutritional support would be appropriate. In patients unable to tolerate tube feedings immediately following their injury, parenteral nutrition can be instituted and a transition made to enteral feedings after 3 to 5 days [41,47] (see Fig. 21-7). Palatable caloric and protein supplements can be added when necessary to allow for the discontinuation of tube feedings. In patients with altered levels of consciousness or persistent gastrointestinal tract dysfunction, enteral feedings may offer a safe, effective, and economic route of nutrition and allow for out-of-hospital patient disposition.

Selection of the enteral formula most appropriate for a given patient requires a familiarity with the products available. In circumstances where normal gastrointestinal function and absorption are present, meal replacement formulas can be utilized most economically [55]. These are based on protein isolates and are usually free of fiber. They generally contain approximately 1000 kcal/L, 30 to 35 percent of which is supplied by fat, and approximately 40 gm/L of protein [27,55]. In calorically adequate volumes, these products meet all of the standard recommended dietary allowances for all nutrients [55]. Some products require tube administration due to poor palatability, while others are in flavored forms that are more acceptable to the patient. There are circumstances in which the protein needs of the trauma patient cannot be met by a tube feeding formula containing 40 gm/L of protein. There are several high-nitrogen formulations for these situations. In addition, there are products that are calorically dense for use in patients with fluid restrictions. Occasionally, the calculated nutritional needs of a given patient will not be met by available enteral products. Nutritional modules can help in the management of these patients by providing extra calories or protein as needed [73].

Elemental or chemically defined diets are more expensive than meal replacement formulas, but less expensive than parenteral solutions [73]. These products are also nutritionally complete but contain food elements in their digested form so that minimal absorptive capacity is required for their assimilation. Some products contain up to 30 percent of the calories as fat with the minimal amount of long-chain triglycerides needed to meet essential fatty acid requirements. Products that provide a portion of the calories as fat utilize medium-chain triglycerides for this purpose. The protein component may be a mixture of whole protein and hydrolyzed protein in peptide form or be composed of crystalline amino acids. Recently, reports have described improved absorption using dipeptide- and tripeptide-based formulas [74].

The use of elemental diets should be limited to clinical settings in which full gastrointestinal function has not returned yet and are best tolerated for feeding into the jejunum, because the secretion of bile and pancreatic enzymes are not necessary for absorption and the low viscosity permits the use of small-caliber catheters [47]. Other uses in trauma patients include pancreatitis, pancreatic fistula, small-bowel fistula, malabsorption secondary to extensive bowel resection or malnutrition, and when minimal colonic residue is desired [73].

Although enteral feedings are safer than parenteral feedings, they are not without their own inherent complications. These can be minimized with adherence to strict protocols [42]. Aspiration can be minimized by placing the tube distal to the ligament of Treitz whenever possible. Furthermore, elevation of the head of the bed to 30 degrees and continuous feedings with a controller pump are recommended [43,57]. When gastric feedings are administered, residuals must be checked frequently to ensure adequate gastric emptying. If the gastric residual exceeds 100 ml, feedings should be held or markedly decreased. If this becomes a persistent problem, consideration should be given to passing the tube into the jejunum so that full support can be resumed [43,57].

Hyperosmolar hyperglycemic, nonketotic dehydration is another complication of enteral feedings [73]. This complication can be avoided by close monitoring of urine and blood sugars in addition to adding water to the feedings as indicated. In situations where blood glucose exceeds 200 mg/dl, insulin therapy and converting to a formula containing more fat will ease patient management.

Diarrhea sometimes complicates enteral feedings and can contribute to dehydration, electrolyte disturbances, and worsening of malnutrition [73]. Potential causes include bacterial overgrowth in the liquid feeding, magnesium deficiency, gut mucosal atrophy with decreased absorptive capacity, hypoalbuminemia, and colonic bacterial overgrowth from antibiotics. Since most trauma patients receive a course of antibiotics, stool cultures and titers for *Clostridium difficile* are appropriate [73].

Parenteral Therapy

The majority of trauma victims will never need hyperalimentation. For patients who are well nourished and sustain mild to moderate injury so that an adequate diet is projected within 5 to 7 days, 100 gm/day of glucose in the form of standard intravenous fluid is considered to be adequate parenteral therapy [26] (see Fig. 21-7).

To deliver adequate nutritional support in appropriate fluid volumes to the severely injured patient, hypertonic solutions must be given through a central venous catheter [27,43]. To minimize complications and facilitate placement, a strictly sterile technique, volume expansion, and placement of the patient in the Trendelenburg position are recommended [75,76]. The presence of a tracheostomy increases the risk of catheter infection and requires that the exit site be tunneled away from the tracheostomy site. Ideal use of the hyperalimentation catheter dictates its exclusive use for total parenteral nutrition (TPN) solutions. In general, no medications should be piggybacked, no blood samples drawn, and no central venous pressure measurements performed using the catheter [43,76]. However, the critically ill patient often presents vascular access problems so that the risk-to-benefit ratio of violating the line must be reassessed on an individual basis [43]. Multilumen catheters may be helpful in that one port can be designated exclusively for hyperalimentation. Subsequently, when access is no longer a problem, the multilumen catheter should be replaced by a single-lumen catheter [66].

Several factors determine what constitutes the length of time that a central hyperalimentation line can remain in place. In our surgical intensive care unit, multilumen catheters are used almost exclusively. The central catheters of infected patients are changed every 3 days, while those of clean patients can remain in place for up to 6 days. When line sepsis is suspected or longer catheterization is desired, a guidewire technique is used to exchange catheters, and the intracutaneous segment of the line that was removed is cultured semiquantitatively [77]. If the culture result is positive, the replaced catheter is removed, and a new line is placed through a new insertion site. If the culture is negative, the replaced catheter can remain in place from 3 to 6 days. This protocol resulted in the salvage of the access site in 80 percent of the patients studied [77]. A second guidewire exchange is not recommended because of the high incidence of positive cultures.

With institution of parenteral nutrition, strict protocols must be followed to avoid metabolic complications. Therapy must begin slowly, with close observation for patient tolerance of fluids, glucose, and protein. There should be strict adherence to calculated values of nutritional requirements [43]. The selection of a formula requires proper consideration be given to volume, cardiopulmonary, renal, hepatic, and hematologic statuses (vida infra) [27]. When hyperalimentation solutions are discontinued, measures should be taken to avoid rebound hypoglycemia. This is most important for patients on insulin therapy. If the solution cannot be weaned over several hours, an infusion of 10% dextrose in water should be instituted for at least 2 to 3 hours [75].

Proper calculation of the amount and concentration of dextrose solution needed requires that caloric needs first be determined as previously outlined. Although oral carbohydrate yields 4 kcal/gm, the dextrose in intravenous form is a monohydrate and yields only 3.4 kcal/gm [27,67] (see Table 21-2). Because glucose that is not oxidized is used to synthesize fat, the following formula is useful to determine whether an excess of glucose calories has been ordered [78]:

$$\frac{\text{Energy intake (kcal)}}{\text{Body weight (kg)}} \leq 40 \text{ kcal/kg}$$

If the calculated ratio approaches 40, an excess of glucose calories is being administered, and fat calories should be used to replace the excess [78].

Controversy surrounds the choice of the most optimal nonprotein fuel source to use in injured and septic patients [14,26,27,33,43,64, 79–82]. Advantages of carbohydrate systems (glucose) include a daily requirement of 125 gm, oxidation by all tissues, ease of administration, and efficient utilization [26,42,67].

Those in favor of mixed fuel systems of carbohydrate and fat point out the benefits of lipid therapy. There is a minimal daily requirement of essential fatty acids, which can be supplied by approximately 100 ml of 10% lipid emulsion [14]. Lipids are an isotonic, concentrated form of calories that are easily given through peripheral veins [26,67]. Furthermore, fats may be the preferred fuel source in stressed and septic patients [32,67,81,82].

The use of a mixed fuel system is most practical when prescribing parenteral nutrition formulas for critically injured patients [14]. By administering 40 percent of the nonprotein calories as fat and only 60 percent of dextrose, adequate support can be provided with a reduction in hyperglycemic complications [15,27,43,83]. Providing support in this fashion is also more physiologic, since it more closely resembles a standard diet [67].

Lipids are available in 10% and 20% emulsions that provide linoleic and linolenic acid [84]. The 10% solution provides 1.1 kcal/ml, while the 20% solution provides 2.0 kcal/ml [85]. The maximum daily dose of fat should not exceed 4 gm/kg body weight and should not be given more rapidly than 0.15 gm/kg/hr [85]. Four hours following the completion of the infusion, the lipids should be cleared and any hyperlipidemia resolved [84]. Adverse reactions that have been reported, primarily with rapid infusion rates, include chest pain, nausea, chills, and fever [84]. Contraindications to the use of lipids include pathologic hyperlipidemia, egg allergy, and pancreatitis secondary to hyperlipidemia [84]. Investigation to improve fat utilization and tolerance includes the administration of L-carnitine in sepsis and the development of fat emulsions that contain medium-chain triglycerides [80,86].

Crystalline synthetic L–amino acid solutions that are 100-percent utilizable as substrate are now available for protein administration and have replaced the inferior protein hydrolysate solutions [26,85,87]. Standard solutions usually contain at least 30 to 40% essential amino acids and will fulfill the requirements of the majority of clinical situations [26]. Recently, however, new "stress formulas" of amino acids have been developed. Approximately 50 percent of the amino acids in these solutions are composed of the branched-chain amino acids (BCAA) leucine, isoleucine, and valine [26,88]. This is in contrast to the standard solutions, which contain approximately 20% BCAA [26]. Branched-chain amino acids are metabolized primarily in muscle, where their deaminated carbon chains enter the tricarboxylic acid cycle and provide energy for oxidative phosphorylation [27,67] (see Fig. 21-6). The demand for BCAA as energy substrate in muscle is increased during periods of stress [15,27]. It has been hypothesized that because of their increased utilization as fuel in stressed conditions, BCAA availability may be rate limiting for protein synthesis [12]. By administering exogenous BCAA, the catabolic rate of muscle may be reduced, and visceral protein synthesis can be maintained [9,27,43,67]. Furthermore, it has been proposed that leucine and its alpha–keto acid metabolite have a modulating effect on the post-traumatic injury response. Both inhibit protein breakdown, while leucine also stimulates protein synthesis in a dose-related fashion [12,26,27,38].

Numerous studies demonstrate improved biochemical and laboratory parameters during stress when using BCAA-enriched solutions [12,15]. Benefits include improved satisfaction of caloric demands, enhanced protein synthesis, normalization of the serum amino acid profile, decreased proteolysis, improved nitrogen retention and nitrogen balance, and improved immunologic parameters [12,15,24,26,27,38,43,88,90,91].

While other studies have challenged these findings, some have validated the findings of increased protein accretion, but have concluded that there was no clinical benefit demonstrable in patient groups where BCAA-enriched solutions were used [92–94]. A recent review of the subject by the American Society of Parenteral and Enteral Nutrition (A.S.P.E.N.) does not endorse the widespread use of BCAA solutions for stressed patients [89].

There are times when polypharmaceutical therapy is necessary in the critically injured patient. Because of fluid limitations, it may be convenient to add certain medications to the TPN solutions. Drugs that can safely be added include heparin, insulin, cimetidine, ranitidine, hydrocortisone, albumin, hydrochloric acid, and iron dextran [43]. Although drugs should not be piggybacked through hyperalimentation lines, occasionally a break in the line is warranted. Drugs that can be given in this fashion are aminophylline, certain antibiotics, dopamine, dobutamine, furosemide, isoproterenol, and lidocaine [43]. Drugs that are absolutely incompatible are amphotericin and ampicillin [43].

Special Circumstances

The care of the trauma patient may provide special circumstances in which the nutritional management of the patient must be adjusted. These situations will range from specific types of injuries to surgical complications and ultimately to organ system failure.

Thermal Injuries

The provision of adequate nutritional support to a major burn victim is essential for survival, since the lethal limits of negative protein and caloric balance can be reached within 3 weeks if support is not provided [30,95,96]. The recommended caloric intake in an adult with a thermal injury varies directly with the percentage of body surface area involved (Fig. 21-8). In the past it was calculated from the following formula [96,97]:

$$\text{Recommended kcal/day} = (25 \times \text{wt in kg}) + (40 \times \%\ \text{burn})$$

However, this formula tends to overestimate caloric needs.

The protein requirements of the thermally injured patient can be estimated by calculating the caloric requirements and then supplying protein so that the calorie-to-nitrogen ratio is approximately 100 : 1 [96]. Nitrogen balance studies can be performed, taking the burn wound protein losses into consideration [96]. It has been reported that the burn wound loses 1 to 3 gm/day of protein for each percentage of body surface area involved [98].

The hypermetabolic state of the burn patient is also associated with increased vitamin and mineral requirements. Twice the daily dosage of a multivitamin supplement is usually sufficient when complemented by additional quantities of vitamin C, vitamin A, potassium, and zinc [96].

With a functioning gastrointestinal tract, enteral support is certainly the best method of nutritional support; however, this issue takes on greater significance in the burn patient because of the increased rate of septic complications accompanying intravenous lines [96]. Nasogastric feedings are often necessary to administer the large volumes of high-protein formulas that are required to meet calculated needs. When anasarca and concomitant bowel edema preclude adequate absorption of meal replacement formulas, elemental formulas may be better assimilated. Lack of gastrointestinal tract availability for any prolonged period of time necessitates the institution of parenteral support [95,99].

Neurosurgical Injuries

The assessment of the metabolic needs of patients with central nervous system injury can be challenging. The caloric requirements of these patients can range from 1.2 to 2.0 times the basal metabolic rate, with an average of 1.7 during the first 12 days following injury [57]. It is important to note that both seizure activity and posturing will increase energy expenditure, while the metabolic rate will decrease sharply during barbiturate coma and neuromuscular blockade [27,57]. In multiple trauma victims with associated head injury, massive amounts of urinary nitrogen are excreted. This condition can persist for as long as 3 weeks in patients who remain vegetative [57]. In the presence of steroid therapy, measured nitrogen losses may be in excess of what would be expected for the extent of injury [57].

Patients with head trauma need to have a nutritional assessment performed on post-injury day 3 as previously outlined. Mixed fuel system parenteral support can be used to avoid the hyperglycemia that commonly occurs in this patient population [57,100,101]. This is relevant in light of recent animal studies demonstrating a detrimental effect of glucose administration prior to hypoxic brain injury [102,103]. Serum glucose levels as low as 180 mg/dl were implicated.

Gastrointestinal Cutaneous Fistulae

Fistulization that occurs as a complication of abdominal trauma has a mortality of 20 percent [42]. The first priority in management is to restore fluid and electrolyte balance, followed by the provision of adequate nutrition while maintaining bowel rest [104]. Parenteral nutritional support can be instituted in hopes of healing the fistula with conservative measures. Adjunctive therapies that can help decrease fistula output include H_2 blockers and antidiarrheals.

Although 90 percent of gastrointestinal fistulae will heal within 1 month with intravenous feedings, several months may be necessary in certain patients [41,104,105]. Because of the risk and expense of long-term parenteral therapy, chemically defined diets have been used in this setting [104]. As long as the fistula output does not increase with elemental feedings, they may be administered proximal to the fistula [104]. Reinstitution of parenteral therapy will be required if fistula output increases significantly. For very proximal fistulae, an elemental formula can be infused distally [104]. A closure rate of 50 percent has been described by Rocchio and associates [105] in the treatment of intestinocutaneous fistulae with elemental diets.

Pancreatitis and Pancreatic Fistula

Blunt or penetrating trauma can result in pancreatic injury with the subsequent development of pancreatitis or pancreatic fistula [43]. Many of these patients will require early institution of nutritional support in the form of parenteral or elemental feedings [43]. If the pancreatic complication had not been anticipated and postinjury nutritional support was withheld, therapy should be started after a total of 5 to 7 days without an adequate diet [41].

With conservative therapy, closure of 80 percent of pancreatic fistulae can be anticipated [106,107]. It is generally felt that stimuli that increase pancreatic secretions should be avoided in patients with pancreatitis or pancreatic fistulae. Parenteral alimentation has been demonstrated to suppress pancreatic secretion in some studies [43,106,108,109]. The addition of lipid infusions does not increase pancreatic fistula volume, serum amylase, or lipase and therefore remains useful in this setting [43,106]. The use of enteral formulas is not contraindicated in this patient population [110,111]. When intestinal function permits, excellent clinical results can be obtained using elemental diets in complicated pancreatitis [108,111].

Renal Failure

Acute renal failure can be seen in the setting of extensive trauma and aggravates underlying metabolic and circulatory disturbances [42,112]. Although renal failure may be the result of renovascular injury, secondary causes such as shock, sepsis, rhabdomyolysis, and drug therapy are more common [43].

The approach to nutritional support in patients with acute renal failure has changed dramatically over the last quarter century [42]. Before dialysis therapy was available, carbohydrate was the only substrate administered [112]. Wilmore and Dudrick were the first to add essential amino acids in limited quantities (approximately 12 gm/day) to hypertonic dextrose solutions in these patients [42,113,114]. These studies demonstrated that nitrogen balance was more positive, and dialysis requirements were decreased. In a similar study, Abel and colleagues demonstrated improved survival rates from acute renal failure in patients receiving essential amino acids [112,113,115]. However, the enthusiasm for the use of these solutions decreased when Baek and coworkers demonstrated similar results using balanced protein solutions [85,116]. Because toxic dosages of the essential amino acids were required to promote positive nitrogen balance, current therapy has shifted to the provision of standard amino acid solutions [43,66,112].

The goals of nutritional therapy in the trauma patient with acute renal failure are twofold. The first is to not worsen the metabolic disturbances of the uremic state, and the second is to optimize nutritional support [112]. The oliguric acute renal failure patient will often require daily dialysis if adequate protein substrate is provided [15,43,112]. Protein therapy can be started at 1.0 to 1.2 gm/kg/day in patients who are without symptoms of uremia and whose BUN is less than 70 mg/dl [66]. If the BUN does not increase and the patient remains stable, the protein can be slowly increased to meet calculated requirements. When the BUN is between 70 and 100 mg/dl, protein administration can be started between 0.8 and 1.0 gm/kg/day [43,66]. If the BUN then rises, more aggressive dialysis will have to be instituted or protein will have to be further restricted. If the BUN exceeds 100 mg/dl or the patient is clinically uremic, protein is usually started at the rate of 0.5 to 0.8 mg/kg/day until better control of the uremia can be achieved.

Due to the protein limitations of the uremic patient, adequate caloric support is necessary to optimize nitrogen balance [55]. If a metabolic cart is not available, a stress factor of at least 1.4 should be assigned or caloric support provided to achieve a calorie-to-nitrogen ratio of at least 150 : 1 [112]. When fluid restrictions exist that cannot be eased by frequent dialysis, calorically dense formulas and lipids should be used to provide nonprotein calories [42,43,75]. Some authors have described infusing parenteral solutions while the patient is on hemodialysis [43,112,117].

Patients with acute renal failure need close monitoring of serum electrolyte and glucose concentrations. Initially, phosphorus, magnesium, potassium, and sodium are usually restricted. However, as refeeding progresses, supplementation of potassium, phosphorus, and magnesium may become necessary as intracellular shifts of these ions occur [42,112]. Because zinc and chromium are normally excreted in the urine, close monitoring of these trace minerals is necessary to prevent toxic levels [14].

Hepatic Failure

Hepatic failure is associated with a peripheral energy deficit, resulting in a state of ongoing catabolism. Branched-chain amino acids are oxidized, and aromatic amino acids accumulate [43,75,118,119]. A minority of patients with hepatic failure will be hypoglycemic, while the majority will be glucose intolerant and require insulin supplementation [43,119]. The decision to use lipids as caloric supplements is dependent on the acuity of the hepatic failure and whether encephalopathy is present. Patients with acute hepatic failure or encephalopathy should not receive lipids [119]. Stable cirrhotics without encephalopathy may be given a maximum of 50 gm/day to provide up to 40 percent of the caloric requirement. It is best to document clearance with triglyceride levels in this clinical setting [119].

Amino acid therapy in sufficient quantities to promote positive nitrogen balance is important in the management of the patient with hepatic failure [120]. Intravenous amino acid therapy has been demonstrated to improve hepatic function and survival in patients with acute alcoholic hepatitis without increasing the incidence of encephalopathy [66,120]. This is in contrast to patients with cirrhosis, who cannot increase hepatic function, so that 50 percent of stable patients will develop encephalopathy with standard amino acid formulas [43,66,120]. Special hepatic formulas are now available that contain more branched-chain and less aromatic amino acids [43,118,121]. They appear to normalize amino acid profiles, increase protein synthesis, decrease muscle catabolism, and improve encephalopathy [43,87,118,122]. Therefore, hepatic amino acid formulas are recommended for patients with hepatic dysfunction and increased protein requirements (1.0–1.5 gm/kg/day) and at a lesser dosage for those with grade II encephalopathy (0.8–1.0 gm/kg/day) [118]. Patients with mild liver impairment and no history of encephalopathy may be started on 0.8 gm/kg/day of a standard amino acid formula [118]. If encephalopathy develops or protein requirements increase, a switch to hepatic formula is recommended [119].

Special enteral formulas are available for the nutritional therapy of encephalopathic patients with gastrointestinal function [43,123]. However, patients with severe chronic liver disease often have mild malabsorption resulting in deficiencies of vitamins, zinc, magnesium, iron, and potassium [119]. If diarrhea develops, it should be controlled with dietary manipulation, administration of pancreatic enzymes, or removal of all lactose-containing products [119]. In general, vegetable protein sources are better tolerated than animal sources [119]. With chronic nutritional therapy, it is important to monitor copper and manganese levels because of impaired hepatic excretion in these patients [14].

Respiratory Failure

Patients with traumatic injury may develop respiratory failure due to primary causes such as pulmonary contusion or flail chest or secondarily from adult respiratory distress syndrome, fat embolism, or pneumonia [43]. Nutritional status and substrate intake may have a profound effect on respiratory function in the marginally compensated patient [124–127]. Nutritional therapy of ventilator-dependent patients with adequate calories and protein has been associated with more successful weaning from postoperative respiratory support [66,124,125].

Just as inadequate nutritional status may exacerbate respiratory failure, overzealous support can also be detrimental [128]. Excessive protein administration should be avoided, since the increase in minute ventilation may increase respiratory effort and precipitate dyspnea [125,126]. The administration of excessive carbohydrate loads results in an increase in catecholamine release, a shift to glucose oxidation, and an increase in carbon dioxide production [6,129]. For this reason, glucose infusions should be limited to 4 to 5 mg/kg/min, with 50 percent of the nonprotein energy provided as lipid [125,130]. Of note, fats have been shown to have no adverse clinical effects on pulmonary diffusion capacity in critically ill patients [43,131]. Phosphate balance must be carefully monitored when providing nutritional support to patients with respiratory failure [43]. Hypophosphatemia results in decreased 2,3-diphosphoglycerate levels, which cause diminished tissue oxygen delivery [125]. In addition, phospholipid metabolism is important in the maintenance of lung surfactant.

Cardiac Failure

Cardiac failure may become manifest in the trauma patient as a result of myocardial contusion, myocardial infarction, or underlying cardiac insufficiency [43]. The resulting decrease in cardiac output leads to a state of cellular hypoxia where glucose is the preferred substrate [43,132].

Sodium and volume restriction is necessary when administering nutritional support to patients with myocardial insufficiency, but it should not preclude adequate feeding [43,132]. Maximally concentrated parenteral and enteral formulas are necessary due to sodium (30–40 mg/day) and volume (1500 ml/day) restrictions [43,66,132,133]. The density of enteral formulas can be increased further by the addition of carbohydrate and protein modules [43]. Body fluid losses should always be replaced with nutritional support solutions [132]. Diuretic therapy may allow for greater volume administration; however, the resulting losses of potassium and magnesium must be aggressively supplemented to prevent life-threatening arrhythmias [132].

Controversy exists over the use of intravenous fat emulsions in this clinical setting. Their caloric density makes them very useful in volume-restricted patients. However, there are reports of adverse hemodynamic effects in cardiac patients when lipids were given [134]. These effects seem to depend on the dosage and rate of administration, so that 20% lipid emulsions may be used if given in small quantities or over longer periods of time [132,135]. For example, the maximum dose that should be given to a 50-kg patient is 500 ml of 20% solution over at least 12 hours.

REFERENCES

1. Sanderson, I., Basi, S. S., and Deitel, M. History of Nutrition in Surgery. In M. Deitel, *Nutrition in Clinical Surgery* (2nd ed.) Baltimore: Williams & Wilkins, 1985. P. 3.
2. Cuthbertson, D. P. Observations in the disturbances of metabolism produced by injury of the limbs. *Q. J. Med.* 25:233, 1932.
3. Cahill, G. F., Jr. Starvation in man. *N. Engl. J. Med.* 282:668, 1970.
4. Kirkpatrick, J. R. Fat and Energy Metabolism. In J. R. Kirkpatrick, *Nutrition and Metabolism in the Surgical Patient.* Mt. Kisco, NY: Futura, 1983. P. 3.
5. Wolfe, R. R. Carbohydrate Metabolism and Requirements. In J. L. Rombeau and M. D. Caldwell, *Clinical Nutrition.* Vol. 2, Parenteral Nutrition. Philadelphia: Saunders, 1986. P. 59.
6. Wolfe, B. M., and Ney, D. M. Lipid Metabolism in Parenteral Nutrition. In J. L. Rombeau and M. D. Caldwell, *Clinical Nutrition.* Vol. 2, Parenteral Nutrition. Philadelphia: Saunders, 1986. P. 72.
7. Burr, G. O., and Burr, M. M. A new deficiency disease produced by the rigid exclusion of fat from the diet. *J. Biol. Chem.* 82:345, 1929.
8. Burr, G. O., and Burr, M. M. On the nature of the role of the fatty acids essential in nutrition. *Biol. Chem.* 86:587, 1930.
9. Blackburn, G. L., Bistrian, B. R., and Homsy, F. N. Protein Metabolism in the Surgical Patient. In J. R. Kirkpatrick, *Nutrition and Metabolism in the Surgical Patient.* Futura, Mount Kisco, New York. 1983. P. 59.
10. Wolfe, B. M., Ruderman, R. L., and Pollard A. Basic Principles of Surgical Nutrition: Metabolic Response to Starvation, Trauma, and Sepsis. In M. Deitel, *Nutrition in Clinical Surgery* (2nd ed.). Baltimore: Williams & Wilkins. 1985. P. 14.
11. Moore, F. *Metabolic Care of the Surgical Patient.* Philadelphia: Saunders, 1959. Chapters 1, 2, 31.
12. Stein, T. P. Protein Metabolism and Parenteral Nutrition. In J. L. Rombeau and M. D. Caldwell, *Clinical Nutrition.* Vol. 2, Parenteral Nutrition. Philadelphia: Saunders, 1986. P. 100.
13. Stein, T. P., and Buzby, G. P. Protein metabolism in surgical patients. *Surg. Clin. North Am.* 61:519, 1981.
14. Elwyn, D. H. Nutritional requirements for adult surgical patients. *Crit. Care Med.* 8:9, 1980.
15. Cerra, F. B. Sepsis and Trauma. In J. R. Kirkpat-

rick, *Nutrition and Metabolism in the Surgical Patient.* Mt. Kisco, NY: Futura, 1983. P. 407.

16. Peters, C., and Fischer, J. E. Studies on calorie to nitrogen ratio for total parenteral nutrition. *Surg. Gynecol. Obstet.* 151:1, 1980.
17. Shizgal, H. M. Energy and Nitrogen Interactions. In J. L. Rombeau and M. D. Caldwell, *Clinical Nutrition.* Vol. 2, Parenteral Nutrition. Philadelphia: Saunders, 1986. P. 21.
18. Owen, O. E., et al. Interrelationships Among Key Tissues in the Utilization of Metabolic Substrates. In H. M. Katzen and R. J. Mahler, *Advances in Modern Nutrition.* Vol. 2, Obesity and Vascular Disease. New York: Wiley, 1978. P. 517.
19. White, A., Handler, P., and Smith, E. Proteins I: Amino Acids and Peptides. In *Principles of Biochemistry* (5th ed.). New York: McGraw-Hill, 1973. P. 89.
20. Rose, W. C. Nutritional significance of amino acids. *Physiol. Rev.* 18:109, 1938.
21. Dahn, M. S. Neuro-Hormonal Regulation in Starvation and Injury. In J. R. Kirkpatrick, *Nutrition and Metabolism in the Surgical Patient.* Mount Kisco, NY: Futura, 1983. P. 89.
22. Gamble, J. L. *Chemical Anatomy, Physiology and Pathology of Extracellular Fluid: A Lecture Syllabus* (5th ed.). Cambridge, Mass.: Harvard University Press, 1947.
23. Cuthbertson, D. P. Post-shock metabolic response. *Lancet* 242:433, 1942.
24. Cerra, F. B., et al. Septic autocannibalism: A failure of exogenous nutritional support. *Ann. Surg.* 192:570, 1980.
25. McMenamy, R. J., et al. Multiple systems organ failure: The basal state. *J. Trauma* 21:99, 1981.
26. Gilder, H. Parenteral nourishment of patients undergoing surgical or traumatic stress. *J.P.E.N.* 10:88, 1986.
27. Bessey, P. Q. Parenteral Nutrition and Trauma. In J. L. Rombeau and M. D. Caldwell, *Clinical Nutrition.* Vol. 2, Parenteral Nutrition. Philadelphia: Saunders, 1986. P. 471.
28. Bistrian, B. R. A simple technique to estimate the severity of stress. *Surg. Gynecol. Obstet.* 148:675, 1979.
29. Dahn, M. S. Carbohydrate Metabolism. In J. R. Kirkpatrick, *Nutrition and Metabolism in the Surgical Patient.* Mt. Kisco, NY: Futura, 1983. P. 29.
30. Wilmore, D. W. Carbohydrate metabolism in trauma. *Clin. Endocrinol. Metab.* 5:731, 1976.
31. Selye, H. *The Stress of Life.* Book II, The Dissection of Stress. New York: McGraw-Hill, 1976. P. 55.
32. Askanazi, J., et al. Influence of total parenteral nutrition on fuel utilization in injury and sepsis. *Ann. Surg.* 191:40, 1980.
33. Black, P. R., et al. Mechanisms of insulin resistance following injury. *Ann. Surg.* 196:420, 1982.
34. Brooks, D. C., et al. Post-traumatic insulin resistance in uninjured forearm tissue. *J. Surg. Res.* 37:100, 1984.
35. Grunert, A. Pathobiochemical functions and their relation to carbohydrate metabolism after trauma. *Acta Chir. Scand.* [*Suppl.*] 498:123, 1980.
36. Gump, F. E., et al. Studies of glucose intolerance in septic and injured patients. *J. Trauma* 14:378, 1974.
37. Wilmore, D. W., et al. Effect of injury and infection on visceral metabolism and circulation. *Ann. Surg.* 192:491, 1980.
38. Blackburn, G. L., et al. Branched chain amino acid administration and metabolism during starvation, injury and infection. *Surgery* 86:307, 1979.
39. Felig, P. The glucose-alanine cycle. *Metabolism* 22:179, 1973.
40. Odessey, R., Khairallah, E. A., and Goldberg, A. L. Origin and possible significance of alanine production by skeletal muscle. *J. Biol. Chem.* 249:7623, 1974.
41. A.S.P.E.N. Board of Directors. Guidelines for use of total parenteral nutrition in the hospitalized adult patient. *J.P.E.N.* 10:441, 1986.
42. Kudsk, K. A., Stone, J. M., and Sheldon, G. F. Nutrition in trauma and burns. *Surg. Clin. North Am.* 62:183, 1982.
43. Abbot, W. C., et al. Nutritional care of the trauma patient. *Surg. Gynecol. Obstet.* 157:585, 1983.
44. Shenkin, A., et al. Biochemical changes associated with severe trauma. *Am. J. Clin. Nutr.* 33:2119, 1980.
45. Curreri, P. W., et al. Burn Injury: Analysis of survival and hospitalization time for 937 patients. *Ann. Surg.* 192:472, 1980.
46. Alexander, J. W., et al. Beneficial effects of aggressive protein feeding in severely burned children. *Ann. Surg.* 192:505, 1980.

47. Moore, E. E., and Jones, T. N. Benefits of immediate jejunostomy feeding after major abdominal trauma: A prospective, randomized study. *J. Trauma* 26:874, 1986.
48. Buzby, G. P., and Mullen, J. L. Nutritional Assessment. In J. L. Rombeau and M. D. Caldwell, *Clinical Nutrition.* Vol. 1, Enteral and Tube Feeding. Philadelphia: Saunders, 1984. P. 127.
49. Dempsey, D. T., Buzby, G. P., and Mullen, J. L. Patient Assessment in Nutritional Support. In J. R. Kirkpatrick, *Nutrition and Metabolism in the Surgical Patient.* Mt. Kisco, NY: Futura, 1983. P. 201.
50. Mullen, J. L., et al. Implications of malnutrition in the surgical patient. *Arch. Surg.* 114:121, 1979.
51. Muller, J. M., et al. Preoperative parenteral feeding in patients with gastrointestinal carcinoma. *Lancet* 1:68, 1982.
52. Blackburn, G. L., et al. Immunological abnormalities in the malnourished trauma patient. *Infect. Surg.* 3:681, 1984.
53. Moore, E. E. Enteral elemental nutrition in major trauma. *Contemp. Surg.* 28:18, 1986.
54. Baker, J. P., et al. Nutritional assessment: A comparison of clinical judgement and objective measurements. *N. Engl. J. Med.* 306:969, 1982.
55. Dudrick, S. J., et al. Nutritional Assessment: Indications for Nutritional Support. In M. Deitel, *Nutrition in Clinical Surgery* (2nd ed.). Baltimore: Williams & Wilkins, 1985. P. 24.
56. Blackburn, G. L., et al. Nutritional and metabolic assessment of the hospitalized patient. *J.P.E.N.* 1:11, 1977.
57. Gadisseux, P., et al. Nutrition and the neurosurgical patient. *J. Neurosurg.* 60:219, 1984.
58. Bistrian, B. R., et al. Therapeutic index of nutritional depletion in hospitalized patients. *Surg. Gynecol. Obstet.* 141:512, 1975.
59. Moore, E. E., et al. Penetrating abdominal trauma index. *J. Trauma* 21:439, 1981.
60. Meakins, J. L., et al. Delayed Hypersensitivity: Indicator of acquired failure of host defenses in sepsis and trauma. *Ann. Surg.* 186:241, 1977.
61. Buzby, G. P., et al. Prognostic nutritional index in gastrointestinal surgery. *Am. J. Surg.* 139:160, 1980.
62. Dunn, E. L., Moore, E. E., and Jones, T. Nutritional assessment following abdominal trauma (Abstract). *J.P.E.N.* 4:584, 1980.
63. Rutten, P., et al. Determination of optimal hyperalimentation infusion rate. *J. Surg. Res.* 18:477, 1975.
64. Goodenough, R. D., and Wolfe, R. R. Effect of total parenteral nutrition on free fatty acid metabolism in burned patients. *J.P.E.N.* 8:357, 1984.
65. Clifton, G. L., Robertson, C. S., and Contant, C. F. Enteral hyperalimentation in head injury. *J. Neurosurg.* 62:186, 1985.
66. Echenique, M. M., Bistrian, B. R., and Blackburn, G. L. Theory and techniques of nutritional support in the ICU. *Crit. Care Med.* 10:546, 0000.
67. Kirkpatrick, J. R. Alternate Methods of Parenteral Nutritional Support. In J. R. Kirkpatrick, *Nutrition and Metabolism in the Surgical Patient.* Mt. Kisco, NY: Futura, 1983. P. 281.
68. Schenk, W. G., and Moylan, J. A. Hypercalciuresis in trauma patients on high-nitrogen enteral and parenteral diets. *J. Trauma* 19:227, 1979.
69. Clark, N. G. Vitamin and Mineral Requirements in the Stressed Patient. In *Current Concepts in Nutritional Support* (Monograph 3). Norwich, NY: Norwich Eaton Pharmaceuticals, Inc., Biomedical Information Corp., 1984.
70. Valentine, R. J., et al. Does nasoenteral feeding afford adequate gastroduodenal stress prophylaxis? *Crit. Care Med.* 14:599, 1986.
71. Page, C. P., et al. Safe, cost-effective postoperative nutrition: Defined formula diet via needle-catheter jejunostomy. *Am. J. Surg.* 138:939, 1979.
72. Hearne, B. E., and Daly, J. M. Enteral Nutrition. In J. R. Kirkpatrick, *Nutrition and Metabolism in the Surgical Patient.* Mt. Kisco, NY: Futura, 1983. P. 223.
73. Deitel, M., et al. Elemental and Liquid Diets in Surgery. In M. Deitel, *Nutrition in Clinical Surgery* (2nd ed.). Baltimore: Williams & Wilkins, 1985. P. 44.
74. Matthews, D. M., and Adibi, S. A. Peptide absorption. *Gastroenterology* 71:151, 1976.
75. Dean, R. E. Total Parenteral Nutrition: Standard Techniques. In J. R. Kirkpatrick, *Nutrition and Metabolism in the Surgical Patient.* Mt. Kisco, NY: Futura, 1983. P. 243.

76. Ryan, J. A., et al. Catheter complications in total parenteral nutrition: A prospective study of 200 consecutive patients. *N. Engl. J. Med.* 290:757, 1974.
77. Civetta, J. M., et al. Utility and efficacy of guidewire changes (Abstract). *Crit. Care Med.* 15:380, 1987.
78. Pursell, T. A Simple Equation for Evaluating Whether Parenteral Glucose Administration is Excessive. ASPEN 11th Clinical Congress, *Nutrition Practice Poster Session.* New Orleans, 1987.
79. Fischer, G. W., et al. Diminished bacterial defences with intralipid. *Lancet* 2:819, 1980.
80. Gibault, J. P., et al. Effects of L-carnitine infusion on intralipid clearance and utilization: Study carried out in septic patients of an intensive care unit. *J.P.E.N.* 12:29, 1988.
81. Long, C. L. Fuel preference in the septic patient: Glucose or lipid? *J.P.E.N.* 11:333, 1987.
82. White, R. H., et al. Hormonal and metabolic responses to glucose infusion in sepsis studied by the hyperglycemic glucose clamp technique. *J.P.E.N.* 11:345, 1987.
83. Wolfe, R. R., et al. Investigation of factors determining the optimal glucose infusion rate in total parenteral nutrition. *Metabolism* 29:892, 1980.
84. Dowling, R. J., Alexander, M. A. J., and Mullen, J. L. Use of Fat Emulsions. In M. Deitel, *Nutrition in Clinical Surgery* (2nd ed.). Baltimore: Williams & Wilkins, 1985. P. 139.
85. Louie, N., and Niemiec, P. W. Parenteral Nutrition Solutions. In J. L. Rombeau and M. D. Caldwell, *Clinical Nutrition.* Vol. 2, Parenteral Nutrition. Philadelphia: Saunders, 1986. P. 272.
86. Dennison, A. R., et al. Total parenteral nutrition using conventional and medium chain triglycerides: Effect on liver function tests, complement, and nitrogen balance. *J.P.E.N.* 12(1):15, 1988.
87. Zlotkin, S. J., and Anderson, G. H. Amino-acid Requirements and Sources During Total Parenteral Nutrition. In M. Dietel, *Nutrition in Clinical Surgery* (2nd ed.) Baltimore: Williams & Wilkins, 1985. P. 131.
88. Cerra, F. B., et al. Branched chain metabolic support: A prospective, randomized, double blind trial in surgical stress. *Ann. Surg.* 199:286, 1984.
89. Brennan, M. F., et al. Report of a research workshop: Branched chain amino acids in stress and injury. *J.P.E.N.* 10:446, 1986.
90. Cerra, F. B., et al. Branched chains support postoperative protein synthesis. *Surgery* 92:192, 1982.
91. Cerra, F. B., et al. The effect of stress level, amino acid formula and nitrogen dose on nitrogen retention in traumatic and septic stress. *Ann. Surg.* 205:282, 1987.
92. Rowlands, B., et al. Intravenous and enteral nutrition with branched chain amino acid enriched products following multiple trauma with closed head injury (Abstract). *J.P.E.N.* 10:4S, 1986.
93. Vander Woude, P., et al. Addition of branched-chain amino acids to parenteral nutrition of stressed critically ill patients. *Crit. Care Med.* 14:685, 1986.
94. Von Meyenfeldt, M. F., et al. Branched chain amino acids enriched TPN solution fails to alter the clinical course of septic and traumatized patients (Abstract). *J.P.E.N.* (Suppl.) 10:3S, 1986.
95. Kirkpatrick, J. R., and Meakins, J. The Burn Patient. In J. R. Kirkpatrick, *Nutrition and Metabolism in the Surgical Patient.* Mt. Kisco, NY: Futura, 1983. P. 425.
96. Ruberg, R. L., and Burdge, J. J. Nutritional Support in the Burn Patient. In M. Deitel, *Nutrition in Clinical Surgery* (2nd ed.). Baltimore: Williams & Wilkins, 1985. P. 366.
97. Curreri, P. W., et al. Dietary requirements of patients with major burns. *J. Am. Diet. Assoc.* 65:415, 1974.
98. Nylen, B., and Wallenius, G. The protein loss via exudation from burns and granulating wound surfaces. *Acta Chir. Scand.* 122:97, 1961.
99. Goodwin, C. W. Parenteral Nutrition in Thermal Injuries. In J. L. Rombeau and M. D. Caldwell, *Clinical Nutrition.* Vol. 2, Parenteral Nutrition. Philadelphia: Saunders, 1986. P. 489.
100. Fell, D., et al. Metabolic profiles in patients with acute neurosurgical injuries. *Crit. Care Med.* 12:649, 1984.
101. Michenfelder, J. D. Current Status of Brain Protection. In P. G. Barash (ed.), *American Society of Anesthesiologists (ASA) Refresher Courses in Anesthesiology.* American Society of Anesthesiologists 15:125, 1987.
102. Lanier, W. L., et al. Effects of I.V. dextrose and

head position on neurologic outcome after complete cerebral ischemia (Abstract). *Anesthesiology* 63:110, 1985.
103. Warner, D. S., Smith, M. L., and Siesjo, B. K. Ischemia in normo- and hyperglycemic rats: Effects on brain water and electrolytes. *Anesthesiol. Rev.* 13:23, 1986.
104. Betzhold, J., and Howard, L. Enteral Nutrition and Gastrointestinal Disease. In J. L. Rombeau and M. D. Caldwell, *Clinical Nutrition.* Vol. 1, Enteral and Tube Feeding. Philadelphia: Saunders, 1984. P. 338.
105. Rocchio, M. A., et al. Use of chemically defined diets in the management of patients with high output gastrointestinal cutaneous fistulas. *Am. J. Surg.* 127:148, 1974.
106. Grundfest, S., et al. The effect of intravenous fat emulsions in patients with pancreatic fistula. *J.P.E.N.* 4:27, 1980.
107. Ragins, H. R., et al. Intrajejunal administration of an elemental diet at neutral pH avoids pancreatic stimulation. *Am. J. Surg.* 126:606, 1973.
108. Blackburn, G. L., et al. New approaches to the management of severe acute pancreatitis. *Am. J. Surg.* 131:114, 1976.
109. Kelly, G. A., and Nahrwold, D. L. Pancreatic secretion in response to an elemental diet and intravenous hyperalimentation. *Surg. Gynecol. Obstet.* 143:87, 1976.
110. Dyck, W. P. Influence of intrajejunal glucose on pancreatic exocrine function in man. *Gastroenterology* 60:864, 1971.
111. Voitk, A., et al. Use of an elemental diet in the treatment of complicated pancreatitis. *Am. J. Surg.* 125:223, 1973.
112. Feinstein, E. I. Nutrition in Acute Renal Failure. In J. L. Rombeau and M. D. Caldwell, *Clinical Nutrition.* Vol. 2, Parenteral Nutrition. Philadelphia: Saunders, 1986. P. 586.
113. Briggs, W. A. Renal Failure. In J. R. Kirkpatrick, *Nutrition and Metabolism in the Surgical Patient.* Mt. Kisco, NY: Futura, 1983. P. 341.
114. Wilmore, D. W., and Dudrick, S. J. Treatment of acute renal failure with intravenous essential L-amino acids. *Arch. Surg.* 99:669, 1969.
115. Abel, R. M., et al. Improved survival from acute renal failure after treatment with intravenous essential L-amino acids and glucose: Results of a prospective double-blind study. *N. Engl. J. Med.* 288:695, 1973.
116. Baek, Se-Min, et al. The influence of parenteral nutrition on the course of acute renal failure. *Surg. Gynecol. Obstet.* 141:405, 1975.
117. Wolfson, M., Jones, M. R., and Kopple, J. D. Amino acid losses during hemodialysis with infusion of amino acids and glucose. *Kidney Int.* 21:500, 1982.
118. Bower, R. H., and Fischer, J. E. Hepatic Indications for Parenteral Nutrition. In J. L. Rombeau and M. D. Caldwell, *Clinical Nutrition.* Vol. 2, Parenteral Nutrition. Philadelphia: Saunders, 1986. P. 602.
119. Ehrinpreis, M. N. Hepatic Failure. In J. R. Kirkpatrick, *Nutrition and Metabolism in the Surgical Patient.* Mt. Kisco, NY: Futura, 1983. P. 357.
120. Nasrallah, S. M., and Galambos, J. T. Amino acid therapy of alcoholic hepatitis. *Lancet* 2:1276, 1980.
121. Okada, A., and Kamata, S. Hepatic Failure (Encephalopathy)—Acute and Chronic. In M. Deitel, *Nutrition in Clinical Surgery* (2nd ed.). Baltimore: Williams & Wilkins, 1985. P. 341.
122. Fischer, J. E., et al. Effects of FO80 in clinical hepatic encephalopathy: Result of Phase I study (Abstract). *Gastroenterology* 75:963, 1978.
123. Keohane, P. P., et al. Nutritional support of malnourished encephalopathic cirrhotic patients using a specially formulated enteral diet (Abstract). *Gastroenterology* 82:1098, 1982.
124. Bassili, H. R., and Dietel, M. Effect of nutritional support on weaning patients off mechanical ventilators. *J.P.E.N.* 5:161, 1981.
125. Deitel, M., Rice, T. W., and Field, S. K. Respiratory Failure and the Ventilator-Dependent Patient. In M. Deitel, *Nutrition in Clinical Surgery* (2nd ed.). Baltimore: Williams & Wilkins, 1985. P. 357.
126. Takala, J., et al. Changes in respiratory control induced by amino acid infusions. *Crit. Care Med.* 16:465, 1988.
127. Weissman, C., et al. Amino acids and respiration. *Ann. Intern. Med.* 98:41, 1983.
128. Askanazi, J., et al. Nutrition for the patient with respiratory failure: Glucose vs. fat. *Anesthesiology* 54:373, 1981.
129. Askanazi, J., et al. Respiratory changes induced by the large glucose loads of total parenteral nutrition. J.A.M.A. 243:1444, 1980.
130. Askanazi, J., et al. Nutrition and the respiratory system. *Crit. Care Med.* 10:163, 1982.

131. Jarnberg, P., Lindholm, M., and Eklund, J. Lipid infusion in critically ill patients: Acute effects on hemodynamics and pulmonary gas exchange. *Crit. Care Med.* 9:27, 1981.
132. Abel, R. M. Nutritional Support and the Cardiac Patient. In J. L. Rombeau and M. D. Caldwell, *Clinical Nutrition.* Vol. 2, Parenteral Support. Philadelphia: Saunders, 1986. P. 575.
133. Abel, R. M., et al. Malnutrition in cardiac surgical patients: Results of a prospective randomized evaluation of early postoperative parenteral nutrition. *Arch. Surg.* 111:45, 1976.
134. Fisch, D., and Abel, R. M. Hemodynamic effects of intravenous fat emulsions in patients with heart disease. *J.P.E.N.* 5:402, 1981.
135. Abel, R. M., Fisch, D., and Grossman, M. L. Hemodynamic effects of intravenous 20% soy oil emulsion following coronary bypass surgery. *J.P.E.N.* 7:534, 1983.

22

Trauma and the Blood Bank

Thomas A. Noto

The importance of blood bank services in the care of trauma patients has been well documented both in war and in civilian life. Although the staff of the hospital blood bank or transfusion service are not involved with the direct care of trauma victims, their expertise plays an indispensable role in the successful management of shock. While the entire organization of this area of the laboratory must be directed to respond to emergency requests in a timely fashion, it is also charged with the duty of providing blood and blood components for a safe transfusion.

The scope of this chapter is to discuss transfusion medicine issues that are relevant to both the trauma surgeon and the hospital transfusion service. As with any other medical specialty, transfusion medicine has also experienced many changes and advances. Some of these affect the manner in which the blood requirements are met for the trauma patient. Consequently, this chapter will discuss current practices of pretransfusion compatibility testing of the recipient, the hemostatic changes brought about by a massive transfusion, and the approach to the management of hemorrhage. One may argue that the progress of procuring a blood sample for pretransfusion testing is elementary and that any discussion pertaining to it might insult the reader. This is neither the case nor the intent. As the reader will see, this procedure is very important and demands careful attention. In addition, it is through the blood sample that the first contact is ordinarily made between the trauma patient and the attending physician with the hospital transfusion service.

Well-established lines of communication should exist between the trauma unit and the hospital transfusion service. Because the care of the bleeding trauma patient requires numerous resources, their availability and possible limitations should be explored and established prior to the organization of a hospital trauma unit. The chief of the trauma division should communicate the anticipated requirements for blood and blood components for the level of trauma care that is to be delivered. This information should be the basis for establishing acceptable response times to requests for blood. Together with the director of the transfusion service, the chief of the trauma service should organize criteria that outline blood ordering practices and the proper utilization of blood and blood components [1].

PROCUREMENT OF BLOOD SAMPLES

The proper and accurate identification of the trauma patient at the time that the blood sample is procured for the transfusion service is the first procedure that ensures a safe transfusion. Because fatal hemolytic transfusion reactions are largely the result of clerical errors in patient identification, strict adherence to the hospital policies in this regard is an absolute necessity. Whatever identification information is available at the time the trauma victim is admitted to the emergency department must be used for labeling tubes of blood samples and the request forms for blood.

In most emergency situations, the patient's identity is unknown. Nevertheless, this does not absolve anyone from using the emergency identification process properly. Whatever emergency identification is available and used must be cross-referenced with the patient's name and identification number when these become established. If this is not done, procurement of a new blood specimen is usually required so that patient identification is maintained accurately. Improper identification of the patient and blood sample ultimately results in transfusion delays. Even in critical emergency situations, individuals performing the pretransfusion compatibility testing should not be expected to assume any responsibility for accepting an improperly labeled tube of blood or a blood specimen from an inaccurately identified patient. Current standards of practice for transfusion services [2] dictate that if there is any discrepancy or any doubt about the identity of a patient, a new blood sample must be collected. These approved standards further emphasize the importance of correct patient identification by stating that it is unacceptable for anyone to rectify an incorrectly labeled specimen.

Normally, blood samples in the emergency room are collected prior to the placement of infusion lines. However, it is permissible to obtain a blood sample from an infusion line through which the patient is receiving intravenous fluids. Proper collection, under these circumstances, requires that the tubing be flushed with saline and the first 5 ml of blood withdrawn be discarded. This prevents the residual fluid in the line from interfering with the pretransfusion serologic tests.

In the acutely bleeding patient, it is often difficult to determine how much blood replacement will be required initially. Clarke and associates [1] provide criteria useful for determining emergency transfusion needs that may be used as guidelines for requesting cross-matched blood. A request for 6 units of blood will be sufficient to manage blood losses of between 2000 and 3000 ml. With more pronounced and continued blood losses, additional units may be readily available because of the current laboratory procedures for providing compatible blood in an emergent situation. These subsequent requests may consist of 4 to 6 additional units, depending on the clinical situation. When the blood loss is moderate and the vital signs are relatively stable, blood requirements should be met by requesting less than 6 units of blood. It is appropriate to use the "type and screen" request when it is uncertain that a patient will require blood transfusions during an impending emergency operative procedure. When using the type and screen request, the patient is tested for ABO and Rh blood groups and for the presence of unexpected erythrocyte alloantibodies. No units of cross-matched blood are reserved for the patient. This latter request option gives the surgeon the flexibility of obtaining blood immediately if an urgent situation should arise later. The use of the type and screen is recommended because of the confirmed unnecessary and overrequesting of cross-matched blood from emergency departments [1].

TRANSFUSION OF UNCROSS-MATCHED BLOOD

The trauma surgeon should be knowledgeable of the options available for obtaining blood to transfuse in desperately urgent situations. Clinically defined criteria should be available justifying the transfusion of blood prior to the completion of tests for detecting red cell antibodies and determining recipient-donor compatibility. Blood for emergency transfusions can be provided as (1) group O, Rh-negative red blood cells or (2) group-specific whole blood or red blood cells. Prior to the administration of uncross-matched blood, a blood sample must be obtained from the patient. This will permit the determination of the hereditary blood group of the patient so that subsequent transfusions may be blood group–specific, when group O blood is initially given.

The plasma of group O whole blood contains anti-A and anti-B, which may cause hemolysis in patients who are group A, B, or AB. Because of this, uncross-matched group O blood must be used as red blood cells rather than as whole blood. The Rh status of both donor and patient must also be considered in emergency situations. While the use of Rh-positive blood poses no immediate threat when transfused to a patient who is Rh-negative, nevertheless alloimmunization, especially of females in the childbearing age, is of prime concern [3]. This is why the use of uncross-matched group O, Rh-positive red blood cells should be restricted to male patients when the supply of group O, Rh-negative blood is limited. It has been our experience that most Rh-negative male trauma patients have no past history of blood transfusions. Consequently, they have no alloantibodies in their plasma to red cell antigens. Within the context of alloimmunization to the Rh factor (the D antigen), the absence of anti-D in most male patients would make this practice safe in life-threatening situations. However, to ensure a safe transfusion, only when the results of the antibody detection test are available should the decision be made to give Rh-positive blood to Rh-negative male individuals or female patients who are not in the childbearing age. If and when the patient develops anti-

D, then only Rh-negative red blood cells must be transfused.

Blood transfusions in the emergency room are given in an environment that is usually tense and hectic. This is particularly true when multiple trauma victims require immediate medical care. In these circumstances, restricting transfusions to group O, Rh-negative red blood cells eliminates errors in patient identification, thereby preventing the foremost cause of an acute hemolytic transfusion reaction as a result of ABO incompatibility. This fact should be considered when physicians develop transfusion criteria for the emergency room management of multiple casualties with severe, hypovolemic shock.

Group-specific uncross-matched blood [4] also has its utility in patients for whom emergency transfusion is indicated. This choice is preferred by some if proper ABO grouping and Rh typing can be accomplished readily. An advantage to the use of group-specific blood is that it may be used as whole blood, thereby making it possible to replace blood volume and red cells simultaneously. Group-specific uncross-matched blood may be used in one of two ways: (1) it may be used in the initial resuscitative measures instead of group O red blood cells, or (2) when group O uncross-matched blood is initially transfused, subsequent transfusions may be given as group-specific blood. Table 22-1 summarizes the advantages and disadvantages associated with the use of each category of transfusion. Whenever group-specific blood is transfused in an emergency setting, pretransfusion identification procedures of the patient and donor blood must be conducted properly without sacrificing any specified details.

The use of uncross-matched blood is a relatively safe procedure not associated with a high incidence of adverse transfusion reactions. Military and civilian experiences, the latter in both adults and children, support this observation [4,5–9]. However, while the use of uncross-matched blood in the emer-

Table 22-1. Advantages and Disadvantages in the Emergency Use of Red Blood Cells and Whole Blood

Blood category	Advantage	Disadvantage
Group O, Rh-negative	Readily available	Must be used as red blood cells
	Issued immediately prior to completion of compatibility tests	May be incompatible if patient is alloimmunized
ABO and Rh group specific	Available in 5 min following determination of ABO and Rh groups	May be incompatible if patient is alloimmunized
	May be used as whole blood	

gency management of trauma patients is an approved clinical practice, its indiscriminate use is not advocated. It is recommended that this practice should be monitored closely by the hospital transfusion committee to prevent its abuse. Not every trauma patient fulfills clinically defined criteria justifying the transfusion of uncross-matched blood [6]. For example, emergency transfusion appears to be of little value in cardiac arrest.

As indicated in Table 22-1, the *potential* for hemolytic transfusion reactions exists in a small number of trauma patients, namely those who have been previously transfused or who have been pregnant. In these patients, the presence of clinically significant alloantibodies may cause destruction of the transfused red cells if the corresponding antigens should be present on the red cells of the uncross-matched blood.

PRETRANSFUSION COMPATIBILITY TESTING—CURRENT PRACTICES

A number of selected serologic tests are essential for the safe transfusion of whole blood and red blood cell components. The extent of pretransfusion compatibility testing and the manner in which these tests are performed will determine the readiness with which blood will be available for transfusion.

The compatibility tests performed on prospective recipients are standard. They include ABO grouping, Rh typing, the detection (screening) test for unexpected serum alloantibodies to red cell antigens, and the major cross match. The procedures for detecting unexpected alloantibodies, other than anti-A and anti-B, in the blood of the recipient and for determining recipient-donor compatibility vary among laboratories. Nevertheless, the methods employed are based on the same principles, namely, that they must be capable of demonstrating clinically significant alloantibodies. These are antibodies that are known to cause a shortened survival of transfused red cells. The antibody screening test includes incubation of the recipient's serum with reagent red cells at 37°C and the antiglobulin test. The complete major cross match involves the testing of the recipient's serum with the red cells of the selected donor(s), requiring incubation at 37°C and the antiglobulin test. The purpose of the cross match is to demonstrate ABO compatibility between recipient and donor and the absence of unexpected alloantibodies against antigens on the donor's red cells.

The approach to the cross match procedure differs significantly today from that practiced for the past 25 years. Based on the data and experience obtained from the use of the type and screen request during the past 10 years, abbreviation of the major cross match is approved and accepted as a safe transfusion practice preventing incompatible blood transfusions [10–14]. The abbreviated cross match eliminates the incubation phase and the antiglobulin test, thus providing not only simplicity in performance but also the immediate availability of compatible blood for any emergency situation. Furthermore, the abbreviated cross match is greater than 99.9 percent safe [11] when the patient has no demonstrable unexpected alloantibodies to erythrocyte antigens. The limited major cross match verifies ABO compatibility. This is an important factor, since ABO incompatibility results in acute and sometimes fatal hemolytic transfusion reactions.

A discrepancy or unexpected finding in any one of the pretransfusion serologic tests presents a problem for the emergency transfusion. These discrepant or unexpected test results should be resolved prior to the transfusion of blood. However, in life-threatening situations, compromises in performing the required laboratory procedures may have to be made. For example, if the recipient's ABO blood group cannot be established accurately, then group O red blood cells may have to be administered.

Depending on the nature of the problem encountered, considerable time and effort are expended to provide blood for a safe transfusion. For example, the presence of single or multiple clinically significant alloantibodies to red cell antigens will require identification of their blood group specificity. Depending on the specificity of the alloantibodies, the selected compatible donor blood units must be phenotyped to ensure absence of the specific antigens. However, when the patient has received a large-volume transfusion, the abbreviated cross match may be used if the donor red cells are typed and lack the corresponding antigen to the identified alloantibody.

Whenever any of these serologic problems causes undue delay in providing blood, the attending physician and the transfusion service director may have to agree to the transfusion of incompatible blood as a lifesaving measure until the problem is resolved satisfactorily. Following the transfusion of incompatible blood, the attending physician should be alert to the clinical and laboratory findings suggestive of a possible hemolytic transfusion reaction. These include an unexplained anemia in the absence of bleeding, a rising serum bilirubin level, and fever, which may present several days following the transfusion. A positive direct antiglobulin test (direct Coombs' test) in the post-transfusion blood sample will verify a hemolytic process.

In a previous section, the conditions for switching an Rh-negative recipient to Rh-positive donor blood were discussed. During a massive transfusion, it may be necessary to switch to a different ABO blood group. Table 22-2 outlines the group-compatible donor blood that may be used for each major ABO group. The change to group-compatible do-

Table 22-2. Selection of Donor ABO Blood Group for the Transfusion of Red Blood Cells (RBCs)

Patient's ABO blood group	First choice of donor blood group	Alternative donor blood group
O	O	None
A	A	O (RBCs)
B	B	O (RBCs)
AB	AB	A, B, O (RBCs)

Table 22-3. Selection of Donor ABO Blood Group for the Transfusion of Fresh Frozen Plasma

Patient's ABO blood group	Acceptable blood group	Antibody in plasma unit
O	O	Anti-A and anti-B
	A	Anti-B
	B	Anti-A
	AB	None
A	A	Anti-B
	AB	None
B	B	Anti-A
	AB	None
AB	AB	None

nor blood requires that the transfusions be limited to red blood cells. Ideally, group-specific fresh frozen plasma is also selected for transfusion. However, circumstances may require the administration of group-compatible plasma, as indicated in Table 22-3. Written policies in the transfusion service should specify acceptable situations for the change of blood types during a massive transfusion.

WHOLE BLOOD AND RED BLOOD CELL TRANSFUSIONS

Trauma victims are prime candidates for a massive transfusion. A massive transfusion is defined as one that approximates the patient's blood volume within a 24-hour interval. However, in many trauma victims, this volume is administered within a shorter time interval. Essential to the definition of a massive transfusion is an understanding of the principles of an exchange transfusion. The administration of large volumes of blood is essentially an exchange of the patient's blood with stored donor blood. The concept of an exchange transfusion will be considered in the next section when alterations of hemostasis in the trauma patient are discussed.

The trauma surgeon is well aware that the primary treatment of hemorrhage involves the control of the bleeding source and the rapid restoration of blood loss. Expansion and maintenance of blood volume is of primary concern [15]. Because the transport of oxygen is usually inadequate in the acutely injured, it is important that restoration of red cell volume also receive attention. In assessing transfusion requirements, the approach must be individualized for each patient by considering the following facts: (1) extent and rate of red cell loss, (2) oxygen requirements, (3) response of the patient's cardiorespiratory system, (4) status of tissue perfusion, and (5) the presence of any preexisting disease.

Hemorrhagic shock is managed with transfusions of either red blood cells or whole blood. The discussion here will focus on the current preservation of red blood cell components. It will also consider the advantages and disadvantages of each in the transfusion of trauma patients.

Whole blood is stored in citrate-phosphate-dextrose anticoagulant-preservative to which adenine is added (CPDA-1). This anticoagulant permits the storage of whole blood for 35 days. During storage, blood undergoes biochemical and cellular changes that reflect the "lesion of storage." These alterations have been adequately described [16,17] and include reduction in pH and depletion of cellular adenosine triphosphate (ATP) and of 2,3-diphosphoglycerate (2,3-DPG). Leakage of intracellular potassium into the plasma occurs. Because of these changes, hyperkalemia, hypocalcemia, and acidosis have in the past been stressed as complications of a massive transfusion, in fact perhaps overemphasized.

Because citrate binds ionized calcium, administration of the anticoagulant present in the transfused donor blood results in a transient decrease of the patient's ionized calcium. This decrease is related directly to the amount of citrate transfused and to the rapid rate of the infusion [18]. The average adult can tolerate transfusion rates of 100 ml/min without demonstrating citrate toxicity [19]. Citrate is rapidly metabolized by nucleated cells in the body; however, hypotension and hypoperfusion may impair this process. To counterbalance the citrate effect, parathyroid hormone is released in an attempt to restore normal levels of ionized calcium. Some investigators [20] have been unable to demonstrate the adverse effects of citrate administration and do not advocate the routine use of calcium salts. In fact, because changes in ionized calcium occur rapidly, the administration of calcium salts may result in hypercalcemia and cardiac arrhythmias.

Another concern of a massive transfusion is the ensuing hyperkalemia. This is more of a theoretical than a real entity. The loss of intracellular potassium during blood storage is the result of a failure of the sodium-potassium pumping mechanism. Whole blood collected in CPDA-1 and stored for 35 days contains 27 mEq/L of plasma potassium, or approximately 7 mEq/unit. The amount of transfused potassium will depend on the number of donor blood units given and on the storage age of the transfused blood. The increment of potassium in the plasma of the patient is transient, since potassium reenters the transfused red cells. This response is influenced by the alkalosis resulting from the metabolism of citrate, which aids the intracellular movement of potassium, and also by the renal excretion of potassium. Consequently, the effect is more often hypokalemia. However, potential potassium toxicity exists for those patients with renal failure or severe acidosis. For most massively transfused patients, hyperkalemia does not pose a real problem.

Even though the plasma of stored whole blood contains the waste products of cellular metabolism, it is a good source of coagulation factors. It is often mistakenly assumed that stored whole blood is devoid of clotting factors. Actually, only factors V and VIII deteriorate significantly [21] during storage. Factor V levels decrease to about 50 percent of normal at 14 days of storage and to 35 percent at 21 days. On the other hand, factor VIII levels fall rapidly to about 50 percent of normal during the first 24 hours of storage, and then the decline is slow [21]. The remainder of the coagulation factors are stable, and their quantity, although hemostatically sufficient, will vary depending on the storage period of the blood. Platelets, on the other hand, decline rapidly during the first 3 days of storage. The clinical implications of these changes will be addressed when hemostasis is discussesd. These findings dispel the myth that stored whole blood is devoid in the quantity of functional plasma coagulation factors.

The advantage to the use of stored whole blood for a massive transfusion is that it contains all of the constituents for correcting hypovolemia and oxygen transport. Thus, a valid indication [21,22] for the transfusion of whole blood is acute blood loss. Excluding the fact that whole blood is platelet-poor, it is useful for replacing deficient plasma coagulation factors if there is a documented need to do so.

Red blood cells, also known as packed cells or red cell concentrate, are currently prepared in one of two ways. In one method, the supernatant plasma from whole blood collected in CPDA-1 is removed by centrifugation; however, about 70 to 80 ml of residual plasma is retained. When prepared in a closed system, this component also has a shelf life of 35 days. The second method provides for the extended storage of red blood cells to 42 days. Whole blood is first collected in CPD anticoagulant, and then the plasma is removed. The contents from an attached satellite bag, 100 ml of an additive solution composed of saline, dextrose, adenine, and mannitol (AS-1; Adsol, Fenwal Laboratories), are added to the packed red cells [23]. A variant of this system consists of collecting whole blood in CP2D, a CPD solution with additional dextrose. After plasma removal, the additive solution as described above, but without the mannitol, is added (AS-2; Nutricel, Cutter Laboratories). With this additive system, red blood cells are stored for 35 days. Red blood cells prepared with additive solutions are essentially devoid of plasma.

When stored in CPDA-1 for 35 days, red blood cells contain approximately 78 mEq/L of plasma potassium. While the products of cellular metabolism appear elevated in this product, the total volume of plasma in these units is only 70 to 80 ml. Therefore, routinely prepared red blood cells carry the same metabolic burden as whole blood. This situation is eliminated only when red blood cells are prepared shortly before transfusion. However, this is neither practical nor essential.

The red blood cells with additive solutions contain less citrate than those products without these second preservatives. However, when stored for 35 days, they have equivalent amounts of extracellular potassium to those preserved in CPDA-1 for the same period of time. The plasma potassium is in the range of 5 to 6 mEq/unit. Another advantage to the use of red blood cells with additive solutions is that they have the same viscosity as whole blood and thus have the flow characteristics of whole blood. Because of this, dilution of this product with normal saline is not necessary prior to administration.

Because of the limited amount of whole blood available in most communities, the majority of massive transfusions are managed with red blood cells, crystalloid solutions, and specific blood components when they are indicated. Some trauma surgeons [24] prefer the use of blood components to the transfusion of whole blood. On the other hand, there are those that advocate the use of whole blood after a designated number of red blood cell units have been transfused. Either approach is acceptable. However, it is not appropriate to transfuse red blood cells in conjunction with fresh frozen plasma to reconstitute whole blood from red cells. While a recent study [25] showed that only a small percentage of red blood cells are given in this manner, other studies [26,27] indicate that there is a tendency to transfuse both concomitantly for volume replacement. This practice is not appropriate and most often not clinically indicated. For example, the use of fresh frozen plasma for volume expansion is not acceptable and should be discouraged. Likewise, the routine supplementation of whole blood with fresh frozen plasma is inappropriate. As mentioned earlier, the plasma of stored whole blood contains adequate levels of the essential clotting factors.

The final note in this section concerns the periodic requests made for "fresh" blood. The definition of "fresh" will vary as to the constituent of whole blood one refers to. For example, red cells may be considered fresh within 7 days of collection, whereas this dating period is inadequate for platelets because of their rapid deterioration. Current blood banking practices and testing requirements of donor blood do not make the availability of fresh blood logistically feasible. Furthermore, hemotherapy utilizing specific blood components does not justify this request. When there appears to be a need for fresh whole blood, it is probably more prudent to consider consulting with either an expert in coagulation or a specialist in transfusion medicine.

ABNORMAL HEMOSTASIS IN TRAUMA

Trauma patients receiving massive transfusions are susceptible of developing coagulation abnormalities. These are usually the result of dilution caused by the transfusion of stored blood components, or they may be consumptive in nature. The management of bleeding secondary to a coagulopathy is challenging and can be a rewarding experience for both the trauma team and transfusion service.

The concept of a dilutional coagulopathy is explained best by the exchange transfusion model alluded to earlier. Based on the kinetics of this model, replacing one blood volume in a 70-kg adult with blood transfusions will leave 25 to 30 percent of the patient's initial blood and cellular elements in the circulation. Approximately 10 percent of the patient's blood elements remain following a transfusion replacement of 2 times the blood volume [19]. This provides a rough guideline for the interpretation of intraoperative laboratory changes when compared to baseline laboratory studies.

There is no doubt that dilution of blood elements takes place during a massive transfusion. However, the clinical significance of this process must address its assumed role in abnormal hemostasis. To accomplish this, in addition to considering the volume of the transfusion, one should consider (1) the type of blood components administered, (2) the coagulation elements in question, and (3) the presence of any preexisting acquired or congenital coagulopathy in the patient.

The transfusion of either stored whole blood or red blood cells may result in thrombocytopenia on the basis of dilution [28–31]. This has been documented in some patients following a massive transfusion when 1.5 times their blood volume has been replaced with transfusions. However, it has been shown recently that dilutional thrombocytopenia may be less common than previously thought [32]. The clinical manifestation of dilutional thrombocytopenia is *diffuse microvascular bleeding.* Intraoperative platelet counts are clinically significant when below 60,000/μl. The transfusion of platelets, based on 1 unit/10 kg of body weight, is effective in providing the quantity of platelets required for effective hemostasis. The efficacy of this transfusion platelet dose is achieved best when surgical bleeding is controlled. To justify the intraoperative transfusion of platelets, two facts should be documented: (1) a low platelet count and (2) the presence of slow, generalized bleeding (oozing) that is typically distinguishable from surgical bleeding.

It is possible for trauma patients to have an adequate number of platelets and manifest a diffuse bleeding diathesis. Data [31,33] are available that indicate that an acquired platelet dysfunction may occur with trauma. This complication has been attributed to tissue injury. The possible coexistence of platelet dysfunction may compound the effects of dilutional thrombocytopenia. On the other hand, it has been observed [33] that despite severe changes in both the number and function of platelets in massive transfusion, microvascular bleeding may not occur. Patients with bleeding because of platelet dysfunction respond to platelet transfusions.

The abuse of platelet therapy in trauma patients is related to their prophylactic administration [32,33]. Often, platelets are transfused on an empiric basis to prevent thrombocytopenia from occurring. However, as stated previously, not all massively transfused patients experience this complication [31]. This observation has been documented recently in a prospective, randomized, double-blind clinical study [32]. The study supports the fact that the development of dilutional thrombocytopenia is often counteracted by the release of endogenous platelets principally from the spleen. Consequently, the prophylactic administration of platelets to prevent this complication is not warranted.

Unfortunately, the dilution of plasma coagulation factors secondary to massive transfusions is not easily dispensed with. Dilution of plasma coagulation factors may occur as a result of a massive transfusion. However, its etiology must first consider the type of red blood cell component given. Secondly, one must question the clinical significance, if any, of the dilutional effect on hemostasis.

As stated previously, whole blood, when stored for at least 3 weeks, has sufficient levels of all plasma coagulation factors except factor VIII. Studies [28] performed with the transfusion of modified whole blood, which mirrors the composition of stored whole blood in that it is platelet-poor and factor VIII–deficient, did not confirm the dilution of clotting factors below hemostatic levels, that is, a plasma level below 30 percent. In like manner, the use of stored whole blood for a massive transfusion should not produce clinically significant dilution of the plasma coagulation factors [34].

On the other hand, the fate of plasma coagulation factor levels in patients receiving large-volume transfusions of red blood cells alone is not definitely known. Theoretically, based on the exchange transfusion model, significant dilution of the plasma coagulation factors may occur depending on the patient's blood volume replaced. Limited data [35] are available showing that surgical patients receiving 7 units of red blood cells and Ringer's lactate during major surgery compared favorably with similar patients transfused with equivalent units of whole blood. The patients in both groups showed no significant alterations in the coagulation tests performed, and more importantly, no episodes of clinical bleeding were observed. Whether patients receiving more than 7 units of red blood cells without fresh frozen plasma might develop a clinically significant dilution of plasma coagulation factors resulting in microvascular bleeding remains to be established [36]. Currently, from the available reports, the degree of dilution of coagulation factors with massive transfusion is poorly predictable.

In defense that the transfusion of large volumes of stored red blood cells rarely causes clinically significant dilution of the patient's plasma coagulation factors is the fact that these factors are replenished by de novo synthesis and released from sites of extravascular distribution to maintain normal hemostasis. Based on this information, it is currently held that dilution of plasma coagulation factors with massive transfusions of stored whole blood or red blood cells is rarely the sole cause of abnormal hemostasis. However, any dilution that does occur may be critically influenced by preexisting diseases, such as congenital coagulopathies or liver disease, that affect synthesis of coagulation proteins [37] or, more commonly in trauma patients, by a consumptive process.

The incidence of acute disseminated intravascular coagulation (DIC) is reported to occur in 5 to 30 percent of trauma patients [28,29,36]. This complication is more apt to occur with severe trauma, so its incidence among trauma units will be influenced by the level of trauma care offered. The cause of DIC is related to such factors as the extent of tissue damage, organ involvement, and the duration of hypovolemic shock. Here, unlike dilutional thrombocytopenia where only the platelets are decreased, there is also derangement of laboratory tests measuring the activity or quantity of plasma coagulation factors. Therefore, the use of such tests as prothrombin time (PT), activated partial thromboplastin time (APTT), fibrinogen level, and platelet count provides a differentiation between a coagulopathy as the result of dilutional thrombocytopenia and acute DIC. Tests determining the presence of fibrin degradation products (FDPs) are not essential for the diagnosis of acute DIC. FDPs are elevated in many situations, especially in surgical patients, and are not specific for DIC. As in dilutional thrombocytopenia, the bleeding associated with acute DIC is slow and diffuse.

Trauma patients with acute DIC should receive prompt correction of the lesions present. Likewise, measures for correcting the hypovolemia and shock should be instituted promptly. In addition, hemotherapy to restore adequate hemostasis [37,38] must be used. Either whole blood or red blood cells and fresh frozen plasma should be transfused. Cryoprecipitate may be given when the plasma fibrinogen level is less than 75 mg/dl. There appears to be no agreement on the amount of these products to administer. For fresh frozen plasma, the initial dose may be based on 10 ml/kg of body weight; for cryoprecipitate, 1 bag/10 kg of body weight. The best approach, however, is to individualize their use based on intraoperative laboratory evaluation and clinical observation. When the thrombocytopenia is severe and the cause of the DIC is reversible, platelets may be given. Unlike dilutional thrombocytopenia, repeat transfusion of platelets is usually indicated. However, subsequent transfusions should be based on the results of intraoperative platelet counts and the persistence of generalized microvascular bleeding. Because platelets contain approximately 50 to 60 ml of plasma, they supply coagulation factors as well. A transfusion dose of 8 units of platelets consists of a volume equivalent to approximately 2 units of fresh frozen plasma. This fact should be considered when indications exist for the transfusion of both blood components.

Table 22-4. Recommended Approach to the Transfusion of Blood Components During Massive Blood Replacement

Blood component	Indications
Platelets	Platelet count of 50,000/μl or less; active bleeding
	Platelet count of 30,000/μl or less; no bleeding, but surgery indicated
Fresh frozen plasma	PT of 15 seconds or greater; active bleeding
	APTT of 50 seconds or greater; active bleeding
Cryoprecipitate	Plasma fibrinogen level ≤75 mg/dl; active bleeding

TRANSFUSION THERAPY GUIDELINES

When administering blood components, it is important to recognize that the patient's level of plasma coagulation factors or platelets do not have to be corrected to the normal range. The goal of hemotherapy is to achieve *hemostatic levels,* quantities that are less than what are normally present in the circulation. This means that the quantity of most plasma coagulation factors should be above 30 percent and the platelets above 60,000/μl. Higher platelet counts are preferred in patients who have sustained brain injury. Plasma coagulation levels at 30 percent will correct the PT and APTT. Overtreatment with blood components should be avoided, especially when the patient is no longer bleeding.

A drawback in the management of a bleeding trauma patient is that the transfusion dose for any blood component is poorly defined. What then should be the approach to the management of hemostasis in this setting? Table 22-4 gives a guideline that conforms to the available current information [17,29]. The decision-making process is based on the results of intraoperative laboratory testing coupled with clinical observation and judgment. In this regard, the surgeon must be able to distinguish microvascular bleeding, as the result of abnormal hemostasis, from surgical bleeding. The latter situation responds best to prompt surgical intervention. It is also important that coagulation studies be obtained regularly so that the selection of the proper blood component and transfusion dose be made appropriately. Because of the logistics involved in performing a template bleeding time to document platelet dysfunction during surgery, this test is not included as a consideration for platelet transfusion.

The use of empiric formulas to transfuse fresh frozen plasma and/or platelets does not help to reduce the incidence of hemostatic abnormalities [17,29] and does not provide for a judicious use of blood components. Coagulation studies and platelet counts should be readily available in any hospital caring for trauma victims. The laboratory evaluation of hemostasis assists in defining the type of coagulopathy, provides information for the use of specific blood components, and simultaneously renders therapeutic regulation of the patient. However, laboratory monitoring of the bleeding patient does not relieve the trauma surgeon from making careful clinical evaluations. Even when the coagulation studies are severely altered and there is no evidence of generalized oozing, the decision not to give platelets and/or fresh frozen plasma is justifiable [33]. This supports the current thinking that prophylactic transfusions of blood components are not warranted. On the other hand, there will be the rare situation when the reverse condition prevails; the coagulation studies are normal, the patient is oozing, and there appears to be no response to the hemotherapy. The solution to such a problem is not easily obtainable. Here, the approach to management should be individualized, and a consultant's recommendations for specialized laboratory studies and additional hemotherapy should be sought.

REFERENCES

1. Clarke, J. R., et al. Optimal blood ordering for emergency department patients. *Ann. Emerg. Med.* 9:2, 1980.
2. Committee on Standards of the American Association of Blood Banks. *Standards for Blood Banks and Transfusion Services* (11th ed.). Arlington, Va.: American Association of Blood Banks, 1984. Pp. 23–24.
3. Sohmer, P. R., et al. Rh sensitization subsequent to transfusion with uncrossmatched Rh positive packed red cells. *Crit. Care Med.* 7:144, 1979.
4. Gervin, A. S., and Fischer, R. P. Resuscitation of trauma patients with type-specific uncrossmatched blood. *J. Trauma* 24:327, 1984.
5. Barnes, A. Transfusion of universal donor and uncrossmatched blood. *Bibl. Haematologica* 46:132, 1980.
6. Blumberg, N., and Bove, J. R. Un-cross-matched blood for emergency transfusion: One year's experience in a civilian setting. *J.A.M.A.* 240:2057, 1978.
7. Gervin, A. S., Dunnington, G. L., and Fischer, R. P. Fatal blood transfusion reactions in trauma. *J. Trauma* 23:639, 1983.
8. Jennings, E. R., and Barnes, A. Emergency blood transfusion. *J.A.M.A.* 253:3465, 1985.
9. Siegel, M. M., et al. Transfusion of uncrossmatched blood in children. *Blood* 52:303, 1978.
10. Boral, L. I., and Henry, J. B. The type and screen: A safe alternative and supplement in selected surgical procedures. *Transfusion* 17:163, 1977.
11. Boral, L. I., et al. The type and antibody screen, revisited. *Am. J. Clin. Pathol.* 71:578, 1979.
12. Heistø, H. Pretransfusion blood group serology: Limited value of the antiglobulin phase of the crossmatch when a careful screening test for unexpected antibodies is performed. *Transfusion* 19:761, 1979.
13. Oberman, H. A., Barnes, B. A., and Friedman, B. A. The risk of abbreviating the major crossmatch in urgent or massive transfusion. *Transfusion* 18:127, 1978.
14. Shulman, I. A., et al. Experience with the routine use of an abbreviated crossmatch. *Am. J. Clin. Pathol.* 82:178, 1984.
15. Sohmer, P. R., and Dawson, R. B. Transfusion therapy in trauma: A review of the principles and techniques used in the MIEMS program. *Am. Surg.* 45:109, 1979.
16. Sohmer, P. R., and Scott, R. L. Metabolic burden of massive transfusion. In J. A. Collins, K. Murawski, and A. W. Shafter (eds.), Massive Trans-

fusion in Surgery and Trauma. *Prog. Clin. Biol. Res.* 108:273, 1982.
17. Sohmer, P. R., and Scott, R. L. Massive transfusion. In B. Myhre (ed.), Symposium on Blood Banking and Hemotherapy. *Clin. Lab. Med.* 2:21, 1982.
18. Howland, W. S., Schweizer, O., and Jascott, D. Factors influencing the ionization of calcium during major surgical procedures. *Surg. Gynecol. Obstet.* 143:895, 1976.
19. Collins, J. A. Massive blood transfusion. *Clin. Haematol.* 5:201, 1976.
20. Howland, W. S., Schweizer, O., and Carlon, G. C. The cardiovascular effects of low levels of ionized calcium during massive transfusion. *Surg. Gynecol. Obstet.* 145:581, 1977.
21. Caggiano, V. Red Blood Cell Transfusions. In H. Silver (ed.), *Blood, Blood Components and Derivatives in Transfusion Therapy.* Arlington, Va.: American Association of Blood Banks, 1980. Pp. 1–28.
22. Schmidt, P. J. Whole blood transfusion. *Transfusion* 24:368, 1984.
23. Heaton, A., et al. Use of Adsol® preservation solution for prolonged storage of low viscosity AS-1 red blood cells. *Br. J. Haematol.* 57:467, 1984.
24. Courcy, P. A., Brotman, S., and Dawson, B. Massive blood transfusion in acute trauma. *Transfusion* 23:404, 1983.
25. Kahn, R. A., et al. Use of plasma products with whole blood and packed RBCs. *J.A.M.A.* 242:2087, 1979.
26. Shaikh, B. S., et al. Transfusion pattern of fresh frozen plasma in a medical school hospital. *Vox Sang.* 48:366, 1985.
27. Snyder, A. J., Gottschall, J. L., and Menitove, J. E. Why is fresh-frozen plasma transfused? *Transfusion* 26:107, 1986.
28. Counts, R. B., et al. Hemostasis in massively transfused trauma patients. *Ann. Surg.* 190:91, 1979.
29. Mannucci, P. M., Federici, A. B., and Sirchia, G. Hemostasis testing during massive blood replacement. *Vox Sang.* 42:113, 1982.
30. Noe, D. A., et al. Platelet counts during rapid massive transfusion. *Transfusion* 22:392, 1982.
31. Slichter, S. J. Identification and management of defects in platelet hemostasis in massively transfused patients. In J. A. Collins, K. Murawski, and A. W. Shafer (eds.), Massive Transfusion in Surgery and Trauma. *Prog. Clin. Biol. Res.* 108:225, 1982.
32. Reed, R. L., II, et al. Prophylactic platelet administration during massive transfusion. *Ann. Surg.* 203:40, 1986.
33. Harrigan, C., et al. Serial changes in primary hemostasis after massive transfusion. *Surgery* 98:836, 1985.
34. Harke, H., and Rahman, S. Haemostatic disorders in massive transfusion. *Bibl. Haematologica* 46:179, 1980.
35. Shackford, S. R., Virgilio, R. W., and Peters, R. M. Whole blood versus packed-cell transfusions. *Ann. Surg.* 193:337, 1981.
36. Braunstein, A. H., and Oberman, H. A. Transfusion of plasma components. *Transfusion* 24:281, 1984.
37. Wolff, G. Fresh frozen plasma: Effects and side effects. *Bibl. Haematologica* 46:189, 1980.
38. Sherman, L. A. DIC in massive transfusion. In J. A. Collins, K. Murawski, and A. W. Shafer (eds.), Massive Transfusion in Surgery and Trauma. *Prog. Clin. Biol. Res.* 108:171, 1982.

23

Trauma and Organ Donation

Martin L. Milgrom

The advent of cyclosporine has dramatically improved the results of organ transplantation in the past several years. It allows for effective immunosuppression without as many unpleasant side effects as were seen in the past. Especially because steroids do not have to be used in very large doses, modern transplant patients usually cannot be discerned from the normal population. These improved results have made kidney transplantation a very desirable alternative to dialysis for most young renal-failure patients. In particular, diabetics have an improved life expectancy and a much better course, with improved vision and limb function, when they are transplanted as opposed to dialyzed. Kidney transplantation is also cost-effective, as transplant patients are much more able to work as productive members of society, and the cost of their medical care is much lower than when on dialysis. In the 1980s, cadaver kidney graft survivals are approximately 90 percent at 1 year and 70 percent at 5 years. Unfortunately, even as 8000 kidney transplants are performed in the United States every year, the demand for kidneys is continuing to outstrip the supply, with 15,000 suitable candidates on a formal waiting list and many others not on a list but in need of a transplant [1]. During the past decade, we have also seen dramatically improving results with liver transplantation and heart transplantation (Table 23-1). The 1-year patient survival is about 80 percent for those recipients. This year, roughly a thousand of each will be performed, providing the only chance the young and otherwise viable patients who get them have for survival. It is very dramatic to see a cardiac cripple transformed into a vital and working member of society as it is to see a jaundiced, bleeding liver-failure patient brought back to his family and the work force. It is just as heartbreaking to see many of these patients die for want of an organ that could

Table 23-1. Transplant Statistics, United States (1981–1986)

Organ and tissue	Transplants performed in the United States						Numbers of people waiting*
	1981	1982	1983	1984	1985	1986*	
Kidneys	4485	5358	6112	6968	7695	10566	10,000
Heart	62	103	172	346	731	430	300
Heart/lung	—	—	—	—	30	42	75
Liver	26	62	164	308	605	925	300
Pancreas	—	35	61	87	133	130	50
Corneas	—	18,500	21,250	24,000	26,326	28,000	5000

*Approximate figures for 1986.
Source: Data from the Medical Council on Transplantation.

be readily available. In addition to the above mentioned organs, corneal transplants restore vision to patients with corneal opacification, bone allografts allow for limb preservation in cancer patients, and skin allografts are effectively used for wound coverage problems in burn patients. Pancreas and isolated islet cell preparations are being transplanted to reverse diabetes. Results in these patients are becoming increasingly encouraging, with a 60-percent 1-year graft survival. Heart-lung transplants are also showing encouraging results in the treatment of irreversible pulmonary failure. To make these lifesaving and life-improving tissues available, there has to be a supply of organ donors. The majority of organ donors come from the trauma victims in this country.

ROLE OF HEALTH CARE PERSONNEL

Health care personnel working in the field of trauma must understand that they have multiple responsibilities to society. The first responsibility, of course, is to the individual patient, whose life should be saved and health restored to premorbid conditions whenever possible. The next responsibility is to the patient's family, who may need comfort and help in coping with a traumatized loved one. There is also a responsibility to society with education programs and lobbying efforts with governing bodies to try to lower the incidence of trauma and to develop networks that can best handle the load of trauma. In this expanded view of the role of the health care provider, one must consider a responsibility to patients awaiting organ transplants. Rather than burying organs that could save lives, all attempts should be made to have the unsalvageable patients, the patients who are brain dead, serve as organ donors to save other people's lives. Aside from the obvious benefits to the transplant patients, the victim's family benefits psychologically from organ donation. Studies have shown that the grief is shorter and that families are better able to cope with the death of their loved one when they see that this person has not died in vain, but rather the death has helped other people to lead healthy and productive lives. These trauma personnel and emergency room personnel should become familiar with their local organ procurement agency (OPA).

ORGAN PROCUREMENT AGENCY

There are OPAs throughout the world. Each hospital falls within the catchment area of an OPA. Good relations and open lines of communication between the hospital and the OPA are necessary to have a smooth operation. Most OPAs provide literature and lectures in an effort to educate and raise the awareness of health care providers to the workings of the transplant community. Trauma personnel should avail themselves of these services. No one should ever hesitate to call the OPA with any question.

Whenever a patient who is a potential donor is brought to the emergency room, the OPA should be called. This policy has two advantages. First, it ensures the greatest possible yield of donors. Second, it maintains contact, rapport, and open lines of communication that allow for future smooth relations. It is far better to mobilize for many potential donors that end up not donating than to miss a good donor.

When it looks apparent that a patient will become brain dead and a good donor, the family should be approached. The family is usually approached by the attending physician, but a clergyman, a nurse, or sometimes a member of the OPA may be more appropriate, depending on the circumstances. Approaching the grieving family can be an extraordinarily difficult process [2]. Most people "are not themselves" at such times and can be very angry and even abusive. Tremendous compassion and patience are needed to be successful. The family needs time to marshall their thoughts and emotions. Whenever the potential donor has a donor card or has discussed his or her feelings before the tragic event, the process is easier. The question should always be raised, "What would ______ have wanted"? It must be understood by everyone that the patient either is or is likely to become brain dead shortly, and that the delivery of care is not influenced by the decision to donate. Once the patient is brain dead, support will be withdrawn. At this point, the patient can be taken either for organ donation or to the morgue.

DONOR CANDIDATES

Most patients who are pronounced brain dead are acceptable candidates for organ donation. The most commonly used patient is one who has sustained a head injury, either from a motor vehicle accident, from a fall, or from a gunshot wound. Other common causes of brain death that have led to organ donation are subarachnoid hemorrhage, cerebrovascular accidents, and primary brain tumors. Patients who have suffered cerebral anoxia from drug overdoses and drowning have been used. Children with sudden infant death syndrome who have been incompletely resuscitated can also be used. In cases where there is a violent or unexplained cause of death, the organ procurement team works closely with the medical examiner's office. The medical examiner is made aware of the potential donor and gives permission for the procedures to take place. The medical examiner may stipulate only certain organs be removed, and in all cases, the procurement team looks carefully for any pathology while performing the procurement procedure. Should any potentially important evidence be found during the procedure, the procedure stops, and consultation with the medical examiner is undertaken.

Some brain-dead patients are not acceptable donors for vital organs. In general, elderly patients are not used for organ donation because the quality of their blood vessels and organs are poor, and the organs do not tolerate ischemia well. There is no arbitrary cutoff of age for patients to be considered elderly, although usually people over the age of 65 are not used as kidney donors, and patients over the age of 45 are not used as heart or liver donors as a rule. For obese patients with cerebrovascular accidents, it would be unusual to take kidneys from anyone over 55 years of age. However, each donor needs to be considered individually, and sometimes patients who have been in very good health and have died a traumatic death, even though they are elderly, do serve as good organ donors.

Patients who come to the emergency room dead on arrival cannot serve as organ donors, but they are acceptable for cornea and bone donation. Patients who are known to have cancer cannot be used as organ donors because the recipient will become cancer-ridden in the face of immunosuppression. The exception to this is that patients with primary brain tumors are accepted because the blood-brain barrier protects systemic spread of tumor in the donor. Patients with transmissible diseases are not good organ donors because these diseases will be spread to the recipient and, in the face of immunosuppression, can become life-threatening. Examples of patients with transmissible diseases include septic patients, patients with meningitis, hepatitis, syphilis, and HIV infections. Patients with preexisting renal disease and patients with long-standing hypertension are not acceptable as organ donors, nor are patients who have had diabetes of more than 5 years' duration.

Health care workers taking care of any potential donor should be encouraged to call the organ procurement center to discuss this patient. If organ donation is not possible, there is certainly no harm done; on the other hand, to miss a potential donor is a major tragedy. This feeling may be manifested by litigation on the part of the victim's families who have not been given the option to donate. Some states now have laws that oblige the physician to approach families of all potential candidates.

PROCEDURE FOR ORGAN HARVEST

The time from pronouncement of death to the time when the donor is taken to the operating room should be kept at a minimum for a variety of reasons. First, the bed and nursing time spent on someone who is already dead should be made available to patients who are salvageable. Second, the donor's family in their time of grief should have the remains made available to the funeral home as soon as possible. Third, there is a potential for cardiovascular collapse or sepsis in these severely injured patients, so with the prolonged wait organs could be lost. Nevertheless, there is usually a period of several hours between the time of pronouncement of death and the time of organ harvest. Often the family needs time to make the decision to donate the organs. The procurement team needs time to organize its members and to get to the donor hospital. The operating room team needs time to set up the room and occasionally needs to delay the case to perform other emergency surgery ahead of the donor surgery. When multiple organs are harvested, additional time is needed to coordinate the centers that will be coming to harvest extrarenal organs and to await their arrival. Thus, there usually will be several hours when the patient will need to be maintained with good organ function while awaiting harvest.

Most brain-dead patients will have been kept volume-depleted to prevent brain swelling while brain death was in doubt. Once brain death has been documented, it becomes desirable to hydrate the patient vigorously so that there is good perfusion to the visceral organs. Large volumes of fluid should be administered to accomplish a high filling pressure and optimally to maintain a urine output of over 100 ml/hr. Most organ donors are on vasopressors to maintain an adequate blood pressure in the face of volume depletion. As the hydration is performed, it is good to wean down the pressor as much as possible [3]. Dopamine is the preferred vasopressor, and it is desirable to get the dose of dopamine down to the 2 to 5 μg/kg/min range if possible. A systolic blood pressure of at least 100 mm Hg should be maintained. Severe head trauma is often associated with diabetes insipidus, and in these patients, pitressin may be used if necessary to maintain adequate hydration. A first-generation cephalosporin should be given prophylactically to help guard against sepsis. Nephrotoxic antibiotics like the aminoglycosides should be discontinued. In the case of a cardiac arrest, prompt resuscitation should be attempted; if a good blood pressure cannot be restored rapidly, the kidneys are not likely to be good and organ donation will be cancelled. However, nonvital tissues, such as bone, skin, and eyes are still usable. Eye care and lubrication should be meticulously carried out so that the corneas will be good for transplantation.

DONOR-RECIPIENT MATCHING

For all organ donors, the organ procurement center will need to know the age, weight, and height of the patient. They will also need to know the results of many tests including blood type, VDRL or RPR, HIV, complete blood count, electrolytes, blood gas, creatinine, blood urea nitrogen, and urinalysis. Blood and urine should be taken for culture. In patients who are potential liver donors, which includes patients up to 45 years of age who are in stable hemodynamic condition requiring minimal pressor support, aspartate aminotransferase, alanine aminotransferase, total bilirubin, direct bilirubin, prothrombin time, partial thromboplastin time, and platelets should be drawn. In patients who are potential heart donors (this would include patients up to 45 years of age with no heart history who are on minimal pressor support), a chest x-ray, creatine kinase, and 12-lead electrocardiogram should be obtained. In addition, it is often desirable to perform an echogram of the heart and obtain a consult by a cardiologist. Although some centers will accept donors with mitral valve prolapse, no other cardiac abnormalities are acceptable in the donor.

When the data become available, the transplant coordinator determines whether the patient is a potential liver or heart donor; if the answer is affirmative, the data are entered into a national computer that helps to determine who the recipient should be. The decision is made according to size, ABO compatibility, urgency of the recipient's condition, and travel distance. The transplant coordinator then makes travel arrangements with the recipient hospital team for a joint effort at the donor's hospital. In almost all cases, the local transplant center will perform the nephrectomy and will either use the kidneys locally or send them to another center with a patient who is a good match for the kidney. Because the kidneys can be preserved for well over a day, there is no rush in accomplishing this. When hearts and livers are taken, the center that uses the heart or the liver usually sends members of its team to take these organs. This is done to minimize the preservation time, which must be short for both of these organs. It is also done because the recipient's life is directly dependent on the quality of the harvest organ. For this reason, as many as three different teams may be working in the operating room simultaneously. Support from anesthesiology is paramount for procurement of well-perfused, high-quality organs [4].

After the transplant patients' courses have been stabilized, most OPAs will inform involved health care providers of the outcomes. At this time, the donor's family is also notified. Almost always, pains are taken to maintain confidentiality for both the donor and the recipients. In all cases, all costs incurred by the donation process and physiologic maintenance of the donor before surgery are paid by the OPA from funds generated by billing recipients. OPAs are always nonprofit organizations. Furthermore, the donor families and people caring for the donors are never paid for donors. The motive for donation is and must remain altruism.

REFERENCES

1. Najarian, J. S. (ed.). The crucial role of the practicing surgeon in securing permission for organ donation. *Am. J. Surg.* 154:253, 1987.
2. Weber, P. The human connection: The role of the nurse in organ donation. *J. Neurosurg. Nurs.* 17(2):119, 1985.
3. Jordan, C. A., and Snyder, J. V. Intensive care and intraoperative management of the brain-dead organ donor. *Transplant. Proc.* 19(Suppl. 3):21, 1987.
4. Wetzel, R. C., Setzer, N., Stiff, J. L., and Rogers, M. C. Hemodynamic responses in brain dead organ donor patients. *Anesth. Analg.* 64:125, 1985.

24

Psychiatric Issues in the Acute Management of the Trauma Patient

Deborah Blacker
George E. Tesar

Central to the meaning of the word *traumatic* is the psychological reaction to the sudden and unexpected change in physical functioning after an accident or injury. But a focus on the psychological effects of trauma fails to take into account the extensive and complex relationship between trauma and psychiatric symptoms and diagnoses. Psychiatric impairment can cause trauma: depression may lead to suicide attempts, intoxication to brawls, and delirium to bizarre accidents. Psychiatric or behavioral changes can also follow in the wake of trauma or its treatment: confusion with head trauma; agitation with hypotension or hypoxia; deliria with anesthetics, narcotics, or corticosteroids; or anxiety with major surgery. Finally, the increased physical and psychological stress imposed by the injury, its treatment, or hospitalization can aggravate existing or activate latent pathology in patients with preexisting psychiatric disorders: alcoholic patients may develop withdrawal, demented patients may "sundown," and personality-disordered patients may act inappropriately or disruptively. The focus here will be on the acute management of the trauma patient, that is, in the emergency room, operating room, intensive care unit, and surgical ward. Prevention of long-term sequelae, such as post-traumatic stress disorder and chronic depression, is discussed elsewhere [1].

WHEN TO CALL A PSYCHIATRIC CONSULT

The severity of the trauma and the nature of associated psychiatric symptoms determine when and whether to call a psychiatric consultant. At the initial presentation, combative-

This chapter is dedicated to the memory of Thomas P. Hackett, M.D., Chief of the Massachusetts General Hospital Psychiatry Service, who died during the preparation of the manuscript.

ness, agitation, or self-destructiveness that might otherwise prompt psychiatric consultation will be ignored or treated with restraint or sedation while urgent care is rendered. When the trauma is less severe, however, or the patient's agitation does not respond to the usual measures, a psychiatrist may assist in the evaluation and treatment of an abnormal mental status. A request for psychiatric consultation may also be indicated when a patient refuses vital diagnostic or therapeutic procedures. The consultant can evaluate the patient's mental status and decide whether further explanation, psychiatric treatment, discharge against advice, or a formal declaration of incompetency is appropriate.

Before the patient leaves the emergency room, the surgeon must be alert to whether the circumstances of the trauma warrant further investigation by a psychiatric consultant. Does the patient's or the family's story about an accident make sense, or is there reason to suspect suicide or foul play? Is there another witness? Is the trauma attributable to a preexisting condition that impaired the patient's judgment and should be attended to by a psychiatrist or neurologist? When the trauma may have occurred as the result of a suicide attempt or some other self-destructive behavior, psychiatric consultation is essential during inpatient surgical care or before discharge from the emergency room.

During the patient's stay in intensive care or on the surgical ward, a number of circumstances may dictate a need for psychiatric consultation. Psychiatric consultation is most often considered because the staff wants help with the management of a "difficult" or agitated patient. The psychiatric consultant can assist in the evaluation of such patients and can offer advice and treatment to help maintain staff and patient safety. Difficulties with pain management and significant depression or anxiety may also benefit from psychiatric consultation. Prior to the patient's discharge, the role of the consultant generally centers around the patient's competency to sign out against medical advice, his ability to care for himself in an independent setting, and the need for referral for outpatient psychiatric care.

NEUROPSYCHIATRIC SYNDROMES IN THE TRAUMA PATIENT

The spectrum of neuropsychiatric syndromes that may be associated with trauma is manifold and can be divided into several broad categories. Delirium or psychosis, pain, mood disturbances such as anxiety and depression, and regressive or troublesome behavior may complicate the management of the trauma patient. Bizarre or troublesome behaviors, like hypotension and pain, are *symptoms*, each with a differential diagnosis.

Delirium and Psychosis

The trauma patient with an altered or bizarre mental state may be suffering from a delirium or psychosis [2–4]. Although these terms are often confused, they have different technical meanings. *Delirium* [5] is a syndrome marked by an acutely clouded sensorium due to an identified or presumed organic cause. In a delirium, the level of consciousness, degree of orientation, quality of mood, and intensity of abnormal motor activity all tend to fluctuate. *Psychosis,* a loss of contact with reality in the form of bizarre thinking, delusions (false beliefs), and/or hallucinations (false perceptions), is often present in a delirium. The classic so-called functional psychoses such as schizophrenia and mania [5] differ from delirium in that a normal sensorium is preserved. In addition, visual, olfactory, and tactile hallucinations, common in delirium, are uncommon in the functional psychoses. Despite these etiologic and phenomenologic differences, the treatment of delirious and psychotic patients is frequently the same.

Any delirious or psychotic patient may become agitated and should be carefully monitored. When agitation occurs, it is vital to ensure the safety of the patient, the staff, and the surroundings. Staff should speak calmly and firmly without frightening the patient. Weapons and other dangerous objects should be removed from the patient and from the surrounding area. A "show of force" assembled from several large, preferably male, staff members may be sufficient to subdue irritable or threatening patients, but, if necessary, the hospital security force can be called to help maintain safety. The use of mechanical restraints may be necessary if agitation persists or if there is reason to suspect that it will recur.

As safety measures are instituted, it is important to review the differential diagnosis of delirium (Table 24-1). Important clues to the etiology of delirium may be evident in the patient's history and presentation, physical findings, laboratory test results, and hospital course. The physical and neurologic examination of a delirious or psychotic patient should include observations of (1) the patient's state of arousal and whether it is stable or fluctuating; (2) the level of motor activity; (3) the orientation to name, place, and time; and (4) the presence or absence of verbal or behavioral clues to a loss of contact with reality. If disorientation or change in arousal is present, the patient is probably delirious and needs a thorough clinical and laboratory evaluation. Pertinent laboratory tests to obtain include electrolytes, renal and liver function tests, amylase, calcium, magnesium, erythrocyte sedimentation rate, complete blood count, and toxic screen. An arterial blood gas determination, computed tomography (CT) scan, electroencephalogram, lumbar puncture, and other more specific tests may be required in certain clinical situations.

Delirium that is present at the time of admission to the emergency room may be either a cause or an effect of the presenting trauma. Deliria produced by drug overdose or toxicity [6], intoxication with alcohol or drugs of abuse [7], or acute central nervous system insults (e.g., strokes, seizures) can lead to falls, auto accidents, fights, or suicide attempts. Conversely, patients with critical hypotension, hypoxia, acidosis, or head injury due to trauma may present with delirium.

Other potential causes of delirium emerge during the hospitalization and treatment of the trauma patient. Factors associated with the evolution of the trauma itself (e.g., intracranial bleed, central nervous system [CNS] infection, or fat embolus), complications of treatment (e.g., renal failure, metabolic imbalance, or pulmonary embolism), and medications (e.g., anesthetics, opiate analgesics, corticosteroids, histamine H_2 receptor antagonists, antiarrhythmics, and psychotropics) are all capable of producing delirium. During

Table 24-1. Common Causes of Delirium

- Medications
  - Anticholinergic drugs (including atropine, tricyclic antidepressants, thioridazine, antihistamines, and over-the-counter hypnotics)
  - Sedative-hypnotic agents (especially those with long half-lives, e.g., flurazepam)
  - Decongestants, antiasthmatics, and other sympathomimetics
  - Cimetidine
  - Digitalis
  - L-Dopa
  - Methyldopa
  - Glucocorticoids
- Drug abuse
  - Amphetamine and cocaine
  - Phencyclidine (PCP)
  - Hallucinogens
  - Inhaled drugs (glue, nitrous oxide)
- Withdrawal syndromes
  - Alcohol, benzodiazepines (especially alprazolam), barbiturates, and other sedative-hypnotics
- Metabolic
  - Hepatic encephalopathy
  - Uremia
  - Hypoglycemia
  - Hypoxia
  - Hyponatremia
  - Hypo- and hypercalcemia
  - Hypo- and hypermagnesemia
  - Acidosis
  - Hyperosmolar states
  - Porphyria
- Vitamin deficiencies
  - Thiamine (Wernicke-Korsakoff syndrome)
  - Vitamin B_{12}
  - Nicotinic acid (pellagra)
- Endocrinopathies
  - Hypo- and hyperthyroidism
  - Hypo- and hyperparathyroidism
  - Cushing's syndrome and Addison's disease
  - Hypopituitarism
- Infections
  - Any systemic infection (e.g., pneumonia) in the elderly, especially with a coexisting dementing process
  - Meningitis, encephalitis, and brain abscess
  - Neurosyphilis
  - AIDS encephalopathy
- Neurologic causes
  - Head injury (postconcussive syndromes, bleeds)
  - Stroke
  - Hypertensive encephalopathy
  - Intracranial neoplasms, especially frontal and temporal
  - Complex partial status epilepticus
  - Postictal states
- Toxins and industrial exposures
  - Carbon monoxide
  - Carbon disulfide
  - Organic solvents
  - Heavy metals
- Others
  - Systemic lupus erythematosus (lupus cerebritis)
  - Cerebral vasculitis (temporal arteritis, polyarteritis nodosa)
  - Paraneoplastic syndromes (limbic encephalitis)
  - Hyperviscosity syndromes

Source: Adapted from S. E. Hyman (ed.), *Manual of Psychiatric Emergencies* (2nd ed.). Boston: Little, Brown, 1988.

confinement in the hospital, Wernicke's encephalopathy and alcohol or sedative-hypnotic withdrawal may also lead to delirium.

The treatment of delirium depends on its etiology and severity. Initially, it is necessary to rule out or treat—presumptively, if necessary—the life-threatening causes of delirium, including hypotension, hypoxia, hypoglycemia, increased intracranial pressure, meningitis or encephalitis, CNS depressant withdrawal syndromes, Wernicke's encephalopathy, and toxins. Other specific causes should be remedied wherever possible: metabolic abnormalities corrected and unnecessary medications stopped. In the absence of a specific or treatable cause of delirium, the patient may require pharmacologic treatment. The type of agent chosen depends on the goal of treatment. When only brief sedation is required (e.g., for a CT scan or lumbar puncture), the short-acting barbiturate methohexital (Brevital) may be given as an IV bolus or a continuous drip (5–10 ml in a 1% solution [50–100 ml]), with respiratory support available. Other, nonbarbiturate agents are preferable when more prolonged treatment is indicated. A benzodiazepine is the treatment of choice if alcohol or sedative-hypnotic withdrawal is suspected. Most often, neuroleptic medication, alone or in combination with a benzodiazepine, is the treatment of choice for a delirious or psychotic patient.

The amount and route of administration of sedating or tranquilizing medication depend on the patient's clinical status and the intensity of associated agitation. Quietly delirious patients are probably better off left to clear without additional medications to cloud the picture. When agitation is minimal, a neuroleptic such as haloperidol (Haldol), may be given orally, 2–5 mg every 6 to 12 hours. For elderly, demented, or retarded patients, the recommended starting dose of haloperidol is 0.5 to 1.0 mg. When agitation is more severe, haloperidol should be used in parenteral form for more rapid and reliable absorption. Dosing should start at 5 to 10 mg IM and can be repeated every 1 to 2 hours, up to 100 mg/day if necessary. Haloperidol offers the advantages of little respiratory or cardiovascular depression and calming with minimal clouding of consciousness. When additional sedation is required, lorazepam (Ativan), 1 to 2 mg every 1 to 2 hours, can be added. Lorazepam should be avoided in patients whose sensorium must be closely monitored or in (unventilated) patients with respiratory compromise. For both haloperidol and lorazepam, the oral dose necessary is roughly twice the intramuscular dose.

After sedation is achieved, the total required dose of sedative medication should be calculated. About half this dose can be used on a daily basis for several days, then gradually tapered to zero (or, if applicable, to the patient's baseline dose). Especially during the initial period, the patient's mental status can be expected to be quite variable; he or she may need to be restrained or observed for safety and should be assessed frequently by the psychiatrist.

Oral or intramuscular neuroleptics carry the risk of extrapyramidal symptoms. Especially in young patients, staff should watch for acute dystonic reactions, manifested by acute neck or limb stiffness, eye deviation, torticolis, or in severe cases, laryngospasm. Immediate treatment with benztropine mesylate (Cogentin), 1 to 2 mg IV or IM, or diphenhydramine, 25 to 50 mg IV or IM, is required. These reactions, as well as the less acute parkinsonian symptoms, can be largely prevented with prophylactic administration of benztropine mesylate, 1 mg PO bid, or diphenhydramine, 25 mg PO tid. However, due to their anticholinergic properties, these agents can produce an abnormal mental status and should be avoided in patients with head injuries and in others at risk for delirium. In such patients, intravenous haloperidol may be preferable. However, since intravenous haloperidol is not approved by the Food and Drug Administration, it may be advantageous to inform the hospital pharmacy and obtain informed consent from relatives prior to its use.

Pain

Careful attention to pharmacology, discussed below, is the cornerstone of the effective treatment of pain. However, a number of factors can complicate the pharmacologic management of pain. Coexistent depression or anxiety can intensify the subjective experience of pain and, if untreated, can contribute to ineffective analgesia and excessive analgesic use. Underlying personality disorder and its associated difficult behavior may also make pain management more difficult. A history of substance abuse also raises a concern for most medical staff. While the concern is real, and patients with a history of substance abuse need more careful monitoring, inadequate treatment of pain often paradoxically focuses the patient on pain medicine and may be more likely to foster addiction. Lastly, patients with opiate addiction present special problems in pain management, which are discussed later.

The effective administration of analgesics depends on matching the schedule, agent, route, and dosage to the needs of the individual patient. Patients with intermittent pain require only "as-needed" medication, given in anticipation of painful procedures like physical therapy or dressing changes or in response to fluctuations in symptoms. Patients with constant pain should receive standing doses of pain medications with a frequency about equal to the half-life of the drug. Standing medications may need to be supplemented with as-needed doses for painful procedures or for titrating the dose during the initial stages of treatment.

The agent and route follow from the dosing schedule. The agent should be chosen on the basis of the half-life and the availability and reliability of absorption of oral and parenteral forms. For round-the-clock coverage, especially for periods longer than several days, long-acting agents like methadone are preferable. Oral agents may be preferable for round-the-clock use; they are absorbed more slowly and maintain more constant levels. As-needed dosing can be chosen from a variety of shorter-acting agents, such as meperidine and morphine. For rapid action, parenteral agents are required; oral as-needed medications are only useful if they are given well in advance of a procedure or for mild to moderate pain. When repeated parenteral dosing is needed for either standing or as-needed usage, the prescription of agents that can be given subcutaneously (e.g., morphine, hydromorphone [Dilaudid]) will minimize muscle damage.

The amount of drug needed depends on the severity of the pain and potency of the drug and route chosen. Of note, some drugs require higher doses when given orally. In the case of meperidine and morphine, oral absorption is so poor that oral dosing should be avoided. For all pain medications, requirements are difficult to predict, and dosing should be adjusted according to the patient's clinical response. If the patient is nonverbal or unreliable, the degree of agitation may be used to set the lower boundary on pain medications, and pupil size and respiratory rate the upper. If adequate analgesia is not obtained with significant dosing, a small amount of neuroleptic (e.g., haloperidol, 1–2 mg bid) or stimulant (methylphenidate [Ritalin], 5–10 mg tid) may potentiate the response.

As the patient's condition improves, pain medications can be gradually tapered. Standing doses should be tapered before as-needed doses, and the patient's clinical status should be assessed to be sure that the taper is not being carried out too rapidly. Ideally, the patient should not be discharged on pain medications, since the risk of addiction increases in an unmonitored setting. If pain medications are required on an outpatient basis, the patient's analgesic requirements should be reassessed at frequent office visits, and accurate and limited numbers of pills should be prescribed.

Fear and Anxiety

Fear and anxiety [2] are common and even expected responses to trauma and the actual or threatened pain, confinement, disability, or death that may follow in its wake. In addition, a number of medical conditions and pharmacologic states, including hypoxia, hypoglycemia, hypotension, alcohol withdrawal, drugs of abuse (especially cocaine and amphetamines), and medications (especially corticosteroids and anticholinergic agents) may exacerbate anxiety. Neuroleptic agents (including metoclopramide [Reglan], droperidol, and prochlorperazine [Compazine]) may produce akathisia, an inner restlessness that is often experienced as anxiety.

After medical and pharmacologic contributors to anxiety are remedied, the treatment of anxiety should focus on the patient's specific, often unarticulated concerns. A psychiatric consultant can explore those concerns with the patient and, in conjunction with the primary physician, can conduct a frank discussion of the patient's current status, the expected treatment, and any expected residual deficits. If anxiety is unresponsive to such measures and is disabling or interferes with care, a benzodiazepine (e.g., lorazepam, 0.5–1.0 mg PO/IM/IV tid–qid) or low-dose neuroleptic (e.g., haloperidol, 1–2 mg PO/IM/IV bid) may prove helpful.

Depression

Like fear and anxiety, depression [2,3] is a common and understandable response to trauma. Depression is particularly likely to occur when the damage sustained in the trauma represents a significant loss of function or self-esteem. If depression is lasting or profound, it may impair the patient's ability to work at recovery and rehabilitation or, more seriously, may result in a risk of suicide [8]. Therefore, any pervasive or prolonged depression warrants psychiatric assessment. In particular, a psychiatric consultant can determine whether the patient has only a depressed mood or has the neurovegetative features—change in appetite or sleep patterns, decreased energy, difficulty concentrating, and apathy—required for a diagnosis of major depression [5].

Based on the clinical evaluation, the psychiatrist may recommend a treatment regimen. All patients may benefit from an opportunity to explore their current losses and their fears for the future. For patients with the symptoms of major depression, one of the biologic therapies, such as tricyclic antidepressants, monoamine oxidase inhibitors, or electroconvulsive therapy, will be recommended as well. For short-term treatment, especially when a rapid effect is needed or when standard treatments are poorly tolerated, a psychostimulant such as dextroamphetamine (Dexedrine) or methylphenidate offers a useful alternative.

Behavioral Disturbances

A variety of troublesome behaviors [2,3] frequently hamper the management of trauma. In extreme cases, difficult behavior takes on the form of agitation or the refusal of treatment, which are discussed elsewhere. More commonly, however, patients may become demanding, whiny, or irritable. Such behaviors are particularly likely among personality-disordered patients, whose impulsivity, substance abuse, and poor judgment ensure their overrepresentation on trauma services. These same characteristics, along with the limited ability to tolerate adverse or stressful circumstances that is a hallmark of personality disorder, can lead to significant behavioral difficulties during the treatment of trauma. The nature of the disturbance may vary with the type of personality disorder. Dependent patients may become whiny and passive, narcissistic patients may become demanding and entitled, and antisocial patients may become devious, threatening, or even violent.

The keys to managing all of these disturbances are firmness, consistency, and clarity. For frankly dangerous behavior such as sabotage of necessary care or threats to staff, clear, enforceable sanctions (e.g., loss of visitation, restraints, sedation, or discharge against advice) are required. For less disturbing behaviors, it is helpful to set firm, consistent policies about medications, guests, smoking, and other potential areas of conflict. Staff communication in the hospital record, in nursing reports, and on doctors rounds is critical to minimize conflicts. A psychiatric consultant can provide helpful guidelines for staff and can work with the patient to minimize such behavior.

CONCERNS WITH SPECIAL POPULATIONS

Certain populations are overrepresented among trauma patients and may present particularly difficult clincal problems or require specific treatments and precautions.

Self-Destructive Patients

Psychiatric consultation is mandatory whenever there is an indication or suspicion that a suicidal threat, gesture, or attempt underlies the trauma or may occur in response to its effects [2,3,8]. The issue of suicidal ideation or intent should be considered in patients with single-vehicle motor vehicle accidents, unusual falls or cuts, obvious depression, or a history of prior suicidal gestures or attempts. On rarer occasions, trauma may be the result of a factitious disorder such as Munchausen syndrome. Suicide precautions in the form of a one-to-one sitter or mechanical restraints are recommended until the patient has been evaluated and cleared by a psychiatric consultant.

A psychiatric consultant evaluates the patient's current status, provides any necessary acute treatment, and assists the patient's final disposition. If a potentially self-destructive patient is ready for discharge from the emergency room, the psychiatrist determines whether outpatient follow-up is adequate or whether psychiatric hospitalization is required. If the patient is to be admitted for further surgical care, the psychiatrist decides whether suicide precautions are needed in the hospital. During the hospitalization, the psychiatrist works with the surgical and nursing staff to develop a treatment plan that addresses suicidal behavior, its underlying causes (e.g., depression or psychosis), and the need for postdischarge inpatient or outpatient psychiatric care.

Intoxicated and Alcoholic Patients

Alcoholism and acute alcohol intoxication are frequently associated with trauma and can complicate trauma management in a number of ways [2,3]. First, intoxicated patients are frequently agitated and sometimes require restraint or even sedation to permit evaluation and treatment of the trauma. Second, the effects of intoxication may delay a search for other, possibly life-threatening sources of altered mental status, notably head trauma. Third, alcohol withdrawal or Wernicke's encephalopathy can lead to the disruption of care, a poor surgical outcome, or death.

Wernicke's encephalopathy, an acute confusional state associated with ophthalmoplegia and ataxia, is caused by an acute depletion of brain thiamine and may develop during the emergency room or inpatient phase of trauma management. Classically, it occurs when a malnourished alcoholic is fed, causing already low brain thiamine stores to be further depleted by acute use in glucose metabolism. Accordingly, alcholic and malnourished patients should receive 100 mg of parenteral thiamine before they are given food or intravenous fluids containing glucose. In addition, Wernicke's encephalopathy should be suspected in any patient with confusion or ophthalmoplegia. All such patients should receive thiamine, 100 mg IV or IM immediately and 100 mg by any route daily for 1 week to replete body stores.

Because alcoholism is so prevalent and so likely to be hidden or denied, all newly admitted trauma patients—from prominent business people with skiing injuries to skid-row alcoholics with frostbite—should be carefully monitored for signs of alcohol withdrawal. The *prophylaxis* of withdrawal with medications that may cause excessive sedation must often be withheld to monitor a patient's level of consciousness. However, patients at risk, particularly if they have a known history of withdrawal seizures or delirium tremens (DTs), should have vital signs monitored frequently and, if necessary, should receive the appropriate agent promptly.

The early symptoms of alcohol withdrawal may occur as soon as the blood alcohol level begins to drop and generally within the first 24 to 72 hours. They include tremulousness, irritability, anxiety, mild confusion, nausea with vomiting and/or diarrhea, and a mild rise in blood pressure, pulse, and temperature. Left untreated, these symptoms can progress to frank confusion, hallucinations, and seizures (rum fits). Delirium tremens, a more severe and potentially lethal syndrome marked by agitation, frank confusion, paranoid delusions, tactile and visual hallucinations, and severe autonomic instability, may occur up to a week after the last drink. Since there is a significant risk of death with DTs, intensive care unit monitoring, meticulous supportive care, and adequate pharmacologic treatment are required.

A benzodiazepine is the treatment for alcohol withdrawal of any degree. The route, amount, and frequency of administration of medication are dependent on the severity of current symptoms. Standard doses of oral medication should be sufficient for early, mild stages and may prevent the progression to more severe symptoms. The full-blown syndrome, especially when confusion or agitation is present, requires parenteral, preferably intravenous treatment. Virtually any benzodiazepine is effective in the treatment of alcohol withdrawal, but in a hospitalized population, lorazepam offers many advantages. It can be given both orally and parenterally, has an intermediate half-life (8–12 hours) with no active metabolites, and is safe even in the presence of mild renal or hepatic impairment. Treatment should start with 1 to 2 mg with an estimate based on the patient's size, consumption history, and tolerance (as assessed by alcohol level and level of consciousness at presentation). This dose should be repeated every 30 minutes to 1 hour until vital signs stabilize. On occasion, doses in the range of 50 mg/day of lorazepam have been required. The total dose required to stabilize vital signs should be repeated every 6 hours for 1 or 2 days and then gradually tapered by about 10 percent per day, with the patient's mental state and vital signs watched carefully.

After the patient is stable, the circumstances of the trauma may provide hospital staff with an opportunity to confront the patient about his or her drinking and its harmful consequences. A psychiatric consultant or, if available, a specialist in alcohol-related disorders can provide assistance in the immediate management of alcoholic patients and in discharge planning. Alcoholics Anonymous meetings are held in many large hospitals, and some patients can be encouraged to attend such meetings before discharge.

Sedative-Hypnotic Users and Abusers

For a variety of reasons, sedative-hypnotic dependence is often hidden. Patients may be unable to give a history, may neglect to mention a prescription for phenobarbital or alprazolam (Xanax) they take regularly, or may willfully conceal their diazepam (Valium), other benzodiazepine, or barbiturate abuse. A toxic screen may not measure some of the newer agents or their metabolites, or the drug may have already cleared by the time the patient arrives in the emergency room. Thus, it is critical to maintain a high index of suspicion, to take a careful history, and to monitor for the signs of sedative-hypnotic withdrawal.

Sedative-hypnotic withdrawal has similar features to alcohol withdrawal, including fever, autonomic instability, agitation, delirium, and seizures, and is similar in potential lethality. However, the latency to onset of symptoms varies with the half-life of the drug in question, occurring within hours of the last dose of rapidly metabolized agents such as alprazolam or pentobarbital and up to a week after the last dose of more slowly metabolized agents such as diazepam.

Benzodiazepines, barbiturates, and alcohol are cross-tolerant, so the treatment of sedative-hypnotic withdrawal is essentially the same as for alcohol withdrawal, with careful adjustment of dosing according to vital signs and mental status. However, particularly with triazolobenzodiazepines (alprazolam and triazolam [Halcion]) and barbiturates, replacement is best accomplished with the agent in question. A pentobarbital challenge test, as described by Hyman [3], can be used to estimate the initial requirement for replacement medication and the rate at which it should be tapered.

Narcotics Users and Abusers

Patients who habitually use narcotics [9] are often poorly tolerated and well remembered by hospital personnel. The main difficulty in management is determining the adequacy of analgesia in patients whose high tolerance means they need high doses, but whose habit means they may seek still higher ones. While these patients may not be trustworthy, their level of consciousness, vital signs, and pupil size are, and these parameters should be used in addition to the patient's report to adjust the dosage of medication. Addiction is not a justification for withholding analgesia, and addicts will be far easier to manage if they are adequately medicated.

As with any patient, opiates should be gradually tapered as the clinical situation warrants. If time permits, the patient should be detoxified in the hospital, with the opiate dose gradually tapered to zero. Since it is generally illegal to prescribe opiates for the treatment of addiction alone, the patient can be offered a more rapid taper in the hospital, transferred to a drug addiction facility, or sent out to withdraw "cold turkey" at home. Opiate withdrawal involves uncomfortable but not dangerous signs of autonomic arousal—large pupils, mild tachycardia and hypertension, sweating, nausea and vomiting and/or diarrhea, and perhaps symptoms of irritability or anxiety.

Elderly, Demented, and Retarded Patients

Elderly, demented, and retarded patients share a predilection for trauma by virtue of physical disabilities and/or perceptual and cognitive impairments. *Dementia,* including but not limited to senile dementia [5], is a chronic and acquired loss of cognitive function in the setting of normal arousal. It may affect orientation when severe and is sometimes accompanied by psychosis, particularly of a paranoid type. *Retardation* [5] is a congenital or developmental disorder that may have similar manifestations.

Cognitive deficits that are new or unexplained should be evaluated and treated if possible. A thorough chart review and discussion with relatives should prevent the unnecessary investigation of a long-standing, previously evaluated problem. However, when indicated, basic screening studies to obtain include serum electrolytes, liver and renal function tests, vitamin B_{12} and folate levels, erythrocyte sedimentation rate, complete blood count, and thyroid function tests. A CT scan is generally considered part of the evaluation of any patient; a lumbar puncture or electroencephalogram may also be indicated. In the high-risk groups, HTLV-III infection (so-called AIDS dementia) may also be a culprit, and blood testing may be warranted.

An understanding of the special problems of elderly and cognitively impaired patients is critical to their management on trauma services. Preexisting CNS compromise renders many in this group more vulnerable to further CNS insults such as hypoxia, electrolyte imbalance, or reduced cerebral blood flow. In fact, mental status changes are sometimes seen with illnesses as minor as urinary tract infections. This group of patients is particularly sensitive to medications, especially those with anticholinergic properties, so psychotropic agents, in particular low-potency neuroleptics, certain antidepressants, and antiparkinsonian agents should be given at lower doses and with closer monitoring.

Elderly and cognitively impaired patients have a limited capacity to cope with changes in their environment and to understand and follow orders. They sometimes become disoriented and frightened in the hospital, particularly at night, and may wander. In more severe cases, they may become combative or agitated. Frequent orientation, along with the use of a clock and calendar in the room, may prevent or resolve mild cases of disorientation. For more significant problems, a low-dose neuroleptic, such as haloperidol, 0.5 to 1.0 mg bid by any route, may be helpful. For combative patients or those whose behavior endangers themselves or others, higher doses of medications and/or restraints may be required.

LEGAL ISSUES

Competency and the Refusal of Treatment

At times, patients refuse treatment initially in the emergency room, refuse a diagnostic or therapeutic procedure, or threaten to sign out of the hospital against medical advice. In many such cases, the need for treatment is so urgent and so obvious that the patient's (verbally or behaviorally) expressed wishes are simply overridden. However, whenever the circumstances permit, the patient's ideas must be explored and his or her wishes must often be heeded, even when they differ from the surgeon's idea of proper treatment. Such cases call for a psychiatric consultation to evaluate both the reason the patient is refusing care and his or her competency to do so [10].

The refusal of treatment can be viewed medically—as a symptom with a differential diagnosis. Some patients are simply complaining and will agree to care after reasonable attention to their underlying concerns. At times, the refusal of treatment is a manifestation of anxiety, inadequate analgesia, incipient alcohol withdrawal, paranoia or other psychotic symptoms, or delirium; the treatment of these underlying symptoms can improve both comfort and compliance. Because these underlying problems can change over time and may respond to treatment, refusal and competency should be assessed on more than one occasion.

If treatment or accommodation is not possible, the refusal of treatment should be viewed legally. The legal issue is to balance patients' rights to determine their own destiny with their expectation that a physician will override their judgment when it is impaired by illness. Touching a patient without consent can be viewed as assault and battery, while ignoring the manifest needs of a patient is negligence. State laws differ, as do the actions of state courts, but in general, assault claims are far more easily defended than those for negligence. There have been few lawsuits and still fewer successful ones against doctors who in good faith overrode a patient's wishes in what they judge to be an emergency.

In nonemergent settings, a formal competency examination is required [11]. The psychiatrist assesses the patient's general mental status, with a focus on his or her ability to understand the risks and benefits of having or not having the proposed test or treatment. Based on the psychiatrist's recommendations, a judge then makes a formal determination of competency and assigns a guardian. In semiurgent cases, when there does not appear to be time to contact a judge, a psychiatrist's opinion may be adequate, but particularly if there is any ambiguity as to the appropriate treatment, the hospital legal department should be consulted. In theory, a competency evaluation and consent by relatives or a judge are equally indicated for potentially delirious or demented patients who accept (or acquiesce to) treatment as well as for those who refuse it, although this standard is more likely to be enforced for major, unusual, or risky procedures.

Abuse and Victimization

When dealing with adult victims of assault, there are several concerns beyond the acute clinical care. The most critical is to ensure the patient's safety from further attack. If a patient is ready for discharge and may not be safe at home, a hospital social worker may be able to help arrange a safer placement. Emergency room personnel should be alert to the difficulties of both male and female rape victims and victims of spouse abuse and, in conjunction with a psychiatric consultant or a counsellor, may be able to help patients deal with their reaction to the acute event and minimize the incidence of long-term psychological sequelae [1]. Hospital staff should also be aware of the local procedures for reporting violent crime; rape in particular usually requires fairly specific documentation procedures. With patients who are too impaired to report on their own behalf, hospital staff should undertake careful documentation of their status on arrival and the nature of the injury and await the patient's decision regarding pressing charges or reporting an accident. Any questions should be referred to the hospital legal department.

When a child is a trauma victim, a thorough evaluation includes consideration of whether the trauma could have resulted from child abuse or parental neglect. Nearly every state requires notification of a social welfare agency whenever hospital staff suspect that a child has been abused or neglected. If the abuse is significant, a hospital social worker should determine on the spot whether the child is safe to return home or whether a state agency should be contacted for emergency placement. The emergency room pediatrician, social worker, or psychiatrist will surely know the local requirements for reporting and may also have the necessary phone numbers or forms. Surgeons who see a significant number of children should familiarize themselves with state regulations. Similar reporting statutes aimed at elder abuse are becoming more common; the hospital social service or legal department can provide information as to local rules and reporting procedures.

REFERENCES

1. Peterson, L. G., and O'Shanick, G. J. (eds.). *Psychiatric Aspects of Trauma.* Advances in Psychosomatic Medicine, Vol. 16. Basel: Karger, 1986.
2. Hackett, T. P., and Cassem, N. H. (eds.). *Massachusetts General Hospital Handbook of General Hospital Psychiatry* (2nd ed.). Littleton, Mass.: PSG, 1987.
3. Hyman, S. E. (ed.). *Handbook of Psychiatric Emergencies* (2nd ed.). Boston: Little, Brown, 1988.
4. Tesar, G. E., and Stern, T. A. Evaluation and treatment of agitation in the intensive care unit. *J. Inten. Care Med.* 1:137, 1986.
5. American Psychiatric Association. *Diagnostic and Statistical Manual of Mental Disorders* (3rd ed., rev.). Washington, D.C.: American Psychiatric Press, 1987.
6. Drugs that Cause Psychiatric Symptoms. *Med. Lett. Drugs Ther.* 28:81, 1986.
7. Acute drug abuse reactions. *Med. Lett. Drugs Ther.* 27:77, 1985.
8. Reich, P., and Kelly, M. J. Suicide attempts by hospitalized medical and surgical patients. *N. Engl. J. Med.* 294:298, 1976.
9. Fultz, J. M., and Senay, E. C. Guidelines for the management of hospitalized narcotic addicts. *Ann. Intern. Med.* 82:815, 1975.
10. Gutheil, T. G., and Appelbaum, P. S. *Clinical Handbook of Psychiatry and the Law.* New York: McGraw-Hill, 1982.
11. Roth, L. H., Meisel, A., and Lidz, C. W. Tests of competency to consent to treatment. *Am. J. Psychiatry* 134:279, 1977.

Index

Italic numbers indicate figures; *t* indicates tables

Index